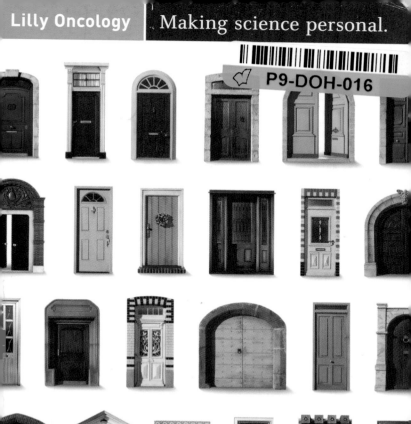

# Every door opened could be a discovery made.

No two cancer patients are alike. That's why Lilly Oncology is committed to developing treatment approaches as individual as the people who need them. We've made many contributions toward improved patient outcomes and—with each door we open—we take another step forward. Our quest to help you provide tailored therapy continues.

*Lilly*
Answers That Matter.

AMERICAN JOINT COMMITTEE ON CANCER

# AJCC CANCER STAGING HANDBOOK

## Seventh Edition

Please visit www.cancerstaging.net for related product information for the *AJCC Cancer Staging Handbook*, including coding updates and important clarifications to the chapters on Purposes and Principles of Staging, Cancer of the Lip and Oral Cavity, Soft Tissue Sarcoma, and Retinoblastoma.

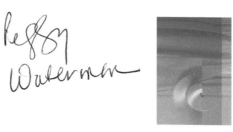

# AJCC CANCER STAGING HANDBOOK

## From the
### *AJCC Cancer Staging Manual,*
### Seventh Edition

AMERICAN JOINT COMMITTEE ON CANCER
Executive Office
633 North Saint Clair Street
Chicago, IL 60611-3211

*This manual was prepared and published through the support of the American Cancer Society, the American College of Surgeons, the American Society of Clinical Oncology, the Centers for Disease Control and Prevention, and the International Union Against Cancer.*

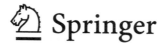 Springer

American Joint Committee on Cancer
Executive Office
633 North Saint Clair Street
Chicago, IL 60611-3211

*Editors*

Stephen B. Edge, M.D., F.A.C.S.
Roswell Park Cancer Institute
Buffalo, NY, USA

David R. Byrd, M.D., F.A.C.S.
University of Washington
School of Medicine
Seattle, WA, USA

Carolyn C. Compton, M.D., ph.D.
National Cancer Institute
Bethesda, MD, USA

April G. Fritz, R.H.I.T., C.T.R.
A. Fritz and Associates
Reno, NV, USA

Frederick L. Greene, M.D., F.A.C.S.
Carolinas Medical Center
Charlotte, NC, USA

Andy Trotti, III, M.D.
H. Lee Moffitt Cancer Center
Tampa, FL, USA

ISBN 978-0-387-88442-4
Springer New York Dordrecht Heidelberg London

Library of Congress Control Number: 2009930461

First to Fifth Editions of the *AJCC Cancer Staging Manual*, and the *AJCC Cancer Staging Handbook*, published by Lippincott Raven Publishers, Philadelphia. PA.

Sixth Edition of the *AJCC Cancer Staging Handbook*, published by Springer-Verlag, New York, NY.

Printed on acid-free paper

(First corrected printing 2009)

Springer is part of Springer Science+Business Media (www.springer.com)

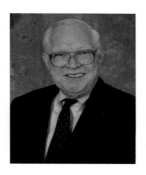

SEVENTH EDITION
Dedicated to Irvin D. Fleming, M.D.

SIXTH EDITION
Dedicated to Robert V. P. Hutter, M.D.

FIFTH EDITION
Dedicated to Oliver Howard Beahrs, M.D.

FOURTH EDITION
Dedicated to the memory of Harvey Baker, M.D.

THIRD EDITION
Dedicated to the memory of W. A. D. Anderson, M.D.
Marvin Pollard, M.D.
Paul Sherlock, M.D.

SECOND EDITION
Dedicated to the memory of Murray M. Copeland, M.D.

## Seventh Edition Dedication

This seventh edition of the *AJCC Cancer Staging Manual* is dedicated to Irvin D. Fleming. Dr. Fleming is a past Chair of the AJCC and a giant in American oncology. The major changes in cancer staging being introduced with this edition are largely the outgrowth of Dr. Fleming's vision in establishing a landmark collaboration between the AJCC and the National Cancer Institute SEER Program, the National Program for Cancer Registries of the CDC, the Commission on Cancer, the National Cancer Registrars Association, and the North American Association of Central Cancer Registries. Dr. Fleming's influence on cancer care and commitment to patients extends well beyond the AJCC as evidenced by his leadership in many organizations, including service as President of the American Cancer Society. For his vision, leadership, friendship, and support, we dedicate this *Manual* in his honor.

# Preface

Cancer staging plays a pivotal role in the battle on cancer. It forms the basis for understanding the changes in population cancer incidence, extent of disease at initial presentation, and the overall impact of improvements in cancer treatment. Staging forms the base for defining groups for inclusion in clinical trials. Most importantly, staging provides those with cancer and their physicians the critical benchmark for defining prognosis and the likelihood of overcoming the cancer and for determining the best treatment approach for their cases.

Refining these standards to provide the best possible staging system is a never-ending process. Toward this end, the American Joint Committee on Cancer (AJCC) has led these efforts in the USA since 1959. A collaborative effort between the AJCC and the International Union for Cancer Control (UICC) maintains the system that is used worldwide. This system classifies the extent of disease based mostly on anatomic information on the extent of the primary tumor, regional lymph nodes, and distant metastases. This classification was developed in the 1940s by Pierre Denoix of France and formalized by the UICC in the 1950s with the formation of the Committee on Clinical Stage Classification and Applied Statistics. The AJCC was founded in 1959 to complement this work. The AJCC published its first cancer staging manual in 1977. Since the 1980s, the work of the UICC and AJCC has been coordinated, resulting in the simultaneous publication of the *TNM Classification of Malignant Tumours* by the UICC and the *AJCC Cancer Staging Manual*. The revision cycle is 6–8 years, a time frame that provides for accommodation of advances in cancer care while allowing cancer registry systems to maintain stable operations.

The work of the AJCC is made possible by the dedicated volunteer effort of hundreds, and perhaps thousands, of committed health professionals including physicians, nurses, population scientists, statisticians, cancer registrars, supporting staff, and others. These volunteers, representing all relevant disciplines, are organized into disease teams chaired by leading clinicians. These teams make recommendations for change in the staging system based on available evidence supplemented with expert consensus. Supporting these teams is a panel of expert statisticians who provide critical support in evaluation of existing data and in analysis of new data when this is available.

The level of data supporting the staging systems varies among disease sites. For some diseases, particularly less common cancers, there are few outcome data available. These staging systems are based on what limited data are available, supplemented by expert consensus. Though potentially imperfect, these disease schemas are critical to allow the collection of standardized data to support clinical care and for future evaluation and refinement of the staging system.

Increasingly, the disease teams of the AJCC and UICC use existing data sets or establish the necessary collaborations to develop new large data sets to provide high-level evidence to support changes in the staging system. Examples of this include the work in melanoma that led to changes in the sixth edition and their refinement in this seventh edition, use of the National Cancer Data Base and Surveillance Epidemiology and End Results (SEER) data base for evaluation of the colorectal staging system, and the use of existing data sets from the USA, Europe, and Asia in gastric cancer. In addition, groups have been established to collect very large international data sets to refine staging. In addition to the melanoma collaborative, the best examples in refining staging for the seventh edition are the collaborative group of the International Association for the Study of Lung Cancer (IASLC) and the Worldwide Esophageal Cancer Collaborative (WECC).

A major challenge to TNM staging is the rapid evolution of understanding in cancer biology and the availability of biologic factors that predict cancer outcome and response to treatment with better accuracy than purely anatomically based staging. This has led some cancer experts to conclude that TNM is obsolete. Although such statements are misguided, the reality is that the anatomic extent of disease only tells part of the story for many cancer patients.

The question of including nonanatomic prognostic factors in *staging* has led to intense debate about the purpose and structure of staging. Beginning with the sixth edition of the *AJCC Cancer Staging Manual*, there was judicious addition of nonanatomic factors to the classifications that modified stage groups. This shift away from purely anatomic information has been extended in the current edition. Relevant markers that are of such importance that they are required for clinicians to make clear treatment decisions have been included in groupings. Examples include the mitotic rate in staging gastrointestinal stromal tumors and prostate-specific antigen and Gleason score in staging prostate cancer. In the future, the discovery of new markers will make it necessary to include these markers in staging and will likely require the development of new strategies beyond the current grouping systems.

That said, it must also be clearly stated that it is critical to maintain the anatomic base to cancer staging. Anatomic extent of disease remains the key prognostic factor in most diseases. In addition, it is necessary to have clear links to past data to assess trends in cancer incidence and the impact of advances in screening and treatment and to be able to apply stage and compare stage worldwide in situations where new nonanatomic factors are not or cannot be collected. Therefore, the staging algorithms in this edition of the *AJCC Cancer Staging Manual* using nonanatomic factors only use them as modifiers of anatomic groupings. These factors are *not* used to define the T, N, and M components, which remain purely anatomic. Where they are used to define groupings, there is always a convention for assigning a group without the nonanatomic factor. These conventions have been established and defined in collaboration with the UICC.

The work for the seventh edition of the *AJCC Cancer Staging Manual* began immediately on publication of the sixth edition. Under the leadership of the Prognostic Factors Task Force of the UICC, an ongoing review of literature relevant to staging was performed and updated annually. A new data collection system that allows capture of nonanatomic information in conjunction with anatomic staging data was developed and implemented in the USA. A number of working groups continued data collection and analysis with the plan to advise AJCC Task Forces. The AJCC provided a competitive grant program to support work to lead to staging revision. An enhanced statistical task force was empanelled. Finally, in 2006, the disease task forces were convened to review available evidence and recommend changes to TNM. After review by the UICC, the changes reflected in this manual were adopted for application to cases diagnosed on or after January 1, 2010.

This work involved many professionals in all fields in the clinical oncology, cancer registry, population surveillance, and statistical communities. It is hard to single out individuals, but certain people were central to this effort. Irvin Fleming, to whom we dedicate this *Manual*, showed the leadership and the vision over a decade ago that led to the development of the Collaborative Stage Data Collection System. Frederick Greene, as senior editor of the sixth edition, paved the way for this work, developed the extremely popular and useful *AJCC Cancer Staging Atlas*, and did the legwork to enhance the collaboration between the UICC and AJCC. The work of our publisher Springer provided the resources to support this work and the patience needed as the Task Forces and editors finished their work. The many cancer registrars and the Collaborative Stage Version 2 Work Group who worked on the disease teams kept us all properly focused. And the AJCC staff, most notably Donna Gress, Karen Pollitt, and Connie Bura provided the glue and the sweat to keep us all together.

We believe that this, the seventh edition of the *AJCC Cancer Staging Manual*, and the electronic and print products built on this manual, will provide strong support to patients and physicians alike as they face the battle with cancer, and we hope that it provides the concepts and the foundation for the future of cancer staging as we move to the era of personalized molecular oncology.

Stephen B. Edge, Buffalo, NY
David R. Byrd, Seattle, WA
Carolyn C. Compton, Bethesda, MD
April G. Fritz, Reno, NV
Frederick L. Greene, Charlotte, NC
Andy Trotti, Tampa, FL

**Brief Contents by Part**

# Contents

# Introduction
# and Historical Overview

The seventh edition of the *AJCC Cancer Staging Manual* is a compendium of all currently available information on the staging of cancer for most clinically important anatomic sites. It has been developed by the American Joint Committee on Cancer (AJCC) in cooperation with the TNM Committee of the International Union Against Cancer (UICC). The two organizations have worked together at every level to create a staging schema that remains uniform throughout. The current climate that allows for consistency of staging worldwide has been made possible by the mutual respect and diligence of those working in the staging area for both the AJCC and the UICC.

Classification and staging of cancer enable the physician and cancer registrar to stratify patients, which leads to better treatment decisions and the development of a common language that aids in the creation of clinical trials for the future testing of cancer treatment strategies. A common language of cancer staging is mandatory in order to realize the important contributions from many institutions throughout the world. This need for appropriate nomenclature was the driving force that led to clinical classification of cancer by the League of Nations Health Organization in 1929 and later by the UICC and its TNM Committee.

The AJCC was first organized on January 9, 1959, as the American Joint Committee for Cancer Staging and End Results Reporting (AJC). The driving force behind the organization of this body was a desire to develop a system of clinical staging for cancer that was acceptable to the American medical profession. The founding organizations of the AJCC are the American College of Surgeons, the American College of Radiology, the College of American Pathologists, the American College of Physicians, the American Cancer Society, and the National Cancer Institute. The governance of the AJCC is overseen by designees from the founding organizations and representatives of the sponsoring organizations including the American Society of Clinical Oncology and the Centers for Disease Control and Prevention. The Medical Director of the Commission on Cancer functions as the Executive Director of the AJCC. Fostering the work of the AJCC has been undertaken by committees called task forces, which have been established for specific anatomic sites of cancer. In preparation for each new edition of the *AJCC Cancer Staging Manual*, the task forces are convened and serve as consensus panels to review scholarly material related to cancer staging and make recommendations to the AJCC regarding potential changes in the staging taxonomy.

During the last 50 years of activity related to the AJCC, a large group of consultants and liaison organization representatives have worked with the AJCC leadership. These representatives have been selected by the American Society of Clinical Oncology, the Centers for Disease Control and Prevention, the American Urological Association, the Association of

American Cancer Institutes, the National Cancer Registrars Association, the Society of Gynecologic Oncologists, the Society of Urologic Oncology, the National Cancer Institute and the SEER Program, the North American Association of Central Cancer Registries (NAACCR), and the American Society of Colon and Rectal Surgeons.

Chairing the AJCC have been Murray Copeland, M.D. (1959–1969), W.A.D. Anderson, M.D. (1969–1974), Oliver H. Beahrs, M.D. (1974–1979), David T. Carr, M.D. (1979–1982), Harvey W. Baker, M.D. (1982–1985), Robert V. P. Hutter, M.D. (1985–1990), Donald E. Henson, M.D. (1990–1995), Irvin D. Fleming, M.D. (1995–2000), Frederick L. Greene, M.D. (2000–2004), David L. Page, M.D. (2004–2005), Stephen B. Edge, M.D. (2005–2008), and currently Carolyn C. Compton, M.D., Ph.D.

The initial work on the clinical classification of cancer was instituted by the League of Nations Health Organization (1929), the International Commission on Stage Grouping and Presentation of Results (ICPR) of the International Congress of Radiology (1953), and the International Union Against Cancer (UICC). The latter organization became most active in the field through its Committee on Clinical Stage Classification and Applied Statistics (1954). This committee was later known as the UICC TNM Committee, which now includes the Chair of the AJCC.

Since its inception, the AJCC has embraced the TNM system in order to describe the anatomic extent of cancer at the time of initial diagnosis and before the application of definitive treatment. In addition, a classification of the stages of cancer was utilized as a guide for treatment and prognosis and for comparison of the end results of cancer management. In 1976 the AJCC sponsored a National Cancer Conference on Classification and Staging. The deliberation at this conference led directly to the development of the first edition of the *Cancer Staging Manual*, which was published in 1977. With the publication of the first edition, the AJCC broadened its scope by recognizing its leadership role in the staging of cancer for American physicians and registrars. The second edition of this manual (1983) updated the earlier edition and included additional sites. This edition also served to enhance conformity with the staging espoused by the TNM Committee of the UICC.

The expanding role of the American Joint Committee in a variety of cancer classifications suggested that the original name was no longer applicable. In June 1980 the new name, the American Joint Committee on Cancer, was selected. Since the early 1980s, the close collaboration of the AJCC and the UICC has resulted in uniform and identical definitions and stage groupings of cancers for all anatomic sites so that a universal system is now available. This worldwide system was espoused by Robert V. P. Hutter, M.D., in his Presidential Address at the combined meeting of the Society of Surgical Oncology and the British Association of Surgical Oncology in London in 1987.

During the 1990s, the importance of TNM staging of cancer in the USA was heightened by the mandatory requirement that Commission on Cancer–approved hospitals use the AJCC-TNM system as the major language for cancer reporting. This requirement has stimulated education of all physicians and registrars in the use of the TNM system, and credit goes to the Approvals Program of the Commission on Cancer for this insightful recognition. The AJCC recognizes that, with this seventh edition of the *AJCC Cancer Staging Manual*, the education of medical students, resident physicians, physicians in practice, and cancer registrars is paramount. As the twenty-first century unfolds, new methods of education will complement the seventh edition of the *AJCC Cancer Staging Manual* and will ensure that all those who care for cancer patients will be trained in the language of cancer staging.

AMERICAN JOINT COMMITTEE ON CANCER

# AJCC CANCER STAGING HANDBOOK

Seventh Edition

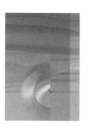

# PART I
# General Information on Cancer Staging and End-Results Reporting

# 1

# Purposes and Principles of Cancer Staging

## INTRODUCTION AND OVERVIEW

The extent or *stage* of cancer at the time of diagnosis is a key factor that defines prognosis and is a critical element in determining appropriate treatment based on the experience and outcomes of groups of prior patients with similar stage. In addition, accurate staging is necessary to evaluate the results of treatments and clinical trials, to facilitate the exchange and comparison of information among treatment centers, and to serve as a basis for clinical and translational cancer research. At a national and international level, the agreement on classifications of cancer cases provides a method of clearly conveying clinical experience to others without ambiguity.

Several cancer staging systems are used worldwide. Differences among these systems stem from the needs and objectives of users in clinical medicine and in population surveillance. The most clinically useful staging system is the tumor node metastasis (TNM) system maintained collaboratively by the American Joint Committee on Cancer (AJCC) and the International Union for Cancer Control (UICC). The TNM system classifies cancers by the size and extent of the primary tumor (T), involvement of regional lymph node (N), and the presence or absence of distant metastases (M), supplemented in recent years by carefully selected nonanatomic prognostic factors. There is a TNM staging algorithm for cancers of virtually every anatomic site and histology, with the primary exception in this manual being staging of pediatric cancers.

**Philosophy of TNM Revision.** The AJCC and UICC periodically modify the TNM system in response to newly acquired clinical data and improved understanding of cancer biology and factors affecting prognosis. Revision is one factor that makes the TNM system the most clinically useful staging system and accounts for its use worldwide. However, changes in staging systems may make it difficult to compare outcomes of current and past groups of patients. Because of this, the organizations only make these changes carefully and based on the best possible evidence.

The revision cycle for TNM staging is 6–8 years. This provides sufficient time for implementation of changes in clinical and cancer registry operations and for relevant examination and discussion of data supporting changes in staging. Table 1.1 shows the publication years for each of the versions of the TNM system up through this current seventh edition of the TNM system. The prior sixth edition was used for cases diagnosed on or after January 1, 2003. The seventh edition published in this manual is effective for cancer cases diagnosed on or after January 1, 2010.

**Anatomic Staging and Use of Nonanatomic Information.** Cancer staging is historically based solely on the anatomic extent of cancer and remains

**TABLE 1.1.** *AJCC Cancer Staging Manual* editions

| Edition | Publication | Dates effective for cancer diagnosed |
|---------|-------------|--------------------------------------|
| 1 | 1977 | 1978–1983 |
| 2 | 1983 | 1984–1988 |
| 3 | 1988 | 1989–1992 |
| 4 | 1992 | 1993–1997 |
| 5 | 1997 | 1998–2002 |
| 6 | 2002 | 2003–2009 |
| 7 | 2009 | 2010– |

primarily anatomic. However, an increasing number of nonanatomic factors about a cancer and its host provide critical prognostic information and may predict the value of specific therapies. Among those factors known to affect patient outcomes and/or response to therapy are the clinical and pathologic anatomic extent of disease, the reported duration of signs or symptoms, gender, age and health status of the patient, the type and grade of the cancer, and the specific biological properties of the cancer. Clinicians use the pure anatomic extent of disease in defining treatment, but in many cases must supplement TNM with other factors in order to counsel patients and make specific treatment recommendations. As more of these factors are fully validated, it will be necessary to develop strategies to incorporate them into prognostic systems for patient management while maintaining the core anatomic structure of staging. The restriction of TNM to anatomic information has led clinicians to develop other prognostic systems and even led some to conclude that TNM is "obsolete" or "anachronistic."

As outlined in this chapter and throughout the *Manual* in many of the revised AJCC staging algorithms, nonanatomic factors are incorporated into stage grouping where needed. This practice started in a limited fashion in prior editions. However, anatomic extent of disease remains central to defining cancer prognosis. Most proposed nonanatomic prognostic factors in use have been validated only for patients with specific types of disease grouped largely on the anatomic stage (e.g., Gleason's score in early stage prostate cancer and genomic profiles that are validated only in women with node-negative breast cancer). Further, it is critical to maintain the ability to report purely anatomic information to allow comparability of patients treated using new prognostic schemas with patients treated in the past using prior anatomic schemas or with current patients for whom new prognostic factors are not obtained because of cost, available expertise, reporting systems, or other logistical issues.

**Defining T, N, M and Timing of Staging Data.** Stage is determined from information on the tumor T, regional nodes N, and metastases M and by grouping cases with similar prognosis. The criteria for defining anatomic extent of disease are specific for tumors at different anatomic sites and of different histologic types. For example, the size of the tumor is a key factor in breast cancer but has no impact on prognosis in colorectal cancer, where the depth of invasion or extent of the cancer is the primary prognostic feature. Therefore, the criteria for T, N, and M are defined separately for each tumor and histologic type. With certain types of tumors, such as Hodgkin and other lymphomas, a different system for designating the extent of disease and prognosis, and for classifying its groupings, is necessary. In these circumstances, other symbols or descriptive criteria are used in place of T, N, and M, and in the case of lymphoma only the *stage group* is defined. The general rules for defining elements of staging are presented later, and the specifics for each type of disease are in the respective chapters.

Beginning with the sixth edition of the *AJCC Cancer Staging Manual*, TNM adopted a change in the rules for timing of staging data collection to coordinate data collection among the major cancer registry organizations in the USA including the North American Central Registry programs [e.g., the NCI Surveillance Epidemiology and End Results Program (SEER) and the National Program of Cancer Registries (NPCR) of the Center for Disease Control and Prevention], and the National Cancer Data Base, and to accommodate changing practice patterns with increased use of sensitive imaging studies that often were applied during the initial diagnostic phase of care, but occurred after surgery. The timing rules state that:

- *Clinical staging* includes any information obtained about the extent of cancer before initiation of definitive treatment (surgery, systemic or radiation therapy, active surveillance, or palliative care) or within 4 months after the date of diagnosis, whichever is *shorter*, as long as the cancer has not clearly progressed during that time frame.
- *Pathologic staging* includes any information obtained about the extent of cancer through completion of definitive surgery as part of first course treatment or identified within 4 months after the date of diagnosis, whichever is *longer*, as long as there is no systemic or radiation therapy initiated or the cancer has not clearly progressed during that time frame.

**TNM Staging Classification: Clinical, Pathologic, Recurrent, Posttreatment, and Autopsy.** Stage may be defined at a number of points in the care of the cancer patient. These include "pretreatment stage" or "clinical stage," and postsurgical or "pathologic stage." In addition, stage may be determined (a) after therapy for those receiving systemic or radiation therapy before surgery (termed neoadjuvant therapy) or as primary treatment without surgery, (b) at the time of recurrence, and (c) for cancers identified at autopsy.

*Clinical stage* (*pretreatment stage*) is the extent of disease defined by diagnostic study before information is available from surgical resection or initiation of neoadjuvant therapy, within the required time frame (see previous discussion). The nomenclature for clinical staging is cT, cN, and cM, and the anatomic stage/prognostic groups based on cTNM are termed the clinical stage groups. Clinical staging incorporates information obtained from symptoms; physical examination; endoscopic examinations; imaging studies of the tumor, regional lymph nodes, and metastases; biopsies of the primary tumor; and surgical exploration without resection. When T is classified only clinically (cT), information from biopsy of single or sentinel lymph nodes may be included in clinical node staging (cN). On occasion, information obtained at the time of surgery may be classified as clinical such as when liver metastases that are identified clinically but not biopsied during a surgical resection of an abdominal tumor.

*Pathologic stage* is defined by the same diagnostic studies used for clinical staging supplemented by findings from surgical resection and histologic examination of the surgically removed tissues. This adds significant additional prognostic information that is more precise than what can be discerned clinically before therapy. This pathologic extent of disease or pathologic stage is expressed as pT, pN, and pM.

*Posttherapy stage* (*yTNM*) documents the extent of the disease for patients whose first course of therapy includes systemic or radiation treatment prior to surgical resection or when systemic therapy or radiation is the primary treatment with no surgical resection. The use of so-called *neoadjuvant* therapy is increasingly common in solid tumors including breast, lung, gastrointestinal, head and neck, and other cancers. Posttherapy stage may be recorded as clinical or pathologic depending on the source of posttreatment information. The extent of disease is classified using the same T, N, and M definitions and identified as posttreatment with a "yc" or "yp" prefix (ycT, ycN, ycTNM; ypT, ypN, ypTNM). Note that American registry systems do not have a data element to record "yc" elements, but these may be recorded in the medical record. The measured response to therapy and/or the extent of cancer after therapy may be prognostic. It is also used to guide subsequent surgery or other therapy.

When a patient receives presurgical treatment and has a posttherapy yc- or yp-TNM stage, the *stage* used for surveillance analysis and for comparison purposes is the clinical stage before the start of therapy. Care should be taken not to record the postneoadjuvant therapy stage as the primary stage for comparison of populations or for clinical trials. This could lead to erroneous reports. For example, a patient with a clinical Stage III breast cancer after chemotherapy could have only residual carcinoma in situ. If the final y stage was used as the original stage, the cancer would be erroneously staged as Stage 0. This would be grossly misleading for a case that in fact presented as a locally advanced Stage III cancer.

Two other staging classifications are defined, though there are no data fields reserved for these stages in most cancer registry systems. The first of these is *"Retreatment" classification* (*rTNM*). This is used because information gleaned from therapeutic procedures and from extent of disease defined clinically may be prognostic for patients with recurrent cancer after a disease-free interval. Clearly the extent of recurrent disease guides therapy, and this should be recorded in the medical record using the TNM classification. It is important to understand that the rTNM classification does not change the original clinical or pathologic staging of the case. The second of these is the *"Autopsy" classification* (*aTNM*) used to stage cases of cancer not recognized during life and only identified postmortem.

**TNM Groupings.** For the purposes of tabulation and analysis of the care of patients with a similar prognosis, T, N, and M are grouped into so-called *anatomic stage/prognostic groups*, commonly referred to as stage groups. Groups are classified by Roman numerals from I to IV with increasing severity of disease. Stage I generally denotes cancers that are smaller or less deeply invasive with negative nodes; Stage II and III define cases with increasing tumor or nodal extent, and Stage IV identifies those who present with distant metastases (M1) at diagnosis. In addition, the term Stage 0 is used to denote carcinoma in situ with no metastatic potential. Stage 0 is almost always determined by pathologic examination.

The primary TNM groupings are purely clinical or pathologic. However, in clinical medicine, it is often expedient to combine clinical and pathologic T, N, and M information to define a mixed stage group for treatment planning. An example of a clinical situation where such "mixed staging" is used clinically is a woman with breast cancer who has had the primary tumor resected providing pathologic T, but for whom there was no lymph node surgery, requiring use of the clinical N. The mixed stage combining clinical and pathologic information is sometimes referred to as *working stage*. However, pure clinical and pathologic stage is still defined for comparative purposes. In addition, clinical M status (M0 or M1) may be mixed with pathologic T and N information to define pathologic stage, and the classification pTis cN0 cM0 may be used to define both clinical and pathologic stage for in situ carcinoma. If there is pathologic evidence of metastases (pM1), it may be used with clinical T and N information to define clinical Stage IV and pathologic Stage IV.

The grouping recommendations in this manual are based primarily on anatomic information. Anatomic extent of disease is supplemented by selected nonanatomic prognostic factors in some disease sites. To denote the significance of this selective use of nonanatomic factors and to underscore the importance of anatomic information, the title of the groupings in the *AJCC Cancer Staging Manual* has been changed to "*Anatomic Stage/ Prognostic Groups.*"

**Recording Cancer Stage in the Medical Record.** All staging classifications, and most importantly clinical and pathologic T, N, and M and stage grouping, should be recorded in the medical record. Clinical stage is used in defining primary therapy (including surgery if surgery is performed), and when surgery is the initial treatment, subsequent systemic or radiation treatment is based on the pathologic stage. Recording clinical stage is also important because it may be the only common denominator among all cancers of a certain anatomic site and histology. Examples include lung cancer, advanced GI tumors, and head and neck cancers where surgery may not be performed, as well as cancers such as prostate cancer and others where surgical resection for limited disease may be omitted. In such scenarios, it may be impossible to compare cases where information is only obtained by clinical means with those where surgical resection is performed. For this reason, clinical stage remains an important component of application of the TNM staging system. This was reinforced in 2008 by the American College of Surgeons Commission on Cancer in its cancer program standards with the requirement that clinical stage be recorded in all cases.

There are many options for recording staging data in the medical record. These include documenting in the initial clinical evaluations, operative reports, discharge summaries, and follow-up reports. Physicians are encouraged to enter the stage of cancer in every record of clinical encounters with the cancer patient. In addition, a paper or electronic staging form may be useful to record stage in the medical record as well as to facilitate communication of staging data to a cancer registry. A simple form for collecting staging data is included for each disease site in this manual.

**The Cancer Registry and the Collaborative Stage Data Collection System.** Recording stage information in a cancer registry allows analysis of treatment effects and longitudinal population studies. Traditionally registries recorded the staging data provided in the medical record or on a staging form by the physician. With the increasing complexity of staging, the potential to incorporate various nonanatomic factors into staging algorithms, and the need to coordinate staging data collection for hospital- and population-based central registries, there was a need for a more standardized data collection tool for staging data. Such a system, termed the Collaborative Stage Data Collection System (CS), was developed by the AJCC and its cancer surveillance and staging partner organizations and implemented in cancer registries in the USA in 2004. It has also been implemented in parts of Canada with the expectation to implement throughout Canada by 2012.

In the CS system, T, N, and M data plus selected nonanatomic factors are recorded and a computer-based algorithm derives TNM stage as defined in the *AJCC Cancer Staging Manual*. The stage derivation uses the nonanatomic factors if they are available and derives a pure anatomic stage if they are not. In addition, the CS algorithm derives Summary Stage 1977 and 2000. In the CS system, the primary data defining T, N, and M are collected and stored in local registries and transmitted to central registries. T is derived from the size and local extension of disease, N from data elements that describe node status and the number of examined and positive nodes, and M from an element that records the presence or absence of metastases. In addition, the CS system includes "site-specific factors" used to record information beyond the anatomic extent of disease. There are two types of site-specific factors: those that are required for deriving the "Anatomic Stage/Prognostic Group" (e.g., Gleason's Score in prostate cancer) and those that are key prognostic or predictive factors for a given disease (e.g., estrogen receptor and HER2/neu status in breast cancer). Anatomic stage/prognostic groups are calculated from the T, N, and M and relevant site-specific factors. Collaborative stage does not assign a "c" or "p" to the stage grouping but only to the TNM elements. The CS system-derived groups are not necessarily purely clinical or pathologic TNM groups, but represent the best stage that combines clinical and pathologic data.

Importantly, the CS system stores the primary data in an interoperable tagged format that may be exported for other purposes including application in prognostic models and nomograms and for research into new prognostic models. The data elements that are collected in the Collaborative Stage Data Collection System are shown in Table 1.2.

The Collaborative Stage Data Collection System has been revised to accommodate this seventh edition of the *AJCC Cancer Staging Manual*. Key revisions are expansion of the site-specific factors to accommodate added prognostic factors and additional data elements necessary to record the clinical stage used for all cases, and the yp stage after neoadjuvant therapy. This will collect information on pretreatment clinical stage prior to the initiation of therapy and the posttreatment pathologic stage (yp) after completion of neoadjuvant therapy in patients who have resection. Detailed information on the CS system and current CS data element standards is available at http://www.cancerstaging.org.

**TABLE 1.2.** Collaborative stage data collection system data elements

| | |
|---|---|
| Tumor | CS tumor size (primary tumor size in mm) |
| | CS extension (direct extension of the primary tumor) |
| | CS tumor size/extension eval (method of evaluating T)[a] |
| Nodes | CS lymph nodes (regional lymph node involvement) |
| | CS lymph nodes eval (method of evaluating N)[a] |
| | Regional nodes positive (number nodes positive) |
| | Regional nodes examined (number nodes examined) |
| Metastases | CS Mets at Dx (distant metastases present at time of diagnosis |
| | CS Mets Eval (method of evaluating M)[a] |
| Site-specific factors | CS site-specific factors (specific number defined by disease)[b] |

[a] Method of evaluation fields: Define source of data – clinical (c) or pathologic (p); response to neoadjuvant therapy utilizing pathologic information (yp).

[b] Site-specific factors: Additional items necessary for (a) defining cancer stage group or (b) key prognostic factors including anatomic disease modifiers and nonanatomic factors (e.g., grade and tumor markers). Most disease sites use only a few of the available site-specific factor fields.

These tumor, node, and metastases fields for best stage are duplicated as needed for pretreatment and posttreatment stages.

For full description of Collaborative Stage Data Collection System, see http://www.cancerstaging.org /cstage/index.html.

## NOMENCLATURE OF THE MORPHOLOGY OF CANCER

Cancer treatment requires assessment of the extent and behavior of the tumor and the status of the patient. The most widely used is TNM based on documentation of the anatomic extent of the cancer and selected related nonanatomic factors. The description of the anatomic factors is specific for each disease site. These descriptors and the nomenclature for TNM have been developed and refined over many editions of the *AJCC Cancer Staging Manual* by experts in each disease and cancer registrars who collect the information, taking into consideration the behavior and natural history of each type of cancer.

An *accurate microscopic diagnosis* is essential to the evaluation and treatment of cancer. The histologic and morphologic characteristics of tumors are generally reported by expert pathologists. This is best accomplished using standardized nomenclature in a structured report such as the synoptic reports or cancer protocols defined by the College of American Pathologists (CAP). In addition, for some cancers measurements of other factors including biochemical, molecular, genetic, immunologic, or functional characteristics of the tumor or normal tissues have become important or essential elements in classifying tumors precisely. Techniques that supplement standard histological evaluation including immunohistochemistry, cytogenetics, and genetic characterization are used to characterize tumors and their potential behavior and response to treatment.

**Related Classifications.** In the interest of promoting international collaboration in cancer research and to facilitate comparison of data among different clinical studies, use of the *WHO International Classification of Tumours* for classification and definition of tumor types, the *International Classifications of Diseases for Oncology* (ICD-0) codes for storage and retrieval of data, CAP protocols for pathology reporting of cancer pathology specimens, and the Collaborative Stage Data Collection System for collecting staging data is recommended. Given here is a summary of relevant related classification and coding systems with source citations.

- *World Health Organization Classification of Tumours, Pathology and Genetics.* Since 1958, the World Health Organization (WHO) has had a program aimed at providing internationally accepted criteria for the histological classification of tumors. The most recent edition is a ten-volume series that contains definitions, descriptions, and illustrations of tumor types and related nomenclature (WHO: World Health Organization Classification of Tumours. Various editions. Lyon, France: IARC Press, 2000–2008).
- *WHO International Classification of Diseases for Oncology (ICD-0), 3rd edition.* ICD-0 is a numerical classification and coding system by topography and morphology (WHO: ICD-O-3 International Classification of Diseases for Oncology. 3rd ed. Geneva: WHO, 2000).
- *Systematized Nomenclature of Medicine (SNOMED).* Published by the CAP, SNOMED provides tumor classification systems compatible with the ICD-O system (http://snomed.org).
- *Collaborative Stage Data Collection System.* This system for collecting cancer staging data was developed through a collaboration of the AJCC and other standard setting organizations. Primary data are recorded on the size and extension of the primary tumor, the status of lymph nodes, and presence of distant metastases and certain "site-specific factors." These data are used to derive TNM stage and Summary Stage (http://www.cancerstaging.org/cstage/index.html).
- *CAP Cancer Protocols.* The CAP publishes standards for pathology reporting of cancer specimens for all cancer types and cancer resection types. These specify the elements necessary for the pathologist to report the extent and characteristics of cancer specimens. These elements are being coordinated with the *Collaborative Stage Data Collection System* to allow direct reporting of pathology elements to cancer registries (http://www.cap.org).
- *caBIG.* The National Cancer Institute of the USA has developed the Cancer Bioinformatics Grid (caBIG) to standardize data elements and integration of these elements for the reporting of information for clinical trials and to annotate biological specimens (http://cabig.cancer.gov).
- *Atlas of Tumor Pathology.* A comprehensive and well-known English language compendium of the macroscopic and microscopic characteristics of tumors and their behavior is the *Atlas of Tumor Pathology* series, published in many volumes by the Armed Forces Institute of Pathology in Washington, DC. These are revised periodically and are used as a basic reference by pathologists throughout the world (*Atlas of Tumor Pathology*, 3rd edition series. Washington, DC: Armed Forces Institute of Pathology, 1991–2002).
- *American College of Radiology Appropriateness Criteria.* The American College of Radiology maintains guidelines and criteria for use of imaging and interventional radiology procedures for many aspects of cancer care. This includes the extent of imaging testing that is recommended for

the diagnostic evaluation of the extent of disease of the primary tumor, nodes, and distant metastases in a number of cancer types. The ACR appropriateness criteria are updated regularly (http://www.acr.org/ac).

- *Practice Guidelines of the National Comprehensive Cancer Network (NCCN).* The NCCN provides practice guidelines for most types of cancers. These guidelines are updated at least annually. They include recommendations for diagnostic evaluation and imaging for the primary tumor and screening for metastases for each cancer type that may be useful to guide staging (http://www.nccn.org).

## GENERAL RULES FOR TNM STAGING

The TNM system classifies and groups cancers primarily by the anatomic extent of the primary tumor, the status of regional draining lymph nodes, and the presence or absence of distant metastases. The system is in essence a shorthand notation for describing the clinical and pathologic anatomic extent of a tumor. In addition, the AJCC recommends collection of key prognostic factors that either are used to define groupings or are critical to prognosis or defining patient care.

T     The T component is defined by the size or contiguous extension of the primary tumor. The roles of the size component and the extent of contiguous spread in defining T are specifically defined for each cancer site.

N     The N component is defined by the absence, or presence and extent of cancer in the regional draining lymph nodes. Nodal involvement is categorized by the number of positive nodes and for certain cancer sites by the involvement of specific regional nodal groups.

M     The M component is defined by the absence or presence of distant spread or metastases, generally in locations to which the cancer spread by vascular channels, or by lymphatics beyond the nodes defined as "regional."

For each of T, N, and M the use of increasing values denotes progressively greater extent of the cancer as shown later. For some disease sites, subdivisions of the main designators are used to provide more specific prognostic information (e.g., T1mi, T1a, T1b, T1c or N2a, N2b in breast cancer or M1a, M1b, M1c for prostate cancer). Specific definitions for each cancer type are provided in the respective chapters. General designators for T, N, and M are shown later and general rules for applying these designators are shown in the tables. For each designator, the prefix of c, p, yc, yp, r, or a may be applied to denote the classification of stage (see later):

| *Primary Tumor (T)* | |
| --- | --- |
| T0 | No evidence of primary tumor |
| Tis | Carcinoma in situ |
| T1, T2, T3, T4 | Increasing size and/or local extension of the primary tumor |
| TX | Primary tumor cannot be assessed (use of TX should be minimized) |

### Regional Lymph Nodes (N)

| | |
|---|---|
| N0 | No regional lymph node metastases |
| N1, N2, N3 | Increasing number or extent of regional lymph node involvement |
| NX | Regional lymph nodes cannot be assessed (use of NX should be minimized) |

### Distant Metastasis (M)

| | |
|---|---|
| M0 | No distant metastases |
| M1 | Distant metastases present |

*Note*: The MX designation has been eliminated from the AJCC/UICC TNM system.

The M1 category may be further specified according to the following notation signifying the location of metastases:

| | |
|---|---|
| Pulmonary | PUL |
| Osseous | OSS |
| Hepatic | HEP |
| Brain | BRA |
| Lymph nodes | LYM |
| Bone marrow | MAR |
| Pleura | PLE |
| Peritoneum | PER |
| Adrenal | ADR |
| Skin | SKI |
| Other | OTH |

**Nonanatomic Prognostic Factors Required for Staging.** In some cancer types, nonanatomic factors are required for assigning the anatomic stage/prognostic group. These are clearly defined in each chapter. These factors are collected separately from T, N, and M, which remain purely anatomic, and are used to assign stage groups. Where nonanatomic factors are used in groupings, there is a definition of the groupings provided for cases where the nonanatomic factor is not available (X) or where it is desired to assign a group ignoring the nonanatomic factor.

**Use of the Unknown X Designation.** The X category is used when information on a specific component is unknown. Cases where T or N is classified as X cannot be assigned a stage (an exception is *Any T* or *Any N M1*, which includes TX or NX, classified as Stage IV – e.g., TX NX M1 or TX N3 M1 are Stage IV). Therefore, the X category for T and N should be used only when absolutely necessary.

The category MX has been eliminated from the AJCC/UICC TNM system. Unless there is clinical or pathologic evidence of distant metastases, the case is classified as clinical M0 (cM0). Because of the requirement for pathologists to assign TNM on cancer pathology reports, and because the pathologist often does not have information to assign M, the CAP has dropped the M component from pathology templates to further discour-

**TABLE 1.3.** General rules for TNM staging

| *General rules for staging* | |
|---|---|
| Microscopic confirmation | Microscopic confirmation required for TNM classification |
| | Rare cases without microscopic confirmation should be analyzed separately |
| | Cancers classified by ICD-O-3 |
| | Recommend pathology reporting using CAP cancer protocols |
| Timing of data eligible for clinical staging | Data obtained before definitive treatment as part of primary treatment or within 4 months of diagnosis, whichever is shorter |
| | The time frame for collecting clinical stage data also ends when a decision is made for active surveillance ("watchful waiting") without therapy |
| Timing data eligible for pathologic staging | Data obtained through definitive surgery as part of primary treatment or within 4 months of diagnosis, whichever is longer |
| Timing of data eligible for staging with neoadjuvant therapy | Stage in cases with neoadjuvant therapy is (a) clinical as defined earlier before initiation of therapy and (b) clinical or pathologic using data obtained after completion of neoadjuvant therapy (ycTNM or ypTNM) |
| Staging in cases with uncertainty among T, N, or M categories | Assign the lower (less advanced) category of T, N, or M, prognostic factor, or stage group |
| Absence of staging-required nonanatomic prognostic factor | Assign stage grouping by the group defined by the lower (less advanced) designation for that factor |
| Multiple synchronous primary tumors in single organ | Stage T by most advanced tumor; use "m" suffix or the number of tumors in parentheses, e.g., pT3(m)N0M0 or pT3(4)N0M0 |
| Synchronous primary tumors in paired organs | Stage and report independently |
| Metachronous primary tumors in single organ (not recurrence) | Stage and report independently |
| T0 staging – unknown primary | Stage based on clinical suspicion of primary tumor (e.g., T0 N1 M0 Group IIA breast cancer) |

age use of MX. The elimination of the code MX is a change in the seventh edition of the *AJCC Cancer Staging Manual* and *UICC TNM Cancer Staging Manual*. See later for rules for M classification.

The following general rules apply to application of T, N, and M for all sites and classifications (Table 1.3):

1. Microscopic confirmation: All cases should be confirmed microscopically for classification by TNM (including clinical classification). Rare cases that do not have any biopsy or cytology of the tumor can be staged, but survival should be analyzed separately. These cases should not be included in overall disease survival analyses.

2. Eligible time period for determination of staging:
    a. *Clinical staging* includes any information obtained about the extent of cancer before initiation of definitive treatment (surgery, systemic or radiation therapy, active surveillance, or palliative care) or within 4 months after the date of diagnosis, whichever is *shorter*, as long as the cancer has not clearly progressed during that time frame.
    b. *Pathologic staging* includes any information obtained about the extent of cancer up through completion of definitive surgery as part of first course treatment or identified within 4 months after the date of diagnosis, whichever is *longer*, as long as there is no systemic or radiation therapy initiated or the cancer has not clearly progressed during that time frame.
3. Staging with neoadjuvant or primary systemic or radiation therapy: Cases with neoadjuvant, or primary systemic or radiation, therapy may have a second stage defined from information obtained after therapy that is recorded using a yc or yp prefix (ycTNM or ypTNM; y must always be modified as yc or yp). However, these patients should also have clinical stage recorded as this is the stage used for comparative purposes. Clinical stage includes only information collected prior to the start of treatment.
4. Progression of disease: In cases where there is documented progression of cancer prior to the initiation of therapy or surgery, only information obtained prior to documented progression is used for staging.
5. If uncertain, classify or stage using the lower category: If there is uncertainty in assigning a T, N, or M classification, a stage modifying factor (i.e., in clinical situations where it is unclear if the lymph nodes are N2 or N1), or anatomic stage/prognostic group, default to the lower (lesser) of the two categories in the uncertain range.
6. Nonanatomic factor not available: If a nonanatomic factor required for grouping is not available, the case is assigned to the group assuming that factor was the lowest or least advanced (e.g., lower Gleason's score in prostate cancer).

**Stage Classifications.** Five stage classifications may be described for each site (Table 1.4):

- Clinical stage/pretreatment stage, designated as cTNM or TNM
- Pathologic stage, designated as pTNM
- Post therapy or postneoadjuvant therapy stage, designated as ycTNM or ypTNM
- Retreatment or recurrence classification, designated as rTNM
- Autopsy classification, designated as aTNM

**Clinical Classification.** Clinical classification is based on evidence acquired before the initiation of primary treatment (definitive surgery, or neoadjuvant radiation or systemic therapy). The clinical stage (pretreatment stage) is essential to selecting primary therapy. In addition, the clinical stage is critical for comparison of groups of cases because differences in the use of primary therapy may make such comparisons based on pathologic assessment impossible, such as in situations where some patients are treated with primary surgery and others are treated with neoadjuvant chemotherapy or with no therapy.

**TABLE 1.4.** Staging classifications

| Classification | Data source | Usage |
|---|---|---|
| Clinical (pretreatment) (cTNM) | Diagnostic data including symptoms, physical examination, imaging, endoscopy; biopsy of primary site; resection of single node/sentinel node(s) with clinical T; surgical exploration without resection; other relevant examinations | Define prognosis and initial therapy<br><br>Population comparisons |
| Pathologic (pTNM) | Diagnostic data and data from surgical resection and pathology | Most precise prognosis estimates<br><br>Define subsequent therapy |
| Post therapy (ycTNM or ypTNM) | Clinical and pathologic data after ystemic or radiation before surgery or as primary therapy denoted with a yc (clinical) or yp (pathologic) prefix | Determine subsequent therapy<br><br>Identify response to therapy |
| Retreatment (rTNM) | Clinical and pathologic data at time of retreatment for recurrence or progression | Define treatment |
| Autopsy (aTNM) | Clinical and pathologic data as determined at autopsy | Define cancer stage on previously undiagnosed cancer identified at autopsy |

Clinical assessment uses information available from clinical history, physical examination, imaging, endoscopy, biopsy of the primary site, surgical exploration, or other relevant examinations. Observations made at surgical exploration where a biopsy of the primary site is performed without resection or where pathologic material is not obtained are classified as clinical, unless the biopsy provides pathologic material on the highest possible T category in which case it is classified at pT (see pathologic staging later). Pathologic examination of a single node in the absence of pathologic evaluation of the primary tumor is classified as clinical (cN) (e.g., if sentinel node biopsy is performed prior to neoadjuvant therapy in breast cancer). Extensive imaging is not necessary to assign clinical classifications. Guides to the generally accepted standards for diagnostic evaluations of individual cancer types include the American College of Radiology Appropriateness Standards (http://www.acr.org/ac) and the NCCN Practice Guidelines (http://www.nccn.org). The clinical (pretreatment) stage assigned on the basis of information obtained prior to cancer-directed treatment is not changed on the basis of subsequent information obtained from the pathologic examination of resected tissue or from information obtained after initiation of definitive therapy. In the case of treatment with palliative care or active surveillance (watchful waiting), the information for staging is that defined prior to making the decision for no active treatment or that which occurs within 4 months of diagnosis, whichever is shorter. Any information obtained after the decision for active surveillance or palliative care may not used in clinical staging. Classification of T, N, and M by clinical means is denoted by use of a lower case c prefix (cT, cN, cM).

Clinical staging of metastases warrants special consideration. A case where there are no symptoms or signs of metastases is classified as clinically M0. There is no MX classification. The only evaluation necessary to classify a case as clinically M0 is history and physical examination. It is not necessary to do extensive imaging studies to classify a case as clinically M0. The optimal extent of testing required in many cancer types is provided in guidelines of the American College of Radiology Appropriateness Criteria (http://www. acr.org/ac) and in the National Comprehensive Cancer Network practice guidelines (http://www.nccn.org). The classification pM0 does not exist and may not be assigned on the basis of a negative biopsy of a suspected metastatic site. Cases with clinical evidence of metastases by examination, invasive procedures including exploratory surgery, and imaging, but without a tissue biopsy confirming metastases are classified as cM1. If there is a positive biopsy of a metastatic site (pM1) and T and N are staged only clinically, then the case may be staged as clinical and pathologic Stage IV.

**Pathologic Classification.** The pathologic classification of a cancer is based on information acquired before treatment supplemented and modified by the additional evidence acquired during and from surgery, particularly from pathologic examination of resected tissues. The pathologic classification provides additional precise and objective data. Classification of T, N, and M by pathologic means is denoted by use of a lower case p prefix (pT, pN, pM).

*Pathologic T.* The pathologic assessment of the *primary tumor (pT)* generally is based on resection of the primary tumor generally from a single specimen (Table 1.5). Resection of the tumor with several partial removals at the same or separate operations necessitates an effort at reasonable estimates of the size and extension of the tumor to assign the correct or highest pT category. Tumor size should be recorded in whole millimeters. If the size is reported in smaller units such as a tenth or hundredth of a millimeter, it should be rounded to the nearest whole millimeter for reporting stage. Rounding is performed as follows: one through four are rounded down, and five through nine are rounded up. For example, a breast tumor

**TABLE 1.5.** T classification rules

| |
|---|
| T determined by site-specific rules based on size and/or local extension |
| Clinical assessment of T (cT) based on physical examination, imaging, endoscopy, and biopsy and surgical exploration without resection |
| Pathologic assessment of T (pT) entails a resection of the tumor or may be assigned with biopsy only if it assigns the highest T category |
| pT generally based on resection in single specimen. If resected in >1 specimen, make reasonable estimate of size/extension. Disease-specific rules may apply |
| Tumor size should be recorded in whole millimeters. If the size is reported in smaller units such as a tenth or hundredth of a millimeter, it should be rounded to the nearest whole millimeter for reporting stage. Rounding is performed as follows: one through four are rounded down, and five through nine are rounded up |
| If not resected, and highest T and N category can be confirmed microscopically; case may be classified by pT or pN without resection |

reported as 1.2 mm in size should be recorded for staging as a 1-mm tumor, and a 1.7-mm tumor should be recorded as a 2-mm tumor. If the tumor is not resected, but a biopsy of the primary tumor is performed that is adequate to evaluate the highest pT category, the pT classification is assigned. Some disease sites have specific rules to guide assignment of pT category in such cases.

***Pathologic N.*** The pathologic assessment of *regional lymph nodes* (pN) ideally requires resection of a minimum number of lymph nodes to assure that there is sufficient sampling to identify positive nodes if present (Table 1.6). This number varies among diseases sites, and the expected number of lymph nodes is defined in each chapter. The recommended number generally does not apply in cases where sentinel node has been accepted as accurate for defining regional node involvement and a sentinel node procedure has been performed. However, in cases where lymph node surgery results in examination of fewer than the ideal minimum number, the N category is still generally classified as pathologic N according to the number of positive nodes and/or location of the most advanced pathologic node resected. At least one node with presence or absence of cancer documented by pathologic examination is required for pathologic staging N. The impact of use of pathologic N classification with fewer than the minimum resected nodes may be subsequently defined by review of the number of resected nodes as recorded in a cancer registry.

Pathologic assessment of T (pT) is generally necessary to assign pathologic assessment of lymph nodes. In conjunction with pT, it is not necessary to have pathologic confirmation of the status of the highest N category to

**TABLE 1.6.** N classification rules

| |
| --- |
| Categorize N by disease-specific rules based on number and location of positive regional nodes |
| Minimum expected number and location of nodes to examine for staging defined by disease type |
| If lymph node surgery is performed, classify N category as pathologic even if minimum number is not examined |
| Pathologic assessment of the primary tumor (pT) is necessary to assign pathologic assessment of nodes (pN) except with unknown primary (T0). If pathologic T (pT) is available, then any microscopic evaluation of nodes is pN |
| In cases with only clinical T in the absence of pT excision of a single node or sentinel node(s) is classified as clinical nodal status (cN) |
| Microscopic examination of a single node or nodes in the highest N category is classified as pN even in the absence of pathologic information on other nodes |
| Sentinel lymph node biopsy is denoted with (sn), e.g., pN0(sn); pN1(sn) |
| Lymph nodes with ITC only generally staged as pN0; disease-specific rules may apply (e.g., melanoma) |
| Direct extension of primary tumor into regional node classified as node positive |
| Tumor nodule with smooth contour in regional node area classified as positive node |
| When size is the criterion for N category, stage by size of metastasis, not size of node when reported (unless specified in disease-specific rules) |

assign pN. However, if N is based on microscopic confirmation of the highest N category, it is pN regardless of whether T is pT or cT. For example, in the case of breast cancer with pT defined by resection, pN may be assigned solely on the basis of resected level I or II nodes, or a level I sentinel node without biopsy of level III or supraclavicular nodes. However, if there is microscopic confirmation of supraclavicular node involvement, the case may also be classified as pN3.

Specialized pathologic techniques such as immunohistochemistry or molecular techniques may identify limited metastases in lymph nodes that may not have been identified without the use of the special diagnostic techniques. Single tumor cells or small clusters of cells are classified as *isolated tumor cells* (ITC). The standard definition for ITC is a cluster of cells not more than 0.2 mm in greatest diameter. The appropriate N classification for cases with nodes only involved by ITC's is defined in the disease site chapters for those cancers where this commonly occurs. In most of such chapters, these cases with ITC only in lymph nodes or distant sites are classified as pN0 or cM0. This rule also generally applies to cases with findings of tumor cells or their components by nonmorphologic techniques such as flow cytometry or DNA analysis. There are specific designators to identify such cases by disease site [e.g., N0 (i+) in breast cancer to denote nodes with ITC only].

***Pathologic M.*** The pathologic assignment of the presence of *metastases* (*pM1*) requires a biopsy positive for cancer at the metastatic site (Table 1.7). Pathologic M0 is an undefined concept and the category pM0 may not be used. Pathologic classification of the absence of distant metastases can only be made at autopsy. However, the assessment of metastases to group a patient by pathologic TNM groupings may be either clinical (cM0 or cM1) or pathologic (pM1) (e.g., pTNM = pT; pN; cM or pM). Cases with a biopsy of a possible metastatic site that shows ITC such as circulating tumor cells (CTCs) or disseminated tumor cells (DTCs), or bone marrow

**TABLE 1.7.** M classification rules

| |
|---|
| Clinical M classification only requires history and examination |
| Imaging of distant organ sites not required to assign cM0 |
| Infer status as clinical M0 status unless known clinical M1 |
| "MX" is not a valid category and may not be assigned |
| Elimination of "MX" is new with AJCC/UICC, 7th edition |
| Pathologic M classification requires a positive biopsy of the metastatic site (pM1) |
| Pathologic M0 ("pM0") is not a valid category and may not be assigned |
| Stage a case with a negative biopsy of suspected metastatic site as cM0 |
| Case with pathologic T and N may be grouped as pathologic TNM using clinical M designator (cM0 or cM1) (e.g., pT1 pN0 cM0 = pathologic stage I) |
| Case with pathologic M1 (pM1) may be grouped as clinical and pathologic Stage IV regardless of "c" or "p" status of T and N (e.g., cT1 cN1 pM1 = clinical or pathologic stage IV) |
| ITC in metastatic sites (e.g., bone marrow) |
| Or circulating or DTCs classified as cM0(i+) |
| Disease-specific rules may apply |

micrometastases detected by IHC or molecular techniques are classified as cM0(i+) to denote the uncertain prognostic significance of these findings and to classify the stage group according to the T and N and M0.

Pathologic staging depends on the proven anatomic extent of disease, whether or not the primary lesion has been completely removed. If a primary tumor cannot be technically removed, or when it is unreasonable to remove it, and if the highest T and N categories or the M1 category of the tumor can be confirmed microscopically, the criteria for pathologic classification and staging have been satisfied without total removal of the primary tumor. Note that microscopic confirmation of the highest T and N does not necessarily require removal of that structure and may entail biopsy only.

***Posttherapy or Postneoadjuvant Therapy Classification (yTNM).*** Cases where systemic and/or radiation therapy are given before surgery (*neoadjuvant*) or where no surgery is performed may have the extent of disease assessed at the conclusion of the therapy by clinical or pathologic means (if resection performed). This classification is useful to clinicians because the extent of response to therapy may provide important prognostic information to patients and help direct the extent of surgery or subsequent systemic and/or radiation therapy. T and N are classified using the same categories as for clinical or pathologic staging for the disease type, and the findings are recorded using the prefix designator y (e.g., ycT; ycN; ypT; ypN). The yc prefix is used for the clinical stage after therapy, and the yp prefix is used for the pathologic stage for those cases that have surgical resection after neoadjuvant therapy. Both the ycTNM and ypTNM may be recorded in the medical record, though cancer registries will in general only record the ypTNM in cases where surgery is performed. The M component should be classified by the M status defined clinically or pathologically prior to therapy. If a biopsy of a metastatic site is positive, the case is classified as clinical and pathologic Stage IV. The estimate of disease prior to therapy is recorded using the clinical designator as described earlier (cTNM). The stage used for case comparisons and population purposes in these cases should be the clinical (cTNM) one.

***Retreatment Classification.*** The retreatment classification (rTNM) is assigned when further treatment is planned for a cancer that recurs after a disease-free interval. The original stage assigned at the time of initial diagnosis and treatment does not change when the cancer recurs or progresses. The use of this staging for retreatment or recurrence is denoted using the r prefix (rTNM). All information available at the time of retreatment should be used in determining the rTNM stage. Biopsy confirmation of recurrent cancer is important if clinically feasible. However, this may not be appropriate for each component, so clinical evidence for the T, N, or M component by clinical, endoscopic, radiologic, or related methods may be used.

***Autopsy Classification.*** TNM classification of a cancer may be performed by postmortem examination for a patient where cancer was not evident prior to death. This autopsy classification (aTNM) is denoted using the a prefix (aTNM) and should include all clinical and pathologic information obtained at the time of death and autopsy.

**Stage Groupings.** Cases of cancers with similar prognosis are grouped based on the assigned cT, cN, and cM and/or pT, pN and c/pM categories, and disease-specific groups of T, N, and M are defined. In select disease sites nonanatomic factors are required to supplement T, N, and M to define these groups. Termed *anatomic stage/prognostic groups*, and commonly referred to as stage groups, these form a reproducible and easily communicated summary of staging information (Table 1.8).

Groups are assigned increasing values that correlate with worsening prognosis. Stage I is usually assigned to tumors confined to the primary site with a better prognosis, stages II and III for tumors with increasing local and regional nodal involvement, and stage IV to cases with distant metastatic disease. In addition, a group termed stage 0 is assigned to cases of carcinoma in situ (CIS). Groupings may be expanded into subsets (e.g., stage II can become stage IIA, stage IIB) for more refined prognostic information.

Generally, a pure clinical group and pure pathologic group are defined for each case, using the classifications discussed earlier. In the clinical setting, it is appropriate to combine clinical and pathologic data when only partial information is available in either the pathologic or clinical classification, and this may be referred to as the *working* stage.

Carcinoma in situ (CIS) is an exception to the stage grouping guidelines. By definition, CIS has not involved any structures in the primary organ that would allow tumor cells to spread to regional nodes or distant sites. Therefore, pTis cN0 cM0 should be reported as both clinical and pathologic stage 0.

The clinical, pathologic, and if applicable, posttherapy and retreatment, groups are recorded in the medical record. Once assigned according to the appropriate rules and timing, the stage group recorded in the medical record does not change. The rule applied to T, N, or M that in cases with uncertainty about the classification the cases are assigned the lower (less advanced) category also applies to grouping. One specific circumstance requires special comment. When there has been a complete pathologic response and the ypTNM is ypT0 ypN0 cM0, this is not a "stage 0" case as this would denote in situ disease, and as in every case, the stage for comparison of cases is the pretreatment clinical stage.

**TABLE 1.8.** Anatomic stage/prognostic grouping rules

| |
|---|
| Define separate clinical and pathologic group for each case |
| May combine clinical and pathologic information as a "working stage" in either the pathologic or clinical classification when only partial information is available – this may be necessary for clinical care |
| Minimize use of TX and NX |
| Use of "X" for any component makes case unstageable |
| Case will not be usable in comparison analyses (exception: any combination of T and N including TX or NX with M1 is stage IV) |
| For groupings that require a nonanatomic factor, if factor is missing, stage using lowest category for that factor |
| Case with pT and pN and cM0 or cM1 staged as pathologic stage group |
| Case with cT and cN and pM1 staged as clinical and pathologic stage group |
| Carcinoma in situ, stage pTis cN0 cM0 as both clinical and pathologic stage 0 |

**Multiple Tumors.** When there are multiple simultaneous tumors of the same histology in one organ, the tumor with the highest T category is the one selected for classification and staging, and the multiplicity or the number of tumors is indicated in parentheses: for example, T2(m) or T2(5). For simultaneous bilateral cancers in paired organs, the tumors are classified separately as independent tumors in different organs. For tumors of the thyroid, liver, and ovary, multiplicity is a criterion of the T classification. Most registry software systems have a mechanism to record the m descriptor.

**Metachronous Primaries.** Second or subsequent primary cancers occurring in the same organ or in different organs are staged as a new cancer using the TNM system described in this manual. Second cancers are not staged using the y prefix unless the treatment of the second cancer warrants this use.

**Unknown Primary.** In cases where there is no evidence of a primary tumor or the site of the primary tumor is unknown, staging may be based on the clinical suspicion of the primary tumor with the T category classified as T0. For example, a case with metastatic adenocarcinoma in axillary lymph nodes that is pathologically consistent with breast cancer, but in which there is no apparent primary breast tumor may be classified as breast cancer – T0 N1 M0 (Table 1.9).

## HISTOPATHOLOGIC TYPE, GRADE, AND OTHER DESCRIPTORS

**Histopathologic Type.** The histopathologic type is a *qualitative* assessment whereby a tumor is categorized according to the normal tissue type or cell type it most closely resembles (e.g., hepatocellular or cholangiocarcinoma, osteosarcoma, squamous cell carcinoma). The *World Health Organization Classification of Tumours* published in numerous anatomic site-specific editions may be used for histopathologic typing. Each chapter in the *AJCC Cancer Staging Manual* includes the applicable ICD-O-3 histopathologic codes expressed as individual codes or ranges of codes. If a specific histology is not listed, the case should not be staged using the AJCC classification in that chapter.

**Grade.** The grade of a cancer is a qualitative assessment of the degree of differentiation of the tumor. Grade may reflect the extent to which a tumor resembles the normal tissue at that site. Historically, histologic stratification of solid tumors has been dominated by the description of differentiation with grade expressed as the overall histologic differentiation of the cancer in numerical grades from the most or well differentiated (grade 1) to the least differentiated (grade 3 or 4). This system is still used in some cancer types. For many cancer types, more precise and reproducible grading systems have been developed. These incorporate more specific and objective criteria based on single or multiple characteristics of the cancers. These factors include such characteristics as nuclear grade, the number of mitoses identified microscopically (mitotic count), measures of histologic differentiation (e.g., tubule formation in breast cancer), and others. For some cancer types these systems have been fully validated and largely

**TABLE 1.9.** Special classification/designator rules

| | | |
|---|---|---|
| ycTNM or ypTNM | Posttherapy classification: "y" prefix to utilize with "c" or "p" for denoting extent of cancer after neoadjuvant or primary systemic and/or radiation therapy | Assess clinical stage prior to initiation of therapy (cTNM) |
| | | Use cTNM for comparison of cases and population surveillance |
| | | Denote posttherapy T and N stage using "y" prefix – ycT; ycN; ypT; ypN |
| | | yc is used for clinical information postprimary therapy systemic or radiation therapy, or postneoadjuvant therapy before surgery |
| | | yp is used for pathologic postneoadjuvant systemic or radiation therapy followed by surgical resection |
| | | Use clinical/pretreatment M status |
| r TNM | Retreatment classification | The original stage assigned at initial diagnosis and treatment should not be changed at the time of recurrence or progression |
| | | Assign for cases where treatment is planned for cancer that recurs after a disease-free interval |
| | | Use all information available at time of retreatment or recurrence (c or p) |
| | | Biopsy confirmation desirable if feasible, but not required |
| a TNM | Autopsy classification | Applied for cases where cancer is not evident prior to death |
| | | Use all clinical and pathologic information obtained at the time of death and at postmortem examination |
| m suffix | Multiple primary tumors | Multiple simultaneous tumors in one organ: Assign T by the tumor with the highest T category. Indicate multiplicity by "(m)" or "(number)" in parentheses – e.g., T2(m) or T2(5) |

implemented worldwide. Examples include the Gleason's scoring system for prostate cancer and the Scarff–Bloom–Richardson (Nottingham) grading system for breast cancer.

The recommended grading system for each cancer type is specified in the site-specific chapters. In general, when there is no specific grading system for a cancer type, it should be noted if a two-grade, three-grade, or four-grade system was used. For some anatomic sites, grade 3 and grade 4 are combined into a single grade – for example, poorly differentiated to undifferentiated (G3–4). The use of grade 4 is reserved for those tumors that show no specific differentiation that would identify the cancer as arising from its site of origin. In some sites, the WHO histologic classification includes undifferentiated carcinomas. For these, the tumor is graded as undifferentiated – grade 4. Some histologic tumor types are by definition listed as grade 4 for staging purposes but are not to be assigned a grade of undifferentiated in ICD-O-3 coding for cancer registry purposes. These include the following:

- Small cell carcinoma, any site
- Large cell carcinoma of lung
- Ewing's sarcoma of bone and soft tissue
- Rhabdomyosarcoma of soft tissue

The grade should be recorded for each cancer. Two data elements should be recorded: the grade and whether a two, three, or four-grade system was used for grading. If there is evidence of more than one grade of level or differentiation of the tumor, the least differentiated (highest grade) is recorded.

**Residual Tumor and Surgical Margins.** The absence or presence of residual tumor after treatment is described by the symbol R. cTNM and pTNM describe the extent of cancer in general without consideration of treatment. cTNM and pTNM can be supplemented by the R classification, which deals with the tumor status after treatment. In some cases treated with surgery and/or with neoadjuvant therapy there will be residual tumor at the primary site after treatment because of incomplete resection or local and regional disease that extends beyond the limit or ability of resection. The presence of residual tumor may indicate the effect of therapy, influence further therapy, and be a strong predictor of prognosis. In addition, the presence or absence of disease at the margin of resection may be a predictor of the risk of recurrent cancer. The presence of residual disease or positive margins may be more likely with more advanced T or N category tumors. The R category is not incorporated into TMM staging itself. However, the absence or presence of residual tumor and status of the margins may be recorded in the medical record and cancer registry.

The absence or presence of residual tumor at the primary tumor site after treatment is denoted by the symbol R. The R categories for the primary tumor site are as follows:

R0    No residual tumor
R1    Microscopic residual tumor
R2    Macroscopic residual tumor
RX    Presence of residual tumor cannot be assessed

The margin status may be recorded using the following categories:

- Negative margins (tumor not present at the surgical margin)
- Microscopic positive margin (tumor not identified grossly at the margin, but present microscopically at the margin)
- Macroscopic positive margin (tumor identified grossly at the margin)
- Margin not assessed

**Lymph-Vascular Invasion.** Indicates whether microscopic lymph-vascular invasion (LVI) is identified in the pathology report. This term includes lymphatic invasion, vascular invasion, or lymph-vascular invasion (synonymous with "lymphovascular").

## ORGANIZATION OF THE *AJCC CANCER STAGING MANUAL* AND ANATOMIC SITES AND REGIONS

In general, the anatomic sites for cancer in this manual are listed by primary site code number according to the International Classification of Diseases for Oncology (ICD-O, third edition, WHO, 2000). Each disease site or region is discussed and the staging classification is defined in a separate chapter. There are a number of new chapters and disease sites in this seventh edition of the *AJCC Cancer Staging Manual.*

Each chapter includes a discussion of information relevant to staging that cancer type, the data supporting the staging, and the specific rationale for changes in staging. In addition, it includes definition of key prognostic factors including those required for staging and those recommended for collection in cancer registries. Each chapter ends with the specific definitions of T, N, M, site-specific factors, and anatomic stage/prognostic groups (Table 1.10).

**TABLE 1.10.** Chapter outline for the seventh edition of the *AJCC Cancer Staging Manual*

| | |
|---|---|
| Staging at a Glance | Summary of anatomic stage/prognostic grouping and major changes |
| Changes in Staging | Table summarizing changes in staging from the 6th edition |
| Introduction | Overview of factors affecting staging and outcome for the disease |
| Anatomic Considerations | Primary tumor |
| | Regional lymph nodes |
| | Metastatic sites |
| Rules for Classification | Clinical |
| | Pathologic |
| Prognostic Features | Identification and discussion of nonanatomic prognostic factors important in each disease |
| Definitions of TNM | T: Primary tumor |
| | N: Regional lymph nodes |
| | M: Distant metastases |
| Anatomic Stage/Prognostic Groups | |
| Prognostic Factors (Site-Specific Factors) | (a) Required for staging |
| | (b) Clinically significant |
| Grade | |
| Histopathologic Type | |
| Bibliography | |
| Staging Form | |

**Cancer Staging Data Form.** Each site chapter includes a staging data form that may be used by providers and registrars to record the TNM classifications and the stage of the cancer. The form provides for entry of data on T, N, M, site-specific prognostic factors, cancer grade, and anatomic stage/prognostic groups. This form may be useful for recording information in the medical record and for communication of information from providers to the cancer registrar.

The staging form may be used to document cancer stage at different points in the course of therapy, including before the initiation of therapy, after surgery and completion of all staging evaluations, or at the time of recurrence. It is best to use a separate form at each point. If all time points are recorded on a single form, the staging basis for each element should be clearly identified.

The cancer staging form is a specific additional document in the patient records. It is not a substitute for documentation of history, physical examination, and staging evaluation, nor for documenting treatment plans or follow-up. The data forms in this manual may be duplicated for individual or institutional use without permission from the AJCC or the publisher. Incorporation of these forms into electronic record systems requires appropriate permission from the AJCC and the publisher.

# Cancer Survival Analysis

Analysis of cancer survival data and related outcomes is necessary to assess cancer treatment programs and to monitor the progress of regional and national cancer control programs. The appropriate use of data from cancer registries for outcomes analyses requires an understanding of the correct application of appropriate quantitative tools and the limitations of the analyses imposed by the source of data, the degree to which the available data represent the population, and the quality and completeness of registry data. In this chapter the most common survival analysis methodology is illustrated, basic terminology is defined, and the essential elements of data collection and reporting are described. Although the underlying principles are applicable to both, the focus of this discussion is on the use of survival analysis to describe data typically available in cancer registries rather than to analyze research data obtained from clinical trials or laboratory experimentation. Discussion of statistical principles and methodology will be limited. Persons interested in statistical underpinnings or research applications are referred to textbooks that explore these topics at length.[1-7]

## BASIC CONCEPTS

A *survival rate* is a statistical index that summarizes the probable frequency of specific outcomes for a group of patients at a particular point in time. A *survival curve* is a summary display of the pattern of survival rates over time. The basic concept is simple. For example, for a certain category of patient, one might ask what proportion is likely to be alive at the end of a specified interval, such as 5 years. The greater the proportion surviving, the lower the *risk* for this category of patients. Survival analysis, however, is somewhat more complicated than it first might appear. If one were to measure the length of time between diagnosis and death or record the vital status when last observed for every patient in a selected patient group, one might be tempted to describe the survival of the group as the proportion alive at the end of the period under investigation. This simple measure is informative only if all of the patients were observed for the same length of time.

In most real situations, not all members of the group are observed for the same amount of time. Patients diagnosed near the end of the study period are more likely to be alive at last contact and will have been followed for less time than those diagnosed earlier. Even though it was not possible to follow these persons as long as the others, their survival might eventually prove to be just as long or longer. Although we do not know the complete survival time for these individuals, we do know a minimum survival time (time from diagnosis to last known contact date), and this information is still valuable in estimating survival rates. Similarly, it is usually not possible to know the outcome status of all of the patients who were in the group at the beginning. People may be lost to follow-up for many reasons: they may move, change names, or change physicians. Some of these individuals may have died and others could be still living. Thus, if a survival rate is to describe the outcomes for an entire group accurately, there must be some means to deal with the fact that different people in the group are observed for different lengths of time and that for others, their vital status is not known at the time of analysis. In the language of survival analysis, subjects who are observed until they reach the endpoint of interest (e.g., recurrence or death) are called *uncensored* cases, and those who survive beyond the end of the follow-up or who are lost to follow-up at some point are termed *censored* cases.

Two basic survival procedures that enable one to determine overall group survival, taking into account both censored and uncensored observations, are the life table method and the Kaplan–Meier method.[8,9] The life table method was the first method generally used to describe cancer survival results, and it came to be known as the actuarial method because of its similarity to the work done by actuaries in the insurance industry. It is most useful when data are only available in grouped categories as described in the next section. The Kaplan–Meier estimate utilizes individual survival times for each patient and is preferable when data are available in this form.

The specific method of computation, that is, life table or Kaplan–Meier, used for a specific study should always be clearly indicated in the report to avoid any confusion associated with the use of less precise terminology. Rates computed by different methods are not directly comparable, and when the survival experiences of different patient groups are compared, the different rates must be computed by the same method.

The concepts of survival analysis are illustrated in this chapter. These illustrations are based on data obtained from the public-use files of the National Cancer Institute's Surveillance, Epidemiology, and End Results (SEER) Program. The cases selected are a 1% random sample of the total number for the selected sites and years of diagnosis. Follow-up of these patients continued through the end of 1999. Thus, for the earliest patients, there can be as many as 16 years of follow-up, but for those diagnosed at the end of the study period, there can be as little as 1 year of follow-up. These data are used both because they are realistic in terms of the actual survival rates they yield and because they encompass a number of cases that might be seen in a single large tumor registry over a comparable number of years. They are intended only to illustrate the methodology and concepts of survival analysis. SEER results from 1973 to 1997 are more fully described elsewhere.[10] These illustrations are not intended and should not be used or cited as an analysis of patterns of survival in breast and lung cancer in the USA.

## THE LIFE TABLE METHOD

The life table method involves dividing the total period over which a group is observed into fixed intervals, usually months or years. For each interval, the proportion surviving to the end of the interval is calculated on the basis of the number known to have experienced the endpoint event (e.g., death) during the interval and the number estimated to have been at risk at the start of the interval. For each succeeding interval, a cumulative survival rate

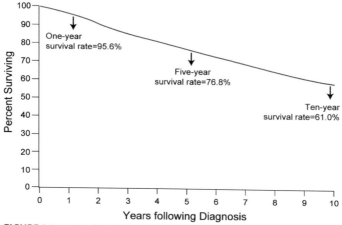

**FIGURE 2.1.** Survival of 2,819 breast cancer patients from the Surveillance, Epidemiology, and End Results Program of the National Cancer Institute, 1983–1998. Calculated by the life table method.

may be calculated. The cumulative survival rate is the probability of surviving the most recent interval multiplied by the probabilities of surviving all of the prior intervals. Thus, if the percent of the patients surviving the first interval is 90% and is the same for the second and third intervals, the cumulative survival percentage is 72.9% ($0.9 \times 0.9 \times 0.9 = 0.729$).

Results from the life table method for calculating survival for the breast cancer illustration are shown in Figure 2.1. Two-thousand eight-hundred nineteen (2,819) patients diagnosed between 1983 and 1998 were followed through 1999. Following the life table calculation method for each year after diagnosis, the 1-year survival rate is 95.6%. The 5-year cumulative survival rate is 76.8%. At 10 years, the cumulative survival is 61.0 %.

The lung cancer data show a much different survival pattern (Figure 2.2). At 1 year following diagnosis, the survival rate is only 41.8%. By 5 years it has fallen to 12.0%, and only 6.8% of lung cancer patients are estimated to have survived for 10 years following diagnosis. For lung cancer patients the *median survival time* is 10.0 months. Median survival time is the point at which half of the patients have experienced the endpoint event and half of the patients remain event-free. If the cumulative survival does not fall below 50% it is not possible to estimate median survival from the data, as is the case in the breast cancer data.

In the case of breast cancer, the 10-year survival rate is important because such a large proportion of patients live more than 5 years past their diagnosis. The 10-year time frame for lung cancer is less meaningful because such a large proportion of this patient group dies well before that much time passes.

An important assumption of all actuarial survival methods is that censored cases do not differ from the entire collection of uncensored cases in

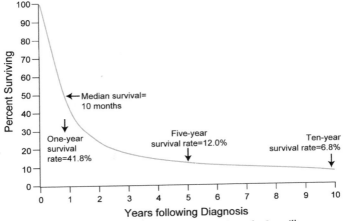

**FIGURE 2.2.** Survival of 2,347 lung cancer patients from the Surveillance, Epidemiology, and End Results Program of the National Cancer Institute, 1983–1998. Calculated by the life table method.

any systematic manner that would affect their survival. For example, if the more recently diagnosed cases in Figure 2.1, that is, those who were most likely not to have died yet, tended to be detected with earlier-stage disease than the uncensored cases or if they were treated differently, the assumption about comparability of censored and uncensored cases would not be met, and the result for the group as a whole would be inaccurate. Thus, it is important, when patients are included in a life table analysis, that one be reasonably confident that differences in the amount of information available about survival are not related to differences that might affect survival.

## THE KAPLAN–MEIER METHOD

If individual patient data are available, these same data can be analyzed using the Kaplan–Meier method.[9] It is similar to the life table method but calculates the proportion surviving to each point that a death occurs, rather than at fixed intervals. The principal difference evident in a survival curve is that the stepwise changes in the cumulative survival rate appear to occur independently of the intervals on the "Years Following Diagnosis" axis. Where available, this method provides a more accurate estimate of the survival curve.

## PATIENT-, DISEASE-, AND TREATMENT-SPECIFIC SURVIVAL

Although overall group survival is informative, comparisons of the overall survival between two groups often are confounded by differences in the patients, their tumors, or the treatments they received. For example, it would be misleading to compare the overall survival depicted in Figure 2.1 for the sample of all breast cancer cases with the overall survival for a sample

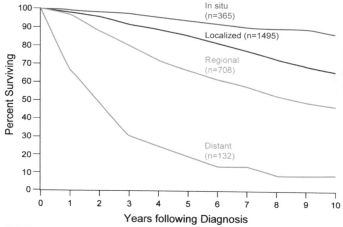

**FIGURE 2.3.** Survival of 2,819 breast cancer patients from the Surveillance, Epidemiology, and End Results Program of the National Cancer Institute, 1983–1998. Calculated by the life table method and stratified by historic stage of disease. *Note*: Excludes 119 patients with unknown stage of disease. SEER uses extent of disease (EOD) staging.

of breast cancer patients who were diagnosed with more advanced disease, whose survival would be presumed to be poorer. The simplest approach to accounting for possible differences between groups is to provide survival results that are specific to the categories of patient, disease, or treatment that may affect results. In most cancer applications, the most important variable by which survival results should be subdivided is the stage of disease. Figure 2.3 shows the *stage-specific* 5-year survival curves of the same breast cancer patients described earlier. These data show that breast cancer patient survival differs markedly according to the stage of the tumor at the time of diagnosis.

Almost any variable can be used to subclassify survival rates, but some are more meaningful than others. For example, it would be possible to provide season-of-diagnosis-specific (i.e., spring, summer, winter, and fall) survival rates, but the season of diagnosis probably has no biologic association with the length of a breast cancer patient's survival. On the other hand, the race-specific and age-specific survival rates shown in Figures 2.4 and 2.5 suggest that both of these variables are related to breast cancer survival. Caucasians have the highest survival rates and African-Americans the lowest. In the case of age, these data suggest that only the oldest patients experience poor survival and that it would be helpful to consider the effects of other causes of death that affect older persons using adjustments to be described.

Although the factors that affect survival may be unique to each type of cancer, it has become conventional that a basic description of survival for a specific cancer should include stage-, age-, and race-specific survival results. Treatment is a factor by which survival is commonly subdivided,

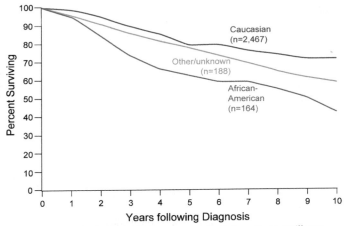

**FIGURE 2.4.** Survival of 2,819 breast cancer patients from the Surveillance, Epidemiology, and End Results Program of the National Cancer Institute, 1983–1998. Calculated by the life table method and stratified by race.

but it must be kept in mind that selection of treatment is usually related to other factors that exert influence on survival. For example, in cancer care the choice of treatment is often dependent on the stage of disease at diagnosis. Comparison of survival curves by treatment is most appropriately accomplished within the confines of randomized clinical trials.

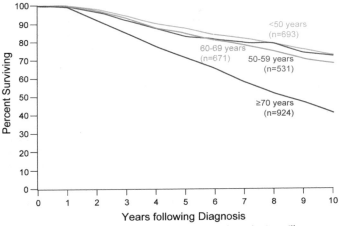

**FIGURE 2.5.** Survival of 2,819 breast cancer patients from the Surveillance, Epidemiology, and End Results Program of the National Cancer Institute, 1983–1998. Calculated by the life table method and stratified by age at diagnosis.

## CAUSE-ADJUSTED SURVIVAL RATE

The survival rates depicted in the illustrations account for all deaths, regardless of cause. This is known as the *observed survival rate*. Although observed survival is a true reflection of total mortality in the patient group, we frequently are interested in describing mortality attributable only to the disease under investigation. In the past, this was most often calculated using the *cause-adjusted survival rate*, defined as the proportion of the initial patient group that escaped death due to a specific cause (e.g., cancer) if no other cause of death was operating. This technique requires that reliable information on cause of death is available and makes an adjustment for deaths due to causes other than the disease under study. This was accomplished by treating patients who died without the disease of interest as censored observations.

## COMPETING RISKS/CUMULATIVE INCIDENCE

The treatment of deaths from other causes as censored is controversial, since statistical methods used in survival analysis settings assume that censoring is independent of outcome. This means that if the patient was followed longer, one could eventually observe the outcome of interest. This makes sense for patients lost to follow-up (if we located them, we might eventually observe their true survival time). However, if a patient dies due to another cause, we will never observe their death due to the cancer of interest. Estimation of the adjusted rate as described previously does not appropriately distinguish between patients who are still alive at last known contact date and those known to have died from another cause. These latter events are called *competing risks*.

When competing risks are present, an alternative to the Kaplan–Meier estimate is the cumulative incidence method. This technique is similar to the Kaplan–Meier estimate in its treatment of censored observations and is identical to the Kaplan–Meier estimate if there are no competing risks. However, in the presence of competing risks, the other causes of death are handled in a different manner.[11]

## RELATIVE SURVIVAL

Information on cause of death is sometimes unavailable or unreliable. Under such circumstances, it is not possible to compute a *cause*-adjusted survival rate. However, it is possible to adjust partially for differences in the risk of dying from causes other than the disease under study. This can be done by means of the *relative survival rate*, which is the ratio of the observed survival rate to the expected rate for a group of people in the general population similar to the patient group with respect to race, sex, and age. The relative survival rate is calculated using a procedure described by Ederer et al.[12]

The relative survival rate represents the likelihood that a patient will not die from causes associated specifically with the cancer at some specified time after diagnosis. It is always greater than the observed survival rate for the same group of patients. If the group is sufficiently large and the patients are roughly representative of the population of the USA (taking race, sex, and age into account), the relative survival rate provides a useful estimate of the probability of escaping death from the specific cancer under study. However, if reliable information on cause of death is available, it is preferable to use the *cause*-adjusted rate. This is particularly true when the series is small or when the patients are largely drawn from a particular socioeconomic segment of the population. Relative survival rates may be derived from life table or Kaplan–Meier results.

## REGRESSION METHODS

Examining survival within specific patient, disease, or treatment categories is the simplest way of studying multiple factors possibly associated with survival. This approach, however, is limited to factors into which patients may be broadly grouped. This approach does not lend itself to studying the effects of measures that vary on an interval scale. There are many examples of interval variables in cancer, such as age, number of positive nodes, cell counts, and laboratory marker values. If the patient population were to be divided up into each interval value, too few subjects would be in each analysis to be meaningful. In addition, when more than one factor is considered, the number of curves that result provides so many comparisons that the effects of the factors defy interpretation.

Conventional multiple regression analysis investigates the joint effects of multiple variables on a single outcome, but it is incapable of dealing with censored observations. For this reason, other statistical methods are used to assess the relationship of survival time to a number of variables simultaneously. The most commonly used is the Cox proportional hazards regression model.[13] This model provides a method for estimating the influence of multiple covariates on the survival distribution from data that include censored observations. Covariates are the multiple factors to be studied in association with survival. In the Cox proportional hazards regression model, the covariates may be categorical variables such as race, interval measures such as age, or laboratory test results.

Specifics of these methods are beyond the scope of this chapter. Fortunately, many readily accessible computer packages for statistical analysis now permit the methods to be applied quite easily by the knowledgeable analyst. Although much useful information can be derived from multivariate survival models, they generally require additional assumptions about the shape of the survival curve and the nature of the effects of the covariates. One must always examine the appropriateness of the model that is used relative to the assumptions required.

## STANDARD ERROR OF A SURVIVAL RATE

Survival rates that describe the experience of the specific group of patients are frequently used to generalize to larger populations. The existence of true population values is postulated, and these values are estimated from the group under study, which is only a sample of the larger population. If a survival rate was calculated from a second sample taken from the same population, it is unlikely that the results would be exactly the same. The difference between the two results is called the sampling variation (chance variation or sampling error). The *standard error* is a measure of the extent to which sampling variation influences the computed survival rate. In repeated observations under the same conditions, the true or population survival rate will lie within the range of two standard errors on either side of the computed rate approximately 95 times in 100. This range is called the *95% confidence interval.*

## COMPARISON OF SURVIVAL BETWEEN PATIENT GROUPS

In comparing survival rates of two patient groups, the statistical significance of the observed difference is of interest. The essential question is, "What is the probability that the observed difference may have occurred by chance?" The standard error of the survival rate provides a simple means for answering this question. If the 95% confidence intervals of two survival rates do not overlap, the observed difference would customarily be considered statistically significant, that is, unlikely to be due to chance. This latter statement is generally true, although it is possible for a formal statistical test to yield a significant difference even with overlapping confidence intervals. Moreover, comparisons at any single time point must be made with care; if a specific time (5 years, for example) is known to be of interest when the study is planned, such a comparison may be valid; however, identification of a time based on inspection of the curves and selection of the widest difference make any formal assessment of difference invalid.

It is possible that the differences between two groups at each comparable time of follow-up do not differ significantly but that when the survival curves are considered in their entirety, the individual insignificant differences combine to yield a significantly different pattern of survival. The most common statistical test that examines the whole pattern of differences between survival curves is the *log rank test.* This test equally weights the effects of differences occurring throughout the follow-up and is the appropriate choice for most situations. Other tests weight the differences according to the numbers of persons at risk at different points and can yield different results depending on whether deaths tend more to occur early or later in the follow-up.

Care must be exercised in the interpretation of tests of statistical significance. For example, if differences exist in the patient and disease characteristics of two treatment groups, a statistically significant difference in survival results may primarily reflect differences between the two patient series, rather than differences in efficacy of the treatment regimens. The more definitive approach to therapy evaluation requires a randomized clinical trial that helps to ensure comparability of the patient characteristics and the disease characteristics of the two treatment groups.

**Definition of Study Starting Point.**  The starting time for determining survival of patients depends on the purpose of the study. For example, the starting time for studying the natural history of a particular cancer might be defined in reference to the appearance of the first symptom. Various reference dates are commonly used as starting times for evaluating the effects of therapy. These include (1) date of diagnosis, (2) date of first visit to physician or clinic, (3) date of hospital admission, (4) date of treatment initiation, date of randomization in a clinical trial evaluating treatment efficacy, and (5) others. The specific reference date used should be clearly specified in every report.

**Vital Status.** At any given time, the vital status of each patient is defined as alive, dead, or unknown (i.e., lost to follow-up). The endpoint of each patient's participation in the study is (1) a specified *terminal event* such as death, (2) survival to the completion of the study, or (3) loss to follow-up. In each case, the observed follow-up time is the time from the starting point to the terminal event, to the end of the study, or to the date of last observation. This observed follow-up may be further described in terms of patient status at the endpoint, such as the following:

- Alive; tumo r-free; no recurrence
- Alive; tumor-free; after recurrence
- Alive with persistent, recurrent, or metastatic disease
- Alive with primary tumor
- Dead; tumor-free
- Dead; with cancer (primary, recurrent, or metastatic disease)
- Dead; postoperative
- Unknown; lost to follow-up

Completeness of the follow-up is crucial in any study of survival, because even a small number of patients lost to follow-up may lead to inaccurate or biased results. The maximum possible effect of bias from patients lost to follow-up may be ascertained by calculating a maximum survival rate, assuming that all lost patients lived to the end of the study. A minimum survival rate may be calculated by assuming that all patients lost to follow-up died at the time they were lost.

**Time Intervals.** The total survival time is often divided into intervals in units of weeks, months, or years. The survival curve for these intervals provides a description of the population under study with respect to the dynamics of survival over a specified time. The time interval used should be selected with regard to the natural history of the disease under consideration. In diseases with a long natural history, the duration of study could be 5–20 years, and survival intervals of 6–12 months will provide a meaningful description of the survival dynamics. If the population being studied has a very poor prognosis (e.g., patients with carcinoma of the esophagus or pancreas), the total duration of study may be 2–3 years, and the survival intervals may be described in terms of 1–3 months. In interpreting survival rates, one must also take into account the number of individuals entering a survival interval.

## SUMMARY

This chapter has reviewed the rudiments of survival analysis as it is often applied to cancer registry data and to the analysis of data from clinical trials. Complex analysis of data and exploration of research hypotheses demand greater knowledge and expertise than could be conveyed herein.

Survival analysis is now performed automatically in many different registry data management and statistical analysis programs available for use on personal computers. Persons with access to these programs are encouraged to explore the different analysis features available to demonstrate for themselves the insight on cancer registry data that survival analysis can provide and to understand the limitations of these analyses and how their validity is affected by the characteristics of the patient cohorts and the quality and completeness of data.

## REFERENCES

1. Cox DR, Oakes D. Analysis of survival data. London: Chapman and Hall; 1984.
2. Fleming TR, Harrington DP. Counting processes and survival analysis. New York: Wiley; 1991.
3. Kalbfleisch JD, Prentice RL. The statistical analysis of failure time data. 2nd ed. New York: Wiley; 2002.
4. Klein JP, Moeschberger ML. Survival analysis: techniques for censored and truncated data. New York: Springer; 1997.
5. Kleinbaum DG. Survival analysis: a self learning text. New York: Springer; 1996.
6. Lee ET. Statistical methods for survival data analysis. New York: Wiley; 1992.
7. Mantel N. Evaluation of survival data and two new rank order statistics arising in its consideration. Cancer Chemother Rep. 1966;50:163–70.
8. Berkson J, Gage RP. Calculation of survival rates for cancer. Proc Staff Meet Mayo Clin. 1950;25:270–86.
9. Kaplan EL, Meier P. Nonparametric estimation from incomplete observations. J Am Stat Assoc. 1958;53:457–81.
10. Ries LAG, Eisner MP, Kosary CL, et al., editors. SEER cancer statistics review, 1973–1997: tables and graphs, National Cancer Institute. Bethesda, MD: National Institutes of Health, NIH Pub. No. 00-2789; 2000.
11. Gooley TA, Leisenring W, Crowley JC, Storer BE. Estimation of failure probabilities in the presence of competing risks; new representations of old estimators. Stat Med. 1999;18:695–706.
12. Ederer F, Axtell LM, Cutler SJ. The relative survival rate: a statistical methodology. Natl Cancer Inst Monogr. 1961;6:101–21.
13. Cox DR. Regression models and life tables. J R Stat Soc B. 1972;34: 187–220.

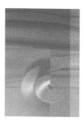

# PART II
# Head and Neck

*General Rules*

---
### SUMMARY OF CHANGES

- The terms "resectable" and "unresectable" are replaced with "moderately advanced" and "very advanced"
- No major changes have been made in the N staging for any sites except that a descriptor has been added. Extracapsular spread (ECS) of disease is added as ECS + or ECS – as a descriptor. These descriptors will not influence nodal staging system
---

## INTRODUCTION

Cancers of the head and neck may arise from any of the lining membranes of the upper aerodigestive tract. The T classifications indicating the extent of the primary tumor are generally similar but differ in specific details for each site because of anatomic considerations. The N classification for cervical lymph node metastasis is uniform for all sites except thyroid, nasopharynx, and skin. The N classification for thyroid and nasopharynx is unique to those sites and is based on tumor behavior and prognosis. The N classification for neck disease from nonmelanoma skin cancers is similar to that for axillary and groin (inguinal) lymph nodes. The staging systems presented in this section are all clinical staging, based on the best possible estimate of the extent of disease before first treatment. Imaging techniques [computed tomography (CT), magnetic resonance imaging (MRI), positron emission tomography (PET), and ultrasonography] may be utilized and, in advanced tumor stages, have added to the accuracy of primary tumor (T) and nodal (N) staging, especially in the nasopharyngeal and paranasal sinuses, primary sites, and regional lymph nodes. Endoscopic evaluation of the primary tumor, when appropriate, is desirable for detailed assessment of the primary tumor for accurate T staging. Fine-needle aspiration biopsy (FNAB) may confirm the presence of tumor and its histopathologic nature, but it cannot rule out the presence of tumor.

Any diagnostic information that contributes to the overall accuracy of the pretreatment assessment should be considered in clinical staging and treatment planning. When surgical treatment is carried out, cancer of the head and neck can be staged [pathologic stage (pTNM)] using all information available from clinical assessment, as well as from the pathologic study of the resected specimen. The pathologic stage does not replace the clinical stage, which should be reported as well.

In reviewing the staging systems, no major changes in the T classifications or stage groupings are made, since they reflect current practices of treatment, clinical relevance, and contemporary data. Uniform T classification for oral cavity, oropharynx, and salivary and thyroid cancers has greatly simplified the system and has improved compliance by clinicians. T4 tumors are subdivided into moderately advanced (T4a) and very advanced (T4b) categories. Regrouping of Stage IV disease for all sites into moderately advanced, local/regional disease (Stage IVa), very advanced local/regional disease (Stage IVb), and distant metastatic disease (Stage IVc) has also simplified stratification of advanced stage disease.

The following chapters present the staging classification for six major head and neck sites: the oral cavity, the pharynx (nasopharynx, oropharynx, and hypopharynx), the larynx, the paranasal sinuses, the salivary glands, and the thyroid gland.

A revised chapter on nonmelanoma skin cancers has also been added to the *Manual* (see Chap. 29). The T and N staging for head and neck skin cancers is consistent with other cutaneous sites in the body. All these chapters apply to epithelial cancers only. Mucosal melanoma warrants separate consideration, and the approach to these lesions is outlined in a separate chapter that addresses mucosal melanoma in all sites of the head and neck (see Chap. 9).

**Regional Lymph Nodes.**  The status of the regional lymph nodes in head and neck cancer is of such prognostic importance that the cervical nodes must be assessed for each patient and tumor. The lymph nodes may be subdivided into specific anatomic subsites and grouped into seven levels for ease of description (Tables 1 and 2 and Figure 1).

Other groups:

Suboccipital
Retropharyngeal
Parapharyngeal
Buccinator (facial)
Preauricular
Periparotid and intraparotid

The pattern of the lymphatic drainage varies for different anatomic sites. However, the location of the lymph node metastases has prognostic significance in patients with squamous cell carcinoma of the head and neck. Survival is significantly worse when metastases involve lymph nodes

**TABLE 1.** Anatomical structures defining the boundaries of the neck levels and sublevels

| Boundary Level | Superior | Inferior | Anterior (medial) | Posterior (lateral) |
|---|---|---|---|---|
| IA | Symphysis of mandible dkfmb | Body of hyoid | Anterior belly of contralateral digastric muscle | Anterior belly of ipsilateral digastric muscle |
| IB | Body of mandible | Posterior belly of diagastric muscle | Anterior belly of digastric muscle | Stylohyoid muscle |
| IIA | Skull base | Horizontal plane defined by the inferior border of the hyoid bone | The stylohyoid muscle | Vertical plane defined by the spinal accessory nerve |
| IIB | Skull base | Horizontal plane defined by the inferior body of the hyoid bone | Vertical plane defined by the spinal accessory nerve | Lateral border of the sternocleido-mastoid muscle |
| III | Horizontal plane defined by the inferior body of hyoid | Horizontal plane defined by the inferior border of the cricoid cartilage | Lateral border of the sternohyoid muscle | Lateral border of the sterno-cleidomastoid or sensory branches of cervical plexus |
| IV | Horizontal plane defined by the inferior border of the cricoid cartilage | Clavicle | Lateral border of the sternohyoid muscle | Lateral border of the sterno-cleidomastoid or sensory branches of cervical plexus |
| VA | Apex of the convergence of the sterno-cleidomastoid and trapezius muscles | Horizontal plane defined by the lower border of the cricoid cartilage | Posterior border of the ster-nocleidomastoid muscle or sensory branches of cervical plexus | Anterior border of the trapezius muscle |
| VB | Horizontal plane defined by the lower border of the cricoid cartilage | Clavicle | Posterior border of the sterno-cleidomastoid muscle | Anterior border of the trapezius muscle |
| VI | Hyoid bone | Suprasternal notch | Common carotid artery | Common carotid artery |
| VII | Suprasternal notch | Innominate artery | Sternum | Trachea, esophagus, and prevertebral fascia |

Modified from Robbins KT, Clayman G, Levine PA, et al. American Head and Neck Society; American Academy of Otolaryngology – Head and Neck Surgery. Neck dissection classification update: revisions proposed by the American Head and Neck Society and the American Academy of Otolaryngology-Head and Neck Surgery. Arch Otolaryngol Head Neck Surg. 2002;128(7):751–8, with permission of the American Medical Association.

**TABLE 2.** Lymph node groups found within the seven levels and sublevels of the neck

| Lymph node group | Description |
|---|---|
| Submental (sublevel IA) | Lymph nodes within the triangular boundary of the anterior belly of the digastric muscles and the hyoid bone. These nodes are at greatest risk for harboring metastases from cancers arising from the floor of mouth, anterior oral tongue, anterior mandibular alveolar ridge, and lower lip. |
| Submandibular (sublevel IB) | Lymph nodes within the boundaries of the anterior and posterior bellies of the digastric muscle, the stylohyoid muscle, and the body of the mandible. It includes the preglandular and the postglandular nodes and the prevascular and postvascular nodes. The submandibular gland is included in the specimen when the lymph nodes within the triangle are removed. These nodes are at greatest risk for harboring mestastases from cancers arising from the oral cavity, anterior nasal cavity, skin, and soft tissue structures of the midface, and submandibular gland. |
| Upper jugular (includes sublevels IIA and IIB) | Lymph nodes located around the upper third of the internal jugular vein and adjacent spinal accessory nerve extending from the level of the skull base (above) to the level of the inferior border of the hyoid bone (below). The anterior (medial) boundary is stylohyoid muscle (the radiologic correlate is the vertical plane defined by the posterior surface of the submandibular gland) and the posterior (lateral) boundary is the posterior border of the sternocleidomastoid muscle. Sublevel IIA nodes are located anterior (medial) to the vertical plane defined by the spinal accessory nerve. Sublevel IIB nodes are located posterior lateral to the vertical plane defined by the spinal accessory nerve. (The radiologic correlate is the lateral border of the internal jugular on a contrast-enhanced CT scan.) The upper jugular nodes are at greatest risk for harboring metastases from cancers arising from the oral cavity, nasal cavity, nasopharynx, oropharynx, hypopharynx, larynx, and parotid gland. |
| Middle jugular (level III) | Lymph nodes located around the middle third of the internal jugular vein extending from the inferior border of the hyoid bone (above) to the inferior border of the cricoid cartilage (below). The anterior (medial) boundary is the lateral border of the sternohyoid muscle, and the posterior (lateral) boundary is the posterior border of the sternocleidomastoid muscle. These nodes are at greatest risk for harboring metastases from cancers arising from the oral cavity, nasophyarynx, oropharynx, hypopharynx, and larynx. |
| Lower jugular (level IV) | Lymph nodes located around the lower third of the internal jugular vein extending from the inferior border of the cricoid cartilage (above) to the clavicle below. The anterior (medial) boundary is the lateral border of the sternohyoid muscle and the posterior (lateral) boundary is the posterior border of the sternocleidomastoid muscle. These nodes are at greatest risk for harboring metatases from cancers arising from the hypopharynx, thyroid, cervical esophagus, and larynx. |

*continued*

**TABLE 2.** Lymph node groups found within the seven levels and sublevels of the neck (continued)

| Lymph node group | Description |
|---|---|
| Posterior triangle group (includes sublevels VA and VB) | This group is composed predominantly of the lymph nodes located along the lower half of the spinal accessory nerve and the transverse cervical artery. The supraclavicular nodes are also included in posterior triangle group. The superior boundary is the apex formed by convergence of the sterno-cleidomastoid and trapezius muscles; the inferior boundary is the clavicle; the anterior (medial) boundary is the posterior border of the sternocleidomastoid muscle, and the posterior (lateral) boundary is the anterior border of the trapezius muscle. Thus, sublevel VA includes the spinal accessory nodes, whereas sublevel VB includes the nodes following the transverse cervical vessels and the supraclavicular nodes, with the exception of the Virchow node, which is located in level IV. The posterior triangle nodes are at greatest risk for harboring metastases from cancers arising from the nasopharynx, oropharynx, and cutaneous structures of the posterior scalp and neck. |
| Anterior compartment group (level VI) | Lymph nodes in this compartment include the pretracheal and paratracheal nodes, precricoid (Delphian) node, and the perithyroidal nodes including the lymph nodes along the recurrent laryngeal nerves. The superior boundary is the hyoid bone; the inferior boundary is the suprasternal notch, and the lateral boundaries are the common carotid arteries. These nodes are at greatest risk for harboring metastases from cancers arising from the thyroid gland, glottic and subglottic larynx, apex of the piriform sinus, and cervical esophagus. |
| Superior mediastinal group (level VII) | Lymph nodes in this group include pretracheal, paratracheal, and esophageal groove lymph nodes, extending from the level of the suprasternal notch cephalad and up to the innominate artery caudad. These nodes are at greatest risk of involvement by thyroid cancer and cancer of the esophagus. |

Modified from Robbins KT, Clayman G, Levine PA, et al. American Head and Neck Society; American Academy of Otolaryngology – Head and Neck Surgery. Neck dissection classification update: revisions proposed by the American Head and Neck Society and the American Academy of Otolaryngology-Head and Neck Surgery. Arch Otolaryngol Head Neck Surg. 2002;128(7):751–8, with permission of the American Medical Association.

beyond the first echelon of lymphatic drainage and, particularly, lymph nodes in the lower regions of the neck, that is, level IV and level VB (supraclavicular region). Consequently, it is recommended that each N staging category be recorded to show whether the nodes involved are located in the upper (U) or lower (L) regions of the neck, depending on their location above or below the lower border of the cricoid cartilage.

Extracapsular spread (ECS) has been recognized to worsen the adverse outcome associated with nodal metastasis. ECS can be diagnosed clinically by a matted mass of nodes adherent to overlying skin, adjacent soft tissue, or clinical evidence of cranial nerve invasion. Radiologic signs of ECS include amorphous, spiculated margins of a metastatic node and stranding of the perinodal soft tissue in previously untreated patients. The absence

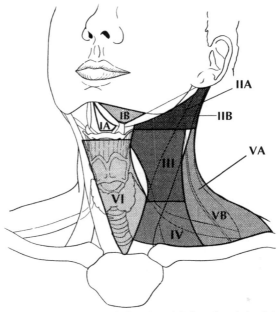

**FIGURE 1.** Schematic indicating the location of the lymph node levels in the neck as described in Table 1.

or presence of clinical/radiologic ECS is designated E− or E+, respectively. Surgically resected metastatic nodes should be examined for the presence and extent of ECS. Gross ECS (Eg) is defined as tumor apparent to the naked eye, beyond the confines of the nodal capsule. Microscopic ECS (Em) is defined as the presence of metastatic tumor beyond the capsule of the lymph node. ECS evident on clinical/radiologic examination is designated E+ or E−, while ECS on histopathologic examination is designated En (no extranodal extension), Em (microscopic ECS), and Eg (gross ECS). These descriptors will not affect current nodal staging.

The natural history and response to treatment of cervical nodal metastases from nasopharynx primary sites are different, in terms of their impact on prognosis, so they justify a different N classification scheme. Regional node metastases from well-differentiated thyroid cancer do not significantly affect the ultimate prognosis in most patients and therefore also justify a unique staging system for thyroid cancers. Nonmelanoma skin cancers in the head and neck have similar behavior as elsewhere in the body. Therefore, nodal staging for these (NMSC) is different than that for mucosal cancers and is similar to that in the axilla and groin for cutaneous cancers.

Histopathologic examination is necessary to exclude the presence of tumor in lymph nodes. No imaging study (as yet) can identify microscopic tumor foci in regional nodes or distinguish between small reactive nodes and small malignant nodes.

When enlarged lymph nodes are detected, the actual size of the nodal mass(es) should be measured. It is recognized that most masses over 3 cm in diameter are not single nodes but are confluent nodes or tumor in soft tissues of the neck. Pathologic examination is necessary for documentation of tumor extent in terms of the location or level of the lymph node(s) involved, the number of nodes that contain metastases, and the presence or absence of ECS of tumor, designated as En (not present), Em (microscopic), or Eg (gross).

**Distant Metastases.** The most common sites of distant spread are in the lungs and bones; hepatic and brain metastases occur less often. Mediastinal lymph node metastases are considered distant metastases, except level VII lymph nodes (anterior superior mediastinal lymph nodes cephalad to the innominate artery).

### Regional Lymph Nodes (N)

| | |
|---|---|
| NX | Regional lymph nodes cannot be assessed |
| N0 | No regional lymph node metastasis |
| N1* | Metastasis in a single ipsilateral lymph node, 3 cm or less in greatest dimension |
| N2* | Metastasis in a single ipsilateral lymph node, more than 3 cm but not more than 6 cm in greatest dimension; or in multiple ipsilateral lymph nodes, none more than 6 cm in greatest dimension; or in bilateral or contralateral lymph nodes, none more than 6 cm in greatest dimension |
| N2a* | Metastasis in single ipsilateral lymph node more than 3 cm but not more than 6 cm in greatest dimension |
| N2b* | Metastasis in multiple ipsilateral lymph nodes, none more than 6 cm in greatest dimension |
| N2c* | Metastasis in bilateral or contralateral lymph nodes, none more than 6 cm in greatest dimension |
| N3* | Metastasis in a lymph node more than 6 cm in greatest dimension |

*Note: A designation of "U" or "L" may be used for any N stage to indicate metastasis above the lower border of the cricoid (U) or below the lower border of the cricoid (L). Similarly, clinical/radiological ECS should be recorded as E− or E+, and histopathologic ECS should be designated En, Em, or Eg.

### Distant Metastasis (M)

| | |
|---|---|
| M0 | No distant metastasis |
| M1 | Distant metastasis |

## OUTCOME RESULTS

The survival curves shown for each anatomic site were constructed using head and neck cancer cases extracted from the National Cancer Data Base (NCDB) for cases diagnosed in 1997 and 1998. Only cases that were staged according to the fifth edition of the AJCC's *Cancer Staging Manual* were included.

The 5-year survival analyses for the different sites were stratified by AJCC *combined* stage, which represents pathologic stage when available and only clinical stage when pathologic stage is not available. The survival methods were performed using SPSS software and included observed survival (death from all causes) as well as relative survival (representing an estimation of death from cancer derived from observed survival rates adjusted for expected deaths based on age, race, and gender). The 95% confidence intervals were provided for each year-5 survival rate to permit analysis of significant differences between the year-5 survival rates of the different stages.

Anatomic sites and histologic types were coded according to the third edition of the International Classification of Diseases for Oncology (ICD-0-3). The subsites included in each analysis were chosen on the basis of those listed in the fifth edition of the AJCC's *Cancer Staging Manual.* Survival analysis for lip, oral cavity, oropharynx, nasopharynx, hypopharynx, and the larynx's subsites was limited to squamous cell carcinomas only (M8050, 8051–8082). Survival analyses for the maxillary sinus and the major salivary glands included all histologic types. Survival analyses for the thyroid gland included papillary adenocarcinoma (M8050, 8260, 8340, 8503-8604), follicular adenocarcinoma (M8330–8332), medullary carcinoma (M8510-M8512), and anaplastic carcinoma (M8021).

## BIBLIOGRAPHY

Beahrs O, Henson DE, Hutter RVP, Kennedy BJ, editors. American Joint Committee on Cancer: manual for staging of cancer. 4th ed. Philadelphia: JB Lippincott; 1992.

Bernier J, Cooper JS. Chemoradiation after surgery for high-risk head and neck cancer patients: how strong is the evidence? Oncologist. 2005;10(3): 215–24.

Cerezo L, Millan I, Torre A, Aragon G, Otero J. Prognostic factors for survival and tumor control in cervical lymph node metastases from head and neck cancer: a multivariate study of 492 cases. Cancer. 1992;69:1224–34.

Cooper JS, Farnan NC, Asbell SO, et al. Recursive partitioning analysis of 2105 patients treated in Radiation Therapy Oncology Group studies of head and neck cancer. Cancer. 1996;77:1905–11.

de Leeuw JR, de Graeff A, Ros WJ, Blijham GH, Hordijk GJ, Winnubst JA. Prediction of depressive symptomatology after treatment of head and neck cancer: the influence of pre-treatment physical and depressive symptoms, coping, and social support. Head Neck. 2000;22(8):799–807.

Deleyiannis FW, Thomas DB, Vaughan TL, et al. Alcoholism: independent predictor of survival in patients with head and neck cancer. J Natl Cancer Inst. 1996;88:542–9.

Dunne AA, Muller HH, Eisele DW, Kessel K, Moll R, Werner JA. Meta-analysis of the prognostic significance of perinodal spread in head and neck squamous cell carcinomas (HNSCC) patients. Eur J Cancer. 2006;42(12): 1863–8.

Faye-Lund H, Abdelnoor M. Prognostic factors of survival in a cohort of head and neck cancer patients in Oslo. Eur J Cancer B Oral Oncol. 1996;2: 83–90.

Gor DM, Langer JE, Loevner LA. Imaging of cervical lymph nodes in head and neck cancer: the basics. Radiol Clin North Am. 2006;44(1):101–10, viii

Grandi C, Alloisio M, Moglia D, et al. Prognostic significance of lymphatic spread in head and neck carcinomas: therapeutic implications. Head Neck Surg. 1985;8:67–73.

Harnsberger HR. Squamous cell carcinoma: nodal staging. In: Handbook of head and neck imaging. 2nd ed. St. Louis: Mosby; 1995. p. 283–298.

Hillsamer PJ, Schuller DE, McGhee RB, et al. Improving diagnostic accuracy of cervical metastases with CT and MRI imaging. Arch Otolaryngol Head Neck Surg. 1990;116:2297–301.

Jones AS, Roland NJ, Field JK, Phillips DE. The level of cervical lymph node metastases: their prognostic relevance and relationship with head and neck squamous carcinoma primary sites. Clin Otolaryngol. 1994;19:63–9.

Kalnins IK, Leonard AG, Sako K, et al. Correlation between prognosis and degree of lymph node involvement in carcinoma of the oral cavity. Am J Surg. 1977;34:450–4.

Kowalski LP, Bagietto R, Lara JR, et al. Prognostic significance of the distribution of neck node metastasis from oral carcinoma. Head Neck. 2000;22:207–14.

Mancuso AA, Harnsberger HR, Muraki AS, et al. Computed tomography of cervical and retropharyngeal lymph nodes: normal anatomy, variants of normal, and application in staging head and neck cancer. II. Pathology. Radiology. 1983;148:715–23.

Medina JE. A rational classification of neck dissections. Otolaryngol Head Neck Surg. 1989;100:169–76.

Percy C, Van Holten V, Muir C, editors. International classification of disease for oncology. 2nd ed. Geneva: World Health Organization; 1990.

Piccirillo JF. Inclusion of comorbidity in a staging system for head and neck cancer. Oncology. 1995;9:831–6.

Richard JM, Sancho-Garnier H, Michaeu C, et al. Prognostic factors in cervical lymph node metastasis in upper respiratory and digestive tract carcinomas: study of 1713 cases during a 15-year period. Laryngoscope. 1987;97:97–101.

Robbins KT, Clayman G, Levine PA, et al. American Head and Neck Society; American Academy of Otolaryngology – Head and Neck Surgery. Neck dissection classification update: revisions proposed by the American Head and Neck Society and the American Academy of Otolaryngology – Head and Neck Surgery. Arch Otolaryngol Head Neck Surg. 2002;128(7):751–8.

Ross GL, Soutar DS, Gordon MacDonald D, Shoaib T, Camilleri I, Roberton AG, et al. Sentinel node biopsy in head and neck cancer: preliminary results of a multicenter trial. Ann Surg Oncol. 2004;11(7):690–6.

Shah JP. Patterns of cervical lymph node metastasis from squamous carcinomas of the upper aerodigestive tract. Am J Surg. 1990;160(4):405–9.

Shah JP, Medina JE, Shaha AR, Schantz SP, Marti JR. Cervical lymph node metastasis. Curr Probl Surg. 1993;30(3):1–335.

Singh B, Bhaya M, Zimbler M, et al. Impact of comorbidity on outcome of young patients with head and neck squamous cell carcinoma. Head Neck. 1998;20:1–7.

Singh B, Alfonso A, Sabin S, et al. Outcome differences in younger and older patients with laryngeal cancer: a retrospective case-control study. Am J Otolaryngol. 2000;21:92–7.

Som PM. Detection of metastasis in cervical lymph nodes: CT and MR criteria and differential diagnosis. Am J Radiol. 1992;158:961–9.

Stell PM, Morton RP, Singh SD. Cervical lymph node metastases: the significance of the level of the lymph node. Clin Oncol. 1983;9:101–7.

Stevens MH, Harnsberger HR, Mancuso AA. Computed tomography of cervical lymph nodes: staging and management of head and neck cancer. Arch Otolaryngol. 1985;111(11):735–9.

Strong EW, Kasdorf H, Henk JM. Squamous cell carcinoma of the head and neck. In: Hermanek P, Gospodarowicz MK, Henson DE, et al., editors. Prognostic factors in cancer, UICC Geneva. Berlin: Springer; 1995. p. 23–27.

Vauterin TJ, Veness MJ, Morgan GJ, Poulsen MG, O'Brien CJ. Patterns of lymph node spread of cutaneous squamous cell carcinoma of the head and neck. Head Neck. 2006;28(9):785–91.

Yousem DM, Som PM, Hackney DB, et al. Central nodal necrosis and extracapsular neoplastic spread in cervical lymph nodes: MR imaging versus CT. Radiology. 1992;182:753–9.

# Lip and Oral Cavity

*(Nonepithelial tumors such as those of lymphoid tissue, soft tissue, bone, and cartilage are not included. Staging for mucosal melanoma of the lip and oral cavity is not included in this chapter – see Chap. 9.)*

## *At-A-Glance*

### SUMMARY OF CHANGES

- T4 lesions have been divided into T4a (moderately advanced local disease) and T4b (very advanced local disease), leading to the stratification of Stage IV into Stage IVA (moderately advanced local/regional disease), Stage IVB (very advanced local/regional disease), and Stage IVC (distant metastatic disease)

### ANATOMIC STAGE/PROGNOSTIC GROUPS

| Stage | T | N | M |
|---|---|---|---|
| Stage 0 | Tis | N0 | M0 |
| Stage I | T1 | N0 | M0 |
| Stage II | T2 | N0 | M0 |
| Stage III | T3 | N0 | M0 |
| | T1 | N1 | M0 |
| | T2 | N1 | M0 |
| | T3 | N1 | M0 |
| Stage IVA | T4a | N0 | M0 |
| | T4a | N1 | M0 |
| | T1 | N2 | M0 |
| | T2 | N2 | M0 |
| | T3 | N2 | M0 |
| | T4a | N2 | M0 |
| Stage IVB | Any T | N3 | M0 |
| | T4b | Any N | M0 |
| Stage IVC | Any T | Any N | M1 |

**ICD-O-3 TOPOGRAPHY CODES**

| | |
|---|---|
| C00.0 | External upper lip |
| C00.1 | External lower lip |
| C00.2 | External lip, NOS |
| C00.3 | Mucosa of upper lip |
| C00.4 | Mucosa of lower lip |
| C00.5 | Mucosa of lip, NOS |
| C00.6 | Commissure of lip |
| C00.8 | Overlapping lesion of lip |
| C00.9 | Lip, NOS |
| C02.0 | Dorsal surface of tongue, NOS |
| C02.1 | Border of tongue |
| C02.2 | Ventral surface of tongue, NOS |
| C02.3 | Anterior two-thirds of tongue, NOS |
| C02.8 | Overlapping lesion of tongue |
| C02.9 | Tongue, NOS |
| C03.0 | Upper gum |
| C03.1 | Lower gum |
| C03.9 | Gum, NOS |
| C04.0 | Anterior floor of mouth |
| C04.1 | Lateral floor of mouth |
| C04.8 | Overlapping lesion of floor of mouth |
| C04.9 | Floor of mouth, NOS |
| C05.0 | Hard palate |

| C05.8 | Overlapping lesion of palate | C06.2 | Retromolar area | ICD-O-3 HISTOLOGY CODE RANGES |
| C05.9 | Palate, NOS | C06.8 | Overlapping lesion of other and unspecified parts of mouth | 8000–8576, 8940–8950, 8980–8981 |
| C06.0 | Cheek mucosa | | | |
| C06.1 | Vestibule of mouth | C06.9 | Mouth, NOS | |

## ANATOMY

**Primary Site.** The oral cavity extends from the skin–vermilion junction of the lips to the junction of the hard and soft palate above and to the line of circumvallate papillae below and is divided into the following specific sites:

**Mucosal Lip.** The lip begins at the junction of the vermilion border with the skin and includes only the vermilion surface or that portion of the lip that comes into contact with the opposing lip. It is well defined into an upper and lower lip joined at the commissures of the mouth.

**Buccal Mucosa.** This includes all the membranous lining of the inner surface of the cheeks and lips from the line of contact of the opposing lips to the line of attachment of mucosa of the alveolar ridge (upper and lower) and pterygomandibular raphe.

**Lower Alveolar Ridge.** This refers to the mucosa overlying the alveolar process of the mandible, which extends from the line of attachment of mucosa in the lower gingivobuccal sulcus to the line of free mucosa of the floor of the mouth. Posteriorly it extends to the ascending ramus of the mandible.

**Upper Alveolar Ridge.** This refers to the mucosa overlying the alveolar process of the maxilla, which extends from the line of attachment of mucosa in the upper gingivobuccal sulcus to the junction of the hard palate. Its posterior margin is the upper end of the pterygopalatine arch.

**Retromolar Gingiva (Retromolar Trigone).** This is the attached mucosa overlying the ascending ramus of the mandible from the level of the posterior surface of the last molar tooth to the apex superiorly, adjacent to the tuberosity of the maxilla.

**Floor of the Mouth.** This is a semilunar space overlying the mylohyoid and hyoglossus muscles, extending from the inner surface of the lower alveolar ridge to the undersurface of the tongue. Its posterior boundary is the base of the anterior pillar of the tonsil. It is divided into two sides by the frenulum of the tongue and contains the ostia of the submandibular and sublingual salivary glands.

**Hard Palate.** This is the semilunar area between the upper alveolar ridge and the mucous membrane covering the palatine process of the maxillary palatine bones. It extends from the inner surface of the superior alveolar ridge to the posterior edge of the palatine bone.

*Anterior Two-Thirds of the Tongue (Oral Tongue).* This is the freely mobile portion of the tongue that extends anteriorly from the line of circumvallate papillae to the undersurface of the tongue at the junction of the floor of the mouth. It is composed of four areas: the tip, the lateral borders, the dorsum, and the undersurface (nonvillous ventral surface of the tongue). The undersurface of the tongue is considered a separate category by the World Health Organization.

**3**

## CHARACTERISTICS OF TUMOR

**Endophytic.** The tumor thickness measurement using an ocular micrometer is taken perpendicular from the surface of the invasive squamous cell carcinoma (A) to the deepest area of involvement (B) and recorded in millimeters. The measurement should not be done on tangential sections or in lesions without a clearly recognizable surface component (Figure 3.1a–c).

**Exophytic.** The measurement that is better characterized as tumor thickness rather than depth of invasion is taken from the surface (A) to the deepest area (B).

**Ulcerated.** The thickness measurement is taken from the ulcer base (A) to the deepest area (B), as well as from the surface of the most lateral extent of the invasive carcinoma (C) to the deepest area (D). Depth of tumor invasion (mm) should be recorded. Depth is *not* used for T staging.

Although the grade of the tumor does not enter into staging of the tumor, it should be recorded. The pathologic description of any lymphadenectomy specimen should describe the size, number, and level of involved lymph node(s) and the presence or absence of extracapsular extension.

**Regional Lymph Nodes.** Mucosal cancer of the oral cavity may spread to regional lymph node(s). Tumors of each anatomic site have their own predictable patterns of regional spread. The risk of regional metastasis is generally related to the T category and, probably more important, to the depth of infiltration of the primary tumor. Cancer of the lip carries a low metastatic risk and initially involves adjacent submental and submandibular nodes, then jugular nodes. Cancers of the hard palate and alveolar ridge likewise have a low metastatic potential and involve buccinator, submandibular, jugular, and occasionally retropharyngeal nodes. Other oral cancers spread primarily to submandibular and jugular nodes and uncommonly to posterior triangle/ supraclavicular nodes. Cancer of the anterior oral tongue may occasionally spread directly to lower jugular nodes. The closer to the midline is the primary, the greater is the risk of bilateral cervical nodal spread. The patterns of regional lymph node metastases are predictable, and sequential progression of disease occurs beyond first echelon lymph nodes. Any previous treatment to the neck, surgical and/or radiation, may alter normal lymphatic drainage

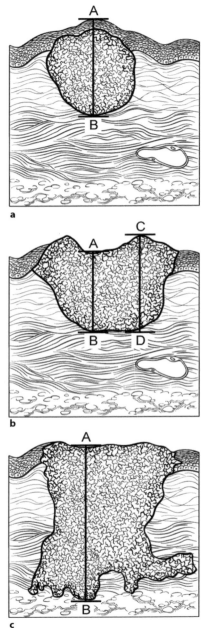

**FIGURE 3.1.** Characteristics of lip and oral cavity tumors. (**a**) Exophytic. (**b**) Ulcerated. (**c**) Endophytic.

patterns, resulting in unusual distribution of regional spread of disease to the cervical lymph nodes. In general, cervical lymph node involvement from oral cavity primary sites is predictable and orderly, spreading from the primary to upper, then middle, and subsequently lower cervical nodes. However, disease in the anterior oral cavity may also spread directly to the mid-cervical lymph nodes. The risk of distant metastasis is more dependent on the N than on the T status of the head and neck cancer. In addition to the components to describe the N category, regional lymph nodes should also be described according to the level of the neck that is involved. It is recognized that the level of involved nodes in the neck is prognostically significant (lower is worse), as is the presence of extracapsular extension of metastatic tumor from individual nodes. Midline nodes are considered ipsilateral. Imaging studies showing amorphous spiculated margins of involved nodes or involvement of internodal fat resulting in loss of normal oval-to-round nodal shape strongly suggest extracapsular (extranodal) tumor spread; however, pathologic examination is necessary for documentation of the extent of such disease. No imaging study (as yet) can identify microscopic foci of cancer in regional nodes or distinguish between small reactive nodes and small malignant nodes (unless central radiographic inhomogeneity is present). For pN, a selective neck dissection will ordinarily include six or more lymph nodes, and a radical or modified radical neck dissection will ordinarily include ten or more lymph nodes. Negative pathologic examination of a lesser number of nodes still mandates a pN0 designation.

Extracapsular spread (ECS) has been recognized to worsen the adverse outcome associated with nodal metastasis. The presence of ECS can be diagnosed clinically by the presence of a "matted" mass of nodes, fixity to overlying skin, adjacent soft tissue, or clinical signs of cranial nerve invasion. Radiologic imaging is capable of detecting clinically undetectable ECS, but histopathologic examination is the only reliable technique currently available for detecting microscopic ECS. Radiologic signs of ECS include amorphous spiculated margins of a metastatic node and stranding of the perinodal soft tissue in previously untreated patients. The absence or presence of clinical/radiologic ECS is designated E− or E+, respectively. Surgically resected metastatic nodes should be examined for the presence and extent of ECS. Gross ECS (Eg) is defined as tumor apparent to the naked eye beyond the confines of the nodal capsule. Microscopic ECS (Em) is defined as the presence of metastatic tumor beyond the capsule of the lymph node with desmoplastic reaction in the surrounding stromal tissue. The absence of ECS on histopathologic examination is designated En.

**Distant Metastases.** The lungs are the commonest site of distant metastases; skeletal and hepatic metastases occur less often. Mediastinal lymph node metastases are considered distant metastases, except level VII lymph nodes (anterior superior mediastinal lymph nodes cephalad to the innominate artery).

## RULES FOR CLASSIFICATION

**Clinical Staging.** The assessment of the primary tumor is based on inspection and palpation of the oral cavity and neck. Physical signs of deep muscle invasion, fixation to bone, and cranial neuropathies should be assessed. Additional studies may include CT, MRI, or ultrasound. Clinical assessment of the extent of mucosal involvement is more accurate than radiographic assessment. The radiographic estimate of deep tissue extent and of regional lymph node involvement is usually more accurate than clinical assessment. MRI is generally more revealing of extent of soft tissue, perivascular and perineural spread, skull base involvement, and intracranial tumor extension. On the other hand, high-resolution CT with contrast will often provide better images of bone and larynx detail and is minimally affected by motion. CT or MRI is useful in evaluation of advanced tumors for assessment of bone invasion (mandible or maxilla) and deep tissue invasion (deep extrinsic tongue muscles, midline tongue, soft tissues of neck). Clinical examination supplemented with dental films or panoramic X-rays may be helpful in determining cortical bone involvement. If CT or MRI is undertaken for primary tumor evaluation, radiologic assessment of nodal involvement should be done simultaneously. For lesions of an advanced extent, appropriate screening for distant metastases should be considered. A PET scan may be useful in this regard. Ultrasonography may be helpful in assessment of major vascular invasion as an adjunctive test. The tumor must be confirmed histologically. All clinical, imaging, and pathologic data available prior to first definitive treatment may be used for clinical staging.

**Pathologic Staging.** Complete resection of the primary site and/or regional nodal dissections, followed by pathologic examination of the resected specimen(s), allows the use of this designation for pT and/or pN, respectively. Specimens that are resected after radiation or chemotherapy need to be identified and considered in context. pT is derived from the actual measurement of the unfixed tumor in the surgical specimen. It should be noted, however, that up to 30% shrinkage of soft tissues may occur in resected specimen after formalin fixation. Pathologic staging represents additional and important information and should be included as such in staging, but it does not supplant clinical staging as the primary staging scheme.

## PROGNOSTIC FEATURES

In addition to the importance of the TNM factors outlined previously, the overall health of these patients clearly influences outcome. An ongoing effort to better assess prognosis using both tumor and nontumor-related factors is underway. Chart abstraction will continue to be performed by cancer registrars to obtain important information regarding specific factors related to prognosis. These data will then be used to further hone the predictive power of the staging system in future revisions.

Comorbidity can be classified by specific measures of additional medical illnesses. Accurate reporting of all illnesses in the patients' medical record is essential to assessment of these parameters. General performance measures are helpful in predicting survival. The AJCC strongly recommends the clinician report performance status using the ECOG, Zubrod, or Karnofsky performance measures along with standard staging information. An interrelationship between each of the major performance tools exists.

## Zubrod/ECOG Performance Scale

0. Fully active, able to carry on all predisease activities without restriction (Karnofsky 90–100)
1. Restricted in physically strenuous activity but ambulatory and able to carry work of a light or sedentary nature. For example, light housework, office work (Karnofsky 70–80)
2. Ambulatory and capable of all self-care but unable to carry out any work activities. Up and about more than 50% of waking hours (Karnofsky 50–60)
3. Capable of only limited self-care, confined to bed or chair 50% or more of waking hours (Karnofsky 30–40)
4. Completely disabled. Cannot carry on self-care. Totally confined to bed (Karnofsky 10–20)
5. Death (Karnofsky 0)

Lifestyle factors such as tobacco and alcohol abuse negatively influence survival. Accurate recording of smoking in pack years and alcohol in number of days drinking per week and number of drinks per day will provide important data for future analysis. Nutrition is important to prognosis and will be indirectly measured by weight loss of >10% of body weight. Depression adversely impacts quality of life and survival. Notation of a previous or current diagnosis of depression should be recorded in the medical record.

Figures 3.2A, B and 3.3A, B show observed and relative survival rates for patients with squamous cell carcinoma of the lip and oral cavity for 1998–1999, classified by the AJCC staging classification.

## DEFINITIONS OF TNM

### Primary Tumor (T)

| | |
|---|---|
| TX | Primary tumor cannot be assessed |
| T0 | No evidence of primary tumor |
| Tis | Carcinoma in situ |
| T1 | Tumor 2 cm or less in greatest dimension |
| T2 | Tumor more than 2 cm but not more than 4 cm in greatest dimension |
| T3 | Tumor more than 4 cm in greatest dimension |
| T4a | Moderately advanced local disease* |
| | (lip) Tumor invades through cortical bone, inferior alveolar nerve, floor of mouth, or skin of face, that is, chin or nose |
| | (oral cavity) Tumor invades adjacent structures only (e.g., through cortical bone [mandible or maxilla] into deep [extrinsic] muscle of tongue [genioglossus, hyoglossus, palatoglossus, and styloglossus], maxillary sinus, skin of face) |
| T4b | Very advanced local disease |
| | Tumor invades masticator space, pterygoid plates, or skull base and/or encases internal carotid artery |

*Note: Superficial erosion alone of bone/tooth socket by gingival primary is not sufficient to classify a tumor as T4.

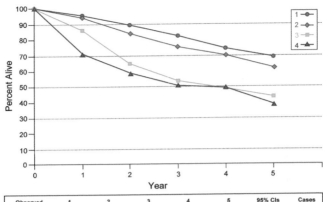

| Observed Survival | 1 | 2 | 3 | 4 | 5 | 95% CIs | Cases |
|---|---|---|---|---|---|---|---|
| 1 | 95.5 | 88.8 | 82.0 | 74.3 | 68.7 | 66.3–71.1 | 2226 |
| 2 | 93.7 | 83.7 | 75.3 | 69.8 | 61.8 | 55.9–67.7 | 370 |
| 3 | 85.5 | 64.4 | 53.1 | 48.3 | 43.1 | 31.0–55.1 | 82 |
| 4 | 71.2 | 58.5 | 50.7 | 49.3 | 38.7 | 28.1–49.4 | 111 |

**A**

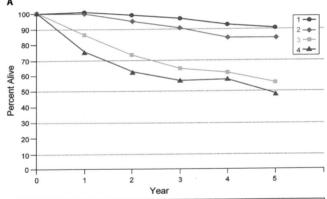

| Relative Survival | 1 | 2 | 3 | 4 | 5 | 95% CIs | Cases |
|---|---|---|---|---|---|---|---|
| 1 | 100 | 98.3 | 95.7 | 91.6 | 89.6 | 86.5–92.7 | 2226 |
| 2 | 99.4 | 94.2 | 89.9 | 83.5 | 83.5 | 75.5–91.5 | 370 |
| 3 | 85.5 | 72.3 | 63.3 | 61.2 | 54.6 | 39.3–69.8 | 82 |
| 4 | 74.6 | 61.3 | 55.8 | 57.0 | 47.2 | 34.2–60.1 | 111 |

**B**

**FIGURE 3.2.** (**A**) Five-year, observed survival by "combined" AJCC stage for squamous cell carcinoma of the lip, 1998–1999. (*95% confidence intervals correspond to year-5 survival rates.). (**B**) Five-year, relative survival by "combined" AJCC stage for squamous cell carcinoma of the lip, 1998–1999. (*95% confidence intervals correspond to year-5 survival rates.)

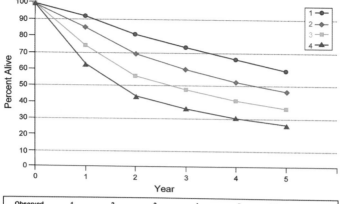

| Observed Survival | 1 | 2 | 3 | 4 | 5 | 95% CIs | Cases |
|---|---|---|---|---|---|---|---|
| 1 | 92.4 | 81.3 | 73.6 | 66.4 | 59.2 | 57.5–60.8 | 4660 |
| 2 | 85.8 | 69.8 | 60.2 | 52.8 | 46.9 | 45.0–48.9 | 3315 |
| 3 | 74.9 | 56.4 | 47.9 | 41.1 | 36.3 | 34.1–38.6 | 2239 |
| 4 | 63.6 | 43.7 | 35.8 | 30.7 | 26.5 | 25.2–27.8 | 5431 |

**A**

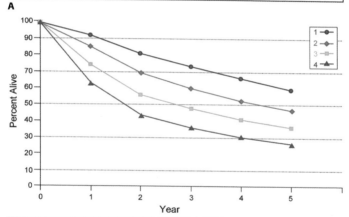

| Relative Survival | 1 | 2 | 3 | 4 | 5 | 95% CIs | Cases |
|---|---|---|---|---|---|---|---|
| 1 | 95.7 | 87.3 | 82.1 | 77.0 | 71.5 | 69.5–73.5 | 4660 |
| 2 | 89.2 | 75.7 | 68.0 | 62.3 | 57.9 | 55.5–60.4 | 3315 |
| 3 | 77.9 | 60.6 | 53.9 | 48.3 | 44.5 | 41.8–47.3 | 2239 |
| 4 | 65.9 | 46.9 | 39.9 | 35.5 | 31.9 | 30.3–33.6 | 5431 |

**B**

**FIGURE 3.3.** (**A**) Five-year, observed survival by "combined" AJCC stage for squamous cell carcinoma of the oral cavity, 1998–1999. (*95% confidence intervals correspond to year-5 survival rates.). (**B**) Five-year, relative survival by "combined" AJCC stage for squamous cell carcinoma of the oral cavity, 1998–1999. (*95% confidence intervals correspond to year-5 survival rates.)

### Regional Lymph Nodes (N)

NX — Regional lymph nodes cannot be assessed

N0 — No regional lymph node metastasis

N1 — Metastasis in a single ipsilateral lymph node, 3 cm or less in greatest dimension

N2 — Metastasis in a single ipsilateral lymph node, more than 3 cm but not more than 6 cm in greatest dimension; or in multiple ipsilateral lymph nodes, none more than 6 cm in greatest dimension; or in bilateral or contralateral lymph nodes, none more than 6 cm in greatest dimension

N2a — Metastasis in single ipsilateral lymph node more than 3 cm but not more than 6 cm in greatest dimension

N2b — Metastasis in multiple ipsilateral lymph nodes, none more than 6 cm in greatest dimension

N2c — Metastasis in bilateral or contralateral lymph nodes, none more than 6 cm in greatest dimension

N3 — Metastasis in a lymph node more than 6 cm in greatest dimension

### Distant Metastasis (M)

M0 — No distant metastasis

M1 — Distant metastasis

### ANATOMIC STAGE/PROGNOSTIC GROUPS

| Stage | T | N | M |
|---|---|---|---|
| Stage 0 | Tis | N0 | M0 |
| Stage I | T1 | N0 | M0 |
| Stage II | T2 | N0 | M0 |
| Stage III | T3 | N0 | M0 |
|  | T1 | N1 | M0 |
|  | T2 | N1 | M0 |
|  | T3 | N1 | M0 |
| Stage IVA | T4a | N0 | M0 |
|  | T4a | N1 | M0 |
|  | T1 | N2 | M0 |
|  | T2 | N2 | M0 |
|  | T3 | N2 | M0 |
|  | T4a | N2 | M0 |
| Stage IVB | Any T | N3 | M0 |
|  | T4b | Any N | M0 |
| Stage IVC | Any T | Any N | M1 |

## PROGNOSTIC FACTORS (SITE-SPECIFIC FACTORS)
### (Recommended for Collection)

| | |
|---|---|
| Required for staging | None |
| Clinically significant | Size of lymph nodes |
| | Extracapsular extension from lymph nodes for head and neck |
| | Head and neck lymph nodes levels I–III |
| | Head and neck lymph nodes levels IV–V |
| | Head and neck lymph nodes levels VI–VII |
| | Other lymph node group |
| | Clinical location of cervical nodes |
| | Extracapsular spread (ECS) clinical |
| | Extracapsular spread (ECS) pathologic |
| | Human papillomavirus (HPV) status |
| | Tumor thickness |

3

## HISTOLOGIC GRADE (G)

Grade is reported in registry systems by the grade value. A two-grade, three-grade, or four-grade system may be used. If a grading system is not specified, generally the following system is used:

| | |
|---|---|
| GX | Grade cannot be assessed |
| G1 | Well differentiated |
| G2 | Moderately differentiated |
| G3 | Poorly differentiated |
| G4 | Undifferentiated |

## HISTOPATHOLOGIC TYPE

The predominant cancer is squamous cell carcinoma. The staging guidelines are applicable to all forms of carcinoma. Mucosal melanoma of the head and neck is very rare but has unique behavior warranting a separate classification discussed in the introductory chapter for the Head and Neck sites. Other nonepithelial tumors such as those of lymphoid tissue, soft tissue, bone and cartilage (i.e., lymphoma and sarcoma) are not included. Histologic confirmation of diagnosis is required. Histopathologic grading of squamous carcinoma is recommended; the grade is subjective and uses a descriptive as well as numerical form, that is, well, moderately well, and poorly differentiated, depending on the degree of closeness to, or deviation from, squamous epithelium in mucosal sites. Also recommended is a quantitative evaluation of depth of invasion of the primary tumor and the presence or absence of vascular invasion and perineural invasion.

## BIBLIOGRAPHY

Byers RM, Weber RS, Andrews T, et al. Frequency and therapeutic implications of "skip metastases" in the neck from squamous carcinoma of the oral tongue. Head Neck. 1997;19:14–9.

Cooper JS, Farnan NC, Asbell SO, et al. Recursive partitioning analysis of 2105 patients treated in Radiation Therapy Oncology Group studies of head and neck cancer. Cancer. 1996;77:1905–11.

Cruse CW, Radocha RF. Squamous carcinoma of the lip. Plast Reconst Surg. 1987;80:787–91.

de Leeuw JRJ, de Graeff A, Ros WJG, et al. Prediction of depressive symptomatology after treatment of head and neck cancer: the influence of pretreatment physical and depressive symptoms, coping, and social support. Head and Neck. 2000;22:799–807.

Deleyiannis FW, Thomas DB, Vaughan TL, et al. Alcoholism: independent predictor of survival in patients with head and neck cancer. J Natl Cancer Inst. 1996;88:542–9.

Evans JF, Shah JP. Epidermoid carcinoma of the palate. Am J Surg. 1981;142:451–5.

Faye-Lund H, Abdelnoor M. Prognostic factors of survival in a cohort of head and neck cancer patients in Oslo. Eur J Cancer B Oral Oncol. 1996;2:83–90.

Franceschi D, Gupta R, Spiro RH, et al. Improved survival in the treatment of squamous carcinoma of the oral tongue. Am J Surg. 1992;166:360–5.

Kaplan MH, Feinstein AR. The importance of classifying initial co-morbidity in evaluating the outcome of diabetes mellitus. J Chron Dis. 1974;27: 387–404.

Karnofsky DA, Abelman WH, Craver LF, Burchenal JH. The use of the nitrogen mustards in the palliative treatment of carcinoma. Cancer. 1948;1:634–56.

Krishnan-Nair M, Sankaranarayanan N, Padmanabhan T. Evaluation of the role of radiotherapy in the management of carcinoma of the buccal mucosa. Cancer. 1988;61:1326–31.

McDaniel JS, Dominique L, Musselman L, et al. Depression in patients with cancer. Psychiatry. 1995;52:89–99.

Mukherji SK, Weeks SM, Castillo M, et al. Squamous cell carcinomas that arise in the oral cavity and tongue base: can CT help predict perineural or vascular invasion? Radiology. 1996;198(1):157–62.

Mukherji SK, Pillsbury HR, Castillo M. Radiology. Imaging squamous cell carcinomas of the upper aerodigestive tract: what clinicians need to know. 1997;205(3):629–46.

Mukherji SK, Isaacs DL, Creager A, et al. CT detection of mandibular invasion by squamous cell carcinoma of the oral cavity. AJR Am J Roentgenol. 2001;177(1):237–43.

Nandapalan V, Roland NJ, Helliwell TR, et al. Mucosal melanoma of the head and neck. Clin Otolaryngol Allied Sci. 1998;23(2):107–16.

Patel SG, Prasad ML, Escrig M, et al. Primary mucosal malignant melanoma of the head and neck. Head Neck. 2002;24(3):247–57.

Petrovich Z, Krusk H, Tobochnik N, et al. Carcinoma of the lip. Arch Otolaryngol. 1979;105:187–91.

Piccirillo JF. Inclusion of comorbidity in a staging system for head and neck cancer. Oncology. 1995;9:831–6.

Rodgers LW, Stringer SP, Mendenhall WH, et al. Management of squamous carcinoma of the floor of the mouth. Head Neck. 1993;15:16–9.

Shah JP. Surgical approaches to the oral cavity primary and neck. Int J Radiat Oncol Biol Phys. 2007;69(2 Suppl):S15–8.

Shaha AR, Spiro RH, Shah JP, et al. Squamous carcinoma of the floor of the mouth. Am J Surg. 1984;148:455–9.

Soo KC, Spiro RH, King W, et al. Squamous carcinoma of the gums. Am J Surg. 1988;156:281–5.

Spiro RH, Huvos AG, Wong GY, et al. Predictive value of tumor thickness in squamous carcinoma confined to the tongue and floor of the mouth. Am J Surg. 1986;152(4):345–50.

Totsuka Y, Usui Y, Tei K, et al. Mandibular involvement by squamous cell carcinoma of the lower alveolus: analysis and comparative study of the histologic and radiologic features. Head Neck. 1991;13:40–50.

Urist M, O'Brien CJ, Soong SJ, et al. Squamous cell carcinoma of the buccal mucosa: analysis of prognostic factors. Am J Surg. 1987;154:411–4.

Wendt CD, Peters LJ, Delclos L, et al. Primary radiotherapy in the treatment of Stage I and II oral tongue cancer: importance of the proportion of therapy delivered with interstitial therapy. Int J Radiat Oncol Biol Phys. 1990;18:1287–92.

3

# Pharynx

*(Nonepithelial tumors such as those of lymphoid
tissue, soft tissue, bone, and cartilage are not
included. Staging of mucosal melanoma of the
pharynx is not included – see Chap. 9.)*

## At-A-Glance

### SUMMARY OF CHANGES

- For nasopharynx, T2a lesions will now be designated T1. Stage IIA will therefore be Stage I. Lesions previously staged T2b will be T2 and therefore Stage IIB will now be designated Stage II. Retropharyngeal lymph node(s), regardless of unilateral or bilateral location, is considered N1

- For oropharynx and hypopharynx only, T4 lesions have been divided into T4a (moderately advanced local disease) and T4b (very advanced local disease), leading to the stratification of Stage IV into Stage IVA (moderately advanced local/regional disease), Stage IVB (very advanced local/regional disease), and Stage IVC (distant metastatic disease)

### ANATOMIC STAGE/PROGNOSTIC GROUPS

*Nasopharynx*

| Stage | T | N | M |
|---|---|---|---|
| Stage 0 | Tis | N0 | M0 |
| Stage I | T1 | N0 | M0 |
| Stage II | T1 | N1 | M0 |
| | T2 | N0 | M0 |
| | T2 | N1 | M0 |
| Stage III | T1 | N2 | M0 |
| | T2 | N2 | M0 |
| | T3 | N0 | M0 |
| | T3 | N1 | M0 |
| | T3 | N2 | M0 |
| Stage IVA | T4 | N0 | M0 |
| | T4 | N1 | M0 |
| | T4 | N2 | M0 |
| Stage IVB | Any T | N3 | M0 |
| Stage IVC | Any T | Any N | M1 |

### ICD-O-3 TOPOGRAPHY CODES

| Code | Description |
|---|---|
| C01.9 | Base of tongue, NOS |
| C02.4 | Lingual tonsil |
| C05.1 | Soft palate, NOS |
| C05.2 | Uvula |
| C09.0 | Tonsillar fossa |
| C09.1 | Tonsillar pillar |
| C09.8 | Overlapping lesion of tonsil |
| C09.9 | Tonsil, NOS |
| C10.0 | Vallecula |
| C10.2 | Lateral wall of oropharynx |
| C10.3 | Posterior pharyngeal wall |
| C10.4 | Branchial cleft |
| C10.8 | Overlapping lesion of oropharynx |
| C10.9 | Oropharynx, NOS |

*Oropharynx, hypopharynx*

| Stage 0 | Tis | N0 | M0 |
|---|---|---|---|
| Stage I | T1 | N0 | M0 |
| Stage II | T2 | N0 | M0 |
| Stage III | T3 | N0 | M0 |
| | T1 | N1 | M0 |
| | T2 | N1 | M0 |
| | T3 | N1 | M0 |
| Stage IVA | T4a | N0 | M0 |
| | T4a | N1 | M0 |
| | T1 | N2 | M0 |
| | T2 | N2 | M0 |
| | T3 | N2 | M0 |
| | T4a | N2 | M0 |
| Stage IVB | T4b | Any N | M0 |
| | Any T | N3 | M0 |
| Stage IVC | Any T | Any N | M1 |

| | |
|---|---|
| C11.0 | Superior wall of nasopharynx |
| C11.1 | Posterior wall of nasopharynx |
| C11.2 | Lateral wall of nasopharynx |
| C11.3 | Anterior wall of nasopharynx |
| C11.8 | Overlapping lesion of nasopharynx |
| C11.9 | Nasopharynx, NOS |
| C12.9 | Pyriform sinus |
| C13.0 | Postcricoid region |
| C13.1 | Hypopharyngeal aspect of aryepiglottic fold |
| C13.2 | Posterior wall of hypopharynx |
| C13.8 | Overlapping lesion of hypopharynx |
| C13.9 | Hypopharynx, NOS |

ICD-O-3 HISTOLOGY
CODE RANGES
8000–8576, 8940–8950,
8980–8981

## ANATOMY

**Primary Sites and Subsites.** The pharynx is divided into three regions: nasopharynx, oropharynx, and hypopharynx (Figure 4.1). Each region is further subdivided into specific sites as summarized in the following:

*Nasopharynx.* The nasopharynx begins anteriorly at the posterior choana and extends along the plane of the airway to the level of the free border of the soft palate. It includes the vault, the lateral walls (including the fossae of Rosenmuller and the mucosa covering the torus tubaris forming the eustachian tube orifice), and the posterior wall. The floor is the superior surface of the soft palate. The posterior margins of the choanal orifices and of the nasal septum are included in the nasal fossa. Nasopharyngeal tumors extending to the nasal cavity or oropharynx in the absence of

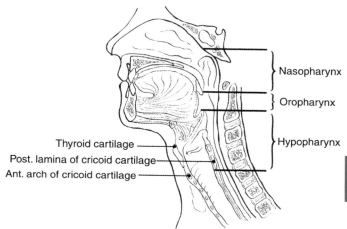

**FIGURE 4.1.** Sagittal view of the face and neck depicting the subdivisions of the pharynx as described in the text.

parapharyngeal space (PPS) involvement do not have significantly worse outcome compared with tumors restricted to the nasopharynx. This edition of the staging system has therefore been updated to reflect the prognostic implication of PPS involvement, which is important in staging nasopharynx cancer.

PPS is a triangular space anterior to the styloid process (prestyloid) that extends from the skull base to the level of the angle of the mandible. The PPS is located lateral to the pharynx and medial to the masticator space and parotid spaces. The PPS contains primarily deep lobe of parotid gland, fat, vascular structures, and small branches of the mandibular division of the fifth cranial nerve. The vascular components include the internal maxillary artery, ascending pharyngeal artery, and the pharyngeal venous plexus. Other less commonly recognized components of the PPS are lymph nodes and ectopic rests of minor salivary gland tissue.

*Poststyloid space* or carotid space (CS) is an enclosed fascial space located posterior to the styloid process and lateral to the retropharyngeal space (RPS) and prevertebral space (PVS). A slip of alar fascia contributes to the medial wall of the CS and helps separate the RPS and PVS from the CS. In the suprahyoid neck, the CS is bordered anteriorly by the styloid process and the PPS, laterally by the posterior belly of the digastric muscle and the parotid space, and medially by the lateral margin of the RPS. The CS contains the internal carotid artery, internal jugular vein, cranial nerves IX–XII, and lymph nodes. The CS extends superiorly to the jugular foramen and inferiorly to the aortic arch.

*Masticator space* primarily consists of the muscles of mastication. Anatomically, the superficial layer of the deep cervical fascia splits to enclose the muscles of mastication to enclose this space. These muscles are the medial and lateral pterygoid, masseter, and temporalis. The contents of the masticator space also include the additional structures encompassed within these fascial boundaries, which include the ramus of the mandible and the third division of the CN V as it passes through foramen ovale into the suprahyoid neck.

*Oropharynx.* The oropharynx is the portion of the continuity of the pharynx extending from the plane of the superior surface of the soft palate to the superior surface of the hyoid bone (or vallecula). It includes the base of the tongue, the inferior (anterior) surface of the soft palate and the uvula, the anterior and posterior tonsillar pillars, the glossotonsillar sulci, the pharyngeal tonsils, and the lateral and posterior pharyngeal walls.

*Hypopharynx.* The hypopharynx is that portion of the pharynx extending from the plane of the superior border of the hyoid bone (or vallecula) to the plane corresponding to the lower border of the cricoid cartilage. It includes the pyriform sinuses (right and left), the lateral and posterior hypopharyngeal walls, and the postcricoid region. The postcricoid area extends from the level of the arytenoid cartilages and connecting folds to the plane of the inferior border of the cricoid cartilage. It connects the two pyriform sinuses, thus forming the anterior wall of the hypopharynx. The pyriform sinus extends from the pharyngoepiglottic fold to the upper end of the esophagus at the lower border of the cricoid cartilage and is bounded laterally by the lateral pharyngeal wall and medially by the lateral surface of the aryepiglottic fold and the arytenoid and cricoid cartilages. The posterior pharyngeal wall extends from the level of the superior surface of the hyoid bone (or vallecula) to the inferior border of the cricoid cartilage and from the apex of one pyriform sinus to the other.

**Regional Lymph Nodes.** The risk of regional nodal spread from cancers of the pharynx is high. Primary nasopharyngeal tumors commonly spread to retropharyngeal, upper jugular, and spinal accessory nodes, often bilaterally. Nasopharyngeal cancer with retropharyngeal lymph node involvement independent of laterality and without cervical lymph node involvement is staged as N1. Oropharyngeal cancers involve upper and mid-jugular lymph nodes and (less commonly) submental/submandibular nodes. Hypopharyngeal cancers spread to adjacent parapharyngeal, paratracheal, and mid- and lower jugular nodes. Bilateral lymphatic drainage is common.

In clinical evaluation, the maximum size of the nodal mass should be measured. Most masses over 3 cm in diameter are not single nodes but, rather, are confluent nodes or tumor in soft tissues of the neck. There are three categories of clinically involved nodes for the nasopharynx, oropharynx, and hypopharynx: N1, N2, and N3. The use of subgroups a, b, and c is required. Midline nodes are considered ipsilateral nodes. Superior mediastinal lymph nodes are considered regional lymph nodes (level VII). In addition to the components to describe the N category, regional lymph nodes should also be described according to the level of the neck that is involved. The level of involved nodes in the neck is prognostically significant (lower is worse), as is the presence of extracapsular spread (ECS) of metastatic tumor from individual nodes. Imaging studies showing amorphous spiculated margins of involved nodes or involvement of internodal fat resulting in loss of normal oval-to-round nodal shape strongly suggest extracapsular (extranodal) spread of tumor. However, pathologic examination is necessary for documentation of such disease extent. No imaging study (as yet) can identify microscopic foci in regional nodes or distinguish between small reactive nodes and small malignant nodes (unless central radiographic inhomogeneity is present).

For pN, a selective neck dissection will ordinarily include six or more lymph nodes, and a radical or modified radical neck dissection will ordinarily include ten or more lymph nodes. Negative pathologic examination of a lesser number of nodes still mandates a pN0 designation.

**Distant Metastases.** The lungs are the commonest site of distant metastases; skeletal or hepatic metastases occur less often. Mediastinal lymph node metastases are considered distant metastases, except level VII lymph nodes.

## RULES FOR CLASSIFICATION

**Clinical Staging.** Clinical staging is generally employed for squamous cell carcinomas of the pharynx. Assessment is based primarily on inspection and on indirect and direct endoscopy. Palpation of sites (when feasible) and of neck nodes is essential. Neurologic evaluation of all cranial nerves is required. Imaging studies are essential in clinical staging of pharynx tumors. Cross-sectional imaging in nasopharyngeal cancer is mandatory to complete the staging process. Magnetic resonance imaging (MRI) often is the study of choice because of its multiplanar capability, superior soft tissue contrast, and sensitivity for detecting skull base and intracranial tumor spread. Computed tomography (CT) imaging with axial and coronal thin section technique with contrast is an alternative. Radiologic nodal staging should be done to assess adequately the retropharyngeal and cervical nodal status.

Cross-sectional imaging in oropharyngeal carcinoma is recommended when the deep tissue extent of the primary tumor is in question. CT or MRI may be employed. Cross-sectional imaging of hypopharyngeal carcinoma is recommended when the extent of the primary tumor is in doubt, particularly its deep extent in relationship to adjacent structures (i.e., larynx, thyroid, cervical vertebrae, and carotid sheath). CT is preferred currently because it entails less motion artifact than MRI. Radiologic nodal staging should be done simultaneously. Complete endoscopy, usually under general anesthesia, is performed after completion of other staging studies, to assess the surface extent of the tumor accurately and to assess deep involvement by palpation for muscle invasion and to facilitate biopsy. A careful search for other primary tumors of the upper aerodigestive tract is indicated because of the incidence of multiple independent primary tumors occurring simultaneously.

**Pathologic Staging.** Pathologic staging requires the use of all information obtained in clinical staging and in histologic study of the surgically resected specimen. The surgeon's evaluation of gross unresected residual tumor must also be included. The pathologic description of any lymph-adenectomy specimen should describe the size, number, and level of any involved nodes and the presence or absence of ECS.

## PROGNOSTIC FEATURES

In addition to the importance of the TNM factors outlined previously, the overall health of these patients clearly influences outcome. An ongoing effort to better assess prognosis using both tumor and nontumor-related factors is underway. Chart abstraction will continue to be performed by cancer registrars to obtain important information regarding specific factors related to prognosis. This data will then be used to further hone the predictive power of the staging system in future revisions.

Comorbidity can be classified by specific measures of additional medical illnesses. Accurate reporting of all illnesses in the patients' medical record is essential to assessment of these parameters. General performance measures are helpful in predicting survival. The AJCC strongly recommends the clinician report performance status using the ECOG, Zubrod or Karnofsky performance measures along with standard staging information. An interrelationship between each of the major performance tools exists.

### Zubrod/ECOG Performance Scale

0. Fully active, able to carry on all predisease activities without restriction (Karnofsky 90–100)
1. Restricted in physically strenuous activity but ambulatory and able to carry work of a light or sedentary nature. For example, light housework, office work (Karnofsky 70–80)
2. Ambulatory and capable of all self-care but unable to carry out any work activities. Up and about more than 50% of waking hours (Karnofsky 50–60)
3. Capable of only limited self-care, confined to bed or chair 50% or more of waking hours (Karnofsky 30–40)
4. Completely disabled. Cannot carry on self-care. Totally confined to bed (Karnofsky 10–20)
5. Death (Karnofsky 0)

Lifestyle factors such as tobacco and alcohol abuse negatively influence survival. Accurate recording of smoking in pack years and alcohol in number of days drinking per week and number of drinks per day will provide important data for future analysis. Nutrition is important to prognosis and will be indirectly measured by weight loss of >10% of body weight. Depression adversely impacts quality of life and survival. Notation of a previous or current diagnosis of depression should be recorded in the medical record.

## MUCOSAL MELANOMA

Mucosal melanoma of all head and neck sites is staged using a uniform classification discussed in Chap. 9.

*Primary Tumor (T)*

TX     Primary tumor cannot be assessed
T0     No evidence of primary tumor
Tis    Carcinoma in situ

*Nasopharynx*

T1     Tumor confined to the nasopharynx, or tumor extends to oropharynx and/or nasal cavity without parapharyngeal extension*
T2     Tumor with parapharyngeal extension*
T3     Tumor involves bony structures of skull base and/or paranasal sinuses
T4     Tumor with intracranial extension and/or involvement of cranial nerves, hypopharynx, orbit, or with extension to the infratemporal fossa/masticator space

*Note*: Parapharyngeal extension denotes posterolateral infiltration of tumor.

*Oropharynx*

T1     Tumor 2 cm or less in greatest dimension
T2     Tumor more than 2 cm but not more than 4 cm in greatest dimension
T3     Tumor more than 4 cm in greatest dimension or extension to lingual surface of epiglottis
T4a    Moderately advanced local disease
       Tumor invades the larynx, extrinsic muscle of tongue, medial pterygoid, hard palate, or mandible*
T4b    Very advanced local disease
       Tumor invades lateral pterygoid muscle, pterygoid plates, lateral nasopharynx, or skull base or encases carotid artery

*Note*: Mucosal extension to lingual surface of epiglottis from primary tumors of the base of the tongue and vallecula does not constitute invasion of larynx.

*Hypopharynx*

T1     Tumor limited to one subsite of hypopharynx and/or 2 cm or less in greatest dimension
T2     Tumor invades more than one subsite of hypopharynx or an adjacent site, or measures more than 2 cm but not more than 4 cm in greatest dimension without fixation of hemilarynx
T3     Tumor more than 4 cm in greatest dimension or with fixation of hemilarynx or extension to esophagus
T4a    Moderately advanced local disease
       Tumor invades thyroid/cricoid cartilage, hyoid bone, thyroid gland, or central compartment soft tissue*
T4b    Very advanced local disease
       Tumor invades prevertebral fascia, encases carotid artery, or involves mediastinal structures

*Note*: Central compartment soft tissue includes prelaryngeal strap muscles and subcutaneous fat.

### Regional Lymph Nodes (N)

*Nasopharynx*
The distribution and the prognostic impact of regional lymph node spread from nasopharynx cancer, particularly of the undifferentiated type, are different from those of other head and neck mucosal cancers and justify the use of a different N classification scheme.

NX    Regional lymph nodes cannot be assessed
N0    No regional lymph node metastasis
N1    Unilateral metastasis in cervical lymph node(s), 6 cm or less in greatest dimension, above the supraclavicular fossa, and/or unilateral or bilateral, retropharyngeal lymph nodes, 6 cm or less, in greatest dimension*
N2    Bilateral metastasis in cervical lymph node(s), 6 cm or less in greatest dimension, above the supraclavicular fossa*
N3    Metastasis in a lymph node(s)* >6 cm and/or to supraclavicular fossa
N3a    Greater than 6 cm in dimension
N3b    Extension to the supraclavicular fossa**

*Note*: Midline nodes are considered ipsilateral nodes.

**Note*: Supraclavicular zone or fossa is relevant to the staging of nasopharyngeal carcinoma and is the triangular region originally described by Ho. It is defined by three points: (1) the superior margin of the sternal end of the clavicle, (2) the superior margin of the lateral end of the clavicle, (3) the point where the neck meets the shoulder (Figure 4.2). Note that this would include caudal portions of levels IV and VB. All cases with lymph nodes (whole or part) in the fossa are considered N3b.

### Regional Lymph Nodes (N)*

*Oropharynx and Hypopharynx*
NX    Regional lymph nodes cannot be assessed
N0    No regional lymph node metastasis
N1    Metastasis in a single ipsilateral lymph node, 3 cm or less in greatest dimension
N2    Metastasis in a single ipsilateral lymph node, more than 3 cm but not more than 6 cm in greatest dimension, or in multiple ipsilateral lymph nodes, none more than 6 cm in greatest dimension, or in bilateral or contralateral lymph nodes, none more than 6 cm in greatest dimension
N2a    Metastasis in a single ipsilateral lymph node more than 3 cm but not more than 6 cm in greatest dimension
N2b    Metastasis in multiple ipsilateral lymph nodes, none more than 6 cm in greatest dimension
N2c    Metastasis in bilateral or contralateral lymph nodes, none more than 6 cm in greatest dimension
N3    Metastasis in a lymph node more than 6 cm in greatest dimension

*Note*: Metastases at level VII are considered regional lymph node metastases.

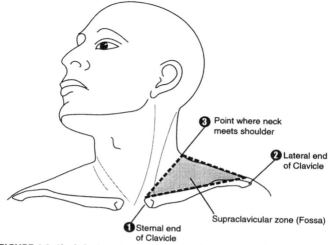

**FIGURE 4.2.** Shaded triangular area corresponds to the supraclavicular fossa used in staging carcinoma of the nasopharynx.

**Labels in figure:**
- ❸ Point where neck meets shoulder
- ❷ Lateral end of Clavicle
- ❶ Sternal end of Clavicle
- Supraclavicular zone (Fossa)

**Distant Metastasis (M)**

M0    No distant metastasis
M1    Distant metastasis

## ANATOMIC STAGE/PROGNOSTIC GROUPS

*Nasopharynx*

| | | | |
|---|---|---|---|
| Stage 0 | Tis | N0 | M0 |
| Stage I | T1 | N0 | M0 |
| Stage II | T1 | N1 | M0 |
| | T2 | N0 | M0 |
| | T2 | N1 | M0 |
| Stage III | T1 | N2 | M0 |
| | T2 | N2 | M0 |
| | T3 | N0 | M0 |
| | T3 | N1 | M0 |
| | T3 | N2 | M0 |
| Stage IVA | T4 | N0 | M0 |
| | T4 | N1 | M0 |
| | T4 | N2 | M0 |
| Stage IVB | Any T | N3 | M0 |
| Stage IVC | Any T | Any N | M1 |

*Oropharynx, hypopharynx*

| Stage | T | N | M |
|-------|-----|--------|-----|
| Stage 0 | Tis | N0 | M0 |
| Stage I | T1 | N0 | M0 |
| Stage II | T2 | N0 | M0 |
| Stage III | T3 | N0 | M0 |
| | T1 | N1 | M0 |
| | T2 | N1 | M0 |
| | T3 | N1 | M0 |
| Stage IVA | T4a | N0 | M0 |
| | T4a | N1 | M0 |
| | T1 | N2 | M0 |
| | T2 | N2 | M0 |
| | T3 | N2 | M0 |
| | T4a | N2 | M0 |
| Stage IVB | T4b | Any N | M0 |
| | Any T | N3 | M0 |
| Stage IVC | Any T | Any N | M1 |

## PROGNOSTIC FACTORS (SITE-SPECIFIC FACTORS)
### (Recommended for Collection)

| | |
|---|---|
| Required for staging | None |
| Clinically significant | Size of lymph nodes |
| | Extracapsular extension from lymph nodes for head and neck |
| | Head and neck lymph nodes levels I–III |
| | Head and neck lymph nodes levels IV–V |
| | Head and neck lymph nodes levels VI–VII |
| | Other lymph nodes group |
| | Clinical location of cervical nodes |
| | ECS clinical |
| | ECS pathologic |
| | Human papillomavirus (HPV) status |

Figures 4.3 through 4.6 show observed and relative survival rates for patients with squamous cell carcinoma of the nasopharynx, oropharynx, hypopharynx, and pharynx (NOS) for 1998–1999, classified by the AJCC staging classification.

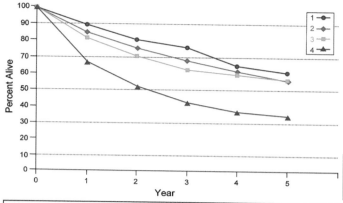

| Observed Survival | 1 | 2 | 3 | 4 | 5 | 95% CIs | Cases |
|---|---|---|---|---|---|---|---|
| 1 | 89.5 | 80.8 | 76.1 | 65.2 | 60.6 | 52.1–69.2 | 170 |
| 2 | 85.3 | 75.2 | 67.8 | 61.6 | 56.2 | 50.1–62.3 | 322 |
| 3 | 81.8 | 70.4 | 61.9 | 59.2 | 55.7 | 50.3–61.0 | 408 |
| 4 | 66.9 | 52.1 | 41.9 | 37.0 | 34.1 | 30.3–37.8 | 759 |

**A**

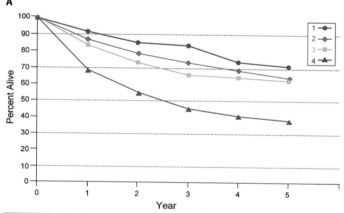

| Relative Survival | 1 | 2 | 3 | 4 | 5 | 95% CIs | Cases |
|---|---|---|---|---|---|---|---|
| 1 | 92.2 | 86.0 | 83.7 | 74.2 | 71.5 | 61.4–81.5 | 170 |
| 2 | 87.3 | 79.0 | 73.1 | 68.4 | 64.2 | 57.2–71.1 | 322 |
| 3 | 83.5 | 73.3 | 65.9 | 64.6 | 62.2 | 56.2–68.2 | 408 |
| 4 | 68.4 | 54.5 | 44.9 | 40.6 | 38.4 | 34.1–42.7 | 759 |

**B**

**FIGURE 4.3.** (**A**) Five-year, observed survival by "combined" AJCC stage for squamous cell carcinoma of the nasopharynx, 1998–1999. (*95% confidence intervals correspond to year-5 survival rates.) (**B**) Five-year, relative survival by "combined" AJCC stage for squamous cell carcinoma of the nasopharynx, 1998–1999. (*95% confidence intervals correspond to year-5 survival rates.)

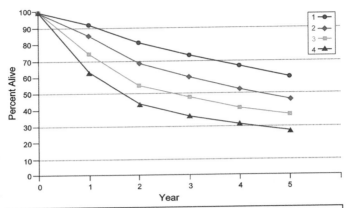

| Observed Survival | 1 | 2 | 3 | 4 | 5 | 95% CIs | Cases |
|---|---|---|---|---|---|---|---|
| 1 | 92.7 | 81.6 | 74.1 | 67.0 | 60.0 | 58.3–61.7 | 4284 |
| 2 | 85.8 | 69.4 | 60.0 | 52.6 | 46.7 | 44.7–48.8 | 2983 |
| 3 | 74.5 | 55.3 | 47.5 | 41.0 | 36.5 | 34.1–38.9 | 1968 |
| 4 | 63.6 | 43.6 | 35.9 | 31.0 | 26.8 | 25.4–28.2 | 5018 |

**A**

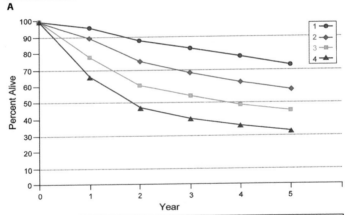

| Relative Survival | 1 | 2 | 3 | 4 | 5 | 95% CIs | Cases |
|---|---|---|---|---|---|---|---|
| 1 | 96.0 | 87.6 | 82.8 | 77.8 | 72.6 | 70.5–74.7 | 4284 |
| 2 | 89.3 | 75.4 | 68.0 | 62.3 | 58.0 | 55.4–60.6 | 2983 |
| 3 | 77.6 | 59.9 | 53.7 | 48.4 | 45.0 | 42.1–48.0 | 1968 |
| 4 | 65.9 | 46.8 | 40.1 | 36.0 | 32.4 | 30.7–34.1 | 5018 |

**B**

**FIGURE 4.4. (A)** Five-year, observed survival by "combined" AJCC stage for squamous cell carcinoma of the oropharynx, 1998–1999. (*95% confidence intervals correspond to year-5 survival rates.) **(B)** Five-year, relative survival by "combined" AJCC stage for squamous cell carcinoma of the oropharynx, 1998–1999. (*95% confidence intervals correspond to year-5 survival rates.)

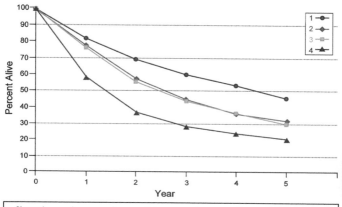

| Observed Survival | 1 | 2 | 3 | 4 | 5 | 95% CIs | Cases |
|---|---|---|---|---|---|---|---|
| 1 | 81.4 | 69.2 | 59.5 | 53.6 | 45.2 | 38.8–51.7 | 297 |
| 2 | 77.1 | 57.4 | 44.4 | 35.9 | 31.1 | 26.6–35.5 | 528 |
| 3 | 75.8 | 55.2 | 43.5 | 36.1 | 29.3 | 25.9–32.7 | 906 |
| 4 | 58.4 | 36.8 | 27.9 | 23.4 | 20.3 | 18.6–22.0 | 2599 |

**A**

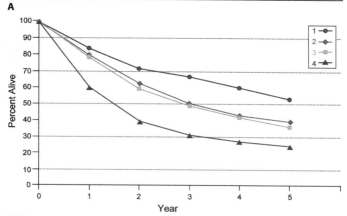

| Relative Survival | 1 | 2 | 3 | 4 | 5 | 95% CIs | Cases |
|---|---|---|---|---|---|---|---|
| 1 | 84.5 | 71.8 | 66.9 | 60.2 | 53.0 | 45.5–60.6 | 297 |
| 2 | 80.5 | 62.6 | 50.8 | 43.2 | 39.3 | 33.7–44.9 | 528 |
| 3 | 78.6 | 59.6 | 48.9 | 42.3 | 36.0 | 31.8–40.1 | 906 |
| 4 | 60.4 | 39.4 | 31.0 | 27.0 | 24.4 | 22.4–26.5 | 2599 |

**B**

**FIGURE 4.5.** (**A**) Five-year, observed survival by "combined" AJCC stage for squamous cell carcinoma of the hypopharynx, 1998–1999. (*95% confidence intervals correspond to year-5 survival rates.) (**B**) Five-year, relative survival by "combined" AJCC stage for squamous cell carcinoma of the hypopharynx, 1998–1999. (*95% confidence intervals correspond to year-5 survival rates.)

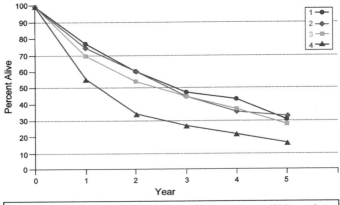

| Observed Survival | 1 | 2 | 3 | 4 | 5 | 95% CIs | Cases |
|---|---|---|---|---|---|---|---|
| 1 | 77.1 | 60.4 | 47.0 | 42.7 | 30.4 | 21.3–39.5 | 121 |
| 2 | 75.0 | 60.2 | 44.9 | 35.3 | 32.5 | 24.2–40.7 | 157 |
| 3 | 69.5 | 54.2 | 44.3 | 36.6 | 27.7 | 20.9–34.5 | 216 |
| 4 | 55.6 | 34.1 | 26.5 | 21.6 | 16.3 | 12.8–19.9 | 536 |

**A**

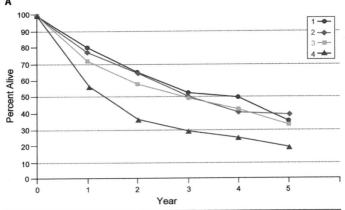

| Relative Survival | 1 | 2 | 3 | 4 | 5 | 95% CIs | Cases |
|---|---|---|---|---|---|---|---|
| 1 | 80.0 | 65.1 | 52.8 | 50.1 | 35.6 | 25.0–46.3 | 121 |
| 2 | 77.7 | 64.7 | 50.2 | 41.1 | 39.5 | 29.5–49.5 | 157 |
| 3 | 72.0 | 58.1 | 49.4 | 42.5 | 33.5 | 25.3–41.7 | 216 |
| 4 | 57.4 | 36.4 | 29.3 | 24.7 | 19.4 | 15.2–23.6 | 536 |

**B**

**FIGURE 4.6.** (**A**) Five-year, observed survival by "combined" AJCC stage for squamous cell carcinoma of the pharynx NOS, 1998–1999. (*95% confidence intervals correspond to year-5 survival rates.) (**B**) Five-year, relative survival by "combined" AJCC stage for squamous cell carcinoma of the pharynx NOS, 1998–1999. (*95% confidence intervals correspond to year-5 survival rates.)

**TABLE 4.1.** Classification of nasopharyngeal carcinoma

| WHO classification | Former terminology |
|---|---|
| Keratinizing squamous cell carcinoma | WHO Type I (squamous cell carcinoma) |
| Nonkeratinizing carcinoma | |
|   Differentiated | WHO Type II (transitional cell carcinoma) |
|   Undifferentiated | WHO Type III (lymphoepithelial carcinoma) |
| Basaloid squamous cell carcinoma | No synonym exists (recently described) |

## HISTOLOGIC GRADE (G)

Grade is reported in registry systems by the grade value. A two-grade, three-grade, or four-grade system may be used. If a grading system is not specified, generally the following system is used:

GX     Grade cannot be assessed
G1     Well differentiated
G2     Moderately differentiated
G3     Poorly differentiated
G4     Undifferentiated

## HISTOPATHOLOGIC TYPE

The predominant cancer type is squamous cell carcinoma for all pharyngeal sites. Mucosal melanoma of the head and neck is very rare but has unique behavior warranting a separate classification discussed in Chap. 9. Other nonepithelial tumors such as those of lymphoid tissue, soft tissue, bone, and cartilage are not included in this system. For nasopharyngeal carcinomas, it is recommended that the World Health Organization (WHO) classification be used (Table 4.1). Histologic diagnosis is necessary to use this classification.

## BIBLIOGRAPHY

Au JSK. In-depth evaluation of the AJCC/UICC 1997 staging system of nasopharyngeal carcinoma: prognostic homogeneity and proposed refinements. Int J Radiat Oncol Biol Phys. 2003;26(2):413–26.

Bolzoni A, Cappiello J, Piazza C, Peretti G, Maroldi R, Farina D, et al. Diagnostic accuracy of magnetic resonance imaging in the assessment of mandibular involvement in oral-oropharyngeal squamous cell carcinoma: a prospective study. Arch Otolaryngol Head Neck Surg. 2004;130(7):837–43.

Boyd TS, Harari PM, Tannehill SP, et al. Planned post-radiotherapy neck dissection in patients with advanced head and neck cancer. Head Neck. 1998;29:132–7.

Chan JKC, Pilch BZ, Kuo TT, Wenig BM, Lee AWM. Tumours of the nasopharynx. In: Eveson BL, JW RP, Sidransky D, editors. World Health Organization classification of tumour, pathology and genetics. Head and neck tumours. Lyon: IARC; 2005. p. 815–97.

Chong V, Mukherji S, Ng S-H, et al. Nasopharyngeal carcinoma; review of how imaging affects staging. J Comput Assist Tomogr. 1999;23:984–93.

Chua D, Sham J, Kwong D, et al: Prognostic value of paranasopharyngeal extension of nasopharyngeal carcinoma. A significant factor in local control and distant metastasis. Cancer 1996;78:202–10.

Colangelo LA, Logemann JA, Pauloski BR, Pelzer JR, Rademaker AW. T stage and functional outcome in oral and oropharyngeal cancer patients. Head Neck. 1996;18:259–68.

Cooper J, Cohen R, Stevens R. A comparison of staging systems for nasopharyngeal carcinoma. Cancer. 1998;83:213–9.

de Leeuw JR, de Graeff A, Ros WJ, Blijham GH, Hordijk GJ, Winnubst JA. Prediction of depressive symptomatology after treatment of head and neck cancer: the influence of pre-treatment physical and depressive symptoms, coping, and social support. Head Neck. 2000;22(8):799–807.

Deleyiannis FW, Weymuller EA Jr, Coltrera MD. Quality of life of disease-free survivors of advanced (Stage III or IV) oropharyngeal cancer. Head Neck. 1997;19:466–73.

Forastiere AA, Trotti A. Radiotherapy and concurrent chemotherapy: a strategy that improves locoregional control and survival in oropharyngeal cancer. J Natl Cancer Inst. 1999;91:2065–6.

Garden AS, Morrison WH, Clayman GL, Ang KK, Peters LJ. Early squamous cell carcinoma of the hypopharynx: outcomes of treatment with radiation alone to the primary disease. Head Neck. 1996;18:317–22.

Gwozdz JT, Morrison WH, Garden AS, Weber RS, Peters LJ, Ang KK. Concomitant boost radiotherapy for squamous carcinoma of the tonsillar fossa. Int J Radiat Oncol Biol Phys. 1997;39:127–35.

Harrison LB, Lee HJ, Pfister DG, Kraus DH, White C, Raben A, et al. Long-term results of primary radiotherapy with/without neck dissection for squamous cell cancer of the base of the tongue. Head Neck. 1998;20:668–73.

Ho J. Stage classification of nasopharyngeal carcinoma, etiology and control, vol. 20. Lyon: IARC Scientific; 1978. p. 99–113.

Hoffman HT, Karnell LH, Shah JP, et al. Hypopharyngeal cancer patient care evaluation. Laryngoscope. 1997;107:1005–17.

Hoffman HT, Karnell LH, Funk GF, Robinson RA, Menck HR. The National Cancer Data Base report on cancer of the head and neck. Arch Otolaryngol Head Neck Surg. 1998;951–62.

Iro H, Waldfahrer F. Evaluation of the newly updated TNM classification of head and neck carcinoma with data from 3, 247 patients. Cancer. 1998;83:2201–7.

King AD. Neck node metastases from nasopharyngeal carcinoma: MR imaging of patterns of disease. Head Neck. 2000;22:275–81.

Kraus DH, Zelefsky MJ, Brock HA, Huo J, Harrison LB, Shah JP. Combined surgery and radiation therapy for squamous cell carcinoma of the hypopharynx. Otolaryngol Head Neck Surg. 1997;116:637–41.

Lee A, Foo W, Law S, et al. N-staging of nasopharyngeal carcinoma: discrepancy between UICC/AJCC and Ho systems. Clin Oncol. 1995;17:377–81.

Lee AWM, Au JS, Teo PM, et al. Staging of nasopharyngeal carcinoma: suggestions for improving the current UICC/AJCC staging system. Clin Oncol. 2004;16:269–76.

Lefebvre JL, Buisset E, Coche-Dequeant B, Van JT, Prevost B, Hecquet B, et al. Epilarynx: pharynx or larynx? Head Neck. 1995;17:377–81.

Lefebvre JL, Chevalier D, Luboinski B, Kirkpatric A, Collette L, Sahmoud T. Larynx preservation in pyriform sinus cancer: preliminary results of a European organization for research treatment of cancer phase III trial. EORTC Head and Neck Cancer Cooperative Group. J Natl Cancer Inst. 1996;88:890–9.

Liu MZ, Tang LL, Zong JF, et al. Evaluation of the sixth edition of AJCC Staging System for nasopharyngeal carcinoma and proposed improvement. Int J Radiat Oncol Biol Phys. 2008;70(4):1115–23.

Low JS, Heng DM, Wee JT. The question of T2a and N3a in the UICC/AJCC (1997) staging system for nasopharyngeal carcinoma. Clin Oncol (R Coll Radiol). 2004;16(8):581–3.

Mendenhall WM, Amdur RJ, Stringer SP, Villaret DB, Cassisi NJ. Stratification of stage IV squamous cell carcinoma of the oropharynx. Head Neck. 2000;22:626–8.

Pauloski BR, Logemann JA, Colangelo LA, Rademaker AW, McConnel FM, Heiser MA, et al. Surgical variables affecting speech in treated patients with oral and oropharyngeal cancer. Laryngoscope. 1998;108:908–16.

Perez CA, Patel MM, Chao KS, Simpson JR, Sessions D, Spector GJ, Haughey B, Lockett MA. Carcinoma of the tonsillar fossa: prognostic factors and long-term therapy outcome. Int J Radiat Oncol Biol Phys 1998;42:1077–84.

Piccirillo JF. Inclusion of comorbidity in a staging system for head and neck cancer. Oncology. 1995;9:831–6.

Prehn RB, Pasic TR, Harari PM, Brown WD, Ford CN. Influence of computed tomography on pretherapeutic tumor staging of head and neck cancer patients. Otolaryngol Head Neck Surg. 1998;199:628–33.

Pugliano FA, Piccirillo JF, Zequeira MR, Emami B, Perez CA, Simpson JR, et al. Clinical-severity staging system for oropharyngeal cancer: five-year survival rates. Arch Otolaryngol Head Neck Surg. 1997;123:1118–24.

Righi PD, Kelley DJ, Ernst R, Deutsch MD, Gaskill-Shipley M, Wilson KM, Gluckman JL. Evaluation of prevertebral muscle invasion by squamous cell carcinoma. Can computed tomography replace open neck exploration? Arch Otolaryngol Head Neck Surg. 1996;122:660–3.

Roh J-L. Nasopharyngeal carcinoma with skull base invasion: a necessity of staging subdivision. Am J Otolaryngol. 2004;25(1):26–32.

Tang LL, Li L, Mao Y, et al. Retropharyngeal lymph node metastasis in nasopharyngeal carcinoma detected by magnetic resonance imaging. Cancer. 2008;113:347–54.

Teresi L, Lufkin R, Vinuela F, et al. MR imaging of the nasopharynx and floor of the middle cranial fossa. II. Malignant tumors. Radiology. 1987;164:817–21.

Thabet HM, Sessions DG, Gado MY, Gnepp DA, Harvey JE, Talaat M. Comparison of clinical evaluation and computed tomographic diagnostic accuracy for tumor of the larynx and hypopharynx. Laryngoscope. 1996;106:589–94.

Veneroni S, Silvestrini R, Costa A, Salvatori P, Faranda A, Monlinari R. Biological indicators of survival in patients treated by surgery for squamous cell carcinoma of the oral cavity and oropharynx. Oral Oncol. 1997;33:408–13.

Wahlberg PC, Andersson KE, Biorklund AT, Moller TR. Carcinoma of the hypopharynx: analysis of incidence and survival in Sweden over a 30-year period. Head Neck. 1998;20:714–9.

Wang MB, Kuber MM, Lee SP, Julliard GF, Abemayor E. Tonsillar carcinoma: analysis of treatment results. J Otolaryngol. 1998;27:263–9.

Weber RS, Gidley P, Morrison WH, Peters LJ, Hankins PD, Wolf P, et al. Treatment selection for carcinoma of the base of the tongue. Am J Surg. 1990;60:415–9.

Zelefsky MJ, Kraus DH, Pfister DG, Raben A, Shah JP, Strong EW, et al. Combined chemotherapy and radiotherapy versus surgical and postoperative radiotherapy for advanced hypopharyngeal cancer. Head Neck. 1996;18:405–11.

**4**

# Larynx

*(Nonepithelial tumors such as those of lymphoid
tissue, soft tissue, bone, and cartilage are
not included)*

## At-A-Glance

### SUMMARY OF CHANGES

• T4 lesions have been divided into T4a (moderately advanced local disease) and T4b (very advanced local disease), leading to the stratification of Stage IV into Stage IVA (moderately advanced local/regional disease), Stage IVB (very advanced local/regional disease), and Stage IVC (distant metastatic disease)

| ANATOMIC STAGE/PROGNOSTIC GROUPS | | | |
|---|---|---|---|
| Stage 0 | Tis | N0 | M0 |
| Stage I | T1 | N0 | M0 |
| Stage II | T2 | N0 | M0 |
| Stage III | T3 | N0 | M0 |
| | T1 | N1 | M0 |
| | T2 | N1 | M0 |
| | T3 | N1 | M0 |
| Stage IVA | T4a | N0 | M0 |
| | T4a | N1 | M0 |
| | T1 | N2 | M0 |
| | T2 | N2 | M0 |
| | T3 | N2 | M0 |
| | T4a | N2 | M0 |
| Stage IVB | T4b | Any N | M0 |
| | Any T | N3 | M0 |
| Stage IVC | Any T | Any N | M1 |

**ICD-O-3 TOPOGRAPHY CODES**

| | |
|---|---|
| C10.1 | Anterior (lingual) surface of epiglottis |
| C32.0 | Glottis |
| C32.1 | Supraglottis (laryngeal surface) |
| C32.2 | Subglottis |
| C32.3 | Laryngeal cartilage |
| C32.8 | Overlapping lesion of larynx |
| C32.9 | Larynx, NOS |

**ICD-O-3 HISTOLOGY CODE RANGES**
8000–8576, 8940–8950, 8980–8981

## ANATOMY

**Primary Site.**  The following anatomic definition of the larynx allows classification of carcinomas arising in the encompassed mucous membranes but excludes cancers arising on the lateral or posterior pharyngeal wall, pyriform fossa, postcricoid area, or base of tongue.

The anterior limit of the larynx is composed of the anterior or lingual surface of the suprahyoid epiglottis, the thyrohyoid membrane, the anterior commissure, and the anterior wall of the subglottic region, which is composed of the thyroid cartilage, the cricothyroid membrane, and the anterior arch of the cricoid cartilage.

The posterior and lateral limits include the laryngeal aspect of the aryepiglottic folds, the arytenoid region, the interarytenoid space, and the posterior surface of the subglottic space, represented by the mucous membrane covering the surface of the cricoid cartilage.

The superolateral limits are composed of the tip and the lateral borders of the epiglottis. The inferior limits are made up of the plane passing through the inferior edge of the cricoid cartilage.

For purposes of this clinical stage classification, the larynx is divided into three regions: supraglottis, glottis, and subglottis. The supraglottis is composed of the epiglottis (both its lingual and laryngeal aspects), aryepiglottic folds (laryngeal aspect), arytenoids, and ventricular bands (false cords). The epiglottis is divided for staging purposes into suprahyoid and infrahyoid portions by a plane at the level of the hyoid bone. The inferior boundary of the supraglottis is a horizontal plane passing through the lateral margin of the ventricle at its junction with the superior surface of the vocal cord. The glottis is composed of the superior and inferior surfaces of the true vocal cords, including the anterior and posterior commissures. It occupies a horizontal plane 1 cm in thickness, extending inferiorly from the lateral margin of the ventricle. The subglottis is the region extending from the lower boundary of the glottis to the lower margin of the cricoid cartilage.

The division of the larynx is summarized as follows:

| Site | Subsite |
|---|---|
| Supraglottis | Suprahyoid epiglottis |
| | Infrahyoid epiglottis |
| | Aryepiglottic folds (laryngeal aspect); arytenoids |
| | Ventricular bands (false cords) |
| Glottis | True vocal cords, including anterior and posterior commissures |
| Subglottis | Subglottis |

**Regional Lymph Nodes.** The incidence and distribution of cervical nodal metastases from cancer of the larynx vary with the site of origin and the T classification of the primary tumor. The true vocal cords are nearly devoid of lymphatics, and tumors of that site alone rarely spread to regional nodes. By contrast, the supraglottis has a rich and bilaterally interconnected lymphatic network, and primary supraglottic cancers are commonly accompanied by regional lymph node spread. Glottic tumors may spread directly to adjacent soft tissues and prelaryngeal, pretracheal, paralaryngeal, and paratracheal nodes, as well as to upper, mid, and lower jugular nodes. Supraglottic tumors commonly spread to upper and midjugular nodes, considerably less commonly to submental or submandibular nodes, and occasionally to retropharyngeal nodes. The rare subglottic primary tumors spread first to adjacent soft tissues and prelaryngeal, pretracheal, paralaryngeal, and paratracheal nodes, then to mid- and lower jugular nodes. Contralateral lymphatic spread is common.

In clinical evaluation, the physical size of the nodal mass should be measured. Most masses over 3 cm in diameter are not single nodes but, rather, are confluent nodes or tumor in soft tissues of the neck. There are three categories of clinically positive nodes: N1, N2, and N3. Midline nodes are considered ipsilateral nodes. In addition to the components to describe the N category, regional lymph nodes should also be described according to the level of the neck that is involved. Pathologic examination is necessary for documentation of such disease extent. Imaging studies showing amorphous spiculated margins of involved nodes or involvement of internodal fat resulting in loss of normal oval-to-round nodal shape strongly suggest extracapsular (extranodal) tumor spread. No imaging study (as yet) can identify microscopic foci in regional nodes or distinguish between small reactive nodes and small malignant nodes without central radiographic inhomogeneity.

**Distant Metastases.** Distant spread is common only for patients who have bulky regional lymphadenopathy. When distant metastases occur, spread to the lungs is most common; skeletal or hepatic metastases occur less often. Mediastinal lymph node metastases are considered distant metastases, except level VII, lymph nodes (in the anterior superior mediastinum, cephalad to the innominate artery).

## RULES FOR CLASSIFICATION

**Clinical Staging.** The assessment of the larynx is accomplished primarily by inspection, using indirect mirror and direct endoscopic examination with a fiberoptic nasolaryngoscope. The tumor must be confirmed histologically, and any other data obtained by biopsies may be included. Cross-sectional imaging in laryngeal carcinoma is recommended when the primary tumor extent is in question on the basis of clinical examination. Radiologic nodal staging should be done simultaneously to supplement clinical examination.

Complete endoscopy under general anesthesia is usually performed after completion of other diagnostic studies to accurately assess, document, and biopsy the tumor. Satisfactory examination of larynx requires the use of microlaryngoscopy and use of telescopes (0°, 30°, 70°, and 120°) to get complete overall assessment.

**Imaging Studies.** Primary site clinical staging for supraglottic carcinoma is based on involvement of various subsites of the supraglottic larynx adjacent regions and vocal cord mobility. Imaging may be helpful to identify occult submucosal transglottic extension. Imaging criteria that define T3 lesions are extension into the preepiglottic space (paralaryngeal fat) or tumors that erode the inner cortex of the thyroid cartilage. Tumors that erode the outer cortex of the thyroid cartilage are defined as T4a tumors.

For T1 and T2 tumors of the glottic larynx, cross-sectional imaging may be used to ensure that the clinical diagnosis of early stage lesions is correct. Imaging may be used as an important adjunct to identify the presence of submucosal extension, especially at the anterior commissure where lesions may spread anteriorly along Broyle's ligament to involve the inner cortex of the thyroid cartilage. Imaging may also identify glottic carcinomas that have occult transglottic or subglottic spread. The normal *paraglottic* space is often difficult to routinely detect at the level of the true vocal cord due to the close apposition of the lateral thyroarytenoid muscle to the inner cortex of the thyroid cartilage. Tumor erosion limited to the inner cortex of the thyroid cartilage indicates a T3 lesion whereas carcinomas that erode the outer cortex of the thyroid cartilage define a T4a tumor. Stage T4 (a and b) is difficult to identify based on clinical examination alone as the majority of the criteria cannot be assessed by endoscopy and palpation.

**Pathologic Staging.** Pathologic staging requires the use of all information obtained in clinical staging and in histologic study of the surgically resected specimen. The surgeon's evaluation of gross unresected residual tumor must also be included. Specimens that are resected after radiation or chemotherapy need to be identified and considered in context. The pathologic description of any lymphadenectomy specimen should describe the size, number, and position of the involved node(s) and the presence or absence of extracapsular spread (ECS).

## MUCOSAL MELANOMA

Mucosal melanoma of all head and neck sites is staged using a uniform classification discussed in Chap. 9.

## DEFINITIONS OF TNM

*Primary Tumor (T)*

| | |
|---|---|
| TX | Primary tumor cannot be assessed |
| T0 | No evidence of primary tumor |
| Tis | Carcinoma in situ |

*Supraglottis*

| | |
|---|---|
| T1 | Tumor limited to one subsite of supraglottis with normal vocal cord mobility |
| T2 | Tumor invades mucosa of more than one adjacent subsite of supraglottis or glottis or region outside the supraglottis (e.g., mucosa of base of tongue, vallecula, medial wall of pyriform sinus) without fixation of the larynx |
| T3 | Tumor limited to larynx with vocal cord fixation and/or invades any of the following: postcricoid area, preepiglottic space, paraglottic space, and/or inner cortex of thyroid cartilage |
| T4a | Moderately advanced local disease |
| | Tumor invades through the thyroid cartilage and/ or invades tissues beyond the larynx (e.g., trachea, soft tissues of neck including deep extrinsic muscle of the tongue, strap muscles, thyroid, or esophagus) |
| T4b | Very advanced local disease |
| | Tumor invades prevertebral space, encases carotid artery, or invades mediastinal structures |

*Glottis*

| | |
|---|---|
| T1 | Tumor limited to the vocal cord(s) (may involve anterior or posterior commissure) with normal mobility |

| T1a | Tumor limited to one vocal cord |
|-----|--------------------------------|
| T1b | Tumor involves both vocal cords |
| T2 | Tumor extends to supraglottis and/or subglottis, and/or with impaired vocal cord mobility |
| T3 | Tumor limited to the larynx with vocal cord fixation and/or invasion of paraglottic space, and/or inner cortex of the thyroid cartilage |
| T4a | Moderately advanced local disease |
| | Tumor invades through the outer cortex of the thyroid cartilage and/or invades tissues beyond the larynx (e.g., trachea, soft tissues of neck including deep extrinsic muscle of the tongue, strap muscles, thyroid, or esophagus) |
| T4b | Very advanced local disease |
| | Tumor invades prevertebral space, encases carotid artery, or invades mediastinal structures |

*Subglottis*

| T1 | Tumor limited to the subglottis |
|----|--------------------------------|
| T2 | Tumor extends to vocal cord(s) with normal or impaired mobility |
| T3 | Tumor limited to larynx with vocal cord fixation |
| T4a | Moderately advanced local disease |
| | Tumor invades cricoid or thyroid cartilage and/or invades tissues beyond the larynx (e.g., trachea, soft tissues of neck including deep extrinsic muscles of the tongue, strap muscles, thyroid, or esophagus) |
| T4b | Very advanced local disease |
| | Tumor invades prevertebral space, encases carotid artery, or invades mediastinal structures |

**Regional Lymph Nodes (N)\***

| NX | Regional lymph nodes cannot be assessed N0; no regional lymph node metastasis |
|----|------------------------------------------------------------------------------|
| N1 | Metastasis in a single ipsilateral lymph node, 3 cm or less in greatest dimension |
| N2 | Metastasis in a single ipsilateral lymph node, more than 3 cm but not more than 6 cm in greatest dimension, or in multiple ipsilateral lymph nodes, none more than 6 cm in greatest dimension, or in bilateral or contralateral lymph nodes, none more than 6 cm in greatest dimension |
| N2a | Metastasis in a single ipsilateral lymph node, more than 3 cm but not more than 6 cm in greatest dimension |
| N2b | Metastasis in multiple ipsilateral lymph nodes, none more than 6 cm in greatest dimension |
| N2c | Metastasis in bilateral or contralateral lymph nodes, none more than 6 cm in greatest dimension |
| N3 | Metastasis in a lymph node, more than 6 cm in greatest dimension |

*\*Note*: Metastases at level VII are considered regional lymph node metastases.

**Distant Metastasis (M)**
M0    No distant metastasis
M1    Distant metastasis

## ANATOMIC STAGE/PROGNOSTIC GROUPS

| | | | |
|---|---|---|---|
| Stage 0 | Tis | N0 | M0 |
| Stage I | T1 | N0 | M0 |
| Stage II | T2 | N0 | M0 |
| Stage III | T3 | N0 | M0 |
| | T1 | N1 | M0 |
| | T2 | N1 | M0 |
| | T3 | N1 | M0 |
| Stage IVA | T4a | N0 | M0 |
| | T4a | N1 | M0 |
| | T1 | N2 | M0 |
| | T2 | N2 | M0 |
| | T3 | N2 | M0 |
| | T4a | N2 | M0 |
| Stage IVB | T4b | Any N | M0 |
| | Any T | N3 | M0 |
| Stage IVC | Any T | Any N | M1 |

## PROGNOSTIC FACTORS (SITE SPECIFIC FACTORS)
### (Recommended for Collection)

Required for staging      None

Clinically significant     Size of lymph nodes
Extracapsular extension from lymph nodes for head and neck
Head and neck lymph nodes levels I–III
Head and neck lymph nodes levels IV–V
Head and neck lymph nodes levels VI–VII
Other lymph nodes group
Clinical location of cervical nodes
Extracapsular spread (ECS) clinical
Extracapsular spread (ECS) pathologic
Human papillomavirus (HPV) status

Figures 5.1 through 5.4 show observed and relative survival rates for patients with squamous cell carcinoma of the larynx, glottis, subglottis, and supraglottis for 1998–1999, classified by the AJCC staging classification.

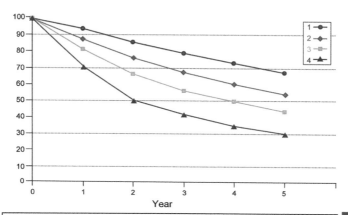

| Observed Survival | 1 | 2 | 3 | 4 | 5 | 95% CIs | Cases |
|---|---|---|---|---|---|---|---|
| 1 | 94.3 | 85.8 | 79.4 | 73.3 | 67.2 | 66.0–68.3 | 8424 |
| 2 | 88.0 | 76.7 | 67.5 | 60.5 | 54.0 | 52.3–55.8 | 4105 |
| 3 | 81.3 | 66.3 | 56.3 | 49.5 | 43.3 | 41.5–45.1 | 3837 |
| 4 | 70.9 | 50.5 | 41.6 | 34.9 | 29.9 | 28.5–31.2 | 5525 |

**A**

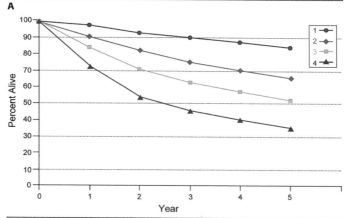

| Relative Survival | 1 | 2 | 3 | 4 | 5 | 95% CIs | Cases |
|---|---|---|---|---|---|---|---|
| 1 | 98.3 | 93.5 | 90.4 | 87.6 | 84.3 | 82.9–85.8 | 8424 |
| 2 | 91.3 | 82.7 | 75.8 | 70.8 | 66.0 | 63.9–68.2 | 4105 |
| 3 | 84.1 | 71.0 | 62.6 | 57.2 | 52.1 | 49.9–54.2 | 3837 |
| 4 | 73.1 | 53.8 | 45.9 | 39.9 | 35.5 | 33.9–37.1 | 5525 |

**B**

**FIGURE 5.1.** (**A**) Five-year, observed survival by "combined" AJCC stage for squamous cell carcinoma of the larynx, 1998–1999. (*95% confidence intervals correspond to year-5 survival rates.). (**B**) Five-year, relative survival by "combined" AJCC stage for squamous cell carcinoma of the larynx, 1998–1999. (*95% confidence intervals correspond to year-5 survival rates.)

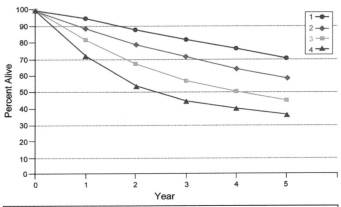

| Observed Survival | 1 | 2 | 3 | 4 | 5 | 95% CIs | Cases |
|---|---|---|---|---|---|---|---|
| 1 | 95.4 | 88.2 | 82.2 | 76.7 | 70.6 | 69.3–71.9 | 6698 |
| 2 | 89.4 | 79.7 | 71.7 | 64.4 | 59.1 | 56.5–61.6 | 1968 |
| 3 | 81.9 | 67.4 | 56.7 | 50.6 | 45.1 | 41.8–48.3 | 1199 |
| 4 | 72.5 | 53.7 | 44.8 | 40.3 | 36.3 | 33.1–39.6 | 1094 |

**A**

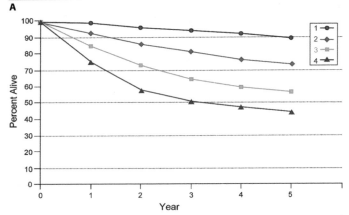

| Relative Survival | 1 | 2 | 3 | 4 | 5 | 95% CIs | Cases |
|---|---|---|---|---|---|---|---|
| 1 | 99.7 | 96.6 | 94.4 | 92.6 | 89.8 | 88.2–91.4 | 6698 |
| 2 | 93.1 | 86.7 | 81.6 | 76.8 | 74.0 | 70.8–77.1 | 1968 |
| 3 | 85.1 | 73.0 | 64.0 | 59.7 | 55.7 | 51.6–59.7 | 1199 |
| 4 | 75.2 | 57.9 | 50.2 | 47.1 | 44.4 | 40.4–48.4 | 1094 |

**B**

**FIGURE 5.2.** (**A**) Five-year, observed survival by "combined" AJCC stage for squamous cell carcinoma of the glottis, 1998–1999. (*95% confidence intervals correspond to year-5 survival rates.). (**B**) Five-year, relative survival by "combined" AJCC stage for squamous cell carcinoma of the glottis, 1998–1999. (*95% confidence intervals correspond to year-5 survival rates.)

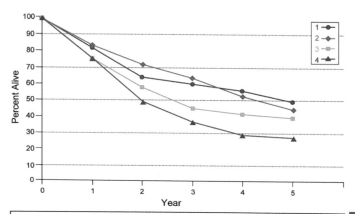

| Observed Survival | 1 | 2 | 3 | 4 | 5 | 95% CIs | Cases |
|---|---|---|---|---|---|---|---|
| 1 | 82.1 | 64.2 | 60.1 | 55.9 | 49.3 | 35.6–62.9 | 59 |
| 2 | 83.9 | 72.1 | 63.8 | 52.4 | 44.6 | 33.2–58.0 | 91 |
| 3 | 75.3 | 58.2 | 44.7 | 41.3 | 39.3 | 27.4–51.2 | 77 |
| 4 | 75.8 | 48.8 | 36.7 | 28.7 | 27.0 | 19.7–34.4 | 170 |

**A**

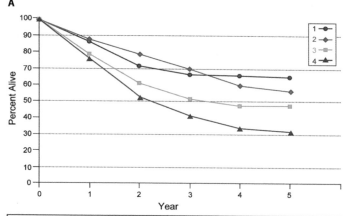

| Relative Survival | 1 | 2 | 3 | 4 | 5 | 95% CIs | Cases |
|---|---|---|---|---|---|---|---|
| 1 | 86.5 | 71.3 | 66.7 | 65.7 | 65.3 | 47.2–83.5 | 59 |
| 2 | 87.5 | 78.6 | 69.5 | 59.8 | 55.9 | 41.6–70.2 | 91 |
| 3 | 78.6 | 60.7 | 51.1 | 47.2 | 47.2 | 32.9–61.5 | 77 |
| 4 | 75.8 | 52.5 | 41.0 | 33.4 | 31.5 | 22.9–40.0 | 170 |

**B**

**FIGURE 5.3.** (**A**) Five-year, observed survival by "combined" AJCC stage for squamous cell carcinoma of the subglottis, 1998–1999. (*95% confidence intervals correspond to year-5 survival rates.). (**B**) Five-year, relative survival by "combined" AJCC stage for squamous cell carcinoma of the subglottis, 1998–1999. (*95% confidence intervals correspond to year-5 survival rates.)

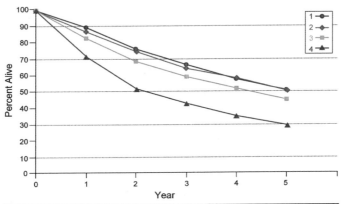

| Observed Survival | 1 | 2 | 3 | 4 | 5 | 95% CIs | Cases |
|---|---|---|---|---|---|---|---|
| 1 | 89.4 | 75.9 | 66.7 | 57.7 | 50.4 | 47.1–53.7 | 1162 |
| 2 | 86.8 | 75.0 | 64.6 | 58.2 | 50.6 | 47.8–53.4 | 1544 |
| 3 | 82.7 | 68.4 | 58.8 | 51.9 | 45.0 | 42.4–47.5 | 1875 |
| 4 | 72.0 | 51.8 | 42.9 | 35.3 | 29.3 | 27.4–31.1 | 3010 |

**A**

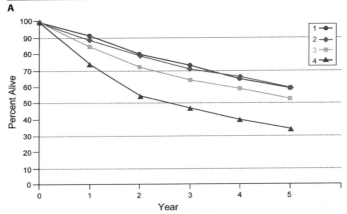

| Relative Survival | 1 | 2 | 3 | 4 | 5 | 95% CIs | Cases |
|---|---|---|---|---|---|---|---|
| 1 | 92.0 | 80.5 | 73.0 | 65.3 | 59.1 | 55.2–63.0 | 1162 |
| 2 | 89.4 | 79.7 | 70.9 | 66.2 | 59.7 | 56.4–63.1 | 1544 |
| 3 | 85.2 | 72.5 | 64.4 | 58.8 | 52.8 | 49.8–55.8 | 1875 |
| 4 | 74.1 | 54.9 | 46.9 | 39.9 | 34.3 | 32.1–36.4 | 3010 |

**B**

**FIGURE 5.4.** (**A**) Five-year, observed survival by "combined" AJCC stage for squamous cell carcinoma of the supraglottis, 1998–1999. (*95% confidence intervals correspond to year-5 survival rates.). (**B**) Five-year, relative survival by "combined" AJCC stage for squamous cell carcinoma of the supraglottis, 1998–1999. (*95% confidence intervals correspond to year-5 survival rates.)

## HISTOLOGIC GRADE (G)

Grade is reported in registry systems by the grade value. A two-grade, three-grade, or four-grade system may be used. If a grading system is not specified, generally the following system is used:

GX     Grade cannot be assessed
G1     Well differentiated
G2     Moderately differentiated
G3     Poorly differentiated
G4     Undifferentiated

## HISTOPATHOLOGIC TYPE

The predominant cancer is squamous cell carcinoma. The staging guidelines are applicable to all forms of carcinoma, including those arising from minor salivary glands. Mucosal melanoma of the head and neck is very rare but has unique behavior warranting a separate classification discussed in Chap. 9. Other nonepithelial tumors such as those of lymphoid tissue, soft tissue, bone, and cartilage (i.e., lymphoma and sarcoma) are not included. Histologic confirmation of diagnosis is required. Histopathologic grading of squamous carcinoma is recommended. The grade is subjective and uses a descriptive as well as numerical form (i.e., well differentiated, moderately differentiated, and poorly differentiated), depending on the degree of closeness to or deviation from squamous epithelium in mucosal sites. Also recommended where feasible is a quantitative evaluation of depth of invasion of the primary tumor and the presence or absence of vascular invasion and perineural invasion. Although the grade of tumor does not enter into the staging of the tumor, it should be recorded. The pathologic description of any lymphadenectomy specimen should describe the size, number, and position of the involved node(s) and the presence or absence of extracapsular spread (ECS).

## BIBLIOGRAPHY

Archer CR, Yeager VL, Herbold DR. CT versus histology of laryngeal cancer: the value in predicting laryngeal cartilage invasion. Laryngoscope. 1983;93: 140–47.

Bonner JA, Harari PM, Giralt J, et al. Radiotherapy plus cetuximab for squamous-cell carcinoma of the head and neck. N Engl J Med. 2006;354(6):567–78.

Cooper JS, Farnan NC, Asbell SO, et al. Recursive partitioning analysis of 2, 105 patients treated in Radiation Therapy Oncology Group studies of head and neck cancer. Cancer. 1996;77:1905–11.

de Leeuw JR, de Graeff A, Ros WJ, et al. Prediction of depressive symptomatology after treatment of head and neck cancer: the influence of pre-treatment physical and depressive symptoms, coping, and social support. Head Neck. 2000;22(8):799–807.

Deleyiannis FW, Thomas DB, Vaughan TL, et al. Alcoholism: independent predictor of survival in patients with head and neck cancer. J Natl Cancer Inst. 1996;88:542–9.

Eibaud JD, Elias EG, Suter CM, et al. Prognostic factors in squamous cell carcinoma of the larynx. Am J Surg. 1989;58:314–7.

Faye-Lund H, Abdelnoor M. Prognostic factors of survival in a cohort of head and neck cancer patients in Oslo. Eur J Cancer B Oral Oncol. 1996;2:83–90.

Forastiere AA, Goepfert H, Maor M, Pajak TF, Weber R, Morrison W, et al. Concurrent chemotherapy and radiotherapy for organ preservation in advanced laryngeal cancer. N Engl J Med. 2003;349(22):2091–8.

Isaacs JJ, Mancuso AA, Mendenhall WM, et al. Deep spread patterns in CT staging of t2–4 squamous cell laryngeal carcinoma. Otolaryngol Head Neck Surg. 1988;99:455–64.

Kaplan MH, Feinstein AR. The importance of classifying initial co-morbidity in evaluating the outcome of diabetes mellitus. J Chron Dis. 1974;37:387–404.

Karnofsky DA, Abelman WH, Craver LF, Burchenal JH. The use of nitrogen mustards in the palliative treatment of carcinoma. Cancer. 1948;1:634–56.

Lefebvre JL, Chevalier D, Luboinski B, Kirkpatric A, Collette L, Sahmoud T. Larynx preservation in pyriform sinus cancer: preliminary results of a European Organization for research treatment of cancer phase III trial. EORTC Head and Neck Cancer Cooperative Group. J Natl Cancer Inst. 1996;88:890–9.

Ljumanovic R, Langendijk JA, van Wattingen M, Schenk B, Knol DL, Leemans CR, et al. MR imaging predictors of local control of glottic squamous cell carcinoma treated with radiation alone. Radiology. 2007;244(1):205–12.

Mafee MF, Schield JA, Valvassori GE, et al. CT of the larynx: correlation with anatomic and pathologic studies in cases of laryngeal carcinoma. Radiology. 1983;147:123–8.

Mendenhall WM, Parsons JT, Stringer SP, et al. Carcinoma of the supraglottic larynx: a basis for comparing the results of radiotherapy and surgery. Head Neck. 1990;12:204–9.

Piccirillo JF. Inclusion of comorbidity in a staging system for head and neck cancer. Oncology. 1995;9:831–6.

Pignon JP, Bourhis J, Domenge C, Designé L. Chemotherapy added to locoregional treatment for head and neck squamous-cell carcinoma: three meta-analyses of updated individual data. MACH-NC Collaborative Group. Meta-Analysis of Chemotherapy on Head and Neck Cancer. Lancet. 2000;355(9208):949–55.

Rozack MS, Maipang T, Sabo K, et al. Management of advanced glottic carcinomas. Am J Surg. 1989;158:318–20.

Singh B, Alfonso A, Sabin S, et al. Outcome differences in younger and older patients with laryngeal cancer: a retrospective case-control study. Am J Otolaryngol. 2000;21:92–7.

Van Nostrand AWP, Brodarec I. Laryngeal carcinoma: modification of surgical techniques based upon an understanding of tumor growth characteristics. J Otolaryngol. 1982;11:186–92.

Veterans Administration Laryngeal Study Group: Induction chemotherapy plus radiation compared to surgery plus radiation in patients with advanced laryngeal cancer. N Engl J Med. 1991;324:1685–90.

# Nasal Cavity and Paranasal Sinuses

*(Nonepithelial tumors such as those of lymphoid tissue, soft tissue, bone, and cartilage are not included. Staging for mucosal melanoma of the nasal cavity and paranasal sinuses is not included in this chapter – see Chap. 9.)*

## *At-A-Glance*

---

### SUMMARY OF CHANGES

- T4 lesions have been divided into T4a (moderately advanced local disease) and T4b (very advanced local disease), leading to the stratification of Stage IV into Stage IVA (moderately advanced local/regional disease), Stage IVB (very advanced local/regional disease), and Stage IVC (distant metastatic disease)

---

**6**

| ANATOMIC STAGE/PROGNOSTIC GROUPS | | | |
|---|---|---|---|
| Stage 0 | Tis | N0 | M0 |
| Stage I | T1 | N0 | M0 |
| Stage II | T2 | N0 | M0 |
| Stage III | T3 | N0 | M0 |
| | T1 | N1 | M0 |
| | T2 | N1 | M0 |
| | T3 | N1 | M0 |
| Stage IVA | T4a | N0 | M0 |
| | T4a | N1 | M0 |
| | T1 | N2 | M0 |
| | T2 | N2 | M0 |
| | T3 | N2 | M0 |
| | T4a | N2 | M0 |
| Stage IVB | T4b | Any N | M0 |
| | Any T | N3 | M0 |
| Stage IVC | Any T | Any N | M1 |

ICD-O-3 TOPOGRAPHY CODES
C30.0    Nasal cavity
C31.0    Maxillary sinus
C31.1    Ethmoid sinus

ICD-O-3 HISTOLOGY CODE RANGES
8000–8576, 8940–8950, 8980–8981

## ANATOMY

**Primary Sites.** Cancer of the maxillary sinus is the most common of the sinonasal malignancies. Ethmoid sinus and nasal cavity cancers are equal in frequency but considerably less common than maxillary sinus cancers. Tumors of the sphenoid and frontal sinuses are rare.

---

The location as well as the extent of the mucosal lesion within the maxillary sinus has prognostic significance. Historically, a plane, connecting the medial canthus of the eye to the angle of the mandible, represented by Ohngren's line, is used to divide the maxillary sinus into an anteroinferior portion (infrastructure), which is associated with a good prognosis, and a posterosuperior portion (suprastructure), which has a poor prognosis (Figure 6.1). The poorer outcome associated with suprastructure cancers reflects early invasion by these tumors to critical structures, including the eye, skull base, pterygoids, and infratemporal fossa.

For the purpose of staging, the nasoethmoidal complex is divided into two sites: nasal cavity and ethmoid sinuses. The ethmoids are further subdivided into two subsites: left and right, separated by the nasal septum (perpendicular plate of ethmoid). The nasal cavity is divided into four subsites: the septum, floor, lateral wall, and vestibule.

| *Site* | *Subsite* |
|---|---|
| Maxillary sinus | Left/right |
| Nasal cavity | Septum |
| | Floor |
| | Lateral wall |
| | Vestibule (edge of naris to mucocutaneous junction) |
| Ethmoid sinus | Left/right |

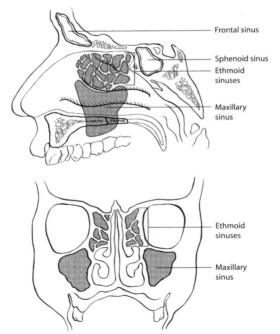

**FIGURE 6.1.** Sites of origin of tumors of the paranasal sinuses.

**Regional Lymph Nodes.** Regional lymph node spread from cancer of nasal cavity and paranasal sinuses is relatively uncommon. Involvement of buccinator, submandibular, upper jugular, and (occasionally) retropharyngeal nodes may occur with advanced maxillary sinus cancer, particularly those extending beyond the sinus walls to involve adjacent structures, including soft tissues of the cheek, upper alveolus, palate, and buccal mucosa. Ethmoid sinus cancers are less prone to regional lymphatic spread. When only one side of the neck is involved, it should be considered ipsilateral. Bilateral spread may occur with advanced primary cancer, particularly with spread of the primary beyond the midline.

In clinical evaluation, the physical size of the nodal mass should be measured. Most masses over 3 cm in diameter are not single nodes but, rather, are confluent nodes or tumor in soft tissues of the neck. There are three categories of clinically positive nodes: N1, N2, and N3. The use of subgroups a, b, and c is required. Midline nodes are considered ipsilateral nodes. In addition to the components to describe the N category, regional lymph nodes should also be described according to the level of the neck that is involved. Pathologic examination is necessary for documentation of such disease extent. Imaging studies showing amorphous spiculated margins of involved nodes or involvement of internodal fat resulting in loss of normal oval-to-round nodal shape strongly suggest extracapsular (extranodal) tumor spread. No imaging study (as yet) can identify microscopic foci in regional nodes or distinguish between small reactive nodes and small malignant nodes without central radiographic inhomogeneity.

For pN, a selective neck dissection will ordinarily include six or more lymph nodes, and a radical or modified radical neck dissection will ordinarily include ten or more lymph nodes. Negative pathologic examination of a lesser number of lymph nodes still mandates a pN0 designation.

**Distant Metastases.** Distant spread usually occurs to lungs but occasionally there is spread to bone.

## RULES FOR CLASSIFICATION

**Clinical Staging.** The assessment of primary maxillary sinus, nasal cavity, and ethmoid tumors is based on inspection and palpation, including examination of the orbits, nasal and oral cavities, and nasopharynx, and neurologic evaluation of the cranial nerves. Nasal endoscopy with rigid or fiberoptic flexible instruments is recommended. Radiologic assessment with magnetic resonance imaging (MRI) or computed tomography (CT) is mandatory for accurate pretreatment staging of malignant tumor of the sinuses. If available, MRI more accurately depicts skull base and intracranial involvement and the differentiation of fluid from solid tumor, and helps define local extension of disease. Neck nodes are assessed by palpation +/− imaging. Imaging for possible nodal metastases is probably unnecessary in the presence of a clinically negative neck. Examinations for distant metastases include appropriate imaging, blood chemistries, blood count, and other routine studies as indicated.

**Pathologic Staging.** Pathologic staging requires the use of all information obtained in clinical staging and histologic study of the surgically resected specimen. The surgeon's evaluation of gross unresected residual tumor must also be included. Specimens that are resected after radiation or chemotherapy need to be identified and considered in context. The pathologic description of the lymphadenectomy specimen should describe the size, number, and level of the involved node(s) and the presence or absence of extracapsular spread (ECS).

## PROGNOSTIC FEATURES

In addition to the importance of the TNM factors outlined previously, the overall health of these patients clearly influences outcome. An ongoing effort to better assess prognosis using both tumor and nontumor related factors is underway. Chart abstraction will continue to be performed by cancer registrars to obtain important information regarding specific factors related to prognosis. This data will then be used to further hone the predictive power of the staging system in future revisions.

Comorbidity can be classified by specific measures of additional medical illnesses. Accurate reporting of all illnesses in the patients' medical record is essential to assessment of these parameters. General performance measures are helpful in predicting survival. The AJCC strongly recommends the clinician report performance status using the ECOG, Zubrod, or Karnofsky performance measures along with standard staging information. An interrelationship between each of the major performance tools exists.

### Zubrod/ECOG Performance Scale

0. Fully active, able to carry on all predisease activities without restriction (Karnofsky 90–100).
1. Restricted in physically strenuous activity but ambulatory and able to carry work of a light or sedentary nature. For example, light housework, office work (Karnofsky 70–80).
2. Ambulatory and capable of all self-care but unable to carry out any work activities. Up and about more than 50% of waking hours (Karnofsky 50–60).
3. Capable of only limited self-care, confined to bed or chair 50% or more of waking hours (Karnofsky 30–40).
4. Completely disabled. Cannot carry on self-care. Totally confined to bed (Karnofsky 10–20).
5. Death (Karnofsky 0).

Lifestyle factors such as tobacco and alcohol abuse negatively influence survival. Accurate recording of smoking in pack years and alcohol in number of days drinking per week and number of drinks per day will provide important data for future analysis. Nutrition is important to prognosis and will be indirectly measured by weight loss of >10% of body weight. Depression adversely impacts quality of life and survival.

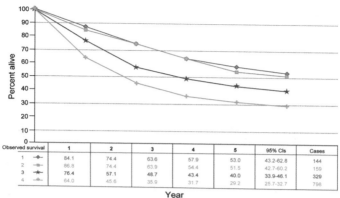

**A**

| Observed survival | 1 | 2 | 3 | 4 | 5 | 95% Cls | Cases |
|---|---|---|---|---|---|---|---|
| 1 | 84.1 | 74.4 | 63.6 | 57.9 | 53.0 | 43.2-62.8 | 144 |
| 2 | 86.8 | 74.4 | 63.9 | 54.4 | 51.5 | 42.7-60.2 | 159 |
| 3 | 76.4 | 57.1 | 48.7 | 43.4 | 40.0 | 33.9-46.1 | 329 |
| 4 | 64.0 | 45.6 | 35.9 | 31.7 | 29.2 | 25.7-32.7 | 798 |

Year

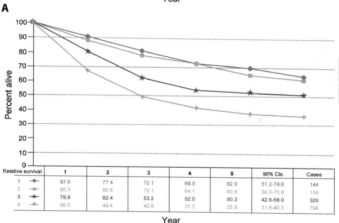

**B**

| Relative survival | 1 | 2 | 3 | 4 | 5 | 95% Cls | Cases |
|---|---|---|---|---|---|---|---|
| 1 | 87.6 | 77.4 | 72.1 | 68.8 | 62.9 | 51.2-74.6 | 144 |
| 2 | 90.3 | 80.6 | 72.1 | 64.1 | 60.6 | 50.3-70.9 | 159 |
| 3 | 79.8 | 62.4 | 53.2 | 52.0 | 50.3 | 42.6-58.0 | 329 |
| 4 | 66.5 | 49.4 | 40.6 | 37.3 | 35.9 | 31.6-40.3 | 798 |

Year

**FIGURE 6.2.** (**A**) Five-year, observed survival by "combined" AJCC stage sinonasal carcinomas (all histologies), 1998–1999. (*95% confidence intervals correspond to year-5 survival rates.) (**B**) Five-year, relative survival by "combined" AJCC stage sinonasal carcinomas (all histologies), 1998–1999. (*95% confidence intervals correspond to year-5 survival rates.)

Notation of a previous or current diagnosis of depression should be recorded in the medical record.

Figure 6.2A, B presents observed and relative survival rates for sinonasal carcinomas (all histologies) for 1998–1999, classified by the AJCC staging classification.

**Mucosal Melanoma.** Mucosal melanoma of all head and neck sites is staged using a uniform classification as discussed in Chap. 9.

## DEFINITIONS OF TNM

### Primary Tumor (T)

TX    Primary tumor cannot be assessed
T0    No evidence of primary tumor
Tis    Carcinoma in situ

#### Maxillary Sinus

T1    Tumor limited to maxillary sinus mucosa with no erosion or destruction of bone
T2    Tumor causing bone erosion or destruction including extension into the hard palate and/or middle nasal meatus, except extension to posterior wall of maxillary sinus and pterygoid plates
T3    Tumor invades any of the following: bone of the posterior wall of maxillary sinus, subcutaneous tissues, floor or medial wall of orbit, pterygoid fossa, ethmoid sinuses
T4a    Moderately advanced local disease
     Tumor invades anterior orbital contents, skin of cheek, pterygoid plates, infratemporal fossa, cribriform plate, sphenoid or frontal sinuses
T4b    Very advanced local disease
     Tumor invades any of the following: orbital apex, dura, brain, middle cranial fossa, cranial nerves other than maxillary division of trigeminal nerve (V2), nasopharynx, or clivus

#### Nasal Cavity and Ethmoid Sinus

T1    Tumor restricted to any one subsite, with or without bony invasion
T2    Tumor invading two subsites in a single region or extending to involve an adjacent region within the nasoethmoidal complex, with or without bony invasion
T3    Tumor extends to invade the medial wall or floor of the orbit, maxillary sinus, palate, or cribriform plate
T4a    Moderately advanced local disease
     Tumor invades any of the following: anterior orbital contents, skin of nose or cheek, minimal extension to anterior cranial fossa, pterygoid plates, sphenoid or frontal sinuses
T4b    Very advanced local disease
     Tumor invades any of the following: orbital apex, dura, brain, middle cranial fossa, cranial nerves other than (V2), nasopharynx, or clivus

### Regional Lymph Nodes (N)

NX    Regional lymph nodes cannot be assessed
N0    No regional lymph node metastasis
N1    Metastasis in a single ipsilateral lymph node, 3 cm or less in greatest dimension
N2    Metastasis in a single ipsilateral lymph node, more than 3 cm but not more than 6 cm in greatest dimension, or in multiple ipsilateral lymph nodes, none more than 6 cm in greatest dimension, or in bilateral or contralateral lymph nodes, none more than 6 cm in greatest dimension

| N2a | Metastasis in a single ipsilateral lymph node, more than 3 cm but not more than 6 cm in greatest dimension |
|---|---|
| N2b | Metastasis in multiple ipsilateral lymph nodes, none more than 6 cm in greatest dimension |
| N2c | Metastasis in bilateral or contralateral lymph nodes, none more than 6 cm in greatest dimension |
| N3 | Metastasis in a lymph node, more than 6 cm in greatest dimension |

**Distant Metastasis (M)**

| M0 | No distant metastasis |
|---|---|
| M1 | Distant metastasis |

## ANATOMIC STAGE/PROGNOSTIC GROUPS

| Stage 0 | Tis | N0 | M0 |
|---|---|---|---|
| Stage I | T1 | N0 | M0 |
| Stage II | T2 | N0 | M0 |
| Stage III | T3 | N0 | M0 |
| | T1 | N1 | M0 |
| | T2 | N1 | M0 |
| | T3 | N1 | M0 |
| Stage IVA | T4a | N0 | M0 |
| | T4a | N1 | M0 |
| | T1 | N2 | M0 |
| | T2 | N2 | M0 |
| | T3 | N2 | M0 |
| | T4a | N2 | M0 |
| Stage IVB | T4b | Any N | M0 |
| | Any T | N3 | M0 |
| Stage IVC | Any T | Any N | M1 |

## PROGNOSTIC FACTORS (SITE-SPECIFIC FACTORS)
### (Recommended for Collection)

| Required for staging | None |
|---|---|
| Clinically significant | Size of lymph nodes |
| | Extracapsular extension from lymph nodes for head and neck |
| | Head and neck lymph nodes levels I–III |
| | Head and neck lymph nodes levels IV–V |
| | Head and neck lymph nodes levels VI–VII |
| | Other lymph nodes group |
| | Clinical location of cervical nodes |
| | Extracapsular spread (ECS) clinical |
| | Extracapsular spread (ECS) pathologic |
| | Human papillomavirus (HPV) status |
| | Tumor thickness |

## HISTOLOGIC GRADE (G)

Grade is reported in registry systems by the grade value. A two-grade, three-grade, or four-grade system may be used. If a grading system is not specified, generally the following system is used:

GX     Grade cannot be assessed
G1     Well differentiated
G2     Moderately differentiated
G3     Poorly differentiated
G4     Undifferentiated

## HISTOPATHOLOGIC TYPE

The predominant cancer is squamous cell carcinoma. The staging guidelines are applicable to all forms of carcinoma. Mucosal melanoma of the head and neck is very rare but has unique behavior warranting a separate classification as discussed in Chap. 9. Other nonepithelial tumors such as those of lymphoid tissue, soft tissue, bone, and cartilage are not included. Histologic confirmation of diagnosis is required. Histopathologic grading of squamous carcinoma is recommended. The grade is subjective and uses a descriptive as well as a numerical form (i.e., well differentiated, moderately differentiated, and poorly differentiated), depending on the degree of closeness to or deviation from squamous epithelium in mucosal sites. Also recommended where feasible is a quantitative evaluation of depth of invasion of the primary tumor and the presence or absence of vascular invasion and perineural invasion. Although the grade of the tumor does not enter into the staging of the tumor, it should be recorded. The pathologic description of any lymphadenectomy specimen should describe the size, number, and level of the involved node(s) and the presence or absence of ECS.

## BIBLIOGRAPHY

Bridger GP, Mendelsohn MS, Baldwinn M, et al. Paranasal sinus cancer. Aust N Z J Surg. 1991;61:290–4.

Cantu G, Solero CL, Mariani L, et al. A new classification for malignant tumors involving the anterior skull base. Arch Otolaryngol Head Neck Surg. 1999;125:1252–7.

de Leeuw JR, de Graeff A, Ros WJ, Blijham GH, Hordijk GJ, Winnubst JA. Prediction of depressive symptomatology after treatment of head and neck cancer: the influence of pre-treatment physical and depressive symptoms, coping, and social support. Head Neck. 2000;22(8):799–807.

Jiang GL, Ang KA, Peters LJ, et al. Maxillary sinus carcinomas: Natural history and results of postoperative radiotherapy. Radiother Oncol. 1991;21:194–200.

Jiang GL, Morrison WH, Garden AS, et al. Ethmoid sinus carcinoma: Natural history and treatment results. Radiother Oncol. 1998;49:21–7.

Kondo M, Horiuchi M, Shiga H, et al. CT of malignant tumors of the nasal cavity and paranasal sinuses. Cancer. 1982;50:226–31.

Le QT, Fu KK, Kaplan M, et al. Treatment of maxillary sinus carcinoma. A comparison of the 1997 and 1977 American Joint Committee on Cancer Staging Systems. Cancer. 1999;86:1700–11.

Nandapalan V, Roland NJ, Helliwell TR, Williams EM, Hamilton JW, Jones AS. Mucosal melanoma of the head and neck. Clin Otolaryngol Allied Sci. 1998;23(2):107–16.

Patel SG, Prasad ML, Escrig M, et al. Primary mucosalmalignant melanoma of the head and neck. Head Neck. 2002;24(3):247–57.

Patel SG, Singh B, Polluri A, et al. Craniofacial surgery for malignant skull base tumors: Report of an international collaborative study. Cancer. 2003;98(6):1179–87.

Paulino AFG, Singh B, Carew J, et al. Epstein-Barr virus in squamous carcinoma of the anterior nasal cavity. Ann Diagn Pathol. 2000;4:7–10.

Piccirillo JF. Inclusion of comorbidity in a staging system for head and neck cancer. Oncology. 1995;9:831–6.

Sisson GA, Toriumi DM, Atiyah RH. Paranasal sinus malignancy: A comprehensive update. Laryngoscope. 1989;99:143–50.

Som PM, Dillon WP, Sze G, et al. Benign and malignant sinonasal lesions with intracranial extension: Differentiation with MRI imaging. Radiology. 1989;172:763–6.

Van Tassel P, Lee YY. GD-DTPA enhanced MR for detecting intracranial extension of sinonasal malignancies. J Comput Assist Tomogr. 1991;15:387–92.

6

## 7

# Major Salivary Glands

*(Parotid, submandibular, and sublingual)*

## *At-A-Glance*

---

### SUMMARY OF CHANGES

- T4 lesions have been divided into T4a (moderately advanced local disease) and T4b (very advanced local disease), leading to the stratification of Stage IV into Stage IVA (moderately advanced local/regional disease), Stage IVB (very advanced local/regional disease), and Stage IVC (distant metastatic disease)

---

### ANATOMIC STAGE/PROGNOSTIC GROUPS

| Stage | T | N | M |
|-------|-----|-------|-----|
| Stage I | T1 | N0 | M0 |
| Stage II | T2 | N0 | M0 |
| Stage III | T3 | N0 | M0 |
| | T1 | N1 | M0 |
| | T2 | N1 | M0 |
| | T3 | N1 | M0 |
| Stage IVA | T4a | N0 | M0 |
| | T4a | N1 | M0 |
| | T1 | N2 | M0 |
| | T2 | N2 | M0 |
| | T3 | N2 | M0 |
| | T4a | N2 | M0 |
| Stage IVB | T4b | Any N | M0 |
| | Any T | N3 | M0 |
| Stage IVC | Any T | Any N | M1 |

**ICD-O-3 TOPOGRAPHY CODES**

| | |
|------|------|
| C07.9 | Parotid gland |
| C08.0 | Submandibular gland |
| C08.1 | Sublingual gland |
| C08.8 | Overlapping lesion of major salivary glands |
| C08.9 | Major salivary gland, NOS |

**ICD-O-3 HISTOLOGY CODE RANGES**

8000–8576, 8940–8950, 8980–8981

## INTRODUCTION

This staging system is based on an extensive retrospective review of the world literature regarding malignant tumors of the major salivary glands. Numerous factors affect patient survival, including the histologic diagnosis, cellular differentiation of the tumor (grade), site, size, degree of fixation or local extension, facial nerve involvement, and the status of regional lymph nodes as well as distant metastases. The classification involves the four dominant clinical variables: tumor size, local extension of the tumor, nodal metastasis, and distant metastasis. The T4 category

*Major Salivary Glands*      **103**

has been divided into T4a and T4b. T4a indicates moderately advanced lesions and T4b reflects very advanced lesions with local extension. Histologic grade, patient age, and tumor site are important additional factors that should be recorded for future analysis and potential inclusion in the staging system.

## ANATOMY

**Primary Site.** The major salivary glands include the parotid, submandibular, and sublingual glands. Tumors arising in minor salivary glands (mucus-secreting glands in the lining membrane of the upper aerodigestive tract) are staged according to the anatomic site of origin (e.g., oral cavity, sinuses, etc.).

Primary tumors of the parotid constitute the largest proportion of salivary gland tumors. Sublingual primary cancers are rare and may be difficult to distinguish with certainty from minor salivary gland primary tumors of the anterior floor of the mouth.

**Regional Lymph Nodes.** Regional lymphatic spread from salivary gland cancer is less common than from head and neck mucosal squamous cancers and varies according to the histology and size of the primary tumor. Most nodal metastases will be clinically apparent on initial evaluation. Low-grade tumors rarely metastasize to regional nodes, whereas the risk of regional spread is substantially higher from high-grade cancers. Regional dissemination tends to be orderly, progressing from intraglandular to adjacent (periparotid, submandibular) nodes, then to upper and midjugular nodes, apex of the posterior triangle (level Va) nodes, and occasionally to retropharyngeal nodes. Bilateral lymphatic spread is rare.

For pathologic reporting (pN), histologic examination of a selective neck dissection will ordinarily include six or more lymph nodes and a radical or modified radical neck dissection will ordinarily include ten or more lymph nodes. Negative pathologic evaluation of a lesser number of nodes still mandates a pN0 designation.

**Distant Metastases.** Distant spread is most frequently to the lungs.

## RULES FOR CLASSIFICATION

**Clinical Staging.** The assessment of primary salivary gland tumors includes a pertinent history (pain, trismus, etc.), inspection, palpation, and evaluation of the cranial nerves. Radiologic studies may add information valuable for staging. The soft tissues of the neck from the skull base to the hyoid bone must be studied, with the lower neck included whenever lymph node metastases are suspected. Images of the intratemporal facial nerve are critical to the identification of perineural spread of tumor in this area. Cancers of the submandibular and sublingual salivary glands merit cross-sectional imaging. Computed tomography (CT) or MRI may be useful in assessing the extent of deep extraglandular tumor, bone invasion, and deep tissue extent (extrinsic tongue muscle and/or soft tissues of the neck).

**Pathologic Staging.** The surgical pathology report and all other available data should be used to assign a pathologic classification to those patients who have resection of the cancer.

## DEFINITIONS OF TNM

*Primary Tumor (T)*

| | |
|---|---|
| TX | Primary tumor cannot be assessed |
| T0 | No evidence of primary tumor |
| T1 | Tumor 2 cm or less in greatest dimension without extraparenchymal extension* |
| T2 | Tumor more than 2 cm but not more than 4 cm in greatest dimension without extraparenchymal extension* |
| T3 | Tumor more than 4 cm and/or tumor having extraparenchymal extension* |
| T4a | Moderately advanced disease |
| | Tumor invades skin, mandible, ear canal, and/or facial nerve |
| T4b | Very advanced disease |
| | Tumor invades skull base and/or pterygoid plates and/or encases carotid artery |

*Note*: Extraparenchymal extension is clinical or macroscopic evidence of invasion of soft tissues. Microscopic evidence alone does not constitute extraparenchymal extension for classification purposes.

**7**

*Regional Lymph Nodes (N)*

| | |
|---|---|
| NX | Regional lymph nodes cannot be assessed |
| N0 | No regional lymph node metastasis |
| N1 | Metastasis in a single ipsilateral lymph node, 3 cm or less in greatest dimension |
| N2 | Metastasis in a single ipsilateral lymph node, more than 3 cm but not more than 6 cm in greatest dimension, or in multiple ipsilateral lymph nodes, none more than 6 cm in greatest dimension, or in bilateral or contralateral lymph nodes, none more than 6 cm in greatest dimension |
| N2a | Metastasis in a single ipsilateral lymph node, more than 3 cm but not more than 6 cm in greatest dimension |
| N2b | Metastasis in multiple ipsilateral lymph nodes, none more than 6 cm in greatest dimension |
| N2c | Metastasis in bilateral or contralateral lymph nodes, none more than 6 cm in greatest dimension |
| N3 | Metastasis in a lymph node, more than 6 cm in greatest dimension |

*Distant Metastasis (M)*

| | |
|---|---|
| M0 | No distant metastasis |
| M1 | Distant metastasis |

| Stage I | T1 | N0 | M0 |
|---------|-----|--------|-----|
| Stage II | T2 | N0 | M0 |
| Stage III | T3 | N0 | M0 |
| | T1 | N1 | M0 |
| | T2 | N1 | M0 |
| | T3 | N1 | M0 |
| Stage IVA | T4a | N0 | M0 |
| | T4a | N1 | M0 |
| | T1 | N2 | M0 |
| | T2 | N2 | M0 |
| | T3 | N2 | M0 |
| | T4a | N2 | M0 |
| Stage IVB | T4b | Any N | M0 |
| | Any T | N3 | M0 |
| Stage IVC | Any T | Any N | M1 |

## PROGNOSTIC FACTORS (SITE-SPECIFIC FACTORS)
### (Recommended for Collection)

| | |
|---|---|
| Required for staging | None |
| Clinically significant | Size of lymph nodes |
| | Extracapsular extension from lymph nodes for head and neck |
| | Head and neck lymph nodes levels I–III |
| | Head and neck lymph nodes levels IV–V |
| | Head and neck lymph nodes levels VI–VII |
| | Other lymph nodes group |
| | Clinical location of cervical nodes |
| | Extracapsular spread (ECS) clinical |
| | Extracapsular spread (ECS) pathologic |

## HISTOLOGIC GRADE (G)

Histologic grading is applicable only to some types of salivary cancer: mucoepidermoid carcinoma, adenocarcinoma not otherwise specified, or when either of these is the carcinomatous element of carcinoma in pleomorphic adenoma.

In most instances, the histologic type defines the grade (i.e., salivary duct carcinoma is high grade; basal cell adenocarcinoma is low grade).

Figure 7.1A, B presents 5-year, observed and relative survival for patients with cancer of the major salivary glands for 1998–1999, classified by the AJCC staging classification.

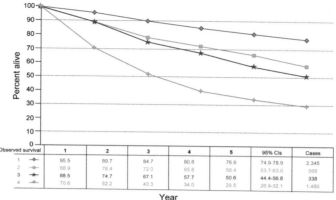

| Observed survival | | 1 | 2 | 3 | 4 | 5 | 95% CIs | Cases |
|---|---|---|---|---|---|---|---|---|
| 1 | ◆ | 95.5 | 89.7 | 84.7 | 80.8 | 76.9 | 74.9-78.9 | 2,345 |
| 2 | ■ | 88.9 | 78.4 | 72.0 | 65.8 | 58.4 | 53.7-63.0 | 568 |
| 3 | ★ | 88.5 | 74.7 | 67.1 | 57.7 | 50.6 | 44.4-56.8 | 338 |
| 4 | ▲ | 70.6 | 52.2 | 40.3 | 34.0 | 29.5 | 26.9-32.1 | 1,460 |

Year

**A**

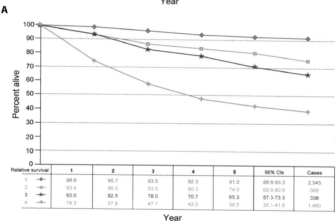

| Relative survival | | 1 | 2 | 3 | 4 | 5 | 95% CIs | Cases |
|---|---|---|---|---|---|---|---|---|
| 1 | ◆ | 98.6 | 95.7 | 93.5 | 92.3 | 91.0 | 88.6-93.3 | 2,345 |
| 2 | ■ | 93.4 | 86.5 | 83.5 | 80.3 | 74.9 | 68.9-80.9 | 568 |
| 3 | ★ | 93.0 | 82.5 | 78.0 | 70.7 | 65.3 | 57.3-73.3 | 338 |
| 4 | ▲ | 74.3 | 57.8 | 47.1 | 42.0 | 38.5 | 35.1-41.9 | 1,460 |

Year

**B**

**FIGURE 7.1.** (**A**) Five-year, observed survival by "combined" AJCC stage for cancer of the major salivary glands, 1998–1999. (*95% confidence intervals correspond to year-5 survival rates.). (**B**) Five-year, relative survival by "combined" AJCC stage for cancer of the major salivary glands, 1998–1999. (*95% confidence intervals correspond to year-5 survival rates.)

## HISTOPATHOLOGIC TYPE

The suggested histopathologic typing is that proposed by the World Health Organization.

Acinic cell carcinoma
Mucoepidermoid carcinoma
Adenoid cystic carcinoma
Polymorphous low-grade adenocarcinoma
Epithelial-myoepithelial carcinoma

Basal cell adenocarcinoma
Sebaceous carcinoma
Papillary cystadenocarcinoma
Mucinous adenocarcinoma
Oncocytic carcinoma
Salivary duct carcinoma
Adenocarcinoma
Myoepithelial carcinoma
Carcinoma in pleomorphic adenoma
Squamous cell carcinoma
Small cell carcinoma
Other carcinomas

## BIBLIOGRAPHY

Batsakis JG, Luna MA. Histopathologic grading of salivary gland neoplasms: I. Mucoepidermoid carcinomas. Ann Otol Rhinol Laryngol. 1990;99: 835–8.

Beckhardt RN, Weber RS, Zane R, et al. Minor salivary gland tumors of the palate: Clinical and pathologic correlates of outcome. Laryngoscope. 1995;105:1155–60.

Calearo C, Pastore A, Storchi OF, et al. Parotid gland carcinoma: analysis of prognostic factors. Ann Otol Rhinol Laryngol. 1998;107:969–73.

Frankenthaler RA, Luna MA, Lee SS, et al. Prognostic variables in parotid gland cancer. Arch Otolaryngol Head Neck Surg. 1991;11:1251–6.

Gallo O, Franchi A, Bottai GV, et al. Risk factors for distant metastases from carcinoma of the parotid gland. Cancer. 1977;80:844–51.

Goepfert H, Luna MA, Lindberg RH, et al. Malignant salivary gland tumors of the paranasal sinuses and nasal cavity. Arch Otolaryngol. 1983;109:662–8.

Hicks MJ, El-Naggar AK, Byers RM, et al. Prognostic factors in mucoepidermoid carcinomas of major salivary glands: a clinicopathologic and flow cytometric study. Eur J Cancer B Oral Oncol. 1994;30B:329–34.

Hoffman HT, Karnell LH, Robinson RA, et al. National Cancer Data Base report on cancer of the head and neck: acinic cell carcinoma. Head Neck. 1999;21:297–309.

Iro H, Waldfahrer F. Evaluation of the newly updated TNM classification of head and neck carcinoma with data from 3, 247 patients. Cancer. 1998;83:2201–7.

Kane WJ, McCaffrey TV, Olsen KD, et al. Primary parotid malignancies: a clinical and pathologic review. Arch Otolaryngol Head Neck Surg. 1991;117: 307–15.

Lopes MA, Santos GC, Kowalski LP. Multivariate survival analysis of 128 cases of oral cavity minor salivary gland carcinomas. Head Neck. 1998;20: 699–706.

Overgaard PD, Sogaard H, Elbrond O, et al. Malignant parotid tumors in 110 consecutive patients: treatment results and prognosis. Laryngoscope. 1992;102:1064–9.

Renehan A, Gleave EN, Hancock BD, et al. Long-term follow-up of over 1, 000 patients with salivary gland tumours treated in a single centre. Br J Surg. 1996;83:1750–4.

Seifert G, Sobin LH. Histological typing of salivary gland tumours. WHO international histological classification of tumours. 2nd ed. Berlin: Springer; 1991.

Spiro RH. Salivary neoplasms: overview of a 35-year experience with 2, 807 patients. Head Neck Surg. 1986;8:177–84.

Spiro RH, Huvos AG. Stage means more than grade in adenoid cystic carcinoma. Am J Surg. 1992;164:623–8.

Spiro RH, Hajdu SI, Strong EW. Tumors of the submaxillary gland. Am J Surg. 1976;132:463–8.

Therkildsen MH, Christensen M, Andersen LJ, et al. Salivary gland carcinomas – prognostic factors. Acta Oncol. 1998;37:701–13.

Vander Poorten VL, Balm AJ, Hilgers FJ, et al. The development of a prognostic score for patients with parotid carcinoma. Cancer. 1999a;85:2057–67.

Vander Poorten VL, Balm AJ, Hilgers FJ, et al. Prognostic factors for long-term results of the treatment of patients with malignant submandibular gland tumors. Cancer. 1999b;85:2255–64.

7

## 8

# Thyroid

## *At-A-Glance*

---

**SUMMARY OF CHANGES**

- Tumor staging (T1) has been subdivided into T1a ( ≤1 cm) and T1b (>1–2 cm) limited to thyroid

- The descriptors to subdivide T categories have been changed to solitary tumor (s) and multifocal tumor (m)

- The terms "resectable" and "unresectable" are replaced with "moderately advanced" and "very advanced"

---

### ANATOMIC STAGE/PROGNOSTIC GROUPS

Separate stage groupings are recommended for papillary or follicular (differentiated), medullary, and anaplastic (undifferentiated) carcinoma

ICD-O-3
TOPOGRAPHY CODE
C73.9    Thyroid gland

ICD-O-3 HISTOLOGY
CODE RANGES
8000–8576, 8940–8950,
8980–8981

*Papillary or follicular (differentiated)*

|  | UNDER 45 YEARS |  |  |
|---|---|---|---|
| Stage I | Any T | Any N | M0 |
| Stage II | Any T | Any N | M1 |
|  | **45 YEARS AND OLDER** |  |  |
| Stage I | T1 | N0 | M0 |
| Stage II | T2 | N0 | M0 |
| Stage III | T3 | N0 | M0 |
|  | T1 | N1a | M0 |
|  | T2 | N1a | M0 |
|  | T3 | N1a | M0 |
| Stage IVA | T4a | N0 | M0 |
|  | T4a | N1a | M0 |
|  | T1 | N1b | M0 |
|  | T2 | N1b | M0 |
|  | T3 | N1b | M0 |
|  | T4a | N1b | M0 |
| Stage IVB | T4b | Any N | M0 |
| Stage IVC | Any T | Any N | M1 |

|  | *Medullary carcinoma* (all age groups) | | |
|---|---|---|---|
| Stage I | T1 | N0 | M0 |
| Stage II | T2 | N0 | M0 |
|  | T3 | N0 | M0 |
| Stage III | T1 | N1a | M0 |
|  | T2 | N1a | M0 |
|  | T3 | N1a | M0 |
| Stage IVA | T4a | N0 | M0 |
|  | T4a | N1a | M0 |
|  | T1 | N1b | M0 |
|  | T2 | N1b | M0 |
|  | T3 | N1b | M0 |
|  | T4a | N1b | M0 |
| Stage IVB | T4b | Any N | M0 |
| Stage IVC | Any T | Any N | M1 |
|  | *Anaplastic carcinoma* | | |
| All anaplastic carcinomas are considered Stage IV | | | |
| Stage IVA | T4a | Any N | M0 |
| Stage IVB | T4b | Any N | M0 |
| Stage IVC | Any T | Any N | M1 |

## INTRODUCTION

Although staging for cancers in other head and neck sites is based entirely on the anatomic extent of disease, it is not possible to follow this pattern for the unique group of malignant tumors that arise in the thyroid gland. Both the *histologic diagnosis* and the *age* of the patient are of such importance in the behavior and prognosis of thyroid cancer that these factors are included in this staging system.

## ANATOMY

**Primary Site.** The thyroid gland ordinarily is composed of a right and a left lobe lying adjacent and lateral to the upper trachea and esophagus. An isthmus connects the two lobes, and in some cases a pyramidal lobe is present extending cephalad anterior to the thyroid cartilage.

**Regional Lymph Nodes.** Regional lymph node spread from thyroid cancer is common but of less prognostic significance in patients with well-differentiated tumors (papillary, follicular) than in medullary cancers. The adverse prognostic influence of lymph node metastasis in patients with differentiated carcinomas is observed, only in the older age group. The first echelon of nodal metastasis consists of the paralaryngeal, paratracheal, and prelaryngeal (Delphian) nodes adjacent to the thyroid gland in the central compartment of the neck generally described as Level VI. Metastases secondarily involve the mid- and lower jugular, the supra-clavicular, and (much less commonly) the upper deep jugular and spinal accessory lymph nodes. Lymph node metastasis to submandibular and submental lymph nodes is very rare. Upper mediastinal (Level VII) nodal spread occurs frequently both anteriorly and posteriorly. Retropharyngeal nodal metastasis may be seen, usually in the presence of extensive lateral cervical metastasis. Bilateral nodal spread is common. The components of the N category are described as follows: first echelon (central compart-ment/Level VI), or N1a, and lateral cervical and/or superior mediastinal or N1b. The lymph node metastasis should also be described according to the level of the neck that is involved. Nodal metastases from medullary thyroid cancer carry a much more ominous prognosis, although they follow a similar pattern of spread.

For pN, histologic examination of a selective neck dissection will ordinarily include six or more lymph nodes, whereas histologic examina-tion of a radical or a modified radical comprehensive neck dissection will ordinarily include ten or more lymph nodes. Negative pathologic evalua-tion of a lesser number of nodes still mandates a pN0 designation.

**Metastatic Sites.**   Distant spread occurs by hematogenous routes – for example to lungs and bones – but many other sites may be involved.

## RULES FOR CLASSIFICATION

**Clinical Staging.**   The assessment of a thyroid tumor depends on inspec-tion and palpation of the thyroid gland and regional lymph nodes. Indi-rect laryngoscopy to evaluate vocal cord motion is essential. A variety of imaging procedures can provide additional useful information. These include radioisotope thyroid scans, ultrasonography, computed tomog-raphy scans (CT), magnetic resonance imaging (MRI) scans, and PET scans. When cross-sectional imaging is utilized, MRI is recommended so as to avoid contamination of the body with the iodinated contrast medium generally used with CT. Iodinated contrast media make it neces-sary to delay the postoperative administration of radioactive iodine-131. The diagnosis of thyroid cancer must be confirmed by needle biopsy or open biopsy of the tumor. Further information for clinical staging may be obtained by biopsy of lymph nodes or other areas of suspected local or distant spread. All information available prior to first treatment should be used.

**Pathologic Staging.**   Pathologic staging requires the use of all information obtained in the clinical staging, as well as histologic study of the surgically resected specimen. The surgeon's description of gross unresected residual tumor must also be included.

8

## DEFINITIONS OF TNM

### Primary Tumor (T)

*Note*: All categories may be subdivided: (s) solitary tumor and (m) multi-focal tumor (the largest determines the classification).

| | |
|---|---|
| TX | Primary tumor cannot be assessed |
| T0 | No evidence of primary tumor |
| T1 | Tumor 2 cm or less in greatest dimension limited to the thyroid |
| T1a | Tumor 1 cm or less, limited to the thyroid |
| T1b | Tumor more than 1 cm but not more than 2 cm in greatest dimension, limited to the thyroid |
| T2 | Tumor more than 2 cm but not more than 4 cm in greatest dimension limited to the thyroid |
| T3 | Tumor more than 4 cm in greatest dimension limited to the thyroid or any tumor with minimal extrathyroid extension (e.g., extension to sternothyroid muscle or perithyroid soft tissues) |
| T4a | Moderately advanced disease<br>Tumor of any size extending beyond the thyroid capsule to invade subcutaneous soft tissues, larynx, trachea, esophagus, or recurrent laryngeal nerve |
| T4b | Very advanced disease<br>Tumor invades prevertebral fascia or encases carotid artery or mediastinal vessels |

*All anaplastic carcinomas are considered T4 tumors*

| | |
|---|---|
| T4a | Intrathyroidal anaplastic carcinoma |
| T4b | Anaplastic carcinoma with gross extrathyroid extension |

### Regional Lymph Nodes (N)

Regional lymph nodes are the central compartment, lateral cervical, and upper mediastinal lymph nodes.

| | |
|---|---|
| NX | Regional lymph nodes cannot be assessed |
| N0 | No regional lymph node metastasis |
| N1 | Regional lymph node metastasis |
| N1a | Metastasis to Level VI (pretracheal, paratracheal, and prelaryngeal/Delphian lymph nodes) |
| N1b | Metastasis to unilateral, bilateral, or contralateral cervical (Levels I, II, III, IV, or V) or retropharyngeal or superior mediastinal lymph nodes (Level VII) |

### Distant Metastasis (M)

| | |
|---|---|
| M0 | No distant metastasis |
| M1 | Distant metastasis |

## ANATOMIC STAGE/PROGNOSTIC GROUPS

Separate stage groupings are recommended for papillary or follicular (differentiated), medullary, and anaplastic (undifferentiated) carcinoma

### Papillary or follicular (differentiated)

UNDER 45 YEARS

| | | | |
|---|---|---|---|
| Stage I | Any T | Any N | M0 |
| Stage II | Any T | Any N | M1 |

45 YEARS AND OLDER

| | | | |
|---|---|---|---|
| Stage I | T1 | N0 | M0 |
| Stage II | T2 | N0 | M0 |
| Stage III | T3 | N0 | M0 |
| | T1 | N1a | M0 |
| | T2 | N1a | M0 |
| | T3 | N1a | M0 |
| Stage IVA | T4a | N0 | M0 |
| | T4a | N1a | M0 |
| | T1 | N1b | M0 |
| | T2 | N1b | M0 |
| | T3 | N1b | M0 |
| | T4a | N1b | M0 |
| Stage IVB | T4b | Any N | M0 |
| Stage IVC | Any T | Any N | M1 |

### Medullary carcinoma (all age groups)

| | | | |
|---|---|---|---|
| Stage I | T1 | N0 | M0 |
| Stage II | T2 | N0 | M0 |
| | T3 | N0 | M0 |
| Stage III | T1 | N1a | M0 |
| | T2 | N1a | M0 |
| | T3 | N1a | M0 |
| Stage IVA | T4a | N0 | M0 |
| | T4a | N1a | M0 |
| | T1 | N1b | M0 |
| | T2 | N1b | M0 |
| | T3 | N1b | M0 |
| | T4a | N1b | M0 |
| Stage IVB | T4b | Any N | M0 |
| Stage IVC | Any T | Any N | M1 |

8

| | *Anaplastic carcinoma* | | |
|---|---|---|---|
| All anaplastic carcinomas are considered Stage IV | | | |
| Stage IVA | T4a | Any N | M0 |
| Stage IVB | T4b | Any N | M0 |
| Stage IVC | Any T | Any N | M1 |

## PROGNOSTIC FACTORS (SITE-SPECIFIC FACTORS)
### (Recommended for Collection)

| | |
|---|---|
| Required for staging | None |
| Clinically significant | Extrathyroid extension |
| | Histology |

Figures 8.1–8.4 show observed and relative survival rates for patients with papillary adenocarcinoma of the thyroid gland (Figure 8.1A, B), follicular adenocarcinoma of the thyroid gland (Figure 8.2A, B), medullary carcinoma of the thyroid gland (Figure 8.3A, B), and Stage 4 anaplastic carcinoma of the thyroid gland (Figure 8.4A, B).

## HISTOLOGIC GRADE (G)

Grade is reported in registry systems by the grade value. A two-grade, three-grade, or four-grade system may be used. If a grading system is not specified, generally the following system is used:

| | |
|---|---|
| GX | Grade cannot be assessed |
| G1 | Well differentiated |
| G2 | Moderately differentiated |
| G3 | Poorly differentiated |
| G4 | Undifferentiated |

## HISTOPATHOLOGIC TYPE

There are four major histopathologic types*:

Papillary carcinoma (including follicular variant of papillary carcinoma)
Follicular carcinoma (including Hurthle cell carcinoma)
Medullary carcinoma
Undifferentiated (anaplastic) carcinoma

*At present, more aggressive variants of differentiated carcinomas like tall cell variant of papillary carcinoma and insular carcinoma are grouped under "differentiated carcinoma."

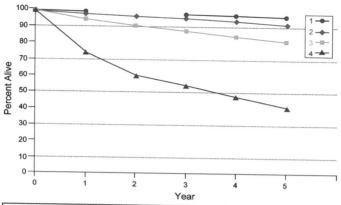

| Observed Survival | 1 | 2 | 3 | 4 | 5 | 95% CIs | Cases |
|---|---|---|---|---|---|---|---|
| 1 | 99.4 | 98.8 | 98.4 | 97.8 | 97.1 | 96.7–97.4 | 14124 |
| 2 | 98.7 | 97.3 | 96.1 | 94.7 | 92.8 | 92.0–93.7 | 4701 |
| 3 | 95.4 | 91.3 | 88.2 | 85.2 | 82.0 | 80.5–83.6 | 2953 |
| 4 | 74.8 | 60.6 | 54.8 | 47.6 | 41.4 | 36.2–46.7 | 412 |

Five-year, observed survival by "combined" AJCC stage papillary adenocarcinoma of the thyroid, 1998-1999

**A**

| Relative Survival | 1 | 2 | 3 | 4 | 5 | 95% CIs | Cases |
|---|---|---|---|---|---|---|---|
| 1 | 99.9 | 99.9 | 99.9 | 99.9 | 99.8 | 99.4–100 | 14124 |
| 2 | 100 | 100 | 100 | 100 | 100 | 100–100 | 4701 |
| 3 | 97.7 | 95.8 | 94.9 | 94.3 | 93.3 | 91.6–95.1 | 2953 |
| 4 | 77.6 | 65.4 | 61.6 | 55.7 | 50.7 | 44.2–57.2 | 412 |

Five-year, relative survival by "combined" AJCC stage papillary adenocarcinoma of the thyroid, 1998-1999

**B**

**FIGURE 8.1.** (**A**) Five-year, observed survival by "combined" AJCC stage for papillary adenocarcinoma of the thyroid gland, 1998–1999. (95% confidence intervals correspond to year-5 survival rates.) (**B**) Five-year, relative survival by "combined" AJCC stage for papillary adenocarcinoma of the thyroid gland, 1998–1999. (95% confidence intervals correspond to year-5 survival rates.)

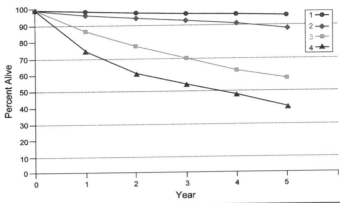

| Observed Survival | 1 | 2 | 3 | 4 | 5 | 95% CIs | Cases |
|---|---|---|---|---|---|---|---|
| 1 | 99.3 | 98.6 | 98.0 | 97.6 | 96.7 | 95.4–97.9 | 1090 |
| 2 | 97.6 | 95.3 | 93.8 | 91.7 | 89.1 | 86.9–91.3 | 1014 |
| 3 | 87.7 | 78.3 | 70.4 | 63.2 | 58.2 | 49.8–66.7 | 160 |
| 4 | 75.6 | 61.3 | 54.9 | 48.4 | 40.6 | 32.7–48.6 | 191 |

Five-year, observed survival by "combined" AJCC stage follicular adenocarcinoma of the thyroid, 1998-1999

**A**

| Relative Survival | 1 | 2 | 3 | 4 | 5 | 95% CIs | Cases |
|---|---|---|---|---|---|---|---|
| 1 | 99.7 | 99.5 | 99.3 | 99.4 | 99.0 | 97.7–100 | 1090 |
| 2 | 99.6 | 99.4 | 100 | 100 | 99.7 | 97.3–100 | 1014 |
| 3 | 91.1 | 84.5 | 79.1 | 74.0 | 71.1 | 60.8–81.4 | 160 |
| 4 | 78.5 | 66.4 | 62.1 | 57.3 | 50.4 | 40.6–60.3 | 191 |

Five-year, relative survival by "combined" AJCC stage follicular adenocarcinoma of the thyroid, 1998-1999

**B**

**FIGURE 8.2.** (**A**) Five-year, observed survival by "combined" AJCC stage for follicular adenocarcinoma of the thyroid gland, 1998–1999. (95% confidence intervals correspond to year-5 survival rates.) (**B**) Five-year, relative survival by "combined" AJCC stage for follicular adenocarcinoma of the thyroid gland, 1998–1999. (95% confidence intervals correspond to year-5 survival rates.)

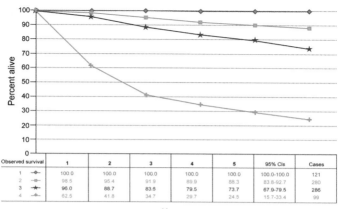

**A**

Five-year, observed survival by "combined" AJCC stage medullary carcinoma of the thyroid, 1998-1999.

| Observed survival | | 1 | 2 | 3 | 4 | 5 | 95% CIs | Cases |
|---|---|---|---|---|---|---|---|---|
| 1 | ◆ | 100.0 | 100.0 | 100.0 | 100.0 | 100.0 | 100.0-100.0 | 121 |
| 2 | ■ | 98.5 | 95.4 | 91.9 | 89.9 | 88.3 | 83.8-92.7 | 280 |
| 3 | ★ | 96.0 | 88.7 | 83.6 | 79.5 | 73.7 | 67.9-79.5 | 286 |
| 4 | ▲ | 62.5 | 41.8 | 34.7 | 29.7 | 24.5 | 15.7-33.4 | 99 |

Year

| Relative survival | | 1 | 2 | 3 | 4 | 5 | 95% CIs | Cases |
|---|---|---|---|---|---|---|---|---|
| 1 | ◆ | 100.0 | 100.0 | 100.0 | 100.0 | 100.0 | 100.0-100.0 | 121 |
| 2 | ■ | 100.0 | 99.2 | 97.6 | 97.5 | 97.9 | 93.0-100.0 | 280 |
| 3 | ★ | 96.0 | 91.9 | 88.2 | 85.6 | 81.0 | 74.6-87.3 | 286 |
| 4 | ▲ | 64.3 | 43.0 | 38.0 | 32.5 | 27.7 | 17.7-37.7 | 99 |

Year

Five-year, relative survival by "combined" AJCC stage medullary carcinoma of the thyroid, 1998-1999.

**B**

**FIGURE 8.3.** (**A**) Five-year, observed survival by "combined" AJCC stage for medullary carcinoma of the thyroid gland, 1985–1991. (95% confidence intervals correspond to year-5 survival rates.) (**B**) Five-year, relative survival by "combined" AJCC stage for medullary carcinoma of the thyroid gland, 1985–1991. (95% confidence intervals correspond to year-5 survival rates.)

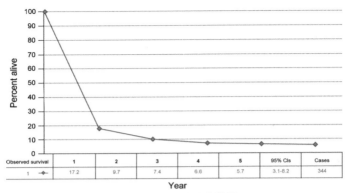

| Observed survival | 1 | 2 | 3 | 4 | 5 | 95% CIs | Cases |
|---|---|---|---|---|---|---|---|
| 1 | 17.2 | 9.7 | 7.4 | 6.6 | 5.7 | 3.1-8.2 | 344 |

Year

Five-year, observed survival by "combined" AJCC stage anaplastic carcinoma of the thyroid, 1996-1999.

**A**

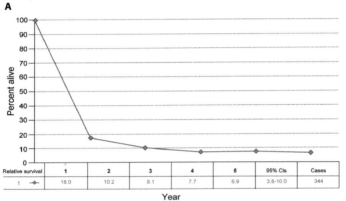

| Relative survival | 1 | 2 | 3 | 4 | 5 | 95% CIs | Cases |
|---|---|---|---|---|---|---|---|
| 1 | 18.0 | 10.2 | 8.1 | 7.7 | 6.9 | 3.8-10.0 | 344 |

Year

Five-year, relative survival by "combined" AJCC stage anaplastic carcinoma of the thyroid, 1996-1999.

**B**

**FIGURE 8.4.** (**A**) Five-year, observed survival by "combined" AJCC stage for Stage 4 anaplastic carcinoma of the thyroid gland, 1985–1991. (95% confidence intervals correspond to year-5 survival rates.) (**B**) Five-year, relative survival by "combined" AJCC stage for Stage 4 anaplastic carcinoma of the thyroid gland, 1985–1991. (95% confidence intervals correspond to year-5 survival rates.)

## BIBLIOGRAPHY

Ain KB. Papillary thyroid carcinoma: etiology, assessment, and therapy. Endocrinol Metab Clin North Am. 1995;24:711–60.

Andersen PE, Kinsella J, Loree TR, Shaha AR, Shah JP. Differentiated carcinoma of the thyroid with extrathyroid extension – risks for failure and patterns of recurrence. Am J Surg. 1995;170:467–70.

Antonacci A, Brierley G, Bacchi F, Consorti C, et al. Thyroid cancer. In: Hermanek P, Gospodarowicz MK, Henson DE, et al., editors. Prognostic factors in cancer. Berlin: Springer; 1995. p. 28–36.

Baloch ZW, LiVolsi VA. Prognostic factors in well-differentiated follicular-derived carcinoma and medullary thyroid carcinoma. Thyroid. 2001;11(7):637–45.

Brierley JD, Asa SL. Thyroid cancer. In: Gospodarowicz MK, O'Sullivan B, Sobin LH, editors. Prognostic factors in cancer. Hoboken, NJ: Wiley; 2006.

Brierley J, Tsang R, Simpson WJ, et al. Medullary thyroid cancer – analyses of survival and prognostic factors and the role of radiation therapy in local control. Thyroid. 1996;6:305–10.

Brierley JD, Panzarella T, Tsang RW, et al. Comparing staging classifications using thyroid cancer as an example. Cancer. 1997;79:2414–3.

Brierley J, Tsang R, Panzarella T, Bana N. Prognostic factors and the effect of treatment with radioactive iodine and external beam radiation on patients with differentiated thyroid cancer seen at a single institution over 40 years. Clin Endocrinol (Oxford). 2005;63(4):418–27.

Cady B, Rossi R, Silverman M, et al. Further evidence of the validity of risk group definition in differentiated thyroid carcinoma. Surgery. 1985;98:1171–8.

Cohn K, Blackdahl M, Forsslund G, et al. Prognostic value of nuclear DNA content in papillary thyroid carcinoma. World J Surg. 1984;8:474–80.

Goutsouliak V, Hay JH. Anaplastic thyroid cancer in British Columbia 1985–1999: a population-based study. Clin Oncol (R Coll Radiol). 2005;17(2):75–8.

Hay ID, Grant CS, Taylor WF, et al. Ipsilateral lobectomy versus bilateral lobar resection in papillary thyroid carcinoma: a retrospective analysis of surgical outcome using a novel prognostic scoring system. Surgery. 1987;102: 1088–95.

Hay ID, McConahey WM, Goellner JR. Managing patients with papillary thyroid carcinoma: insights gained from the Mayo Clinic's experience of treating 2,512 consecutive patients during 1940 through 2000. Trans Am Clin Climatol Assoc. 2002a;113:241–60.

Hay ID, Thompson GB, Grant CS, et al. Papillary thyroid carcinoma managed at the Mayo Clinic during six decades (1940–1999): temporal trends in initial therapy and long-term outcome in 2,444 consecutively treated patients. World J Surg. 2002b;26(8):879–85.

Hedinger C. Histological typing of thyroid tumours: WHO international histological classification of tumours. 2nd ed. Berlin: Springer; 1988.

Hundahl SA, Cady B, Cunningham MP, et al. (United States and German Thyroid Cancer Study Group): initial results from a prospective cohort of 5, 583 cases of thyroid carcinoma treated in the United States during 1996. Cancer. 2000;89:202–17.

Ito Y, Tomoda C, Uruno T, et al. Prognostic significance of extrathyroid extension of papillary thyroid carcinoma: massive but not minimal extension affects the relapse-free survival. World J Surg. 2006;30(5):780–6.

LiVolsi VA. Surgical pathology of the thyroid. Philadelphia, PA: WB Saunders; 1990.

Mazzaferri EL, Jhiang S. Long-term impact of initial surgical and medical therapy on papillary and follicular thyroid cancer. Am J Med. 1994;97: 418–28.

McConahey WM, Hay ID, Woolner LB, et al. Papillary thyroid cancer treated at the Mayo Clinic 1946–1970: initial manifestations, pathological findings, therapy and outcome. Mayo Clinic Proc. 1986;61:978–96.

McIver B, Hay ID, Giuffrida DF, Dvorak CE, Grant CS, Thompson GB, et al. Anaplastic thyroid carcinoma: a 50-year experience at a single institution. Surgery. 2001;130(6):1028–34.

Randolph GW, Maniar D. Medullary carcinoma of the thyroid. Cancer Control. 2000;7(3):253–61.

Rosai J, Carcangiu L, DeLellis RA. Tumors of the thyroid gland, 3rd series. Washington, DC: Armed Forces Institute of Pathology; 1992.

**8**

Rossi R. Prognosis of undifferentiated carcinoma and lymphoma of the thyroid. Am J Surg. 1978;135:589–96.

Saad MF, Ordonez NG, Rashid RK, et al. Medullary carcinoma of the thyroid: a study of the clinical features and prognostic factors in 161 patients. Medicine. 1984;63:319–42.

Shah JP, Loree TR, Dharker D, et al. Prognostic factors in differentiated carcinoma of the thyroid gland. Am J Surg. 1992;1645:658–61.

Shaha AR. Implications of prognostic factors and risk groups in the management of differentiated thyroid cancer. Laryngoscope. 2004;114(3):393–402.

Shaha AR. TNM classification of thyroid carcinoma. World J Surg. 2007;31(5): 879–87.

Shaha AR, Loree TR, Shah JP. Prognostic factors and risk group analysis in follicular carcinoma of the thyroid. Surgery. 1995;118:1131–8.

Shaha AR, Shah JP, Loree TR. Risk group stratification and prognostic factors in papillary carcinoma of the thyroid. Ann Surg Oncol. 1996;3:534–8.

Shoup M, Stojadinovic A, Nissan A, Ghossein RA, Freedman S, Brennan MF, et al. Prognostic indicators of outcomes in patients with distant metastases from differentiated thyroid carcinoma. J Am Coll Surg. 2003;197(2):191–7.

Simpson WL, Panzarella T, Carruthers JS, et al. Papillary and follicular thyroid cancer: impact of treatment in 1, 578 patients. Int J Radiat Oncol Biol Phys. 1988;14:1063–75.

Young RL, Mazzaferri EL, Rahea J, et al. Pure follicular thyroid carcinoma: impact of therapy in 214 patients. J Nucl Med. 1980;21:733–7.

# 9

# Mucosal Melanoma of the Head and Neck

## *At-A-Glance*

---

### SUMMARY OF CHANGES

• This is a new chapter for classification of this rare tumor

---

| ANATOMIC STAGE/PROGNOSTIC GROUPS | | | |
|---|---|---|---|
| Stage III | T3 | N0 | M0 |
| Stage IVA | T4a | N0 | M0 |
| | T3–T4a | N1 | M0 |
| Stage IVB | T4b | Any N | M0 |
| Stage IVC | Any T | Any N | M1 |

ICD-O-3 TOPOGRAPHY CODES

For a complete description of codes, refer to the appropriate anatomic site chapter based on the location of the mucosal melanoma (see Chapters 3–6)

Additionally, mucosal melanomas are staged for the following topography codes; however, no staging exists for nonmucosal melanoma in the same anatomic site:

| C14.0 | Pharynx, NOS |
|---|---|
| C14.2 | Waldeyer's ring |
| C14.8 | Overlapping lesion of lip, oral cavity and pharynx |

The following topography codes are excluded:

| C07.9 | Parotid gland | C30.1 | Middle ear |
|---|---|---|---|
| C08.0 | Submandibular gland | C73.9 | Thyroid |
| C08.1 | Sublingual gland | | |
| C08.8 | Overlapping lesion of major salivary glands | **ICD-O-3 HISTOLOGY CODE RANGES** | |
| C08.9 | Major salivary glands, NOS | 8020–8090 | |

## INTRODUCTION

Mucosal melanoma is an aggressive neoplasm that warrants separate consideration. Approximately two-thirds of these lesions arise in the nasal cavity and paranasal sinuses; one quarter are found in the oral cavity and the remainder occur only sporadically in other mucosal sites of the head and neck. Even small cancers behave aggressively with high rates of recurrence and death. To reflect this aggressive behavior, primary cancers limited to the mucosa are considered T3 lesions. Advanced mucosal melanomas are classified as T4a and T4b. The anatomic extent criteria to define *moderately advanced* (T4a) and *very advanced* (T4b) disease are given below. In situ mucosal melanomas are excluded from staging, as they are extremely rare.

## ANATOMY

Mucosal melanomas occur throughout the mucosa of the upper aerodigestive tract. For a description of anatomy, refer to the appropriate anatomic site chapter based on the location of the mucosal melanoma.

## RULES FOR CLASSIFICATION

Mucosal melanomas occur throughout the mucosa of the upper aerodigestive tract. For the rules for classification, refer to the appropriate anatomic site chapter based on the location of the mucosal melanoma.

## DEFINITIONS OF TNM

*Primary Tumor*

| | |
|---|---|
| T3 | Mucosal disease |
| T4a | Moderately advanced disease |
| | Tumor involving deep soft tissue, cartilage, bone, or overlying skin |
| T4b | Very advanced disease |
| | Tumor involving brain, dura, skull base, lower cranial nerves (IX, X, XI, XII), masticator space, carotid artery, prevertebral space, or mediastinal structures |

*Regional Lymph Nodes*

| | |
|---|---|
| NX | Regional lymph nodes cannot be assessed |
| N0 | No regional lymph node metastases |
| N1 | Regional lymph node metastases present |

*Distant Metastasis*

| | |
|---|---|
| M0 | No distant metastasis |
| M1 | Distant metastasis present |

## ANATOMIC STAGE/PROGNOSTIC GROUPS

| Stage III | T3 | N0 | M0 |
|---|---|---|---|
| Stage IVA | T4a | N0 | M0 |
| | T3–T4a | N1 | M0 |
| Stage IVB | T4b | Any N | M0 |
| Stage IVC | Any T | Any N | M1 |

## PROGNOSTIC FACTORS (SITE-SPECIFIC FACTORS)
### (Recommended for Collection)

| | |
|---|---|
| Required for staging | None |
| Clinically significant | Size of lymph nodes |
| | Extracapsular extension from lymph node for head and neck |
| | Head and neck lymph nodes levels I–III |
| | Head and neck lymph nodes levels IV–V |
| | Head and neck lymph nodes levels VI–VII |
| | Other lymph node group |
| | Clinical location of cervical nodes |
| | Extracapsular spread (ECS) clinical |
| | Extracapsular spread (ECS) pathologic |
| | Tumor thickness |

## HISTOLOGIC GRADE (G)

Grade is reported in registry systems by the grade value. A two-grade, three-grade, or four-grade system may be used. If a grading system is not specified, generally the following system is used:

| | |
|---|---|
| GX | Grade cannot be assessed |
| G1 | Well differentiated |
| G2 | Moderately differentiated |
| G3 | Poorly differentiated |
| G4 | Undifferentiated |

## BIBLIOGRAPHY

Medina JE, Ferlito A, Pellitteri PK, Shaha AR, Khafif A, Devaney KO, et al. Current management of mucosal melanoma of the head and neck. J Surg Oncol. 2003;83:116–22.

Patel SG, Prasad ML, Escrig M, Singh B, Shaha AR, Kraus DH, et al. Primary mucosal malignant melanoma of the head and neck. Head Neck. 2002;24:247–57.

Temam S, Mamelle G, Marandas P, Wibault P, Avril MF, Janot F, et al. Postoperative radiotherapy for primary mucosal melanoma of the head and neck. Cancer. 2005;103:313–9.

Teppo H, Kervinen J, Koivunen P, Alho OP. Incidence and outcome of head and neck mucosal melanoma – a population-based survey from Northern Finland. Int J Circumpolar Health. 2006;65:443–7.

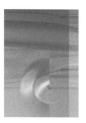

# PART III
# Digestive System

# Esophagus and Esophagogastric Junction

*(Nonmucosal cancers are not included)*

## *At-A-Glance*

---

### SUMMARY OF CHANGES

- Tumor location is simplified, and esophagogastric junction and proximal 5 cm of stomach are included
- Tis is redefined and T4 is subclassified
- Regional lymph nodes are redefined. N is subclassified according to the number of regional lymph nodes containing metastasis
- M is redefined
- Separate stage groupings for squamous cell carcinoma and adenocarcinoma
- Stage groupings are reassigned using T, N, M, and G classifications

---

### ANATOMIC STAGE/PROGNOSTIC GROUPS

*Squamous Cell Carcinoma\**

| Stage | T | N | M | Grade | Tumor Location |
|-------|-----|-----|-----|-------|----------------|
| 0 | T is (HGD) | N0 | M0 | 1, X | Any |
| IA | T1 | N0 | M0 | 1, X | Any |
| IB | T1 | N0 | M0 | 2–3 | Any |
|  | T2–3 | N0 | M0 | 1, X | Lower, X |
| IIA | T2–3 | N0 | M0 | 1, X | Upper, middle |
|  | T2–3 | N0 | M0 | 2–3 | Lower, X |
| IIB | T2–3 | N0 | M0 | 2–3 | Upper, middle |
|  | T1–2 | N1 | M0 | Any | Any |
| IIIA | T1–2 | N2 | M0 | Any | Any |
|  | T3 | N1 | M0 | Any | Any |
|  | T4a | N0 | M0 | Any | Any |
| IIIB | T3 | N2 | M0 | Any | Any |
| IIIC | T4a | N1–2 | M0 | Any | Any |
|  | T4b | Any | M0 | Any | Any |
|  | Any | N3 | M0 | Any | Any |
| IV | Any | Any | M1 | Any | Any |

\*Or mixed histology including a squamous component or NOS.

### ICD-O-3 TOPOGRAPHY CODES

| | |
|---|---|
| C15.0 | Cervical esophagus |
| C15.1 | Thoracic esophagus |
| C15.2 | Abdominal esophagus |
| C15.3 | Upper third of esophagus |
| C15.4 | Middle third of esophagus |
| C15.5 | Lower third of esophagus |
| C15.8 | Overlapping lesion of esophagus |
| C15.9 | Esophagus, NOS |
| C16.0 | Cardia, esophagogastric junction |
| C16.1 | Fundus of stomach, proximal 5 cm only\* |

*Adenocarcinoma*

| Stage | T | N | M | Grade |
|---|---|---|---|---|
| 0 | Tis (HGD) | N0 | M0 | 1, X |
| IA | T1 | N0 | M0 | 1–2, X |
| IB | T1 | N0 | M0 | 3 |
| | T2 | N0 | M0 | 1–2, X |
| IIA | T2 | N0 | M0 | 3 |
| IIB | T3 | N0 | M0 | Any |
| | T1–2 | N1 | M0 | Any |
| IIIA | T1–2 | N2 | M0 | Any |
| | T3 | N1 | M0 | Any |
| | T4a | N0 | M0 | Any |
| IIIB | T3 | N2 | M0 | Any |
| IIIC | T4a | N1–2 | M0 | Any |
| | T4b | Any | M0 | Any |
| | Any | N3 | M0 | Any |
| IV | Any | Any | M1 | Any |

C16.2   Body of stomach, proximal 5 cm only*

*Note*: If gastric tumor extends to or above esophagogastric junction.

ICD-O-3 HISTOLOGY CODE RANGES
8000–8576, 8940–8950, 8980–8981 (C15 only)
8000–8152, 8154–8231, 8243–8245, 8250–8576, 8940–8950, 8980–8981 (C16 only)

# INTRODUCTION

Previous stage groupings of esophageal cancer were based on a simple, orderly arrangement of increasing pathologic anatomic T, then N, and then M classifications. In contrast, this revision is data driven, based on a risk-adjusted random-survival-forest analysis of worldwide data. The previous system was neither consistent with these data nor biologically plausible. Some explanations for the discrepancy relate to the interplay among T, N, and M, histopathologic type, biologic activity of the tumor (histologic grade), and location.

The unique lymphatic anatomy of the esophagus links N to T, permitting lymph node metastases from superficial cancers (pT1); this renders prognosis similar to that of more advanced (higher pT) N0 cancers. Similarly, advanced cancers (higher pT) with a few positive nodes may have a similar prognosis to those of less advanced cancers (lower pT) with more positive nodes. Biologic activity of the cancer, reflected by histologic grade (G), modulates stage such that prognosis of well-differentiated (G1) higher-pT cancers is similar to that of less well-differentiated (G2–G4) lower-pT cancers. Previous staging recommendations ignored histopathologic type, but availability of data on a large mixture of adenocarcinoma and squamous cell carcinomas from around the world has permitted assessing the association of histopathologic type with survival.

Although at first glance these multiple trade-offs seem to create a less orderly arrangement of cancer classifications within and among stage groupings compared with previous stage groupings, when viewed from the perspective of the interplay of these important prognostic factors, the new staging system becomes biologically compelling and consistent with a number of other cancers.

A limitation of this data-driven approach is that staging is based only on pTNM from esophageal cancers treated by esophagectomy alone, without induction or postoperative chemotherapy or radiotherapy; patients not offered operation, deemed inoperable, or undergoing exploratory surgery without esophagectomy were not represented in the data. In addition, patients undergoing surgery alone with pT4 and pM1 cancers represent a select population; placing them into stage groups, therefore, required either combining some classifications or using literature as a supplement. Patients with cervical esophageal cancer, sometimes treated as a head-and-neck tumor, were also poorly represented.

## ANATOMY

**Primary Site.** The location of the primary tumor is defined by the position of the upper end of the cancer in the esophagus. This is best expressed as the distance from the incisors to the proximal edge of the tumor and conventionally by its location within broad regions of the esophagus. ICD coding recognizes three anatomic compartments traversed by the esophagus: cervical, thoracic, and abdominal. It also arbitrarily divides the esophagus into equal thirds: upper, middle, and lower (Table 10.1). However, clinical importance of primary site of esophageal cancer is less related to its position in the esophagus than to its relation to adjacent structures (Figure 10.1).

*Cervical Esophagus.* Anatomically, the cervical esophagus lies in the neck, bordered superiorly by the hypopharynx and inferiorly by the thoracic inlet, which lies at the level of the sternal notch. It is subtended by the trachea, carotid sheaths, and vertebrae. Although length of the esophagus differs somewhat with body habitus, gender, and age, typical endoscopic measurements for the cervical esophagus measured from the incisors are from 15 to <20 cm (Figure 10.1). If esophagoscopy is not available, location can be assessed by computed tomography (CT). If thickening of the esophageal wall begins above the sternal notch, the location is cervical.

*Upper Thoracic Esophagus.* The upper thoracic esophagus is bordered superiorly by the thoracic inlet and inferiorly by the lower border of the azygos vein. Anterolaterally, it is surrounded by the trachea, arch vessels, and great veins, and posteriorly by the vertebrae. Typical endoscopic measurements from the incisors are from 20 to <25 cm (Figure 10.1). CT location of an upper thoracic cancer is esophageal wall thickening that begins between the sternal notch and the azygos vein.

*Middle Thoracic Esophagus.* The middle thoracic esophagus is bordered superiorly by the lower border of the azygos vein and inferiorly by the inferior pulmonary veins. It is sandwiched between the pulmonary hilum

**TABLE 10.1.** Primary site of esophageal cancer based on proximal edge of tumor

| Anatomic name | Compartment ICD-O-3 | ICD-O-3 | Esophageal location Name | Anatomic boundaries | Typical esophagectomy |
|---|---|---|---|---|---|
| Cervical | C15.0 | C15.3 | Upper | Hypopharynx to sternal notch | 15 to <20 cm |
| Thoracic | C15.1 | C15.3 | Upper | Sternal notch to azygos vein | 20 to <25 cm |
| | | C15.4 | Middle | Lower border of azygos vein to inferior pulmonary vein | 25 to <30 cm |
| | | C15.5 | Lower | Lower border of inferior pulmonary vein to esophagogastric junction | 30 to <40 cm |
| Abdominal | C15.2 | C15.5 | Lower | Esophagogastric junction to 5 cm below esophagogastric junction | 40–45 cm |
| | | C16.0 | Esophagogastric junction/cardia | Esophagogastric junction to 5 cm below esophagogastric junction | 40–45 cm |

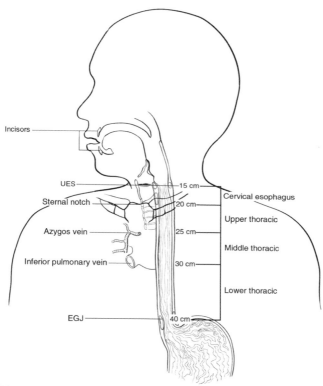

**FIGURE 10.1.** Anatomy of esophageal cancer primary site, including typical endoscopic measurements of each region measured from the incisors. Exact measurements are dependent on body size and height.

anteriorly, descending thoracic aorta on the left, and vertebrae posteriorly; on the right, it lies freely on the pleura. Typical endoscopic measurements from the incisors are from 25 to <30 cm (Figure 10.1). CT location is wall thickening that begins between the azygos vein and the inferior pulmonary vein.

***Lower Thoracic Esophagus/Esophagogastric Junction.*** The lower thoracic esophagus is bordered superiorly by the inferior pulmonary veins and inferiorly by the stomach. Because it is the end of the esophagus, it includes the esophagogastric junction (EGJ). It is bordered anteriorly by the pericardium, posteriorly by vertebrae, and on the left by the descending thoracic aorta. It normally passes through the diaphragm to reach the stomach, but there is a variable intra-abdominal portion, and because of hiatal hernia, this portion may be absent. Typical endoscopic measurements from the incisors are from 30 to 40 cm (Figure 10.1). CT location is wall thickening that begins below the inferior pulmonary vein. The abdominal esophagus is included in the lower thoracic esophagus.

The arbitrary 10-cm segment encompassing the distal 5 cm of the esophagus and proximal 5 cm of the stomach, with the EGJ in the middle, is an area of contention. Cancers arising in this segment have been variably staged as esophageal or gastric tumors, depending on orientation of the treating physician. In this edition, cancers whose epicenter is in the lower thoracic esophagus, EGJ, or within the proximal 5 cm of the stomach (cardia) that extend into the EGJ or esophagus (Siewert III) are stage grouped similar to adenocarcinoma of the esophagus. Although Siewert and colleagues subtype EGJ cancers (types I, II, III), not only do their data support a single-stage grouping scheme across this area, but also they demonstrate that prognosis depends on cancer classification (T, N, M, G) and not Siewert type. All other cancers with an epicenter in the stomach greater than 5 cm distal to the EGJ, or those within 5 cm of the EGJ but not extending into the EGJ or esophagus, are stage grouped using the gastric (non-EGJ) cancer staging system (see Chap. 11).

**Esophageal Wall.** The esophageal wall has three layers: mucosa, submucosa, and muscularis propria (Figure 10.2). The *mucosa* is composed of epithelium, lamina propria, and muscularis mucosae. A basement membrane isolates the mucosa from the rest of the esophageal wall. In the columnar-lined esophagus the muscularis mucosae may be a two-layered structure. The mucosal division can be classified as m1 (epithelium), m2 (lamina propria), or m3 (muscularis mucosae). The *submucosa* has no landmarks, but some divide it into inner (sm1), middle (sm2), and outer thirds (sm3). The *muscularis propria* has inner circular and outer longitudinal muscle layers. There is no serosa; rather, *adventitia* (periesophageal connective tissue) lies directly on the muscularis propria.

**Adjacent Structures.** In close proximity to the esophagus lie pleura-peritoneum, pericardium, and diaphragm. Cancers invading these structures may be resectable (T4a). Aorta, carotid vessels, azygos vein, trachea, left

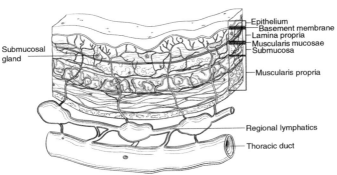

**FIGURE 10.2.** Esophageal wall.

main bronchus, and vertebral body also are in close proximity, but cancers invading these structures are usually unresectable (T4b).

**Lymphatics.** Esophageal lymphatic drainage is intramural and longitudinal (Figure 10.2). Although a lymphatic network is concentrated in the submucosa, lymphatic channels are present in the lamina propria, an arrangement that permits lymphatic metastases early in the course of the disease from superficial cancers that are otherwise confined to the mucosa. Lymphatic drainage of the muscularis propria is more limited, but lymphatic channels pierce this layer to drain into regional lymphatic channels and lymph nodes in the periesophageal fat. Up to 43% of autopsy dissections demonstrate direct drainage from the submucosal plexus into the thoracic duct, which facilitates systemic metastases. The longitudinal nature of the submucosal lymphatic plexus permits lymphatic metastases orthogonal to the depth of tumor invasion. Implications of the longitudinal nature of lymphatic drainage are that the anatomic site of the cancer and the nodes to which lymphatics drain from that site may not be the same.

Regional lymph nodes extend from periesophageal cervical nodes to celiac nodes (Figures 10.3A–D and 10.4). For radiotherapy, fields of treatment may not be constrained within this definition of regional node.

The data demonstrate that the number of regional lymph nodes containing metastases (positive nodes) is the most important prognostic factor. In classifying N, the data support convenient coarse groupings of the number of positive nodes (0, 1–2, 3–6, 7 or more). These have been designated N1 (1–2), N2 (3–6), and N3 (7 or more). Nevertheless, there are no sharp cut-points; rather, each additional positive node increases risk. Clinical determination of positive lymph node number is possible and correlated with survival. Thus, the staging recommendations apply to both clinical and pathologic staging. The data do not support lymph node ratio (number positive divided by number sampled) as a useful measure of lymph node burden. The number of sampled nodes, the denominator of the ratio, is highly variable, distorting the magnitude of lymph node burden.

Data demonstrate that in general, the more lymph nodes resected, the better the survival. This may be due to either improved N classification or a therapeutic effect of lymphadenectomy. On the basis of worldwide data, it was found that optimum lymphadenectomy depends on T classification: For pT1, approximately ten nodes must be resected to maximize survival; for pT2, 20 nodes and for pT3 or pT4, 30 nodes or more. On the basis of different data and analysis methods that focus on maximizing sensitivity, others have suggested that an adequate lymphadenectomy requires resecting 12–22 nodes. Thus, one should resect as many regional lymph nodes as possible, balancing the extent of lymph node resection with morbidity of radical lymphadenectomy.

**Distant Metastatic Sites.** Sites of distant metastases are those that are not in direct continuity with the esophagus and include nonregional lymph nodes (M1). The previous M1a and M1b subclassification has not been found useful.

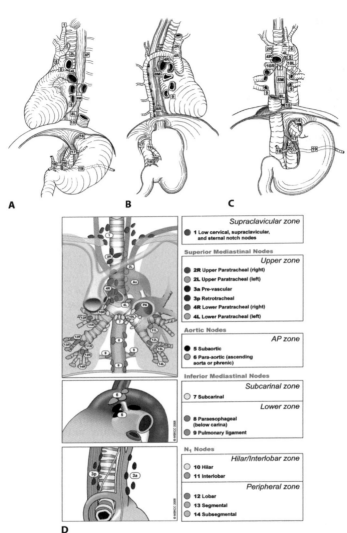

**FIGURE 10.3.** (A–C) Lymph node maps for esophageal cancer. Regional lymph node stations for staging esophageal cancer, from front (**A**) and side (**B**). 1, Supraclavicular nodes; above suprasternal notch and clavicles. 2R, Right upper paratracheal nodes; between intersection of caudal margin of innominate artery with trachea and the apex of the lung. 2L, Left upper paratracheal nodes; between the top of aortic arch and apex of the lung. 3P, Posterior mediastinal nodes; upper paraesophageal nodes, above tracheal bifurcation. 4R, Right lower paratracheal nodes; between intersection of caudal margin of innominate artery with trachea and cephalic border of azygos vein. 4L, Left lower paratracheal nodes; between top of aortic arch and carina. 5, Aortopulmonary nodes; subaortic and para-aortic nodes lateral

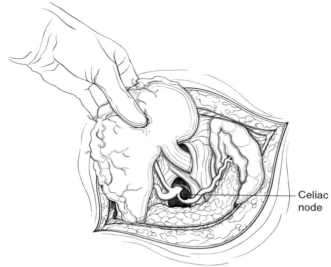

**FIGURE 10.4.** Celiac lymph node.

## NONANATOMIC TUMOR CHARACTERISTICS

This staging of cancer of the esophagus is based on cancers arising from its epithelium, squamous cell carcinoma, and adenocarcinoma. Nonmucosal cancers arising in the wall should be classified according to their cell of origin.

Highest histologic grade on biopsy or resection specimen is the required data for stage grouping. Because the data indicate that squamous cell carcinoma has a poorer prognosis than adenocarcinoma, if a tumor is of mixed histopathologic type or is not otherwise specified, it shall be recorded as squamous cell carcinoma. If grade is not available, it should

---

**FIGURE 10.3.** (Continued) to the ligamentum arteriosum. 6, Anterior mediastinal nodes; anterior to ascending aorta or innominate artery. 7, Subcarinal nodes; caudal to the carina of the trachea. 8M, Middle paraesophageal lymph nodes; from the tracheal bifurcation to the caudal margin of the inferior pulmonary vein. 8L, Lower paraesophageal lymph nodes; from the caudal margin of the inferior pulmonary vein to the esophagogastric junction. 8R, 9, Pulmonary ligament nodes; within the inferior pulmonary ligament. 10R, Right tracheobronchial nodes; from cephalic border of azygos vein to origin of RUL bronchus. 10L, Left tracheobronchial nodes; between carina and LUL bronchus. 15, Diaphragmatic nodes; lying on the dome of the diaphragm and adjacent to or behind its crura. 16, Paracardial nodes; immediately adjacent to the gastroesophageal junction. 17, Left gastric nodes; along the course of the left gastric artery. 18, Common hepatic nodes; along the course of the common hepatic artery. 19, Splenic nodes; along the course of the splenic artery. 20, Celiac nodes; at the base of the celiac artery. (**D**) The IASLC lymph node map. (**D**, © Memorial Sloan-Kettering Cancer Center, 2009.)

**10**

be recorded as GX and stage grouped as G1 cancer. G4, undifferentiated cancers, should be recorded as such and stage grouped similar to G3 squamous cell carcinoma.

## RULES FOR CLASSIFICATION

**Clinical Staging (c, yc).** Clinical classification (c) is based on evidence before primary treatment. It involves esophagoscopy with biopsy, endoscopic esophageal ultrasound (EUS), EUS-directed fine-needle aspiration (EUS-FNA), fused computed tomography (CT), 2[$^{18}$F]fluoro-2-deoxy-D-glucose positron emission tomography (PET/CT) for assessment of T, N, M, and G classifications, and histopathologic type. These may be supplemented by cervical lymph node biopsy, bronchoscopy, endoscopic bronchial ultrasound (EBUS) and EBUS-FNA, mediastinoscopy, thoracoscopy, laparoscopy, and ultrasound- or CT-directed percutaneous biopsy. Clinical reclassification during or following chemotherapy and/or radiotherapy is designated by the prefix yc.

**Pathologic Staging (p, yp).** Pathologic classification uses evidence acquired before treatment, supplemented or modified by additional evidence acquired during and from surgery, particularly from pathologic evaluation of the surgical specimen. Pathologic reclassification during and following surgery that has been preceded by chemotherapy and/or radiotherapy is designated by the prefix yp.

## DEFINITIONS OF TNM*

| *Primary Tumor (T)*** | |
|---|---|
| TX | Primary tumor cannot be assessed |
| T0 | No evidence of primary tumor |
| Tis | High-grade dysplasia*** |
| T1 | Tumor invades lamina propria, muscularis mucosae, or submucosa |
| T1a | Tumor invades lamina propria or muscularis mucosae |
| T1b | Tumor invades submucosa |
| T2 | Tumor invades muscularis propria |
| T3 | Tumor invades adventitia |
| T4 | Tumor invades adjacent structures |
| T4a | Resectable tumor invading pleura, pericardium, or diaphragm |
| T4b | Unresectable tumor invading other adjacent structures, such as aorta, vertebral body, trachea, etc. |

*See Figure 10.5.

**(1) At least maximal dimension of the tumor must be recorded and (2) multiple tumors require the T(m) suffix.

***High-grade dysplasia includes all noninvasive neoplastic epithelia that was formerly called carcinoma in situ, a diagnosis that is no longer used for columnar mucosae anywhere in the gastrointestinal tract.

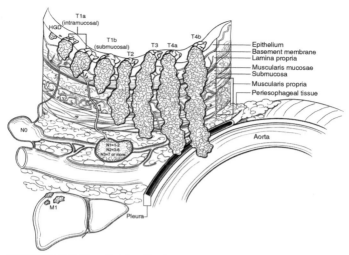

**FIGURE 10.5.** T, N, and M classifications. Primary tumor (T) is classified by depth of tumor invasion. Regional lymph node classifications are determined by metastatic burden. Distant metastatic sites are designated M1.

### Regional Lymph Nodes (N)*

| | |
|---|---|
| NX | Regional lymph nodes cannot be assessed |
| N0 | No regional lymph node metastasis |
| N1 | Metastasis in 1–2 regional lymph nodes |
| N2 | Metastasis in 3–6 regional lymph nodes |
| N3 | Metastasis in seven or more regional lymph nodes |

*Number must be recorded for total number of regional nodes sampled and total number of reported nodes with metastases.

### Distant Metastasis (M)

| | |
|---|---|
| M0 | No distant metastasis |
| M1 | Distant metastasis |

**10**

### ANATOMIC STAGE/PROGNOSTIC GROUPS

*Squamous Cell Carcinoma* (Figure 10.6)*

| Stage | T | N | M | Grade | Tumor Location** |
|---|---|---|---|---|---|
| 0 | Tis (HGD) | N0 | M0 | 1, X | Any |
| IA | T1 | N0 | M0 | 1, X | Any |
| IB | T1 | N0 | M0 | 2–3 | Any |
| | T2–3 | N0 | M0 | 1, X | Lower, X |

*Squamous Cell Carcinoma* (Figure 10.6)*

| Stage | T | N | M | Grade | Tumor Location** |
|-------|-----|-----|-----|-------|-------------------|
| IIA | T2–3 | N0 | M0 | 1, X | Upper, middle |
|     | T2–3 | N0 | M0 | 2–3 | Lower, X |
| IIB | T2–3 | N0 | M0 | 2–3 | Upper, middle |
|     | T1–2 | N1 | M0 | Any | Any |
| IIIA | T1–2 | N2 | M0 | Any | Any |
|      | T3 | N1 | M0 | Any | Any |
|      | T4a | N0 | M0 | Any | Any |
| IIIB | T3 | N2 | M0 | Any | Any |
| IIIC | T4a | N1–2 | M0 | Any | Any |
|      | T4b | Any | M0 | Any | Any |
|      | Any | N3 | M0 | Any | Any |
| IV | Any | Any | M1 | Any | Any |

*Or mixed histology including a squamous component or NOS.

**Location of the primary cancer site is defined by the position of the upper (proximal) edge of the tumor in the esophagus.

*Adenocarcinoma* (Figure 10.7)

| Stage | T | N | M | Grade |
|-------|-----------|-----|-----|-------|
| 0 | Tis (HGD) | N0 | M0 | 1, X |
| IA | T1 | N0 | M0 | 1–2, X |
| IB | T1 | N0 | M0 | 3 |
|    | T2 | N0 | M0 | 1–2, X |
| IIA | T2 | N0 | M0 | 3 |
| IIB | T3 | N0 | M0 | Any |
|     | T1–2 | N1 | M0 | Any |
| IIIA | T1–2 | N2 | M0 | Any |
|      | T3 | N1 | M0 | Any |
|      | T4a | N0 | M0 | Any |
| IIIB | T3 | N2 | M0 | Any |
| IIIC | T4a | N1–2 | M0 | Any |
|      | T4b | Any | M0 | Any |
|      | Any | N3 | M0 | Any |
| IV | Any | Any | M1 | Any |

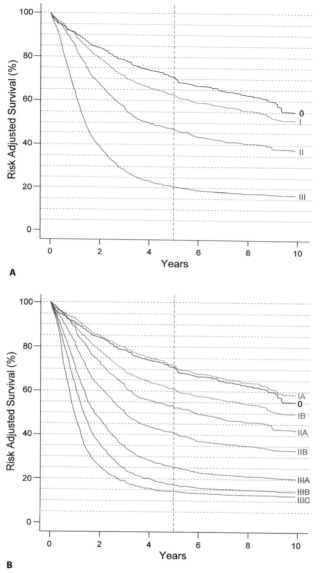

**A**

**B**

**FIGURE 10.6.** (**A**) Survival after esophagectomy only for squamous cell carcinoma stratified by stage groupings, based on worldwide esophageal cancer collaboration (WECC) data. Condensed stage groupings. (**B**) Survival after esophagectomy only for squamous cell carcinoma stratified by stage groupings, based on worldwide esophageal cancer collaboration (WECC) data. Expanded stage groupings.

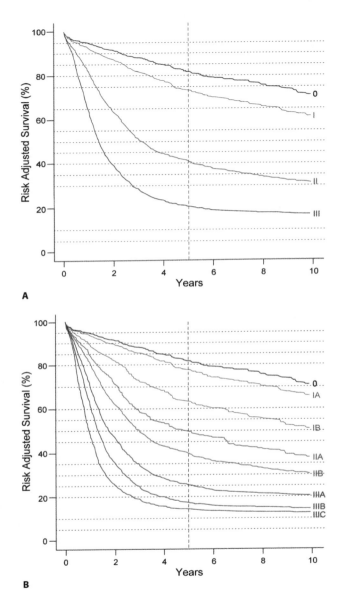

**A**

**B**

**FIGURE 10.7.** (**A**) Survival after esophagectomy only for adenocarcinoma stratified by stage groupings, based on worldwide esophageal cancer collaboration (WECC) data. Condensed stage groupings. (**B**) Survival after esophagectomy only for adenocarcinoma stratified by stage groupings, based on worldwide esophageal cancer collaboration (WECC) data. Expanded stage groupings.

## PROGNOSTIC FACTORS (SITE-SPECIFIC FACTORS)
(Recommended for Collection)

### Squamous Cell Carcinoma

| | |
|---|---|
| Required for staging | Location – based on the position of the upper (proximal) edge of the tumor in the esophagus (upper or middle – cancers above lower border of inferior pulmonary vein; lower – below inferior pulmonary vein) |
| | Grade |
| Clinically significant | Distance to proximal edge of tumor from incisors |
| | Distance to distal edge of tumor from incisors |
| | Number of regional nodes with extracapsular tumor |

### Adenocarcinoma

| | |
|---|---|
| Required for staging | Grade |
| Clinically significant | Distance to proximal edge of tumor from incisors |
| | Distance to distal edge of tumor from incisors |
| | Number of regional nodes with extracapsular tumor |

## HISTOLOGIC GRADE (G)

| | |
|---|---|
| GX | Grade cannot be assessed – stage grouping as G1 |
| G1 | Well differentiated |
| G2 | Moderately differentiated |
| G3 | Poorly differentiated |
| G4 | Undifferentiated – stage grouping as G3 squamous |

## HISTOPATHOLOGIC TYPE

Squamous cell carcinoma
Adenocarcinoma

## BIBLIOGRAPHY

Akiyama H, Tsurumaru M, Kawamura T, Ono Y. Principles of surgical treatment for carcinoma of the esophagus: analysis of lymph node involvement. Ann Surg. 1981;194:438–46.

American Joint Committee on Cancer. AJCC Cancer Staging Manual. 6th ed. New York: Springer-Verlag; 2002.

Chen J, Xu R, Hunt GC, Krinsky ML, Savides TJ. Influence of the number of malignant regional lymph nodes detected by endoscopic ultrasonography on survival stratification in esophageal adenocarcinoma. Clin Gastroenterol Hepatol. 2006;4:573–9.

Choi JY, Lee KH, Shim YM, Lee KS, Kim JJ, Kim SE, et al. Improved detection of individual nodal involvement in squamous cell carcinoma of the esophagus by FDG PET. J Nucl Med. 2000;41:808–15.

Feith M, Stein HJ, Siewert JR. Adenocarcinoma of the esophagogastric junction: surgical therapy based on 1602 consecutive resected patients. Surg Oncol Clin North Am. 2006;15:751–64.

10

Ishwaran H, Blackstone EH, Apperson-Hansen C, et al. A novel approach to cancer staging: application to esophageal cancer. Biostatistics. 2009;Jun 5 [epub ahead of print].

Kodama M, Kakegawa T. Treatment of superficial cancer of the esophagus: a summary of responses to a questionnaire on superficial cancer of the esophagus in Japan. Surgery. 1998;123:432–9.

Kuge K, Murakami G, Mizobuchi S, Hata Y, Aikou T, Sasaguri S. Submucosal territory of the direct lymphatic drainage system to the thoracic duct in the human esophagus. J Thorac Cardiovasc Surg. 2003;125:1343–9.

Murakami G, Sato I, Shimada K, Dong C, Kato Y, Imazeki T. Direct lymphatic drainage from the esophagus into the thoracic duct. Surg Radiol Anat. 1994;16:399–407.

Natsugoe S, Yoshinaka H, Shimada M, Sakamoto F, Morinaga T, Nakano S, et al. Number of lymph node metastases determined by presurgical ultrasound and endoscopic ultrasound is related to prognosis in patients with esophageal carcinoma. Ann Surg. 2001;234:613–8.

Peyre CG, Hagen JA, DeMeester SR, et al. The number of lymph nodes removed predicts survival in esophageal cancer: an international study on the impact of extent of surgical resection. Ann Surg. 2008;248:549–56.

Rice TW, Zuccaro G Jr, Adelstein DJ, Rybicki LA, Blackstone EH, Goldblum JR. Esophageal carcinoma: depth of tumor invasion is predictive of regional lymph node status. Ann Thorac Surg. 1998;65:787–92.

Rice TW, Blackstone EH, Goldblum JR, DeCamp MM, Murthy SC, Falk GW, et al. Superficial adenocarcinoma of the esophagus. J Thorac Cardiovasc Surg. 2001;122:1077–90.

Rice TW, Blackstone EH, Rybicki LA, Adelstein DJ, Murthy SC, DeCamp MM, et al. Refining esophageal cancer staging. J Thorac Cardiovasc Surg. 2003;125:1103–13.

Rice TW, Rusch VW, Apperson-Hansen C, et al. Worldwide esophageal cancer collaboration. Dis Esophagus. 2009;22:1–8.

Riquet M, Saab M, Le Pimpec Barthes F, Hidden G. Lymphatic drainage of the esophagus in the adult. Surg Radiol Anat. 1993;15:209–11.

Rizk NP, Ishwaran H, Rice TW, et al. Optimum lymphadenectomy for esophageal cancer. Ann Surg. 2009;250:1–5.

Siewert JR, Stein HJ. Classification of adenocarcinoma of the oesophagogastric junction. Br J Surg. 1998;85:1457–9.

Siewert JR, Stein HJ, Feith M, Bruecher BL, Bartels H, Fink U. Histologic tumor type is an independent prognostic parameter in esophageal cancer: lessons from more than 1,000 consecutive resections at a single center in the Western world. Ann Surg. 2001;234:360–7; discussion 8–9.

# Stomach

*(Lymphomas, sarcomas, and carcinoid tumors [low-grade neuroendocrine tumors] are not included)*

## At-A-Glance

### SUMMARY OF CHANGES

- Tumors arising at the esophagogastric junction, or arising in the stomach ≤5 cm from the esophagogastric junction and crossing the esophagogastric junction are staged using the TNM system for esophageal adenocarcinoma (see Chap. 10)

- T categories have been modified to harmonize with T categories of the esophagus and small and large intestine

  - T1 lesions have been subdivided into T1a and T1b

  - T2 is defined as a tumor that invades the muscularis propria

  - T3 is defined as a tumor that invades the subserosal connective tissue

  - T4 is defined as a tumor that invades the serosa (visceral peritoneum) or adjacent structures

- N categories have been modified, with N1 = 1–2 positive lymph nodes, N2 = 3–6 positive lymph nodes, N3 = 7 or more positive lymph nodes

- Positive peritoneal cytology is classified as M1

- Stage groupings have been changed

| ANATOMIC STAGE/PROGNOSTIC GROUPS | | | |
|---|---|---|---|
| Stage 0 | Tis | N0 | M0 |
| Stage IA | T1 | N0 | M0 |
| Stage IB | T2 | N0 | M0 |
| | T1 | N1 | M0 |
| Stage IIA | T3 | N0 | M0 |
| | T2 | N1 | M0 |
| | T1 | N2 | M0 |
| Stage IIB | T4a | N0 | M0 |
| | T3 | N1 | M0 |
| | T2 | N2 | M0 |
| | T1 | N3 | M0 |
| Stage IIIA | T4a | N1 | M0 |
| | T3 | N2 | M0 |
| | T2 | N3 | M0 |

ICD-O-3
TOPOGRAPHY
CODES

C16.1  Fundus of stomach*
C16.2  Body of stomach*
C16.3  Gastric antrum
C16.4  Pylorus
C16.5  Lesser curvature of stomach, NOS

*Note: See first statement in Summary of Changes.

**11**

| ANATOMIC STAGE/PROGNOSTIC GROUPS (CONTINUED) | | | | C16.6 | Greater curvature of stomach, NOS |
|---|---|---|---|---|---|
| Stage IIIB | T4b | N0 | M0 | C16.8 | Overlapping lesion of stomach |
| | T4b | N1 | M0 | | |
| | T4a | N2 | M0 | C16.9 | Stomach, NOS |
| | T3 | N3 | M0 | | |
| Stage IIIC | T4b | N2 | M0 | | |
| | T4b | N3 | M0 | | |
| | T4a | N3 | M0 | | |
| Stage IV | Any T | Any N | M1 | | |

C16.6 Greater curvature of stomach, NOS

C16.8 Overlapping lesion of stomach

C16.9 Stomach, NOS

ICD-O-3 HISTOLOGY CODE RANGES
8000–8152, 8154–8231,
8243–8245, 8250–8576,
8940–8950, 8980–8990

## INTRODUCTION

Gastric cancer remains the fourth most common cancer worldwide and the second leading cause of cancer deaths (700,000 deaths annually worldwide). The highest rates of this disease continue to be in areas of Asia and Eastern Europe. Although gastric adenocarcinoma has declined significantly in the USA over the past 70 years, during the early twenty-first century an estimated 22,000 patients develop the disease each year, and of these patients, 13,000 will die, mainly because of nodal and metastatic disease present at the time of initial diagnosis. Trends in survival rates from the 1970s to the 1990s have unfortunately shown very little improvement. During the 1990s, 20% of gastric carcinoma cases were diagnosed while localized to the gastric wall, whereas 30% had evidence of regional nodal disease. Disease resulting from metastasis to other solid organs within the abdomen, as well as to extraabdominal sites, represents 35% of all cases. Although overall 5-year survival is approximately 15–20%, the 5-year survival is approximately 55% when disease is localized to the stomach (Figure 11.1). The involvement of regional nodes reduces the 5-year survival to approximately 20%.

A notable shift in the site of gastric cancer reflects a proportionate increase in disease of the proximal stomach over the past several decades. Previously, there was a predominance of distal gastric cancers presenting as mass lesions or ulceration. Although other malignancies occur in the stomach, approximately 90% of all gastric neoplasms are adenocarcinomas. Tumors of the esophagogastric junction (EGJ) may be difficult to stage as either a gastric or an esophageal primary, especially in view of the increased incidence of adenocarcinoma in the esophagus that presumably results from acid reflux disease.

## ANATOMY

**Primary Site.** The stomach is the first division of the abdominal portion of the alimentary tract, beginning at the esophagogastric junction and extending to the pylorus. The proximal stomach is located immediately below the diaphragm and is termed the cardia. The remaining portions are the fundus and body of the stomach, and the distal portion of the stomach

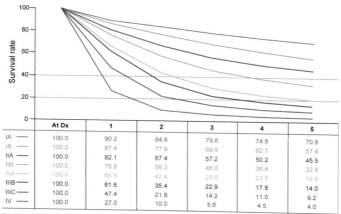

| | At Dx | 1 | 2 | 3 | 4 | 5 |
|---|---|---|---|---|---|---|
| IA — | 100.0 | 90.2 | 84.8 | 79.8 | 74.8 | 70.8 |
| IB — | 100.0 | 87.4 | 77.9 | 69.9 | 62.7 | 57.4 |
| IIA — | 100.0 | 82.1 | 67.4 | 57.2 | 50.2 | 45.5 |
| IIB — | 100.0 | 76.8 | 58.3 | 46.0 | 38.4 | 32.8 |
| IIIA — | 100.0 | 66.5 | 42.4 | 29.9 | 23.5 | 19.8 |
| IIIB — | 100.0 | 61.6 | 35.4 | 22.9 | 17.8 | 14.0 |
| IIIC — | 100.0 | 47.4 | 21.8 | 14.2 | 11.0 | 9.2 |
| IV — | 100.0 | 27.0 | 10.0 | 5.6 | 4.5 | 4.0 |

**FIGURE 11.1.** Observed survival rates for 10,601 surgically resected gastric adenocarcinomas. Data from the SEER 1973–2005 Public Use File diagnosed in years 1991–2000. Stage IA includes 1,194; Stage IB, 655; Stage IIA, 1,161; Stage IIB, 1,195; Stage IIIA, 1,031; Stage IIIB, 1,660; Stage IIIC, 1,053; and Stage IV, 6,148.

is known as the antrum. The pylorus is a muscular ring that controls the flow of food content from the stomach into the first portion of the duodenum. The medial and lateral curvatures of the stomach are known as the lesser and greater curvatures, respectively. Histologically, the wall of the stomach has five layers: mucosal, submucosal, muscular, subserosal, and serosal.

The arbitrary 10-cm segment encompassing the distal 5 cm of the esophagus and proximal 5 cm of the stomach (cardia), with the EGJ in the middle, is an area of contention. Cancers arising in this segment have been variably staged as esophageal or gastric tumors, depending on orientation of the treating physician. In this edition, cancers whose midpoint is in the lower thoracic esophagus, EGJ, or within the proximal 5 cm of the stomach (cardia) that extend into the EGJ or esophagus (Siewert III) are staged as adenocarcinoma of the esophagus (see Chap. 10). All other cancers with a midpoint in the stomach lying more than 5 cm distal to the EGJ, or those within 5 cm of the EGJ but not extending into the EGJ or esophagus, are staged using the gastric (non-EGJ) cancer staging system (Figure 11.2).

Staging of primary gastric adenocarcinoma is dependent on the depth of penetration of the primary tumor. The T1 designation has been subdivided into T1a (invasion of the lamina propria or muscularis mucosae) and T1b (invasion of the submucosa). T2 designation has been changed to invasion of the muscularis propria, and T3 to invasion of the subserosal connective tissue without invasion of adjacent structures or the serosa (visceral peritoneum). T4 tumors penetrate the serosa (T4a) or invade adjacent structures (T4b). These T categories have been changed to harmonize with those of other gastrointestinal sites.

**11**

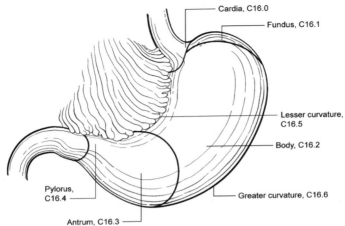

**FIGURE 11.2.** Anatomic location for subsets of gastric cancer.

**Regional Lymph Nodes.** Several groups of regional lymph nodes drain the wall of the stomach. These perigastric nodes are found along the lesser and greater curvatures. Other major nodal groups follow the main arterial and venous vessels from the aorta and the portal circulation. Adequate nodal dissection of these regional nodal areas is important to ensure appropriate designation of the pN determination. Although it is suggested that at least 16 regional nodes be assessed pathologically, a pN0 determination may be assigned on the basis of the actual number of nodes evaluated microscopically.

Involvement of other intra-abdominal lymph nodes, such as the hepatoduodenal, retropancreatic, mesenteric, and para-aortic, is classified as distant metastasis. The specific nodal areas are as follows:

*Greater Curvature of Stomach.* Greater curvature, greater omental, gastroduodenal, gastroepiploic, pyloric, and pancreaticoduodenal

*Pancreatic and Splenic Area.* Pancreaticolienal, peripancreatic, splenic

*Lesser Curvature of Stomach.* Lesser curvature, lesser omental, left gastric, cardioesophageal, common hepatic, celiac, and hepatoduodenal

*Distant Nodal Groups.* Retropancreatic, para-aortic, portal, retroperitoneal, mesenteric

**Metastatic Sites.** The most common metastatic distribution is to the liver, peritoneal surfaces, and nonregional or distant lymph nodes. Central nervous system and pulmonary metastases occur but are less frequent. With large, bulky lesions, direct extension may occur to the liver, transverse colon, pancreas, or undersurface of the diaphragm. Positive peritoneal cytology is classified as metastatic disease.

# RULES FOR CLASSIFICATION

**Clinical Staging.** Designated as cTNM, clinical staging is based on evidence of extent of disease acquired before definitive treatment is instituted. It includes physical examination, radiologic imaging, endoscopy, biopsy, and laboratory findings. All cancers should be confirmed histologically.

**Pathologic Staging.** Pathologic staging depends on data acquired clinically, together with findings on subsequent surgical exploration and examination of the pathologic specimen if resection is accomplished. Pathologic assessment of the regional lymph nodes entails their removal and histologic examination to evaluate the total number, as well as the number that contain metastatic tumor. Metastatic nodules in the fat adjacent to a gastric carcinoma, without evidence of residual lymph node tissue, are considered regional lymph node metastases, but nodules implanted on peritoneal surfaces are considered distant metastases. If there is uncertainty concerning the appropriate T, N, or M assignment, the lower (less advanced) category should be assigned, in accordance with the general rules of staging.

# PROGNOSTIC FEATURES

Treatment is a major prognostic factor for gastric cancer. Patients who are not resected have a poor prognosis, with survival ranging from 3 to 11 months. Depth of invasion into the gastric wall (T) correlates with reduced survival, but regional lymphatic spread is probably the most powerful prognostic factor. For those patients undergoing complete resection, the factors that affect prognosis include the location of the tumor in the stomach, histologic grade, and lymphovascular invasion. The prognosis for proximal gastric cancer is less favorable than for distal lesions. Asian race, female sex, and younger age are predictive of a better outcome, while high preoperative serum levels for tumor markers CEA and CA 19– 9 have been associated with a less favorable outcome.

# DEFINITIONS OF TNM

### Primary Tumor (T)

| | |
|---|---|
| TX | Primary tumor cannot be assessed |
| T0 | No evidence of primary tumor |
| Tis | Carcinoma in situ: intraepithelial tumor without invasion of the lamina propria |
| T1 | Tumor invades lamina propria, muscularis mucosae, or submucosa |
| T1a | Tumor invades lamina propria or muscularis mucosae |
| T1b | Tumor invades submucosa |
| T2 | Tumor invades muscularis propria* |
| T3 | Tumor penetrates subserosal connective tissue without invasion of visceral peritoneum or adjacent structures**,*** |

11

## Primary Tumor (T) (continued)

| | |
|---|---|
| T4 | Tumor invades serosa (visceral peritoneum) or adjacent structures**,*** |
| T4a | Tumor invades serosa (visceral peritoneum) |
| T4b | Tumor invades adjacent structures |

*Note: A tumor may penetrate the muscularis propria with extension into the gastrocolic or gastrohepatic ligaments, or into the greater or lesser omentum, without perforation of the visceral peritoneum covering these structures. In this case, the tumor is classified T3. If there is perforation of the visceral peritoneum covering the gastric ligaments or the omentum, the tumor should be classified T4.

**The adjacent structures of the stomach include the spleen, transverse colon, liver, diaphragm, pancreas, abdominal wall, adrenal gland, kidney, small intestine, and retroperitoneum.

***Intramural extension to the duodenum or esophagus is classified by the depth of the greatest invasion in any of these sites, including the stomach.

## Regional Lymph Nodes (N)

| | |
|---|---|
| NX | Regional lymph node(s) cannot be assessed |
| N0 | No regional lymph node metastasis* |
| N1 | Metastasis in 1–2 regional lymph nodes |
| N2 | Metastasis in 3–6 regional lymph nodes |
| N3 | Metastasis in seven or more regional lymph nodes |
| N3a | Metastasis in 7–15 regional lymph nodes |
| N3b | Metastasis in 16 or more regional lymph nodes |

*Note: A designation of pN0 should be used if all examined lymph nodes are negative, regardless of the total number removed and examined.

## Distant Metastasis (M)

| | |
|---|---|
| M0 | No distant metastasis |
| M1 | Distant metastasis |

## ANATOMIC STAGE/PROGNOSTIC GROUPS

| Stage 0 | Tis | N0 | M0 |
|---|---|---|---|
| Stage IA | T1 | N0 | M0 |
| Stage IB | T2 | N0 | M0 |
| | T1 | N1 | M0 |
| Stage IIA | T3 | N0 | M0 |
| | T2 | N1 | M0 |
| | T1 | N2 | M0 |
| Stage IIB | T4a | N0 | M0 |
| | T3 | N1 | M0 |
| | T2 | N2 | M0 |
| | T1 | N3 | M0 |

| Stage IIIA | T4a | N1 | M0 |
|---|---|---|---|
|  | T3 | N2 | M0 |
|  | T2 | N3 | M0 |
| Stage IIIB | T4b | N0 | M0 |
|  | T4b | N1 | M0 |
|  | T4a | N2 | M0 |
|  | T3 | N3 | M0 |
| Stage IIIC | T4b | N2 | M0 |
|  | T4b | N3 | M0 |
|  | T4a | N3 | M0 |
| Stage IV | Any T | Any N | M1 |

## PROGNOSTIC FACTORS (SITE-SPECIFIC FACTORS) (Recommended for Collection)

| Required for staging | None |
|---|---|
| Clinically significant | Tumor location |
|  | Serum carcinoembryonic antigen |
|  | Serum CA19.9 |

## HISTOLOGIC GRADE (G)

Grade is reported in registry systems by the grade value. A two-grade, three-grade, or four-grade system may be used. If a grading system is not specified, generally the following system is used:

GX   Grade cannot be assessed
G1   Well differentiated
G2   Moderately differentiated
G3   Poorly differentiated
G4   Undifferentiated

## HISTOPATHOLOGIC TYPE

The staging recommendations apply only to carcinomas. Lymphomas, sarcomas, and carcinoid tumors (well-differentiated neuroendocrine tumors) are not included. Adenocarcinomas may be divided into the general subtypes listed later. In addition, the histologic terms intestinal, diffuse, and mixed may be applied. Mixed glandular/neuroendocrine carcinomas should be staged using the gastric carcinoma staging system as described in this chapter, not the staging system for well-differentiated gastrointestinal neuroendocrine tumors.

11

The histologic subtypes are as follows:

Adenocarcinoma
Papillary adenocarcinoma
Tubular adenocarcinoma
Mucinous adenocarcinoma
Signet ring cell carcinoma

Adenosquamous carcinoma
Squamous cell carcinoma
Small cell carcinoma
Undifferentiated carcinoma

## BIBLIOGRAPHY

Abbas SM, Booth MW. Correlation between the current TNM staging and long-term survival after curative D1 lymphadenectomy for stomach cancer. Langenbecks Arch Surg. 2005;390(4):294–9.

Al-Refaie WB, Tseng JF, Gay G, et al. The impact of ethnicity on the presentation and prognosis of patients with gastric adenocarcinoma. Results from the National Cancer Data Base. Cancer. 2008;113(3):461–9.

An JY, Baik YH, Choi MG, Noh JH, Sohn TS, Kim S. Predictive factors for lymph node metastasis in early gastric cancer with submucosal invasion: analysis of a single institutional experience. Ann Surg. 2007;246:749–53.

Baxter NN, Tuttle TM. Inadequacy of lymph node staging in gastric cancer patients: a population-based study. Ann Surg Oncol. 2005;12(12):981–7.

Bentrem D, Wilton A, Mazumdar M, Brennan M, Coit D. The value of peritoneal cytology as a preoperative predictor in patients with gastric carcinoma undergoing a curative resection. Ann Surg Oncol. 2005;12(5):347–53.

de Gara CJ, Hanson J, Hamilton S. A population-based study of tumor-node relationship, resection margins, and surgeon volume on gastric cancer survival. Am J Surg. 2003;186(1):23–7.

Fenoglio-Preiser C, Arneiro F, Correa P, et al. Gastric carcinoma. In: Hamilton SR, Aaltonen LA, editors. World Health Organization classification of tumours. Pathology and genetics of tumours of the digestive system. Lyon: IARC; 2000.

Fotia G, Marrelli D, De Stefano A, Pinto E, Roviello F. Factors influencing outcome in gastric cancer involving muscularis and subserosal layer. Eur J Surg Oncol. 2004;30(9):930–4.

Kooby DA, Suriawinata A, Klimstra DS, Brennan MF, Karpeh MS. Biologic predictors of survival in node-negative gastric cancer. Ann Surg. 2003;237(6):828–35; discussion 835–7.

Nakamura Y, Yasuoka H, Tsujimoto M, et al. Importance of lymph vessels in gastric cancer: a prognostic indicator in general and a predictor for lymph node metastasis in early stage cancer. J Clin Pathol. 2006;59(1):77–82.

Parkin MD, Bray F, Ferlay J, Pisani P. Global cancer statistics, 2002. CA Cancer J Clin. 2005;55:74–108.

Pisters PWT, Kelsen DP, Powell SM, Tepper JE. Cancer of the stomach. In: DeVita VT, Hellman S, Rosenberg SA, editors. Cancer: principles and practice of oncology. 7th ed. Philadelphia, PA: Lippincott Williams & Wilkins; 2005.

Rohatgi PR, Mansfield PF, Crane CH, et al. Surgical pathology stage by American Joint Commission on Cancer criteria predicts patient survival after preoperative chemoradiation for localized gastric carcinoma. Cancer. 2006;107(7):1475–82.

Siewert JR, Stein HJ. Classification of adenocarcinoma of the oesophagogastric junction. Br J Surg. 1998;85:1457–9.

Smith DD, Schwarz RR, Schwarz RE. Impact of total lymph node count on staging and survival after gastrectomy for gastric cancer: data from a large US-population database. J Clin Oncol. 2005;23(28):7114–24.

Talamonti MS, Kim SP, Yao KA, et al. Surgical outcomes of patients with gastric carcinoma: the importance of primary tumor location and microvessel invasion. Surgery. 2003;134(4):720–7.

# Small Intestine

*(Lymphomas, carcinoid tumors, and visceral
sarcomas are not included)*

## At-A-Glance

---

### SUMMARY OF CHANGES

- T1 lesions have been divided into T1a (invasion of lamina propria) and T1b (invasion of submucosa) to facilitate comparison with tumors of other gastrointestinal sites

- Stage II has been subdivided into Stage IIA and Stage IIB

- The N1 category has been changed to N1 (1–3 positive lymph nodes) and N2 (four or more positive lymph nodes), leading to the division of Stage III into Stage IIIA and Stage IIIB

---

### ANATOMIC STAGE/PROGNOSTIC GROUPS

| | | | |
|---|---|---|---|
| Stage 0 | Tis | N0 | M0 |
| Stage I | T1 | N0 | M0 |
| | T2 | N0 | M0 |
| Stage IIA | T3 | N0 | M0 |
| Stage IIB | T4 | N0 | M0 |
| Stage IIIA | Any T | N1 | M0 |
| Stage IIIB | Any T | N2 | M0 |
| Stage IV | Any T | Any N | M1 |

**ICD-O-3 TOPOGRAPHY CODES**

| | |
|---|---|
| C17.0 | Duodenum |
| C17.1 | Jejunum |
| C17.2 | Ileum |
| C17.8 | Overlapping lesion of small intestine |
| C17.9 | Small intestine, NOS |

**ICD-O-3 HISTOLOGY CODE RANGES**
8000–8152, 8154–8231, 8243–8245, 8250–8576, 8940–8950, 8980–8981

## INTRODUCTION

Although the small intestine accounts for one of the largest surface areas in the human body, it is one of the least common cancer sites in the digestive system, accounting for less than 2% of all malignant tumors of the gastrointestinal tract. A variety of tumors occur in the small intestine, with approximately 25–50% of the primary malignant tumors being adenocarcinomas, depending upon the population surveyed. At the beginning of the twenty-first century, approximately 5,600 new cases of cancer involving the small intestine are seen annually in the USA. The 1,100 deaths predicted to occur from small intestinal cancer are divided almost equally between men and women. Over 60% of tumors occur in the duodenum, followed by jejunum (20%) and ileum (15%). An increased incidence of second malignancies has been noted in patients with primary small bowel adenocarcinoma, a finding related in part to the significantly increased risk for this malignancy in patients with hereditary nonpolyposis colorectal cancer. Crohn's disease and celiac disease are also associated with an increased risk for small intestinal carcinomas and lymphomas.

The patterns of local, regional, and metastatic spread for adenocarcinomas of the small intestine are comparable to those of similar histologic malignancies in other areas of the gastrointestinal tract. The classification and stage grouping described in this chapter are used for both clinical and pathologic staging of carcinomas of the small bowel and do not apply to other types of malignant small bowel tumors. Well-differentiated neuroendocrine tumors (carcinoid tumors) arising in the small intestine are staged according to the system described in Chap. 17.

## ANATOMY

**Primary Site.** This classification applies to carcinomas arising in the duodenum, jejunum, and ileum. It does not apply to carcinomas arising in the ileocecal valve or to carcinomas that may arise in Meckel's diverticulum. Carcinomas arising in the ampulla of Vater are staged according to the system described in Chap. 23.

**Duodenum.** About 25 cm in length, the duodenum extends from the pyloric sphincter of the stomach to the jejunum. It is usually divided anatomically into four parts, with the common bile duct and pancreatic duct opening into the second part at the ampulla of Vater.

**Jejunum and Ileum.** The jejunum (8 ft in length) and ileum (12 ft in length) extend from the junction with the duodenum proximally to the ileocecal valve distally. The division point between the jejunum and the ileum is arbitrary. As a general rule, the jejunum includes the proximal 40% and the ileum includes the distal 60% of the small intestine, exclusive of the duodenum.

**General.** The jejunal and ileal portions of the small intestine are supported by a fold of the peritoneum containing the blood supply and the regional lymph nodes, the mesentery. The shortest segment, the duodenum, has no real mesentery and is covered only by peritoneum anteriorly. The wall of all parts of the small intestine has five layers: mucosal, submucosal, muscular, subserosal, and serosal. A very thin layer of smooth muscle cells, the muscularis mucosae, separates the mucosa from the submucosa. The small intestine is entirely ensheathed by peritoneum, except for a narrow strip of bowel that is attached to the mesentery and that part of the duodenum that is located retroperitoneally.

**Regional Lymph Nodes.** For pN, histologic examination of a regional lymphadenectomy specimen will ordinarily include a representative number of lymph nodes distributed along the mesenteric vessels extending to the base of the mesentery. Histologic examination of a regional lymph-adenectomy specimen will ordinarily include six or more lymph nodes. If the lymph nodes are negative, but the number ordinarily examined is not met, pN0 should be assigned. The number of lymph nodes sampled and the number of involved lymph nodes should be recorded.

*Duodenum*
> Duodenal
> Hepatic
> Pancreaticoduodenal
> Infrapyloric
> Gastroduodenal
> Pyloric
> Superior mesenteric
> Pericholedochal
> Regional lymph nodes, NOS

*Ileum and Jejunum*
> Cecal (terminal ileum only)
> Ileocolic (terminal ileum only)
> Superior mesenteric
> Mesenteric, NOS
> Regional lymph nodes, NOS

**Metastatic Sites.** Cancers of the small intestine can metastasize to most organs, especially the liver, or to the peritoneal surfaces. Involvement of regional lymph nodes and invasion of adjacent structures are most common. Involvement of the celiac nodes is considered M1 disease for carcinomas of the duodenum, jejunum, and ileum. The presence of distant metastases and the presence of residual disease (R) have the most influence on survival.

## RULES FOR CLASSIFICATION

**Clinical Staging.** Imaging studies such as CT and MRI play a major role in clinical staging. Metastatic disease is assessed by routine chest films and chest CT. Intraoperative assessment plays a role in clinical evaluation, especially when tumor cannot be resected. Metastatic involvement of the liver may be evaluated by intraoperative ultrasonography.

**Pathologic Staging.** The primary tumor is staged according to its depth of penetration and the involvement of adjacent structures or distant sites. Lateral spread within the duodenum, jejunum, or ileum is not considered in this classification. Only the depth of tumor penetration in the bowel wall and spread to other structures defines the pT stage.

Although the two are similar, differences between this staging system and that of the colon should be noted. In the colon, pTis applies to intra-epithelial (in situ) as well as to intramucosal lesions. In the small intestine, intramucosal spread is listed as pT1 instead of pTis. In this regard, the pT1 definition for the small bowel is essentially the same as the pT1 defined for stomach lesions. Invasion through the wall is classified the same as for colon

**12**

cancer. Discontinuous hematogenous metastases or peritoneal metastases are coded as M1.

## PROGNOSTIC FEATURES

The anatomic extent of the tumor is the strongest indicator of outcome when the tumor can be resected. Prognosis after incomplete removal or for those patients who do not undergo cancer-directed surgery is poor. The presence of Crohn's disease and patients' age greater than 75 years are also associated with poorer outcome.

The pathologic extent of tumor, in terms of the depth of invasion through the bowel wall, is a significant prognostic factor, as is regional lymphatic spread. Histologic grade has not emerged as a significant predictor of outcome in multivariate analysis. There are insufficient data to assess the impact of other more sophisticated pathologic factors and serum tumor markers, but it is logical to believe that the effect of those factors would be similar to that observed with colorectal cancer.

## DEFINITIONS OF TNM

### Primary Tumor (T)

| | |
|---|---|
| TX | Primary tumor cannot be assessed |
| T0 | No evidence of primary tumor |
| Tis | Carcinoma in situ |
| T1a | Tumor invades lamina propria |
| T1b | Tumor invades submucosa* |
| T2 | Tumor invades muscularis propria |
| T3 | Tumor invades through the muscularis propria into the subserosa or into the nonperitonealized perimuscular tissue (mesentery or retroperitoneum) with extension 2 cm or less* |
| T4 | Tumor perforates the visceral peritoneum or directly invades other organs or structures (includes other loops of small intestine, mesentery, or retroperitoneum more than 2 cm, and abdominal wall by way of serosa; for duodenum only, invasion of pancreas or bile duct) |

*Note: The nonperitonealized perimuscular tissue is, for jejunum and ileum, part of the mesentery and, for duodenum in areas where serosa is lacking, part of the interface with the pancreas.

### Regional Lymph Nodes (N)

| | |
|---|---|
| NX | Regional lymph nodes cannot be assessed |
| N0 | No regional lymph node metastasis |
| N1 | Metastasis in 1–3 regional lymph nodes |
| N2 | Metastasis in four or more regional lymph nodes |

### Distant Metastasis (M)

| | |
|---|---|
| M0 | No distant metastasis |
| M1 | Distant metastasis |

## ANATOMIC STAGE/PROGNOSTIC GROUPS

| | | | |
|---|---|---|---|
| Stage 0 | Tis | N0 | M0 |
| Stage I | T1 | N0 | M0 |
| | T2 | N0 | M0 |
| Stage IIA | T3 | N0 | M0 |
| Stage IIB | T4 | N0 | M0 |
| Stage IIIA | Any T | N1 | M0 |
| Stage IIIB | Any T | N2 | M0 |
| Stage IV | Any T | Any N | M1 |

## PROGNOSTIC FACTORS (SITE-SPECIFIC FACTORS)
### (Recommended for Collection)

| | |
|---|---|
| Required for staging | None |
| Clinically significant | Presurgical carcinoembryonic antigen (CEA) |
| | Microsatellite instability (MSI) |
| | Presence of Crohn's disease |

Figure 12.1 shows observed 5-year survival rates for adenocarcinoma of the small intestine.

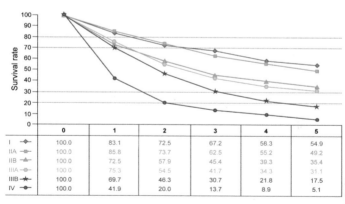

| | 0 | 1 | 2 | 3 | 4 | 5 |
|---|---|---|---|---|---|---|
| I | 100.0 | 83.1 | 72.5 | 67.2 | 58.3 | 54.9 |
| IIA | 100.0 | 85.8 | 73.7 | 62.5 | 55.2 | 49.2 |
| IIB | 100.0 | 72.5 | 57.9 | 45.4 | 39.3 | 35.4 |
| IIIA | 100.0 | 75.3 | 54.5 | 41.7 | 34.3 | 31.1 |
| IIIB | 100.0 | 69.7 | 46.3 | 30.7 | 21.8 | 17.5 |
| IV | 100.0 | 41.9 | 20.0 | 13.7 | 8.9 | 5.1 |

Years from diagnosis

**FIGURE 12.1.** Observed survival rates for 3,086 cases with adenocarcinoma of the small intestine. Data from the National Cancer Data Base (Commission on Cancer of the American College of Surgeons and the American Cancer Society) diagnosed in years 1998–2002. Stage I includes 328; Stage IIA, 685; Stage IIB, 304; Stage IIIA, 715; Stage IIIB, 328; and Stage IV, 726.

12

## HISTOLOGIC GRADE (G)

Grade is reported in registry systems by the grade value. A two-grade, three-grade, or four-grade system may be used. If a grading system is not specified, generally the following system is used:

GX     Grade cannot be assessed
G1     Well differentiated
G2     Moderately differentiated
G3     Poorly differentiated
G4     Undifferentiated

## HISTOPATHOLOGIC TYPE

This staging classification applies only to carcinomas, including mixed carcinoma/well-differentiated neuroendocrine tumors, arising in the small intestine. Lymphomas, pure carcinoid tumors, and visceral sarcomas are not included. The three major histopathologic types are carcinomas (such as adenocarcinoma), well-differentiated neurodendocrine tumors (carcinoid tumors), and lymphomas. Primary lymphomas of the small intestine are staged as extranodal lymphomas. Neuroendocrine tumors (carcinoid tumors) of the small intestine are staged as described in Chap. 17; size, depth of invasion, regional lymph node status, and distant metastasis are considered significant prognostic factors. Less common malignant tumors include gastrointestinal stromal tumors and leiomyosarcoma. The malignant GIST lesions are classified using TNM nomenclature as described in Chap. 16.

## BIBLIOGRAPHY

Dabaja BS, Suki D, Pro B, Bonnen M, Ajani J. Adenocarcinoma of the small bowel: presentation, prognostic factors, and outcome of 217 patients. Cancer. 2005;101:518–26.

Hatzaras I, Palesty JA, Abir F, Sullivan P, Kozol RA, Dudrick SJ, et al. Small-bowel tumors: epidemiologic and clinical characteristics of 1260 cases from the Connecticut tumor registry. Arch Surg. 2007;142:229–35.

Howe JR, Karnell LH, Menck HR, Scott-Conner C. Adenocarcinoma of the small bowel: review of the National Cancer Data Base, 1985–1995. Cancer. 1999;86:2693–706.

Jemal A, Siegel R, Ward E, Murray T, Xu J, Thun MJ. Cancer statistics, 2007. CA Cancer J Clin. 2007;57:43–66.

Jess T, Loftus EV Jr, Velayos FS, et al. Risk of intestinal cancer in inflammatory bowel disease: a population-based study from Olmsted County, Minnesota. Gastroenterology. 2006;130:1039–46.

Schulmann K, Brasch FE, Kunstmann E, et al. HNPCC-associated small bowel cancer: clinical and molecular characteristics. Gastroenterology. 2005;128:590–9.

Ugurlu M, Asoglu O, Potter DD, Barnes SA, Harmsen WS, Donohue JH. Adenocarcinoma of the jejunum and ileum: a 25-year experience. J Gastrointest Surg. 2005;9:1182–8.

Verma D, Stroehlein JR. Adenocarcinoma of the small bowel: a 60-yr perspective derived from M. D. Anderson Cancer Center tumor registry. Am J Gastroenterol. 2006;101:1647–54.

Zeh HJ III. Cancer of the small intestine. In: DeVita VT, Hellman S, Rosenberg SA, editors. Cancer: principles and practice of oncology. Philadelphia, PA: Lippincott-Raven; 2005. p. 1035–49.

12

# Appendix

*(Carcinomas and carcinoid tumors of the appendix
are included, but separately categorized)*

## *At-A-Glance*

---

### SUMMARY OF CHANGES

**Appendiceal Carcinomas**

- In the seventh edition, appendiceal carcinomas are separately classified. In the sixth edition, appendiceal carcinomas were classified according to the definitions for colorectal tumors

- Appendiceal carcinomas are now separated into mucinous and non-mucinous types. Histologic grading is considered of particular importance for mucinous tumors. This is reflected in the staging considerations for metastatic tumors. The change is based on published data and analysis of NCDB data

- In the seventh edition, the T4 category is divided into T4a and T4b as in the colon and is reflected in the subdivision of Stage II

- M1 is divided into M1a and M1b where pseudomyxoma peritonei, M1a, is separated from nonperitoneal metastasis, M1b

- Regional lymph node metastasis is unchanged from the sixth edition, in contrast to the subdivision of N for colorectal tumors, as there are no data justifying such a division for the appendiceal tumors. Therefore, Stage III for the appendix is unchanged from the sixth edition

- In the seventh edition, Stage IV is subdivided on the basis of N, M, and G status, unlike colorectal carcinomas

- Clinically significant prognostic factors are identified for collection in cancer registries including pretreatment CEA and CA 19.9, the number of tumor deposits in the mesentery, and where available, the presence of Microsatellite instability and 18q loss of heterozygosity

**Appendiceal Carcinoids**

- A new classification is added for carcinoid tumors that were not classified previously by TNM. This is a new classification. There are substantial differences between the classification schemes of appendiceal carcinomas and carcinoids and between appendiceal carcinoids and other well-differentiated gastrointestinal neuroendocrine tumors (carcinoids) (see chapters of the digestive system for staging of other gastrointestinal carcinoids)

- Serum chromogranin A is identified as a significant prognostic factor

---

## ANATOMIC STAGE/PROGNOSTIC GROUPS

*Carcinoma*

| Stage | | | | |
|---|---|---|---|---|
| Stage 0 | Tis | N0 | M0 | |
| Stage I | T1 | N0 | M0 | |
| | T2 | N0 | M0 | |
| Stage IIA | T3 | N0 | M0 | |
| Stage IIB | T4a | N0 | M0 | |
| Stage IIC | T4b | N0 | M0 | |
| Stage IIIA | T1 | N1 | M0 | |
| | T2 | N1 | M0 | |
| Stage IIIB | T3 | N1 | M0 | |
| | T4 | N1 | M0 | |
| Stage IIIC | Any T | N2 | M0 | |
| Stage IVA | Any T | N0 | M1a | G1 |
| Stage IVB | Any T | N0 | M1a | G2, 3 |
| | Any T | N1 | M1a | Any G |
| | Any T | N2 | M1a | Any G |
| Stage IVC | Any T | Any N | M1b | Any G |

*Carcinoid*

| Stage | | | |
|---|---|---|---|
| Stage I | T1 | N0 | M0 |
| Stage II | T2, T3 | N0 | M0 |
| Stage III | T4 | N0 | M0 |
| | Any T | N1 | M0 |
| Stage IV | Any T | Any N | M1 |

ICD-O-3
TOPOGRAPHY
CODES
C18.1     Appendix

ICD-O-3 HISTOLOGY
CODE RANGES
8000–8576, 8940–8950,
8980–8981

# INTRODUCTION

**Carcinoma.** Mucinous adenocarcinomas are a major form of appendiceal carcinoma. Metastasis limited to the peritoneal cavity is a particular form of spread of these tumors. Mucinous appendiceal carcinomas and cystadenocarcinomas make up about 50% of appendiceal adenocarcinoma (vs. 10% of colonic carcinomas). The 5-year survival of appendiceal mucinous carcinomas with distant metastasis is around 40–50% (vs. 10% for other appendiceal carcinomas), justifying separation of mucinous from nonmucinous adenocarcinomas and division of M1 into M1a and M1b, the former being amenable to debulking surgery.

Mucinous appendiceal carcinoma with peritoneal involvement limited to the right lower quadrant is much less aggressive than tumor that has gone beyond the RLQ, justifying a T4 designation rather than M1. Grading of mucinous adenocarcinomas is important even when assessing pseudomyxoma peritonei as low-grade tumors may be indolent despite extensive involvement of the peritoneum.

Goblet cell carcinoids are classified according to the criteria of adenocarcinomas because their behavior appears closer to them rather than to appendiceal carcinoids.

**Carcinoid Tumor.** Appendiceal carcinoid tumors, though neuroendocrine in nature, are separately classified because of their greater frequency, variety of subtypes, and behavioral differences compared with other gastrointestinal tract neuroendocrine tumors. Separate staging criteria for appendiceal carcinoids are needed because appendiceal carcinoids have no apparent in situ state, may arise in deep mucosa or submucosa, and the tumor size is considered more important than depth of invasion as a major criterion of aggressiveness for a localized tumor.

## ANATOMY

**Primary Site.** The appendix is a tubular structure that arises from the base of the cecum. Its length varies but is about 10 mm. It is connected to the ileal mesentery by the mesoappendix, through which its blood supply passes from the ileocolic artery.

**Regional Lymph Nodes.** Lymphatic drainage passes into the ileocolic chain of lymph nodes.

**Metastatic Sites.** Mucinous adenocarcinomas commonly spread along the peritoneal surfaces even in the absence of lymph node metastasis. The pattern of spread of nonmucinous adenocarcinomas, in contrast, resembles cecal (colonic) tumors. Appendiceal carcinoids also tend to spread, like cecal tumors, to regional lymph nodes and the liver. Goblet cell carcinoids appear to have a predilection for metastasis to ovary.

## RULES FOR CLASSIFICATION

**Clinical Staging.** Clinical assessment is based on medical history, physical examination, and imaging. Examinations designed to demonstrate the presence of extra-appendiceal metastasis (M) include chest films, computed tomography (CT; abdomen, pelvis, chest), magnetic resonance imaging (MRI), and PET (positron emission tomography) or fused PET/CT scans. In cases of carcinoids, determination of elevated urinary 5-HIAA may indicate liver metastasis.

**Pathologic Staging.** *Appendiceal carcinomas* are usually staged after surgical exploration of the abdomen and pathologic examination of the resected specimen.

T4 lesions are subdivided into T4a (tumor penetrates the visceral peritoneum) and T4b (tumor directly invades other organs or structures).

**13**

Mucinous peritoneal tumor within the right lower quadrant is considered T4a; peritoneal spread beyond the right lower quadrant, including pseudomyxoma peritonei, is classified M1a.

Histological grading, particularly of mucinous tumors (those with over 50% of the tumor mass consisting of extracellular mucus) is needed to separate stages IVA and IVB tumors.

Lymph nodes are classified N1 or N2 according to the number involved with metastatic tumor. Involvement of 1–3 nodes is pN1, and the presence of four or more nodes involved with tumor metastasis is considered pN2.

A satellite peritumoral nodule or tumor deposit (TD) in the periappendiceal adipose tissue of a primary carcinoma without histologic evidence of residual lymph node in the nodule may represent discontinuous spread (T3), venous invasion with extravascular spread (T3, V1/2), or a totally replaced lymph node (N1/2). Replaced nodes should be counted as positive nodes while discontinuous spread or venous invasion should be counted in the site-specific factor TD.

Histological examination of a regional lymphadenectomy specimen ordinarily includes 12 or more lymph nodes. If the resected lymph nodes are negative, but the number of 12 nodes ordinarily examined is not met, the case should still be classified as pN0.

*Appendiceal carcinoids* are usually staged after laparoscopic or open surgical exploration of the abdomen (often for appendicitis) and pathologic examination of the resected specimen.

Classical carcinoid (well-differentiated neuroendocrine tumor), including tubular carcinoid, and atypical carcinoids (well-differentiated neuroendocrine carcinomas), a type seen much more commonly in the lung than in the appendix, also should be separately staged (a mitotic count of 2–10 per 10 hpf and focal necrosis are features of atypical carcinoids).

Goblet cell carcinoids are classified according to the criteria for adenocarcinomas because their behavior appears closer to them than to appendiceal carcinoids.

Lymph nodes with carcinoid are classified N1 regardless of the number of nodes involved.

**Restaging.** For either appendiceal carcinomas or carcinoid tumors, the *r* prefix is used for recurrent tumor status (rTNM) following a disease-free interval posttreatment.

## PROGNOSTIC FEATURES

**Carcinoma.** Appendiceal mucinous carcinomas that spread to the peritoneum have a much better prognosis than nonmucinous tumors (Figure 13.1). Mucus that has spread beyond the right lower quadrant is a poor prognostic factor as is the presence of epithelial cells in the peritoneal cavity outside the appendix. Poor prognosis in pseudomyxoma peritonei is associated with high histological grade and/or invasion deep to the peritoneal surface. Debulking of peritoneal mucus can prolong survival, particularly in low-grade tumors. Cytological and DNA flow cytometry studies

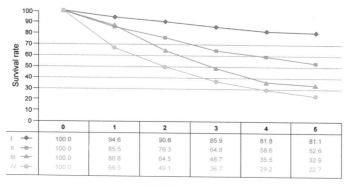

| | 0 | 1 | 2 | 3 | 4 | 5 |
|---|---|---|---|---|---|---|
| I | 100.0 | 94.6 | 90.6 | 85.9 | 81.8 | 81.1 |
| II | 100.0 | 85.5 | 76.3 | 64.8 | 58.6 | 52.6 |
| III | 100.0 | 86.8 | 64.5 | 48.7 | 35.5 | 32.9 |
| IV | 100.0 | 66.5 | 49.1 | 36.7 | 29.2 | 22.7 |

Years from diagnosis

**FIGURE 13.1.** Observed survival rates for 931 cases with carcinoma of the appendix. Data from the SEER 1973–2005 Public Use File diagnosed in years 1991–2000. Stage I includes 150; Stage II, 369; Stage III, 76; and Stage IV, 346.

on aspirated mucus in pseudomyxoma peritonei cases are not helpful for prognostic purposes.

**Carcinoid.** There is controversy about the prognostic significance of mesoappendiceal invasion by a carcinoid. Tumor size appears to be the dominant local criterion for aggressive behavior. Neural invasion is commonly seen in appendiceal carcinoids and does not appear to have prognostic significance. Tubular carcinoids are typically indolent. Goblet cell carcinoids are considered more aggressive than are other appendiceal carcinoids and are classified according to the criteria for appendiceal carcinomas (see previous discussion). They tend to grow in a concentric manner along the longitudinal axis of the appendix without appearing as an easily measurable tumor mass and may even extend imperceptively into the cecum. Therefore, the line of resection is very important in assessing residual tumor. The carcinoid syndrome is typically associated with carcinoids that are metastatic to the liver. An elevated level of serum chromogranin A is considered a poor prognostic indicator for patients with metastatic carcinoid.

## DEFINITIONS OF TNM

### Carcinoma

| *Primary Tumor (T)* | |
|---|---|
| TX | Primary tumor cannot be assessed |
| T0 | No evidence of primary tumor |
| Tis | Carcinoma in situ: intraepithelial or invasion of lamina propria* |
| T1 | Tumor invades submucosa |
| T2 | Tumor invades muscularis propria |
| T3 | Tumor invades through muscularis propria into subserosa or into mesoappendix |

**13**

| | |
|---|---|
| T4 | Tumor penetrates visceral peritoneum, including mucinous peritoneal tumor within the right lower quadrant and/or directly invades other organs or structures**,*** |
| T4a | Tumor penetrates visceral peritoneum, including mucinous peritoneal tumor within the right lower quadrant |
| T4b | Tumor directly invades other organs or structures |

*Tis includes cancer cells confined within the glandular basement membrane (intraepithelial) or lamina propria (intramucosal) with no extension through muscularis mucosae into submucosa.

**Direct invasion in T4 includes invasion of other segments of the colorectum by way of the serosa, e.g., invasion of ileum.

***Tumor that is adherent to other organs or structures, grossly, is classified cT4b. However, if no tumor is present in the adhesion, microscopically, the classification should be pT1-3 depending on the anatomical depth of wall invasion.

### Regional Lymph Nodes (N)

| | |
|---|---|
| NX | Regional lymph nodes cannot be assessed |
| N0 | No regional lymph node metastasis |
| N1 | Metastasis in 1–3 regional lymph nodes |
| N2 | Metastasis in four or more regional lymph nodes |

*Note*: A satellite peritumoral nodule or tumor deposit (TD) in the periappendiceal adipose tissue of a primary carcinoma without histologic evidence of residual lymph node in the nodule may represent discontinuous spread (T3), venous invasion with extravascular spread (T3, V1/2), or a totally replaced lymph node (N1/2). Replaced nodes should be counted as positive nodes while discontinuous spread or venous invasion should be counted in the site-specific factor TD.

### Distant Metastasis (M)

| | |
|---|---|
| M0 | No distant metastasis |
| M1 | Distant metastasis |
| M1a | Intraperitoneal metastasis beyond the right lower quadrant, including pseudomyxoma peritonei |
| M1b | Nonperitoneal metastasis |

*pTNM Pathologic Classification.* The pT, pN, and pM categories correspond to the T, N, and M categories.

*pN0.* Histological examination of a regional lymphadenectomy specimen will ordinarily include 12 or more lymph nodes. If the lymph nodes are negative, but the number ordinarily examined is not met, classify as pN0.

**Carcinoid**

### Primary Tumor (T)

| | |
|---|---|
| TX | Primary tumor cannot be assessed |
| T0 | No evidence of primary tumor |
| T1 | Tumor 2 cm or less in greatest dimension |
| T1a | Tumor 1 cm or less in greatest dimension |
| T1b | Tumor more than 1 cm but not more than 2 cm |
| T2 | Tumor more than 2 cm but not more than 4 cm or with extension to the cecum |
| T3 | Tumor more than 4 cm or with extension to the ileum |
| T4 | Tumor directly invades other adjacent organs or structures, e.g., abdominal wall and skeletal muscle* |

*Note*: Tumor that is adherent to other organs or structures, grossly, is classified cT4. However, if no tumor is present in the adhesion, microscopically, the classification should be classified pT1-3 depending on the anatomical depth of wall invasion.

*Penetration of the mesoappendix does not seem to be as important a prognostic factor as the size of the primary tumor and is not separately categorized.

### Regional Lymph Nodes (N)

| | |
|---|---|
| NX | Regional lymph nodes cannot be assessed |
| N0 | No regional lymph node metastasis |
| N1 | Regional lymph node metastasis |

### Distant Metastasis (M)

| | |
|---|---|
| M0 | No distant metastasis |
| M1 | Distant metastasis |

**pTNM Pathologic Classification.** The pT, pN, and pM categories correspond to the T, N, and M categories except that pM0 does not exist as a category.

**pN0.** Histological examination of a regional lymphadenectomy specimen will ordinarily include 12 or more lymph nodes. If the lymph nodes are negative, but the number ordinarily examined is not met, classify as pN0.

### ANATOMIC STAGE/PROGNOSTIC GROUPS

*Carcinoma*

| | | | |
|---|---|---|---|
| Stage 0 | Tis | N0 | M0 |
| Stage I | T1 | N0 | M0 |
| | T2 | N0 | M0 |
| Stage IIA | T3 | N0 | M0 |
| Stage IIB | T4a | N0 | M0 |
| Stage IIC | T4b | N0 | M0 |

**13**

*Carcinoma*

| | | | | |
|---|---|---|---|---|
| Stage IIIA | T1 | N1 | M0 | |
| | T2 | N1 | M0 | |
| Stage IIIB | T3 | N1 | M0 | |
| | T4 | N1 | M0 | |
| Stage IIIC | Any T | N2 | M0 | |
| Stage IVA | Any T | N0 | M1a | G1 |
| Stage IVB | Any T | N0 | M1a | G2, 3 |
| | Any T | N1 | M1a | Any G |
| | Any T | N2 | M1a | Any G |
| Stage IVC | Any T | Any N | M1b | Any G |

## PROGNOSTIC FACTORS (SITE-SPECIFIC FACTORS)
### (Recommended for Collection)

| | |
|---|---|
| Required for staging | Grade |
| Clinically significant | Preoperative/pretreatment carcinoembryonic antigen (CEA) |
| | Preoperative/pretreatment CA 19-9 |
| | Tumor deposits (TD) |
| | Microsatellite instability (MSI) |
| | 18q Loss of Heterozygosity (LOH) |

ANATOMIC STAGE/PROGNOSTIC GROUPS

*Carcinoid*

| | | | |
|---|---|---|---|
| Stage I | T1 | N0 | M0 |
| Stage II | T2, T3 | N0 | M0 |
| Stage III | T4 | N0 | M0 |
| | Any T | N1 | M0 |
| Stage IV | Any T | Any N | M1 |

## PROGNOSTIC FACTORS (SITE-SPECIFIC FACTORS)
### (Recommended for Collection)

| | |
|---|---|
| Required for staging | None |
| Clinically significant | Serum chromogranin A |

## HISTOLOGIC GRADE (G)

**Carcinoma**

| | | |
|---|---|---|
| GX | Grade cannot be assessed | |
| G1 | Well differentiated | Mucinous low grade |
| G2 | Moderately differentiated | Mucinous high grade |
| G3 | Poorly differentiated | Mucinous high grade |
| G4 | Undifferentiated | |

Histologic grading, particularly of mucinous tumors (those with over 50% of the tumor consisting of extracellular mucus) is needed to separate stages IVA and IVB.

**Carcinoid.** Histologic grading is not carried out for carcinoid tumors, but a mitotic count of 2–10 per 10 hpf and/or focal necrosis are features of atypical carcinoids (well-differentiated neuroendocrine carcinomas), a type seen much more commonly in the lung than in the appendix.

Goblet cell carcinoids are classified according to the carcinoma scheme.

## HISTOPATHOLOGIC TYPE

**Carcinoma.** This staging classification applies to carcinomas that arise in the appendix. The histologic types include the following:

Adenocarcinoma in situ*
Adenocarcinoma
Medullary carcinoma
Mucinous carcinoma (colloid type) (greater than 50% mucinous carcinoma)
Signet ring cell carcinoma (greater than 50% signet ring cell)
Squamous cell (epidermoid) carcinoma
Adenosquamous carcinoma
Small cell carcinoma
Undifferentiated carcinoma
Carcinoma, NOS

*The term "high-grade dysplasia" may be used as a synonym for in situ carcinoma. These cases should be assigned pTis.

**Carcinoid.** This staging classification applies to carcinoids that arise in the appendix. The histologic types include the following:

Carcinoid tumor
Well-differentiated neuroendocrine tumor
Tubular carcinoid
Goblet cell carcinoid
Adenocarcinoid
Atypical carcinoid

Well-differentiated neuroendocrine carcinoma after resection (relevant to resection margins that are macroscopically involved by tumor)

## RESIDUAL TUMOR (R)

### Carcinoma and Carcinoid

R0    Complete resection, margins histologically negative; no residual tumor left after resection

**13**

| R1 | Incomplete resection, margins histologically involved, microscopic tumor remains after resection of gross disease (relevant to resection margins that are microscopically involved by tumor) |
| R2 | Incomplete resection, margins involved or gross disease remains |

## BIBLIOGRAPHY

Anderson JR, Wilson BG. Carcinoid tumours of the appendix. Br J Surg. 1985;72: 545–6.

Anderson NH, Somerville JE, Johnston CF, et al. Appendiceal goblet cell carcinoids: a clinicopathological and immunohistochemical study. Histopathology. 1991;18:61–5.

Bradley RF, Stewart JH IV, Russell GB, Levine EA, Geisinger KR. Pseudomyxoma peritonei of appendiceal origin: a clinicopathologic analysis of 101 patients uniformly treated at a single institution, with literature review. Am J Surg Pathol. 2006;30:551–9.

Burke AP, Sobin LH, Federspiel BH, et al. Appendiceal carcinoids: correlation of histology and immunohistochemistry. Mod Pathol. 1989;2:630–7.

Burke AP, Sobin LH, Federspiel BH, et al. Goblet cell carcinoids and related tumors of the appendix. Am J Clin Pathol. 1990;94:27–35.

Butler JA, Houshiar A, Lin F, et al. Goblet cell carcinoid of the appendix. Am J Surg. 1994;168:685–7.

Capella C, Solcia E, Sobin LH, Arnold R. Endocrine tumours of the appendix. In: Hamilton SR, Aaltonen LA, editors. World Health Organization classification of tumors. Pathology and genetics of tumors of the digestive system. Lyon: IARC; 2000. p. 99–101.

Carr NJ, Sobin LH. Neuroendocrine tumors of the appendix. Semin Diagn Pathol. 2004;21:108–19.

Carr NJ, McCarthy WF, Sobin LH. Epithelial noncarcinoid tumors and tumor-like lesions of the appendix. A clinicopathologic study of 184 cases with a multivariate analysis of prognostic factors. Cancer. 1995;75:757–68.

Carr NJ, Arends MJ, Deans GT, Sobin LH. Adenocarcinoma of the appendix. In: Hamilton SR, Aaltonen LA, editors. World Health Organization classification of tumors. Pathology and genetics of tumors of the digestive system. Lyon: IARC; 2000. p. 95–8.

Costa MJ. Pseudomyxoma peritonei. Histological predictors of patient survival. Arch Pathol Lab Med. 1994;118:1215–9.

Goddard MJ, Lonsdale RN. The histogenesis of appendiceal carcinoid tumours. Histopathology. 1992;20:345–9.

Gough DB, Donohue JH, Schutt AJ, et al. Pseudomyxoma peritonei. Long-term patient survival with an aggressive regional approach. Ann Surg. 1994;219: 112–9.

Hinson FL, Ambrose NS. Pseudomyxoma peritonei. Br J Surg. 1998;85:1332–9.

McCusker ME, Coté TR, Clegg LX, Sobin LH. Primary malignant neoplasms of the appendix: a population-based study from the surveillance, epidemiology and end-results program, 1973–1998. Cancer. 2002;94:3307–12.

Misdraji J, Yantiss RK, Graeme-Cook FM, et al. Appendiceal mucinous neoplasms: a clinicopathologic analysis of 107 cases. Am J Surg Pathol. 2003;27:1089–103.

Moertel CG, Weiland LH, Nagorney DM, et al. Carcinoid tumor of the appendix: treatment and prognosis. N Engl J Med. 1987;317:1699–701.

Park K, Blessing K, Kerr K, et al. Goblet cell carcinoid of the appendix. Gut. 1990;31:322–4.

Roggo A, Wood WC, Ottinger LW. Carcinoid tumors of the appendix. Ann Surg. 1993;217:385–90.

Rossi G, Valli R, Bertolini F, et al. Does mesoappendix infiltration predict a worse prognosis in incidental neuroendocrine tumors of the appendix? Am J Clin Pathol. 2003;120:706–11.

Smith JW, Kemeny N, Caldwell C, et al. Pseudomyxoma peritonei of appendiceal origin. The Memorial Sloan Kettering Cancer Center experience. Cancer. 1992;70:396–401.

Sugarbaker PH, Alderman R, Edwards G, et al. Prospective morbidity and mortality assessment of cytoreductive surgery plus perioperative intraperitoneal chemotherapy to treat peritoneal dissemination of appendiceal mucinous malignancy. Ann Surg Oncol. 2006;13:635–44.

Talbot IC, Ritchie S, Leighton MH, et al. The clinical significance of invasion of veins by rectal cancer. Br J Surg. 1980;67:439–42.

Talbot IC, Ritchie S, Leighton MH, et al. Spread of rectal cancer within veins: histologic features and clinical significance. Am J Surg. 1981;141:15–7.

Tepper JE, O'Connell MJ, Niedzwiecki D, et al. Impact of number of nodes retrieved on outcome in patients with rectal cancer. J Clin Oncol. 2001;19:157–63.

Thomas RM, Sobin LH. Gastrointestinal cancer: incidence and prognosis by histologic type. SEER population-based data: 1973–1987. Cancer. 1995;75:154–70.

Wong JH, Severino R, Honnebier MB, et al. Number of nodes examined and staging accuracy in colorectal carcinoma. J Clin Oncol. 1999;17:2896–900.

Yan TD, Bijelic L, Sugarbaker PH. Critical analysis of treatment failure after complete cytoreductive surgery and perioperative intraperitoneal chemotherapy for peritoneal dissemination from appendiceal mucinous neoplasms. Ann Surg Oncol. 2007;14:2289–99.

13

# Colon and Rectum

*(Sarcomas, lymphomas, and carcinoid tumors
of the large intestine are not included)*

## *At-A-Glance*

### SUMMARY OF CHANGES

- In the sixth edition, Stage II was subdivided into IIA and IIB on the basis of whether the primary tumor was T3N0 or T4N0, respectively, and Stage III was subdivided into IIIA (T1-2N1M0), IIIB (T3-4N1M0), or IIIC (any TN2M0). In the seventh edition, further substaging of Stage II and III has been accomplished, based on survival and relapse data that was not available for the prior edition

- Expanded data sets have shown differential prognosis within T4 lesions based on extent of disease. Accordingly T4 lesions are subdivided as T4a (Tumor penetrates the surface of the visceral peritoneum) and as T4b. (Tumor directly invades or is histologically adherent to other organs or structures)

- The potential importance of satellite tumor deposits is now defined by the new site-specific factor Tumor Deposits (TD) that describe their texture and number. T1-2 lesions that lack regional lymph node metastasis but have tumor deposit(s) will be classified in addition as N1c

- The number of nodes involved with metastasis influences prognosis within both N1 and N2 groups. Accordingly N1 will be subdivided as N1a (metastasis in 1 regional node) and N1b (metastasis in 2–3 nodes), and N2 will be subdivided as N2a (metastasis in 4–6 nodes) and N2b (metastasis in 7 or more nodes)

- Stage Group II is subdivided into IIA (T3N0), IIB (T4aN0) and IIC (T4bN0)

- Stage Group III:

  - A category of N1 lesions, T4bN1, that was formerly classified as IIIB was found to have outcomes more akin to IIIC and has been reclassified from IIIB to IIIC

  - Similarly, several categories of N2 lesions formerly classified as IIIC have outcomes more akin to other stage groups; therefore, T1N2a has been reclassified as IIIA and T1N2b, T2N2a-b, and T3N2a have all been reclassified as IIIB

- M1 has been subdivided into M1a for single metastatic site vs. M1b for multiple metastatic sites

## ANATOMIC STAGE/PROGNOSTIC GROUPS

| Stage | T | N | M | Dukes* | MAC* |
|-------|---|---|---|--------|------|
| 0 | Tis | N0 | M0 | – | – |
| I | T1 | N0 | M0 | A | A |
|  | T2 | N0 | M0 | A | B1 |
| IIA | T3 | N0 | M0 | B | B2 |
| IIB | T4a | N0 | M0 | B | B2 |
| IIC | T4b | N0 | M0 | B | B3 |
| IIIA | T1–T2 | N1/N1c | M0 | C | C1 |
|  | T1 | N2a | M0 | C | C1 |
| IIIB | T3–T4a | N1/N1c | M0 | C | C2 |
|  | T2–T3 | N2a | M0 | C | C1/C2 |
|  | T1–T2 | N2b | M0 | C | C1 |
| IIIC | T4a | N2a | M0 | C | C2 |
|  | T3–T4a | N2b | M0 | C | C2 |
|  | T4b | N1–N2 | M0 | C | C3 |
| IVA | Any T | Any N | M1a | – | – |
| IVB | Any T | Any N | M1b | – | – |

*Note*: cTNM is the clinical classification, pTNM is the pathologic classification. The y prefix is used for those cancers that are classified after neoadjuvant pretreatment (e.g., ypTNM). Patients who have a complete pathologic response are ypT0N0cM0 that may be similar to Stage Group 0 or I. The r prefix is to be used for those cancers that have recurred after a disease-free interval (rTNM).

*Dukes B is a composite of better (T3 N0 M0) and worse (T4 N0 M0) prognostic groups, as is Dukes C (Any TN1 M0 and Any T N2 M0). MAC is the modified Astler-Coller classification.

### ICD-O-3 TOPOGRAPHY CODES

| | |
|---|---|
| C18.0 | Cecum |
| C18.2 | Ascending colon |
| C18.3 | Hepatic flexure of colon |
| C18.4 | Transverse colon |
| C18.5 | Splenic flexure of colon |
| C18.6 | Descending colon |
| C18.7 | Sigmoid colon |
| C18.8 | Overlapping lesion of colon |
| C18.9 | Colon, NOS |
| C19.9 | Rectosigmoid junction |
| C20.9 | Rectum, NOS |

### ICD-O-3 HISTOLOGY CODE RANGES

8000–8152, 8154–8231, 8243–8245, 8250–8576, 8940–8950, 8980–8981

## INTRODUCTION

The TNM classification for carcinomas of the colon and rectum provides more detail than other staging systems. Compatible with the Dukes' system, the TNM adds greater precision in the identification of prognostic subgroups. TNM staging is based on the depth of tumor invasion into or beyond the wall of the colorectum (T), invasion of or adherence to adjacent organs or structures (T), the number of regional lymph nodes involved (N), and the presence or absence of distant metastasis (M). The TNM classification applies to both clinical and pathologic staging. Most cancers of the colon and many cancers of the rectum are staged after pathologic examination of a resected specimen. However, patients with high-risk rectal cancers are commonly receiving preoperative adjuvant treatment prior to surgical resection and pathological stage annotation should employ the y prefix in such cases. This staging system applies to all carcinomas arising in the colon or rectum. Adenocarcinomas of the vermiform appendix are classified according to the TNM staging system for appendix (see Chap. 13), whereas cancers that occur in the anal canal are staged according to the classification used for the anus (see Chap. 15). Well-differentiated neuroendocrine carcinomas (carcinoid tumors) of the colorectum are classified according to the TNM staging system for gastric, small bowel, and colonic and rectal carcinoid tumors (well-differentiated neuroendocrine tumors and well-differentiated neuroendocrine carcinomas) as described in Chap. 17.

## ANATOMY

The divisions of the colon and rectum are as follows:

Cecum
Ascending colon
Hepatic flexure
Transverse colon
Splenic flexure
Descending colon
Sigmoid colon
Rectosigmoid junction
Rectum

**Primary Site.** The large intestine (colorectum) extends from the terminal ileum to the anal canal. Excluding the rectum and vermiform appendix, the colon is divided into four parts: the right or ascending colon, the middle or transverse colon, the left or descending colon, and the sigmoid colon. The sigmoid colon is continuous with the rectum which terminates at the anal canal.

The cecum is a large, blind pouch that arises from the proximal segment of the right colon. It measures 6–9 cm in length and is covered with a visceral peritoneum (serosa). The ascending colon measures 15–20 cm in length. The posterior surface of the ascending (and descending) colon lacks peritoneum and thus is in direct contact with the retroperitoneum. In contrast, the anterior and lateral surfaces of the ascending (and descending) colon have serosa and are intraperitoneal. The hepatic flexure connects the ascending colon with the transverse colon, passing just inferior to the liver and anterior to the duodenum.

The transverse colon is entirely intraperitoneal, supported on a mesentery that is attached to the pancreas. Anteriorly, its serosa is continuous with the gastrocolic ligament. The splenic flexure connects the transverse colon to the descending colon, passing inferior to the spleen and anterior to the tail of the pancreas. As noted above, the posterior aspect of the descending colon lacks serosa and is in direct contact with the retroperitoneum, whereas the lateral and anterior surfaces have serosa and are intraperitoneal. The descending colon measures 10–15 cm in length. The colon becomes completely intraperitoneal once again at the sigmoid colon, where the mesentery develops at the medial border of the left posterior major psoas muscle and extends to the rectum. The transition from sigmoid colon to rectum is marked by the fusion of the taenia of the sigmoid colon to the circumferential longitudinal muscle of the rectum. This occurs roughly 12–15 cm from the dentate line.

Approximately 12 cm in length, the rectum extends from the fusion of the taenia to the puborectalis ring. The rectum is covered by peritoneum in front and on both sides in its upper third and only on the anterior wall in its middle third. The peritoneum is reflected laterally from the rectum to form the perirectal fossa and, anteriorly, the uterine or rectovesical fold. There is no peritoneal covering in the lower third, which is often known as the rectal ampulla.

The anal canal, which measures 3–5 cm in length, extends from the superior border of the puborectalis sling to the anal verge. The superior border of the puborectalis sling is the proximal portion of the palpable anorectal ring on digital rectal examination and is approximately 1–2 cm proximal to the dentate line.

**Regional Lymph Nodes.**  Regional nodes are located (1) along the course of the major vessels supplying the colon and rectum, (2) along the vascular arcades of the marginal artery, and (3) adjacent to the colon – that is, located along the mesocolic border of the colon. Specifically, the regional lymph nodes are the pericolic and perirectal nodes and those found along the ileocolic, right colic, middle colic, left colic, inferior mesenteric artery, superior rectal (hemorrhoidal), and internal iliac arteries.

In the assessment of pN, the number of lymph nodes sampled should be recorded. The number of nodes examined from an operative specimen has been reported to be associated with improved survival, possibly because of increased accuracy in staging. It is important to obtain at least 10–14 lymph nodes in radical colon and rectum resections in patients without neoadjuvant therapy, but in cases in which tumor is resected for palliation or in patients who have received preoperative radiation, fewer lymph nodes may be removed or present. In all cases, however, it is essential that the total number of regional lymph nodes recovered from the resection specimen be described since that number is prognostically important (Tables 14.1–14.7; Figures 14.1 and 14.2; see section "Prognostic Features"). A pN0 determination is assigned when these nodes are histologically negative, even though fewer than the recommended number of nodes has been analyzed. However, when fewer than the number of nodes recommended by the College of American Pathologists (CAP) have been found, it is important that the pathologist report the degree of diligence of their efforts to find lymph nodes in the specimen.

**TABLE 14.1.** Impact of node and tumor category on survival and relapse: Rectal cancer pooled analysis 1[a]

| Category | Overall survival[a] | | | Disease-free survival[a] | | | Local recurrence[b] | | Distant metastasis[b] | |
|---|---|---|---|---|---|---|---|---|---|---|
| | No. | 5-Year (%) | p Value | No. | 5-Year (%) | p Value | 5-Year (%) | p Value | 5-Year (%) | p Value |
| N0T3 | 668 | 74 | 0.046 | 664 | 66 | 0.05 | 8 | 0.04 | 19 | 0.04 |
| T4 | 95 | 65 | | 95 | 54 | | 15 | | 28 | |
| N1T1-2 | 225 | 81 | <0.001 | 225 | 74 | <0.001 | 6 | 0.002 | 15 | <0.001 |
| T3 | 544 | 61 | | 536 | 50 | | 11 | | 34 | |
| T4 | 59 | 33 | | 59 | 30 | | 22 | | 39 | |
| N2T1-2 | 180 | 69 | <0.001 | 180 | 62 | <0.001 | 8 | 0.14 | 26 | <0.001 |
| T3 | 663 | 48 | | 659 | 39 | | 15 | | 45 | |
| T4 | 84 | 38 | | 84 | 30 | | 19 | | 50 | |

Modified from Gunderson LL, Sargent DJ, Tepper JE, et al. Impact of T and N substage on survival and disease relapse in adjuvant rectal cancer: A pooled analysis. Int J Radiat Oncol Biol Phys. 2002;54:386–96, with permission of Elsevier.

[a] Unadjusted Kaplan–Meier survival estimates.

[b] Cumulative incidence rates.

14

**TABLE 14.2.** Impact of node and tumor category on survival and relapse: US GI Intergroup 0144

| Category | Overall survival[a] | | | Disease-free survival[b] | | | Local recurrence[b] | | Distant metastasis[b] | |
|---|---|---|---|---|---|---|---|---|---|---|
| | No. | 5-Year (%) | p Value | No. | 5-Year (%) | p Value | 5-Year (%) | p Value | 5-Year (%) | p Value |
| N0T3 | 503 | 86 | 0.14 | 503 | 79 | 0.25 | 4 | 0.77 | 12 | 0.66 |
| T4 | 45 | 71 | | 45 | 64 | | 7 | | 18 | |
| N1T1-2 | 223 | 82 | <0.001 | 223 | 75 | <0.001 | 5 | 0.035 | 18 | 0.002 |
| T3 | 482 | 67 | | 482 | 57 | | 10 | | 31 | |
| T4 | 40 | 63 | | 40 | 55 | | 13 | | 25 | |
| N2T1-2 | 83 | 69 | <0.001 | 83 | 62 | <0.001 | 5 | 0.009 | 30 | 0.02 |
| T3 | 403 | 48 | | 403 | 39 | | 11 | | 49 | |
| T4 | 33 | 36 | | 33 | 24 | | 24 | | 42 | |

Modified from Smalley SR, et al. Phase III trial of fluorouracil-based chemotherapy regimens plus radiotherapy in postoperative adjuvant rectal cancer: GI INT 0144. J Clin Oncol. 2006;24:3542–7, with permission of ASCO; updated Aug (2007) by Benedetti J, et al., Personal communication.

[a] Unadjusted Kaplan–Meier survival estimates.

[b] Cumulative incidence rates.

**TABLE 14.3.** Survival and relapse rates by risk for relapse category: Rectal cancer pooled analysis[1]

| Risk for relapse | Stage[a] TN | Stage[a] MAC | Survival, 5-year[b] OS (%) | Survival, 5-year[b] DFS (%) | Relapse Local (%) | Relapse Distant (%) | Stage Dukes[d] | Stage TNM[c] |
|---|---|---|---|---|---|---|---|---|
| Low[d] | T1N0 | A | ~90 | ~90 | ≤5 | ~10 | A | I |
| | T2N0 | B1 | ~90 | ~90 | ≤5 | ~10 | A | II |
| Intermediate | T1-2N1 | C1 | 81 | 74 | 6 | 15 | C | IIIA |
| | T3N0 | B2 | 74 | 66 | 8 | 19 | B | II |
| Moderately high | T1-2N2 | C1 | 69 | 62 | 8 | 26 | C | IIIC |
| | T4N0 | B3 | 65 | 54 | 15 | 28 | B | IIB |
| | T3N1 | C2 | 61 | 50 | 11 | 34 | C | IIIB |
| High | T3N2 | C2 | 48 | 39 | 15 | 45 | C | IIIC |
| | T4N1 | C3 | 33 | 30 | 22 | 39 | C | IIIB |
| | T4N2 | C3 | 38 | 30 | 19 | 50 | C | IIIC |

Modified from Gunderson LL, Sargent DJ, Tepper JE, et al. Impact of T and N substage on survival and disease relapse in adjuvant rectal cancer: a pooled analysis. Int I Radiat Oncol Biol Phys. 2002;54:386–96, with permission of Elsevier.

[a] Stage of disease based on surgical and pathological findings at the time of resection.

[b] Survival – Unadjusted Kaplan–Meier estimates; OS overall survival and DFS disease-free survival.

[c] AJCC 6th edition.

[d] Data derived from prior publications, as low-risk patients were not eligible for the three phase III trials in the pooled analysis.

**TABLE 14.4.** Rectal cancer: Changes in AJCC substaging for stage III

| Category[a] | Pooled Analysis #1 Survival, 5-year(%)[b] | | US GI INT 0144 Survival, 5-year(%)[c] | | TNM stage 6th ed | TNM stage 7th ed[d] | SEER[e] Survival, 5-year relative (%) | Survival, 5-year observed (%) |
|---|---|---|---|---|---|---|---|---|
| TN | OS | DFS | OS | DFS | | | | |
| T1-2N0 | – | – | – | – | I | I | 93.6 | 77.6 |
| T3N0 | 74 | 66 | 86 | 79 | IIA | IIA | 78.7 | 64.0 |
| T4N0 | 65 | 54 | 71 | 64 | IIB | IIB | 61.6 | 50.5 |
| T1-2N1 | 81 | 74 | 82 | 75 | IIIA | IIIA | 85.1 | 72.1 |
| T1-2N2 | 69 | 62 | 69 | 62 | IIIC | **IIIB** | 64.9 | 56.1 |
| T3N1 | 61 | 50 | 67 | 57 | IIIB | IIIB | 63.1 | 52.4 |
| T3N2 | 48 | 39 | 48 | 39 | IIIC | IIIC | 44.1 | 37.5 |
| T4N1 | 33 | 30 | 63 | 55 | IIIB | **IIIC** | 44.9 | 37.4 |
| T4N2 | 38 | 30 | 36 | 24 | IIIC | IIIC | 31.2 | 26.4 |

Bold print and gray screen indicate change from AJCC 6th edition.

[a] Stage of disease based on surgical and pathological findings at the time of resection.

[b] Modified from Gunderson LL, Sargent D), Tepper JE, et al. Int J Radiat Oncol Biol Phys. 2002;54:386-96.

[c] Modified from Smalley SR, et al. J Clin Oncol. 2006;24:3542-7, with permission of ASCO; updated Aug (2007) by Benedetti J, et al., Personal communication.

[d] Change in substaging of Stage III (bold type and gray-screened items) based on outcomes in Rectal Pooled Analyses, INT 0144, SEER data.

[e] SEER relative and observed survival data; modified from Gunderson LL, Jessup JM, Sargent D, et al. J Clin Oncol, in press.

**TABLE 14.5.** Rectal cancer: Expanded changes in AJCC substaging for stage II and III based on expanded SEER data

| Category | SEER | | | | SEER | |
|---|---|---|---|---|---|---|
| TN | Relative Survival, 5-year (%) | SE% | TNM stage, 6th ed | TNM stage, 7th ed[a] | Observed Survival, 5-year (%) | SE (%) |
| T1N0 | 96.6 | 0.9 | I | I | 81.4 | 0.8 |
| T2N0 | 92.1 | 0.7 | I | I | 75.7 | 0.6 |
| T3N0 | 78.7 | 0.7 | IIA | IIA | 64.0 | 0.5 |
| T4aN0 | 69.2 | 2.4 | IIB | IIB | 55.7 | 1.9 |
| T4bN0 | 53.6 | 2.5 | IIB | IIC | 44.7 | 2.1 |
| T1-2N1 | 85.1 | 1.4 | IIIA | IIIA | 72.1 | 1.2 |
| T1N2a | 82.7 | 7.0 | IIIC | IIIA | 73.8 | 6.2 |
| T2N2a[b] | 67.7 | 4.0 | IIIC | IIIB | 58.2 | 3.4 |
| T3N1a | 66.9 | 1.4 | IIIB | IIIB | 55.4 | 1.1 |
| T4aN1a | 65.6 | 4.6 | IIIB | IIIB | 53.2 | 3.7 |
| T3N1b | 59.7 | 1.3 | IIIB | IIIB | 49.7 | 1.1 |
| T1N2b | 59.3 | 14.6 | IIIC | IIIB | 53.2 | 13.0 |
| T4aN2a[c] | 53.1 | 4.8 | IIIC | IIIC | 44.3 | 4.0 |
| T4aN1b | 52.6 | 4.1 | IIIB | IIIB | 43.9 | 3.4 |
| T3N2a | 49.9 | 1.5 | IIIC | IIIB | 42.5 | 1.3 |
| T2N2b | 46.2 | 5.8 | IIIC | IIIB | 41.7 | 5.0 |
| T3N2b | 37.5 | 1.5 | IIIC | IIIC | 32.0 | 1.3 |

*continued*

14

**TABLE 14.5.** Rectal cancer: Expanded changes in AJCC substaging for stage II and III based on expanded SEER data (continued)

| Category | SEER | | | | SEER | |
|---|---|---|---|---|---|---|
| TN | Relative Survival, 5-year (%) | SE% | TNM stage, 6th ed | TNM stage, 7th ed[a] | Observed Survival, 5-year (%) | SE (%) |
| T4aN2b | 28.5 | 4.0 | IIIC | IIIC | 24.5 | 3.4 |
| **T4bN1** | 28.5 | 2.9 | IIIB | **IIIC** | 24.3 | 2.5 |
| T4bN2a | 22.1 | 4.3 | IIIC | IIIC | 18.5 | 3.6 |
| T4bN2b | 14.1 | 4.0 | IIIC | IIIC | 12.3 | 3.5 |

Bold print and gray screen indicate change from AJCC 6th edition.

[a]Change in substaging of stages II/III (bold type and gray-screened items) based on expanded outcomes in SEER data analyses.

[b]T2N2a rectal lesions did worse than colon T2N2a lesions, both categories placed in Stage IIIB.

[c]T4aN2a rectal lesions did better than colon T4aN2a lesions, both categories placed in Stage IIIC.

**TABLE 14.6.** Colon cancer: Changes in AJCC substaging for stage III

| Category[a] | SEER[b] | | | | SEER[b] | NCDB[d] |
|---|---|---|---|---|---|---|
| TN | Survival, 5-year Relative | TNM stage 6th ed | | TNM stage 7th ed[c] | Survival, 5-year Observed | Survival, 5-year Observed |
| T1-2N0 | 97.1 | I | | I | 76.3 | 71 |
| T3N0 | 87.5 | IIA | | IIA | 66.7 | 61.5 |
| T4N0 | 71.5 | IIB | | IIB | 55.0 | 47 |
| T1-2N1 | 87.7 | IIIA | | IIIA | 71.1 | 67.4 |
| **T1-2N2** | 75.0 | IIIC | | **IIIB** | 61.5 | 51.2 |
| T3N1 | 68.7 | IIIB | | IIIB | 54.9 | 53.1 |
| T3N2 | 47.3 | IIIC | | IIIC | 38.1 | 37.3 |
| **T4N1** | 50.5 | IIIB | | **IIIC** | 39.6 | 34.1 |
| T4N2 | 27.1 | IIIC | | IIIC | 21.7 | 22.4 |

Bold print and gray screen indicate change from AJCC 6th edition.

[a] Stage of disease based on surgical and pathological findings at the time of resection.

[b] SEER relative and observed survival data; modified from Gunderson LL, Jessup JM, Sargent D, et al. J. Clin Oncol., in press.

[c] Change in substaging of stage III (bold type and gray-screened items) based on outcomes in SEER and NCDB data analyses.

[d] NCDB observed survival; Modified from Stewart A, Greene R. Personal communication, May 2007.

The regional lymph nodes for each segment of the large bowel are designated as follows:

| Segment | Regional Lymph Nodes |
|---|---|
| Cecum | Pericolic, anterior cecal, posterior cecal, ileocolic, right colic |
| Ascending colon | Pericolic, ileocolic, right colic, middle colic |
| Hepatic flexure | Pericolic, middle colic, right colic |
| Transverse colon | Pericolic, middle colic |
| Splenic flexure | Pericolic, middle colic, left colic, inferior mesenteric |
| Descending colon | Pericolic, left colic, inferior mesenteric, sigmoid |
| Sigmoid colon | Pericolic, inferior mesenteric, superior rectal (hemorrhoidal), sigmoidal, sigmoid mesenteric |
| Rectosigmoid | Pericolic, perirectal, left colic, sigmoid mesenteric, sigmoidal, inferior mesenteric, superior rectal (hemorrhoidal), middle rectal (hemorrhoidal) |
| Rectum | Perirectal, sigmoid mesenteric, inferior mesenteric, lateral sacral presacral, internal iliac, sacral promontory, internal iliac, superior rectal (hemorrhoidal), middle rectal (hemorrhoidal), inferior rectal (hemorrhoidal) |

**Metastatic Sites.** Although carcinomas of the colon and rectum can metastasize to almost any organ, the liver and lungs are most commonly affected. Seeding of other segments of the colon, small intestine, or peritoneum also can occur.

**TABLE 14.7.** Colon cancer: Expanded changes in AJCC substaging for stage II and III based on expanded SEER data

| Category[a] TN | SEER Relative Survival, 5-year | SE | TNM Stage, 6th ed | TNM stage, 7th ed[b] | SEER Observed Survival, 5-year | SE |
|---|---|---|---|---|---|---|
| T1N0 | 97.4 | 0.6 | I | I | 78.7 | 0.5 |
| T2N0 | 96.8 | 0.6 | I | I | 74.3 | 0.4 |
| T3N0 | 87.5 | 0.4 | IIA | IIA | 66.7 | 0.3 |
| T4aN0 | 79.6 | 1.0 | IIB | IIB | 60.6 | 0.8 |
| **T4bN0** | 58.4 | 1.3 | IIB | **IIC** | 45.7 | 1.0 |
| T1-2N1a | 90.7 | 1.5 | IIIA | IIIA | 73.7 | 1.2 |
| T1-2N1b | 83.0 | 2.0 | IIIA | IIIA | 67.2 | 1.6 |
| **T1-2N2a**[a] | 79.0 | 3.6 | IIIC | **IIIA/IIIB**[a] | 64.7 | 3.0 |
| T3N1a | 74.2 | 0.8 | IIIB | IIIB | 58.2 | 0.6 |
| T4aN1a | 67.6 | 2.0 | IIIB | IIIB | 52.2 | 1.5 |
| T3N1b | 65.3 | 0.8 | IIIB | IIIB | 51.7 | 0.6 |
| **T1-2N2b** | 62.4 | 6.5 | IIIC | **IIIB** | 51.8 | 5.3 |
| T4aN1b | 54.0 | 1.9 | IIIB | IIIB | 42.1 | 1.5 |
| **T3N2a** | 53.4 | 1.0 | IIIC | **IIIB** | 42.8 | 0.8 |
| T4aN2a[c] | 40.9 | 2.1 | IIIC | IIIC | 32.5[c] | 1.7 |
| T3N2b | 37.3 | 1.2 | IIIC | IIIC | 30.4 | 0.9 |
| **T4bN1a** | 38.5 | 2.2 | IIIB | **IIIC** | 30.6 | 1.8 |
| **T4bN1b** | 31.2 | 2.0 | IIIB | **IIIC** | 25.4 | 1.6 |
| T4bN2a | 23.3 | 2.1 | IIIC | IIIC | 18.3 | 1.6 |
| T4aN2b | 21.8 | 2.2 | IIIC | IIIC | 17.5 | 1.7 |
| T4bN2b | 15.7 | 1.9 | IIIC | IIIC | 12.9 | 1.5 |

Bold print and gray screen indicate change from AJCC 6th edition.

[a] T2N2a colon lesions did better than rectal T2N2a (both categories placed in stage IIIB).

[b] Change in substaging of stages II/III (bold type and gray-screened items) based on expanded outcomes in SEER data analyses.

[c] T4aN2a colon lesions did worse than rectal T4aN2a (both categories placed in Stage IIIC).

## RULES FOR CLASSIFICATION

**Clinical Staging.** Clinical assessment is based on medical history, physical examination, sigmoidoscopy, and colonoscopy with biopsy. Examinations designed to demonstrate the presence of extrarectal or extracolonic metastasis (M) may include chest radiographic films, computed tomography (CT; abdomen, pelvis, chest), magnetic resonance imaging (MRI), and positron emission tomography (PET) or fused PET/CT scans.

For patients with rectal cancer, the pelvic extent of disease (TN categories) combined with the absence of extrapelvic metastasis (M) determines whether or not preoperative adjuvant treatment is appropriate. The primary imaging modalities to assess the preoperative pelvic extent of disease are endoscopic ultrasound (EUS), pelvic CT, and pelvic MRI alone or with endorectal coil. To improve the accuracy of nodal staging, EUS may be augmented with fine-needle aspiration of lymph nodes suspicious for metastasis. It is especially important that patients who will receive preoperative adjuvant treatment should be assigned a clinical stage based on disease extent prior to the initiation of treatment (cTNM).

**Pathologic Staging.** Most cancers of the colon and many cancers of the rectum are pathologically staged after surgical exploration of the abdomen, cancer-directed surgical resection, and pathologic examination of the resected specimen (pTNM). For patients who were given a clinical stage (cTNM) prior to initiating preoperative adjuvant treatment, a modified pathologic stage is generated after surgical resection annotated by the y prescript (ypTNM).

The definition of in situ carcinoma – pTis – includes cancer cells confined within the glandular basement membrane (intraepithelial) or lamina propria (intramucosal) with no extension through the muscularis mucosae

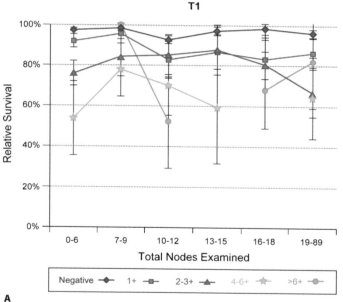

**A**

**FIGURE 14.1.** (A–E) Interaction among T and N classifications and total nodes examined on 5-year survival in colon cancer. Relative survival for pT1-4 by N1a (1 positive node), N1b (2–3 positive nodes), N2a (4–6 positive nodes), and N2b (7 or more positive nodes) on 171,006 patients, SEER analysis. The effect of the total number of nodes examined is categorized along the abscissa. Relative survival increases for most combinations of T and N classification as the number of nodes examined increases. Data are mean ± standard error of the mean 5-year survival for each data point (From ssp://seerstat.cancer. gov:2038).

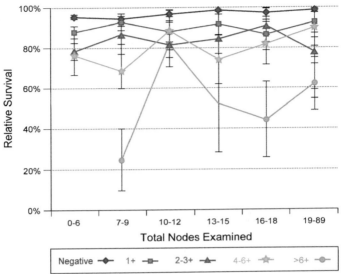

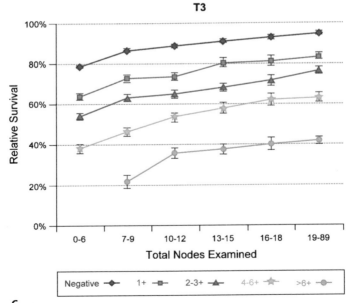

**C**

**FIGURE 14.1.** (Continued)

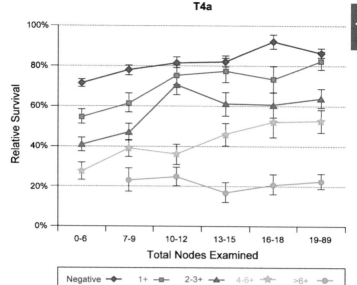

**D**

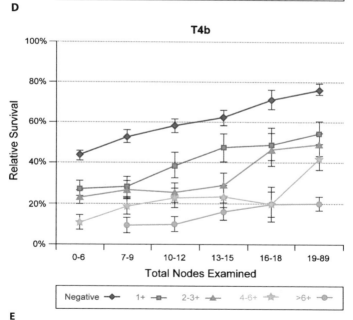

**E**

**FIGURE 14.1.** (Continued)

into the submucosa. Neither intraepithelial nor intramucosal carcinomas of the large intestine are associated with risk for metastasis.

Carcinoma in a polyp is classified according to the pT definitions adopted for colorectal carcinomas. For instance, carcinoma that is limited to the lamina propria is classified as pTis, whereas tumor that has invaded through the muscularis mucosae and entered the submucosa of the polyp head or stalk is classified as pT1.

Tumor that has penetrated the visceral peritoneum as a result of direct extension through the wall and subserosa of the colon or proximal rectum is assigned to the pT4 category, as is tumor that directly invades or is histologically adherent to other organs or structures, whether or not it penetrates a serosal surface. For both colon and rectum, expanded data sets have shown different outcomes for tumors within the pT4 category based on extent of disease (see section "Prognostic Factors"; Tables 14.4–14.7). Therefore, T4 lesions have been subdivided into pT4a (tumor penetrates to the surface of the visceral peritoneum) and pT4b (tumor directly invades or is adherent to other organs or structures). Tumors that clinically appear

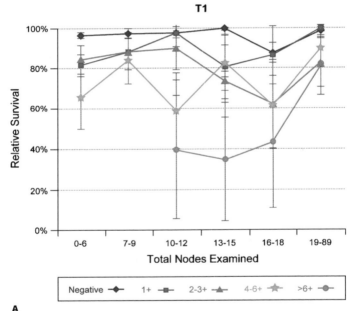

**A**

**FIGURE 14.2.** (A–E) Interaction among T and N classifications and total nodes examined on 5-year survival in rectal cancer. Relative survival for pT1-4 by N1a (1 positive node), N1b (2–3 positive nodes), N2a (4–6 positive nodes) and N2b (7 or more positive nodes) on 70,131 patients, SEER analysis. The effect of the total number of nodes examined is categorized along the abscissa. Relative survival increases for most combinations of T and N classification as the number of nodes examined increases. Data are mean ± standard error of the mean 5-year survival for each data point (From ssp://seerstat.cancer.gov:2038).

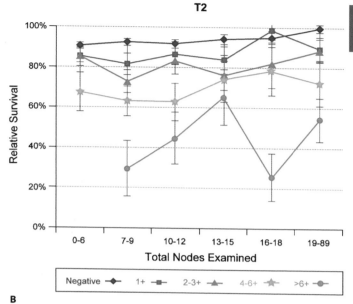

**B**

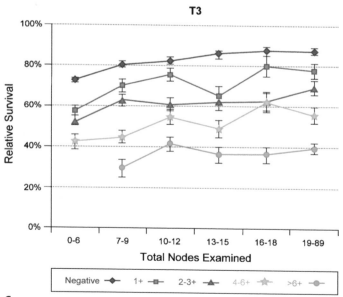

**C**

**FIGURE 14.2.** (Continued)

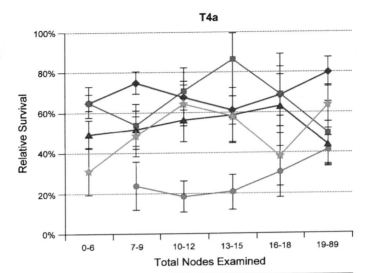

**T4a**

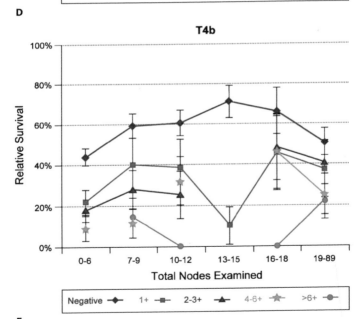

**T4b**

E

**FIGURE 14.2.** (Continued)

adherent to another organ or structure should be resected en bloc as standard of practice. However, if on microscopic review the adhesion is secondary to inflammation and the carcinoma does not actually involve the adjacent structure or organ, then the lesion is classified as either pT3 or pT4a, as appropriate.

Regional lymph nodes are classified as N1 or N2 according to the number involved by metastatic tumor. Involvement of 1–3 nodes by metastasis is pN1; involvement of 4 or more nodes by tumor metastasis is pN2. The number of nodes involved with metastasis influences outcome within both the N1 and the N2 groups (see section "Prognostic Features"; Tables 14.1–14.7; Figures 14.1 and 14.2). Accordingly pN1 has been subdivided into pN1a (metastasis in 1 regional lymph node) and pN1b (metastasis in 2–3 regional lymph nodes), and pN2 has been subdivided into pN2a (metastasis in 4–6 regional lymph nodes) and pN2b (metastasis in 7 or more regional lymph nodes).

Discrete foci of tumor found in the pericolic or perirectal fat or in adjacent mesentery (mesocolic fat) away from the leading edge of the tumor and showing no evidence of residual lymph node tissue but within the lymph drainage area of the primary carcinoma are considered to be peritumoral deposits or satellite nodules, and their number should be recorded in the site-specific Prognostic Markers on the staging form as Tumor Deposits (TD). Such tumor deposits may represent discontinuous spread, venous invasion with extravascular spread (V1/2), or a totally replaced lymph node (N1/2). If tumor deposits are observed in lesions that would otherwise be classified as T1 or T2, then the primary tumor classification is not changed, but the nodule is recorded in the TD category and as a N1c positive node.

Metastasis to only one site (e.g., liver, lung, ovary, nonregional node) should be recorded as M1a. Metastasis to multiple sites or the peritoneal surface is M1b. The absence of metastasis in any specific site or sites examined pathologically is not pM0. The designation of M0 should never be assigned by the pathologist, because M0 is a global designation referring to the absence of detectable metastasis anywhere in the body. Therefore, "pM0" would connote pathological documentation of the absence of distance metastasis throughout the body, a determination that could only be made at autopsy (and would be annotated as aM0).

If the tumor recurs at the site of surgery, it is anatomically assigned to the proximal segment of the anastomosis (unless that segment is the small intestine, in which case the colonic or rectal segment should be designated as appropriate) and restaged by the TNM classification. The r prefix is used for the recurrent tumor stage (rTNM).

## PROGNOSTIC FEATURES

Seven new prognostic factors that are clinically significant are included for collection, in addition to the prior notation of serum CEA levels. The new site-specific factors include: tumor deposits (TD, the number of satellite tumor deposits discontinuous from the leading edge of the carcinoma and that lack evidence of residual lymph node); a tumor regression grade that enables the pathologic response to neoadjuvant therapy to be graded, the circumferential resection margin (CRM, measured in mm from the edge of tumor to the nearest dissected margin of the surgical resection); microsatellite instability (MSI), an important but controversial prognostic factor especially for colon cancer; and perineural invasion (PN, histologic evidence of invasion of regional nerves) that may have a similar prognosis as lymphovascular invasion. KRAS mutation status will also be collected since recent analyses indicate that mutation in KRAS is associated with lack of response to treatment with monoclonal antibodies directed against the epidermal growth factor receptor (EGFR) in patients with metastatic colorectal carcinoma. The 18q LOH assay has been validated, and there is work to qualify this as a prognostic marker that would suggest the need for adjuvant therapy in stage II colon cancer.

**Tumor Regression Grade.** The pathologic response to preoperative adjuvant treatment should be recorded according to the CAP guidelines for recording the tumor regression grade (see CAP Protocol for the examination of Specimens from Patients with Carcinomas of the Colon and Rectum) because neoadjuvant chemoradiation in rectal cancer is often associated with significant tumor response and down-staging. Although the data are not definitive, complete eradication of the tumor, as detected by pathologic examination of the resected specimen, may be associated with a better prognosis and, conversely, failure of the tumor to respond to neoadjuvant treatment appears to be an adverse prognostic factor. Therefore, specimens from patients receiving neoadjuvant chemoradiation should be thoroughly examined at the primary tumor site, in regional nodes and for peritumoral satellite nodules or deposits in the remainder of the specimen. The degree of tumor response may correlate with prognosis. Those patients with minimal or no residual disease after therapy may have a better prognosis than gross residual disease. Whereas a number of different grading systems for tumor regression have been advocated, a four-point tumor regression grade will be used to assess response that is similar to that of Ryan et al. except that the complete absence of viable tumor will be recorded as a Grade 0 (Table 14.8).

**Circumferential Resection Margins.** It is essential that accurate pathologic evaluation of the CRM adjacent to the deepest point of tumor invasion be performed. The CRM is the surgically dissected nonperitonealized surface of the specimen. It corresponds to any aspect of the colorectum that is not covered by a serosal layer of mesothelial cells and must be dissected from the retroperitoneum or subperitoneum in order to remove the viscus. In contradistinction, serosalized surfaces of the colorectum are not dissected; they are naturally occurring anatomic structures and are not pathologic surgical margins. The circumferential surface of surgical resection

**TABLE 14.8.** Tumor regression grade

| Description | Tumor regression grade |
| --- | --- |
| No viable cancer cells | 0 (Complete response) |
| Single cells or small groups of cancer cells | 1 (Moderate response) |
| Residual cancer outgrown by fibrosis | 2 (Minimal response) |
| Minimal or no tumor kill; extensive residual cancer | 3 (Poor response) |

specimens of ascending colon, descending colon, or upper rectum is only partially peritonealized, and the demarcation between the peritonealized surface and the nonperitonealized surface (corresponding to the CRM) of such specimens is not always easily appreciated on pathologic examination. Therefore, the surgeon is encouraged to mark the peritoneal reflection and/or the area of deepest tumor penetration adjacent to a nonperitonealized surface with a clip or suture so that the pathologist may accurately identify and evaluate the CRM.

For mid and distal rectal cancers (subperitoneal location), the entire surface of the resection specimen corresponds to a CRM (anterior, posterior, medial, lateral). For proximal rectal or retroperitoneal colon cancers (ascending, descending, possibly cecum), surgically dissected margins will include those that lie in a retroperitoneal or subperitoneal location as described above (Figure 14.3). For segments of the colon that are entirely covered by a visceral peritoneum (transverse, sigmoid, possibly cecum), the only specimen margin that is surgically dissected is the mesenteric margin, unless the cancer is adherent to or invading an adjacent organ or structure. Therefore, for cancers of the cecum, transverse or sigmoid colon that extends to the cut edge of the mesentery, assignment of a positive CRM is appropriate.

For rectal cancer, the quality of the surgical technique is likely a key factor in the success of surgical outcomes relative to local recurrence and possibly long-term survival. Numerous nonrandomized studies have demonstrated that total mesorectal excision (TME) with adequate surgical clearance around the penetrating edge of the tumor decreases the rate of local relapse. The TME technique entails precise sharp dissection within the areolar plane of loose connective tissue outside (lateral to) the visceral mesorectal fascia in order to remove the rectum. With this approach, all mesorectal soft tissues encasing the rectum, which includes the mesentery

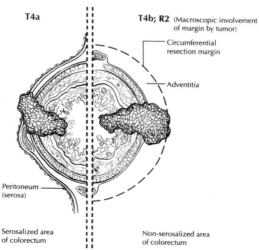

**FIGURE 14.3.** Circumferential resection margin.

and all regional nodes, are removed intact. Thus, the circumferential surface (CRM) of TME resection specimens is the mesorectal or Waldeyer's fascia. Rectal resection performed by less precise techniques may be associated with incomplete excision of the mesorectum. It is critical that the analysis of the surgical specimen follows the CAP guidelines that refer to examination of the TME specimen. In addition, it is essential that the distance between the closest leading edge of the tumor and the CRM (known as the surgical clearance) be measured pathologically and recorded in mm in the CRM field on the staging form. A margin of greater than 1 mm is required with TME to be considered a negative margin because surgical clearance of 1 mm or less is associated with a significantly increased risk of local recurrence and should be classified as positive (Figure 14.3).

**Residual Tumor (R).** The completeness of resection is largely dependent on the status of the CRM, although the designation is global and would include the transverse margins and other disease observed but not removed at surgery. The resection (R) codes should be given for each procedure:

- R0—Complete tumor resection with all margins histologically negative
- R1—Incomplete tumor resection with microscopic surgical resection margin involvement (margins grossly uninvolved)
- R2—Incomplete tumor resection with gross residual tumor that was not resected (primary tumor, regional nodes, macroscopic margin involvement)

**Isolated Tumor Cells and Molecular Node Involvement.** As technology progresses and sentinel node biopsy or other procedures may become feasible in colon and rectal surgery, the issue of interpretation of very small amounts of detected tumor in regional lymph nodes will continue to be classified as pN0, and the universal terminology for these isolated tumor cells (ITC) will follow the terminology referenced in Chap. 1. The prognostic significance of ITCs, defined as single malignant cells or a few tumor cells in microclusters, identified in regional lymph nodes that otherwise would be considered to be negative is still unclear. Therefore, ITC identified the collection of data on ITC that may be generated by pathologists who use special immunohistochemical stains or molecular analysis procedures to identify ITC in nodes that might otherwise be considered negative for metastasis by standard hematoxylin and eosin (H&E). It should be noted that isolated tumor cells identified on H&E stains alone are also classified as ITC and are annotated in the same fashion as ITC seen on immunohistochemical stains (i.e., pN0(i+); "i" = "isolated tumor cells").

**KRAS.** Analysis of multiple recent clinical trials has shown that the presence of a mutation in either codon 12 or 13 of KRAS (abnormal or "mutated" KRAS) is strongly associated with a lack of response to treatment with anti-EGFR antibodies in patients with metastatic colorectal carcinoma. It is recommended that patients with advanced colorectal carcinoma be tested for the presence of mutations in KRAS if treatment will include an anti-EGFR antibody. Where the status of KRAS is known, it should be recorded as a site-specific factor as either Normal ("Wild Type") or Abnormal ("Mutated").

**Anatomic Boundary.** The boundary between the rectum and anal canal most often has been equated with the dentate line, which is identified pathologically. However, with advances in sphincter-preservation surgery, defining the boundary between the rectum and the anus as the anorectal ring, which corresponds to the proximal border of the puborectalis muscle palpable on digital rectal examination, is more appropriate.

**TNM Stage of Disease.** Since publication of the sixth edition, new prognostic data with regard to survival and disease relapse justifies further substaging of both Stages II and III (Tables 14.1–14.7) by anatomic criteria. Differential prognosis has been shown for patients with T4 lesions based on the extent of disease in SEER analyses for both rectal cancer (Tables 14.4 and 14.5) and colon cancer (Tables 14.6 and 14.7). Accordingly, for the seventh edition of AJCC, T4 lesions have been subdivided as T4a (tumor penetrates to the surface of the visceral peritoneum) and T4b (tumor directly invades or is adherent to other organs or structures). In addition, the number of nodes involved by metastasis has been shown to influence prognosis within both N1 and N2 groups, in separate analyses of SEER (rectal cancer, Tables 14.4–14.5, Figure 14.2; colon cancer, Tables 14.4–14.7; Figure 14.1). For the SEER analyses, both relative and observed survival are listed by TN category of disease (relative survival is survival corrected by age-related comorbidity; see Chap. 2 for more information). Also the total number of nodes examined has an important impact on survival in colon and rectal cancer (Figures 14.1 and 14.2). The impact of increased nodes examined in the resected specimen is clearly associated with better outcome in colon cancer for all combinations of T and N (Figure 14.1) whereas the association holds in T1–T3 lesions in rectal cancer but appears to be less important in T4a and T4b lesions, perhaps because of the greater use of preoperative radiation or concurrent chemoradiation of the smaller number of patients in the rectal carcinoma subgroups (Figure 14.2).

Stage Group II has been further subdivided into IIA (T3N0), IIB (T4aN0), and IIC (T4bN0), based on differential survival prognosis. These differences are shown in the SEER analyses for both rectal cancer (Tables 14.4 and 14.5) and colon cancer (Tables 14.6 and 14.7).

Within Stage III, a number of changes have been made based on differential prognosis found in the rectal cancer pooled analyses (Tables 14.1–14.3), the SEER rectal and colon cancer analyses (Tables 14.4–14.7), and the NCDB colon cancer analysis (Table 14.6). A category of N1 tumors has prognosis more akin to IIIC (T4bN1) and has been shifted from Stage IIIB to IIIC. In addition, several categories of N2 tumors have prognosis more akin to IIIA (the T1N2a group) or IIIB (the T1N2b, T2N2a-b, and T3N2a groups) and have been shifted out of Stage IIIC accordingly.

Figures 14.4 and 14.5 present observed survival rates for 28,491 cases with adenocarcinoma of the colon from 1998 to 2000 and observed survival rates for 9,860 cases with adenocarcinoma of the rectum from 1998 to 2000.

**Independent Prognostic Factors and Molecular Markers.** In addition to the TNM, independent prognostic factors that are generally used in patient management and are well supported in the literature include residual disease, histologic type, histologic grade, serum carcinoembryonic antigen and cytokine levels, extramural venous invasion, and submucosal vascular

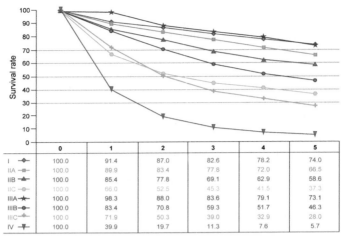

| | 0 | 1 | 2 | 3 | 4 | 5 |
|---|---|---|---|---|---|---|
| I ◆ | 100.0 | 91.4 | 87.0 | 82.6 | 78.2 | 74.0 |
| IIA ■ | 100.0 | 89.9 | 83.4 | 77.8 | 72.0 | 66.5 |
| IIB ▲ | 100.0 | 85.4 | 77.8 | 69.1 | 62.9 | 58.6 |
| IIC ● | 100.0 | 66.0 | 52.5 | 45.3 | 41.5 | 37.3 |
| IIIA ★ | 100.0 | 98.3 | 88.0 | 83.6 | 79.1 | 73.1 |
| IIIB ● | 100.0 | 83.4 | 70.8 | 59.3 | 51.7 | 46.3 |
| IIIC ▲ | 100.0 | 71.9 | 50.3 | 39.0 | 32.9 | 28.0 |
| IV ▼ | 100.0 | 39.9 | 19.7 | 11.3 | 7.6 | 5.7 |

Years from diagnosis

**FIGURE 14.4.** Observed survival rates for 28,491 cases with adenocarcinoma of the colon. Data from the SEER 1973–2005 Public Use File diagnosed in years 1998–2000. Stage I includes 7,417; Stage IIA, 9,956; Stage IIB, 997; Stage IIC, 725; Stage IIIA, 868; Stage IIIB, 1,492; Stage IIIC, 2,000; and Stage IV, 5,036.

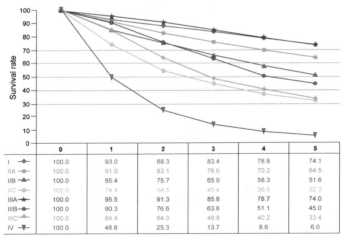

| | 0 | 1 | 2 | 3 | 4 | 5 |
|---|---|---|---|---|---|---|
| I ◆ | 100.0 | 93.0 | 88.3 | 83.4 | 78.8 | 74.1 |
| IIA ■ | 100.0 | 91.0 | 83.1 | 76.6 | 70.2 | 64.5 |
| IIB ▲ | 100.0 | 85.4 | 75.7 | 65.9 | 58.3 | 51.6 |
| IIC ● | 100.0 | 74.4 | 54.5 | 45.4 | 36.8 | 32.3 |
| IIIA ★ | 100.0 | 95.5 | 91.3 | 85.8 | 78.7 | 74.0 |
| IIIB ● | 100.0 | 90.3 | 76.6 | 63.6 | 51.1 | 45.0 |
| IIIC ▲ | 100.0 | 84.4 | 64.0 | 48.8 | 40.2 | 33.4 |
| IV ▼ | 100.0 | 48.8 | 25.3 | 13.7 | 8.6 | 6.0 |

Years from diagnosis

**FIGURE 14.5.** Observed survival rates for 9,860 cases with adenocarcinoma of the rectum. Data from the SEER 1973–2005 Public Use File diagnosed in years 1998–2000. Stage I includes 3,470; Stage IIA, 2,752; Stage IIB, 165; Stage IIC, 268; Stage IIIA, 595; Stage IIIB, 615; Stage IIIC, 761; and Stage IV, 1,234.

invasion by carcinomas arising in adenomas. Small cell carcinomas, signet ring cell carcinomas, and undifferentiated carcinomas have a less favorable outcome than other histologic types. In contrast, medullary carcinoma is more favorable prognostically. Submucosal vascular invasion by carcinomas arising in adenomas is associated with a greater risk of regional lymph node involvement. Lymphatic, venous, and perineural invasion also have been shown to have a less favorable outcome. A number of these independent prognostic factors are currently being evaluated in nomograms that also include TNM stage of disease (see below).

In the future, the intratumoral expression of specific molecules, e.g., Deleted in Colorectal Cancer (DCC) or 18q loss of heterozygosity (LOH), $p27^{Kip1}$, DNA microsatellite instability, KRAS mutation, or thymidylate synthase, may be proven to be associated either with prognosis or response to therapy that is independent of TNM stage group or histologic grade. Currently, these molecular markers are not part of the staging system, but it is recommended that they be recorded if available and especially if studied within the context of a clinical trial. Furthermore, it is now clear that there is interaction between the T and N designations that is likely to rely on the expression of specific molecules within the cancer. Thus, by the time of the next edition of TNM staging it may be possible to add molecular profiling information to the TNM information to enhance the precision of predicting prognosis or even response to therapy. Finally, it is important to consider that other factors such as age, gender, race/ethnicity are important factors that affect response to therapy and disease outcome. Although these factors are not included in the TNM Summary or Working Stages at this time, several groups are studying the interaction of these clinicopathological factors with TNM and other prognostic factors in various nomograms such as those at http://www.nomograms.org. In order to determine the optimal way to integrate these various clinical, pathologic, and molecular factors with TNM, collection of the appropriate information prior to the next edition must be carried out.

## DEFINITIONS OF TNM

The same classification is used for both clinical and pathologic staging.

### Primary Tumor (T)

| | |
|---|---|
| TX | Primary tumor cannot be assessed |
| T0 | No evidence of primary tumor |
| Tis | Carcinoma in situ: intraepithelial or invasion of lamina propria* |
| T1 | Tumor invades submucosa |
| T2 | Tumor invades muscularis propria |
| T3 | Tumor invades through the muscularis propria into pericolorectal tissues |
| T4a | Tumor penetrates to the surface of the visceral peritoneum** |
| T4b | Tumor directly invades or is adherent to other organs or structures**,*** |

*Note: Tis includes cancer cells confined within the glandular basement membrane (intraepithelial) or mucosal lamina propria (intramucosal) with no extension through the muscularis mucosae into the submucosa.

**Note*: Direct invasion in T4 includes invasion of other organs or other segments of the colorectum as a result of direct extension through the serosa, as confirmed on microscopic examination (for example, invasion of the sigmoid colon by a carcinoma of the cecum) or, for cancers in a retroperitoneal or subperitoneal location, direct invasion of other organs or structures by virtue of extension beyond the muscularis propria (i.e., respectively, a tumor on the posterior wall of the descending colon invading the left kidney or lateral abdominal wall; or a mid or distal rectal cancer with invasion of prostate, seminal vesicles, cervix, or vagina).

***Note*: Tumor that is adherent to other organs or structures, grossly, is classified cT4b. However, if no tumor is present in the adhesion, microscopically, the classification should be pT1-4a depending on the anatomical depth of wall invasion. The V and L classifications should be used to identify the presence or absence of vascular or lymphatic invasion whereas the PN site-specific factor should be used for perineural invasion.

### Regional Lymph Nodes (N)

| | |
|---|---|
| NX | Regional lymph nodes cannot be assessed |
| N0 | No regional lymph node metastasis |
| N1 | Metastasis in 1–3 regional lymph nodes |
| N1a | Metastasis in one regional lymph node |
| N1b | Metastasis in 2–3 regional lymph nodes |
| N1c | Tumor deposit(s) in the subserosa, mesentery, or nonperitonealized pericolic or perirectal tissues without regional nodal metastasis |
| N2 | Metastasis in four or more regional lymph nodes |
| N2a | Metastasis in 4–6 regional lymph nodes |
| N2b | Metastasis in seven or more regional lymph nodes |

*Note*: A satellite peritumoral nodule in the pericolorectal adipose tissue of a primary carcinoma without histologic evidence of residual lymph node in the nodule may represent discontinuous spread, venous invasion with extravascular spread (V1/2), or a totally replaced lymph node (N1/2). Replaced nodes should be counted separately as positive nodes in the N category, whereas discontinuous spread or venous invasion should be classified and counted in the Site-Specific Factor category Tumor Deposits (TD).

### Distant Metastasis (M)

| | |
|---|---|
| M0 | No distant metastasis |
| M1 | Distant metastasis |
| M1a | Metastasis confined to one organ or site (e.g., liver, lung, ovary, nonregional node) |
| M1b | Metastases in more than one organ/site or the peritoneum |

## ANATOMIC STAGE/PROGNOSTIC GROUPS

| Stage | T | N | M | Dukes* | MAC* |
|-------|---|---|---|--------|------|
| 0 | Tis | N0 | M0 | – | – |
| I | T1 | N0 | M0 | A | A |
| | T2 | N0 | M0 | A | B1 |
| IIA | T3 | N0 | M0 | B | B2 |
| IIB | T4a | N0 | M0 | B | B2 |
| IIC | T4b | N0 | M0 | B | B3 |
| IIIA | T1–T2 | N1/N1c | M0 | C | C1 |
| | T1 | N2a | M0 | C | C1 |
| IIIB | T3–T4a | N1/N1c | M0 | C | C2 |
| | T2–T3 | N2a | M0 | C | C1/C2 |
| | T1–T2 | N2b | M0 | C | C1 |
| IIIC | T4a | N2a | M0 | C | C2 |
| | T3–T4a | N2b | M0 | C | C2 |
| | T4b | N1–N2 | M0 | C | C3 |
| IVA | Any T | Any N | M1a | – | – |
| IVB | Any T | Any N | M1b | – | – |

*Note*: cTNM is the clinical classification, pTNM is the pathologic classification. The y prefix is used for those cancers that are classified after neoadjuvant pretreatment (e.g., ypTNM). Patients who have a complete pathologic response are ypT0N0cM0 that may be similar to Stage Group 0 or I. The r prefix is to be used for those cancers that have recurred after a disease-free interval (rTNM).

*Dukes B is a composite of better (T3 N0 M0) and worse (T4 N0 M0) prognostic groups, as is Dukes C (Any TN1 M0 and Any T N2 M0). MAC is the modified Astler-Coller classification.

## PROGNOSTIC FACTORS (SITE-SPECIFIC FACTORS)
### (Recommended for Collection)

| | |
|--|--|
| Required for staging | None |
| Clinically significant | Preoperative or pretreatment carcinoembryonic antigen (CEA) (ng/ml) |
| | Tumor deposits (TD) |
| | Circumferential resection margin (CRM) |
| | Perineural invasion (PN) |
| | Microsatellite instability (MSI) |
| | Tumor regression grade (with neoadjuvant therapy) |
| | KRAS gene analysis |

## HISTOLOGIC GRADE (G)

GX     Grade cannot be assessed
G1     Well differentiated
G2     Moderately differentiated
G3     Poorly differentiated
G4     Undifferentiated (corresponds to the histologic type "undifferentiated carcinoma" as below)

It is recommended that the terms "low-grade" (G1–G2) and "high-grade" (G3–G4) be applied, because data indicate that low and high grade may be associated with outcome independently of TNM stage group for both colon and rectum adenocarcinoma. Some authors suggest that G4 lesions be identified separately because they may represent a small subgroup of carcinomas that are very aggressive. However, these tumors would be designated as "undifferentiated" carcinomas within the classification histologic types shown previously.

## RESIDUAL TUMOR (R)

R0     Complete resection, margins histologically negative, no residual tumor left after resection (primary tumor, regional nodes)
R1     Incomplete resection, margins histologically involved, microscopic tumor remains after resection of gross disease (primary tumor, regional nodes)
R2     Incomplete resection, margins macroscopically involved or gross disease remains after resection (e.g., primary tumor, regional nodes, or liver metastasis)

## HISTOPATHOLOGIC TYPE

This staging classification applies to carcinomas that arise in the colon or rectum. The classification does not apply to sarcomas, to lymphomas, or to carcinoid tumors of the large intestine or appendix. The histologic types include:

> Adenocarcinoma in situ*
> Adenocarcinoma
> Medullary carcinoma
> Mucinous carcinoma (colloid type) (greater than 50% mucinous carcinoma)
> Signet ring cell carcinoma (greater than 50% signet ring cell)
> Squamous cell (epidermoid) carcinoma
> Adenosquamous carcinoma
> Small cell carcinoma
> Undifferentiated carcinoma
> Carcinoma, NOS

*The terms "high grade dysplasia" and "severe dysplasia" may be used as synonyms for in situ adenocarcinoma and in situ carcinoma. These cases should be assigned pTis.

---

# BIBLIOGRAPHY

Adam IJ, Mohamdee MO, Martin IG, et al. Role of circumferential margin involvement in the local recurrence of rectal cancer. Lancet. 1994;344:707–11.

Allegra CJ, Jessup JM, Somerfield MR, et al. American Society of Clinical Oncology provisional clinical opinion: testing for KRAS gene mutations in patients with metastatic colorectal carcinoma to predict response to anti-epidermal growth factor receptor monoclonal antibody therapy. J Clin Oncol. 2009;27(12):2091–6.

Amado RG, Wolf M, Peeters M, et al. Wild-type KRAS is required for panitumumab efficacy in patients with metastatic colorectal cancer. J Clin Oncol. 2008;26:1626–34.

Arbman G, Nilsson E, Hallböök O, Sjödahl R. Can total mesorectal excision reduce the local recurrence rate in rectal surgery? Br J Surg. 1996;83:375–9.

Astler VB, Coller FA. The prognostic significance of direct extension of carcinoma of the colon and rectum. Ann Surg. 1954;139:846–52.

Bast RC, Desch CE, Ravdin P, et al. Clinical practice guidelines for the use of tumor markers in breast and colorectal cancer: report of the American Society of Clinical Oncology Expert Panel. J Clin Oncol. 1996;14:2843–77.

Bauer K, Bagwell C, Giaretti W, et al. Consensus review of the clinical utility of DNA flow cytometry in colorectal cancer. Cytometry. 1993;14:486–91.

Belluco C, Esposito G, Bertorelle R, et al. Absence of the cell cycle inhibitor p27Kip1 protein predicts poor outcome in patients with stage I–III colorectal cancer. Ann Surg Oncol. 1999;6:19–25.

Belluco C, Frantz M, Carnio S, et al. IL-6 blood level is associated with circulating CEA and prognosis in patients with colorectal cancer. Ann Surg Oncol. 2000;7:133–8.

Benvenuti S, Sartore-Bianchi A, Di Nicolantonio F, et al. Oncogenic activation of the RAS/RAF signaling pathway impairs the response of metastatic colorectal cancers to anti-epidermal growth factor receptor antibody therapies. Cancer Res. 2007;67:2643–8.

Bokemeyer C, Bondarenko I, Hartmann JT, et al. KRAS status and efficacy of first-line treatment of patients with metastatic colorectal (metastatic CRC) with FOLFOX with or without cetuximab: The OPUS experience. J Clin Oncol. 2008;26. May 20 Suppl; Abstr 4000.

Caplin S, Cerottini JP, Bosman FT, et al. For patients with Dukes' B (TNM Stage II) colorectal carcinoma, examination of six or fewer lymph nodes is related to poor prognosis. Cancer. 1998;83:666–72.

Coia LR, Gunderson LL, Haller D, et al. Outcomes of patients receiving radiation for carcinoma of the rectum. Results of the 1988–1989 patterns of care study. Cancer. 1999;86:1952–8.

Compton CC. Updated protocol for the examination of specimens removed from patients with colorectal carcinoma. Arch Pathol Lab Med. 2000;124:1016–25.

Compton CC. Colorectal cancer. In: Gospodarowicz MK, O'Sullivan F, Sobin LH, editors. Prognostic factors in cancer. 3rd ed. Hoboken: Wiley; 2006. p. 133–8. UICC.

Compton CC, Fenoglio-Prieser CM, Pettigrew N, Fielding LP. American joint committee on cancer prognostic factors consensus conference: Colorectal working group. Cancer. 2000a;88:1739–57.

Compton CC, Fielding LP, Burgart LJ, et al. Prognostic factors in colorectal cancer: College of American Pathologists Consensus Statement 1999. Arch Pathol Lab Med. 2000b;124:979–94.

Compton CC, Greene FL. The staging of colorectal cancer: 2004 and beyond. CA Cancer J Clin. 2004;54:295–308.

Copeland EM, Miller LD, Jones RS. Prognostic factors in carcinoma of the colon and rectum. Am J Surg. 1968;116:875–81.

De Roock W, Piessevaux H, De Schutter J, et al. KRAS wild-type state predicts survival and is associated to early radiological response in metastatic colorectal cancer treated with cetuximab. Ann Oncol. 2008;19:508–15.

Di Fiore F, Blanchard F, Charbonnier F, et al. Clinical relevance of KRAS mutation detection in metastatic colorectal cancer treated by Cetuximab plus chemotherapy. Br J Cancer. 2007;96:1166–9.

Dukes CE. Cancer of the rectum: an analysis of 1000 cases. J Pathol Bacteriol. 1940;50:527–39.

Gavioli M, Luppi G, Losi L, et al. Incidence and clinical impact of sterilized disease and minimal residual disease after preoperative radiochemotherapy for rectal cancer. Dis Colon Rectum. 2005;48:1851–7.

Gill S, Loprinzi CL, Sargent DK, et al. Pooled analysis of fluorouracil-based adjuvant therapy for Stage II and III colon cancer: who benefits and by how much? J Clin Oncol. 2004;22:1–10.

Goldstein NS. Lymph node recoveries from 2,427 pT3 colorectal resection specimens spanning 45 years: recommendation for a minimum number of recovered lymph nodes based on predictive probabilities. Am J Surg Pathol. 2002;26:179–89.

Goldstein NS, Turner JR. Pericolonic tumor deposits in patients with T3N + M0 colon adenocarcinomas: a marker for reduced disease-free survival and intra-abdominal metastasis. Cancer. 2000;88:2228–38.

Goldstein NS, Sanford W, Coffey M, Layfield LJ. Lymph node recovery from colorectal resection specimens removed for adenocarcinoma. Trends over time and a recommendation for a minimum number of lymph nodes to be recovered. Am J Clin Pathol. 1997;106:209–16.

Gosens MJ, van Krieken JH, Marijnen CA, et al. Cooperative clinical investigators and the pathology review committee. Improvement of staging by combining tumor and treatment parameters: the value for prognostication in rectal cancer. Clin Gastroenterol Hepatol. 2007;5:997–1003.

Greene FL, Stewart AK, Norton HJ. A new TNM staging strategy for node-positive (Stage III) colon cancer: an analysis of 50,042 patients. Ann Surg. 2002;236:416–21.

Greene FL, Stewart AK, et al. New tumor-node-metastasis for node-positive (Stage III) rectal cancer: an analysis. J Clin Oncol. 2004;22:1778–84.

Gunderson LL, Jessup JM, Sargent DJ, et al. Revised TN categorization for colon cancer based on national survival outcomes data. J Clin Oncol., in press.

Gunderson LL, Jessup JM, Sargent DJ, et al. Revised TN categorization for rectal cancer based on SEER and rectal pooled analysis outcomes. J Clin Oncol., in press.

Gunderson LL, Sosin H. Areas of failure found at reoperation (second or symptomatic look) following "curative surgery" for adenocarcinoma of the rectum. Clinicopathologic correlation and implications for adjuvant therapy. Cancer. 1974;34:1278–92.

Gunderson LL, Sargent DJ, Tepper JE, et al. Impact of T and N substage on survival and disease relapse in adjuvant rectal cancer: a pooled analysis. Int J Radiat Oncol Biol Phys. 2002;54:386–96.

Gunderson LL, Sargent DJ, Tepper JE, et al. Impact of T and N stage and treatment on survival and relapse in adjuvant rectal cancer: a pooled analysis. J Clin Oncol. 2004;22:1785–96.

Hall NR, Finan PJ, al-Jaberi T, et al. Circumferential margin involvement after mesorectal excision of rectal cancer with curative intent: predictor of survival but not local recurrence? Dis Colon Rectum. 1998;41:979–83.

Halling KC, French AJ, McDonnell SK, et al. Microsatellite imbalance in stage B2 and C colorectal cancers. J Natl Cancer Inst. 1999;91:1295–303.

Hamilton SR, Vogelstein B, Kudo S, et al. Carcinoma of the colon and rectum. In: Hamilton SR, Aaltonen LA, editors. World Health Organization classification of tumors. Pathology and genetics of tumors of the digestive system. Lyon: IARC; 2000. p. 105–19.

Harrison JC, Dean PJ, El-Zeky F, Vander Zwaag R. From Dukes through Jass. Pathological prognostic indicators in rectal cancer. Hum Pathol. 1994;25:498–505.

Harrison JC, Dean PJ, El-Zeky F, Vander Zwaag R. Impact of the Crohn's-like lymphoid reaction on staging of right-sided colon cancer: results of a multivariate analysis. Hum Pathol. 1995;26:31–8.

Herrera-Ornelas L, Justiniano J, Castillo N, et al. Metastases in small lymph nodes from colon cancer. Arch Surg. 1987;122:1253–6.

Hobday TJ, Erlichman C. Colorectal cancer. In: Gospodarowicz MK, Henson DE, Hutter RVP, et al., editors. Prognostic factors in cancer. 2nd ed. New York: Wiley; 2001. p. 267–79.

Hoskins RB, Gunderson LL, Dosoretz DE, et al. Adjuvant postoperative radiotherapy in carcinoma of the rectum and rectosigmoid. Cancer. 1985;55:61–71.

Jass JR, Atkin WS, Cuzick J, et al. The grading of rectal cancer: historical perspectives and a multivariate analysis of 447 cases. Histopathology. 1986;10:437–59.

Jass JR, Love SB, Northover JMA. A new prognostic classification of rectal cancer. Lancet. 1987;1:1303–6.

Jen J, Kim H, Piantidosi S, et al. Allelic loss of chromosome 18q and prognosis in colorectal cancer. N Eng J Med. 1994;331:213–21.

Jessup JM, Stewart A, Greene FL, Minsky BD. Adjuvant chemotherapy for stage III colon cancer: implications of race/ethnicity, age, and differentiation. J Am Med Assoc. 2005;294:2703–11.

Joseph NE, Sigurdson ER, Hanlon AL, et al. Accuracy of determining nodal negativity in colorectal cancer on the basis of the number of nodes retrieved on resection. Ann Surg Oncol. 2003;10:213–8.

Kapiteijn E, Marijnen CAM, Nagtegaal ID, et al. Preoperative radiotherapy combined with total mesorectal excision for resectable rectal cancer. N Engl J Med. 2001;345:638–46.

Karapetis CS, Khambata-Ford S, Jonker DJ, et al. K-ras mutations and benefit from cetuximab in advanced colorectal cancer. N Engl J Med. 2008;359:1757–65.

Khambata-Ford S, Garrett CR, Meropol NJ, et al. Expression of epiregulin and amphiregulin and K-ras mutation status predict disease control in metastatic colorectal cancer patients treated with cetuximab. J Clin Oncol. 2007;25:3230–7.

Kokal W, Sheibani K, Terz J, et al. Tumor DNA content in the prognosis of colorectal carcinoma. J Am Med Assoc. 1986;255:3123–7.

Kotanagi H, Fukuoka T, Shibata Y, et al. Blood vessel invasions in metastatic nodes for development of liver metastasis in colorectal cancer. Hepato-Gastroenterology. 1995;42:771–4.

Le Voyer TE, Sigurdson ER, Hanlon AL, et al. Colon cancer survival is associated with increasing number of lymph nodes analyzed. A secondary survey of Intergroup Trial Int-0089. J Clin Oncol. 2003;21:2912–9.

Lievre A, Bachet JB, Boige V, et al. KRAS mutations as an independent prognostic factor in patients with advanced colorectal cancer treated with cetuximab. J Clin Oncol. 2008;26:374–9.

Lindmark G, Gerdin B, Sundberg C, et al. Prognostic significance of the microvascular count in colorectal cancer. J Clin Oncol. 1996;14:461–6.

Lipper S, Kahn LB, Ackerman LV. The significance of microscopic invasive cancer in endoscopically removed polyps of the large bowel: a clinicopathologic study of 51 cases. Cancer. 1983;52:1691.

Locker GY, Hamilton S, Harris J, et al. ASCO 2006 update of recommendations for the use of tumor markers in gastrointestinal cancer. J Clin Oncol. 2006;24:5313–27.

Loda M, Cukor B, Tam SW, et al. Increased proteasome-dependent degradation of the cyclin-dependent kinase inhibitor p27 in aggressive colorectal carcinomas. Nature Medicine. 1997;3:231–4.

Marijnen CA, Nagtegaal ID, Kapiteijn E, et al. Radiotherapy does not compensate for positive resection margins in rectal cancer patients: report of a multicenter randomized trial. Int J Radiat Oncol Biol Phys. 2003;55:1311–20.

Minsky BD, Mies C, Rich TA, et al. Lymphatic vessel invasion is an independent prognostic factor for survival in colorectal cancer. Int J Radiat Oncol. 1989;17:311–8.

Nagtegaal ID, Marijnen CAM, Kranenbarg EKM, et al. Circumferential margin involvement is still an important predictor of local recurrence in rectal carcinoma: not one millimeter but two millimeters is the limit. Am J Surg Pathol. 2002;26:350–7.

Nagtegaal ID, Quirke P. Colorectal tumour deposits in the mesorectum and pericolon; a critical review. Histopathology. 2007;51:141–9.

Newland RC, Chapuis PH, Pheils MT, et al. The relationship of survival to staging and grading of colorectal carcinoma: a prospective study of 503 cases. Cancer. 1981;47:1424–9.

Ondero H, Maetani S, Nishikawa T, et al. The reappraisal of prognostic classifications for colorectal cancer. Dis Colon Rectum. 1989;32:609–14.

Petersen VC, Baxter KJ, Love SB, Shepherd NA. Identification of objective pathological prognostic determinants and models of prognosis in Dukes' B colon cancer. Gut. 2002;51:65–9.

Phillips RKS, Hittinger R, Blesovsky L, et al. Large bowel cancer: surgical pathology and its relationship to survival. Br J Surg. 1984;71:604–10.

Pocard M, Panis Y, Malassagne B, et al. Assessing the effectiveness of mesorectal excision in rectal cancer: prognostic value of the number of lymph nodes found in resected specimens. Dis Colon Rectum. 1998;41:839–45.

Punt CJ, Tol J, Rodenburg CJ, et al. Randomized phase III study of capecitabine, oxaliplatin, and bevacizumab with or without cetuximab in advanced colorectal cancer (ACC), the CAIRO2 study of the Dutch Colorectal Cancer Group (DCCG). J Clin Oncol. 2008;26. May 20 Suppl; Abstr LBA4011.

Puppa G, Maisonneuve P, Sonzogni A, et al. Pathological assessment of pericolonic tumor deposits in advanced colonic carcinoma: relevance to prognosis and tumor staging. Mod Pathol. 2007;20:843–55.

Qizilbash AH. Pathologic studies in colorectal cancer: a guide to the surgical pathology examination of colorectal specimens and review of features of prognostic significance. Pathol Annu. 1982;17(1):1–46.

Quirke P, Williams GT, Ectors N, et al. The future of the TNM staging system in colorectal cancer: time for a debate? Lancet Oncol. 2007;8:651–7.

Ratto C, Sofo L, Ippoliti M, et al. Accurate lymph-node detection in colorectal specimens resected for cancer is of prognostic significance. Dis Colon Rectum. 1999;42:143–54.

Ratto C, Ricci R, Rossi C, et al. Mesorectal microfoci adversely affect the prognosis of patients with rectal cancer. Dis Colon Rectum. 2002;45:733–42.

Ratto C, Ricci R, Valentini V, et al. Neoplastic mesorectal microfoci (MMF) following neoadjuvant chemoradiotherapy: clinical and prognostic implications. Ann Surg Oncol. 2007;14:853–61.

Rich T, Gunderson LL, Lew R, et al. Patterns of recurrence of rectal cancer after potentially curative surgery. Cancer. 1983;52:1317–29.

Ruo L, Tickoo S, Klimstra DS, et al. Long-term prognostic significance of extent of rectal cancer response to preoperative radiation and chemotherapy. Ann Surg. 2002;236:75–81.

Ryan R, Gibbons D, Hyland JMP, et al. Pathological response following long-course neoadjuvant chemoradiotherapy for locally advanced rectal cancer. Histopathology. 2005;47:141–6.

Schild SE, Martenson JA Jr, Gunderson LL, et al. Postoperative adjuvant therapy of rectal cancer: an analysis of disease control, survival, and prognostic factors. Int J Radiat Oncol Biol Phys. 1989;17:55–62.

Scott KWM, Grace RH. Detection of lymph node metastases in colorectal carcinoma before and after fat clearance. Br J Surg. 1989;76:1165–7.

Scott NA, Rainwater LM, Wieland HS, et al. The relative prognostic value of flow cytometric DNA analysis and conventional clinicopathologic criteria in patients with operative rectal carcinoma. Dis Colon Rectum. 1987;30:513–20.

Shepherd N, Baxter K, Love S. The prognostic importance of peritoneal involvement in colonic cancer: a prospective evaluation. Gastroenterology. 1997;112:1096–102.

Shepherd NA, Saraga EP, Love SB, et al. Prognostic factors in colonic cancer. Histopathology. 1989;14:613–20.

Shibata D, Reale MA, Lavin P, et al. The DCC protein and prognosis in colorectal cancer. N Engl J Med. 1996;335:1727–32.

Steinberg SM, Barkin JS, Kaplan RS, et al. Prognostic indicators of colon tumors: the gastrointestinal tumor study group experience. Cancer. 1986;57:1866–70.

Stewart A, Greene F. NCDB colon cancer data, Personal communication. May 2007.

Stocchi L, Nelson H, Sargent DJ, et al. Impact of surgical and pathological variables in rectal cancer: a United States community and cooperative group report. J Clin Oncol. 2001;19:3895–902.

Swanson RS, Compton CC, Stewart AK, Bland KI. The prognosis of T3N0 colon cancer is dependent upon the number of lymph nodes examined. Ann Surg Oncol. 2003;10:65–71.

Talbot IC, Ritchie S, Leighton MH, et al. The clinical significance of invasion of veins by rectal cancer. Br J Surg. 1980;67:439–42.

Surveillance, Epidemiology, and End Results (SEER) Program (http://www.seer.cancer.gov) SEER*Stat Database: Incidence – SEER 17 Regs Limited-Use, Nov 2005 Sub (1973–2003 varying) – Linked To County Attributes – Total U.S., 1969–2003 Counties, National Cancer Institute, DCCPS, Surveillance Research Program, Cancer Statistics Branch. Released April 2006, based on the November 2005 submission.

Talbot IC, Ritchie S, Leighton MH, et al. Spread of rectal cancer within veins: histologic features and clinical significance. Am J Surg. 1981;141:15–7.

Tepper JE, O'Connell MJ, Niedzwiecki D, et al. Impact of number of nodes retrieved on outcome in patients with rectal cancer. J Clin Oncol. 2001;19:157–63.

Tepper JE, O'Connell MJ, Niedzwiecki D, et al. Adjuvant therapy in rectal cancer: analysis of stage, sex and local control – final report of Intergroup 0114. J Clin Oncol. 2002;20:1744–50.

Ueno H, Mochizuki H, Hashiguchi Y, et al. Extramural cancer deposits without nodal structure in colorectal cancer. Am J Clin Pathol. 2007;127:287–94.

Van Cutsem E, Lang I, D'haens G, et al. KRAS status and efficacy in the first-line treatment of patients with metastatic colorectal cancer (metastatic CRC) treated with FOLFIRI with or without cetuximab: The CRYSTAL experience. J Clin Oncol. 2008;26. May 20 Suppl; Abstr 2.

Willett CG, Badizadegan K, Ancukiewica M, Shellito PC. Prognostic factors in stage T3N0 rectal cancer: do all patients require postoperative pelvic irradiation and chemotherapy? Dis Colon Rectum. 1999;42:167–73.

Williams NS, Durdey P, Qwihe P, et al. Pre-operative staging of rectal neoplasm and its impact on clinical management. Br J Surg. 1985;72:868–74.

Wittekind C, Compton CC, Greene FL, Sobin LH. TNM residual tumor classification revisited. Cancer. 2002;94:2511–9.

Wittekind C, Greene FL, Henson DE, Hutter RVP, Sobin LH, editors. TNM supplement: a commentary on uniform use. 3rd ed. New York: Wiley; 2003.

Wolmark N, Fisher B, Wieand HS. The prognostic value of the modifications of the Dukes C class of colorectal cancer: an analysis of the NSABP clinical trials. Ann Surg. 1986;203:115–22.

Wolmark N, Fisher ER, Wieand HS, et al. The relationship of depth of penetration and tumor size to the number of positive nodes in Dukes C colorectal cancer. Cancer. 1984;53:2707–12.

Wong JH, Bowles BJ, Bueno R, Shimizu D. Impact of the number of negative nodes on disease-free survival in colorectal cancer. Dis Colon Rectum. 2002;45:1341–8.

Wong JH, Severino R, Honnebier MB, et al. Number of nodes examined and staging accuracy in colorectal carcinoma. J Clin Oncol. 1999;17:2896–900.

Wright CM, Dent OF, Barker M, et al. Prognostic significance of extensive microsatellite instability in sporadic clinicopathological stage C colorectal cancer. Br J Surg. 2000;87:1197–202.

# Anus

*(The classification applies to carcinomas only; melanomas, carcinoid tumors, and sarcomas are not included.)*

## *At-A-Glance*

---

**SUMMARY OF CHANGES**

* The definitions of TNM and the stage groupings for this chapter have not changed from the sixth edition

* The descriptions of both the boundaries of the anal canal and anal carcinomas have been clarified

* The collection of the reported status of the tumor for the presence of human papilloma virus is included

---

**ANATOMIC STAGE/PROGNOSTIC GROUPS**

| | | | |
|------|-------|-------|-----|
| 0 | Tis | N0 | M0 |
| I | T1 | N0 | M0 |
| II | T2 | N0 | M0 |
| | T3 | N0 | M0 |
| IIIA | T1 | N1 | M0 |
| | T2 | N1 | M0 |
| | T3 | N1 | M0 |
| | T4 | N0 | M0 |
| IIIB | T4 | N1 | M0 |
| | Any T | N2 | M0 |
| | Any T | N3 | M0 |
| IV | Any T | Any N | M1 |

**ICD-O-3 TOPOGRAPHY CODES**

| | |
|-------|---|
| C21.0 | Anus, NOS |
| C21.1 | Anal canal |
| C21.2 | Cloacogenic zone |
| C21.8 | Overlapping lesion of rectum, anus, and anal canal |

**ICD-O-3 HISTOLOGY CODE RANGES**

8000–8152, 8154–8231, 8243–8245, 8250–8576, 8940–8950, 8980–8981

## INTRODUCTION

The proximal region of the anus encompasses true mucosa of three different histologic types: glandular, transitional, and squamous (proximal to distal, respectively). Distally, the squamous mucosa transitions into the perianal skin (true epidermis) at the point that historically has been called the anal verge. Thus, two distinct categories of tumors arise in the anal region. Tumors that develop from mucosa (of any of the three types) are termed anal canal cancers, whereas those that arise within the skin at or distal to the squamous mucocutaneous junction are termed perianal cancers. The boundary between the mucosa-lined anal canal and the skin of the perianal zone is indistinct on macroscopic examination and, anatomically, its location may vary with the patient's body habitus but in general may coincide with the intersphincteric groove. Radially, the squamous mucosa transitions into the perianal zone ends approximately 5–6 cm from the squamous mucocutaneous junction (intersphincteric groove) in the majority of adults.

Anal canal tumors are staged using the classification system described and illustrated herein. Perianal tumors are biologically comparable to other skin tumors and therefore are staged according to the parameters described in Chap. 29. However, the regional nodal drainage (relevant to the N category) of the perianal skin is specific to this anatomic site, as described later.

The primary management of carcinomas of the anal canal has shifted from surgical resection to nonoperative treatment, precluding pathologic staging in most cases. Therefore, carcinomas of the anal canal are typically staged clinically according to the size and extent of the untreated primary tumor. Patients with cancer of the anal canal are typically staged at the time of presentation with inspection, palpation and biopsy of the mass, palpation (and biopsy as needed) of regional lymph nodes, and radiologic imaging of the chest, abdomen, and pelvis.

In contrast, the management of perianal carcinomas remains primarily operative, and nonoperative treatments are used selectively based on involvement of adjacent structures and tumor size. Complete pathologic staging is often possible for a primary tumor at this location. The remainder of the staging of the regional lymph nodes and distant disease is as described for anal cancers.

## ANATOMY

**Primary Site.** The anatomic subsites of the anal canal are illustrated in Figure 15.1. The anal canal begins where the rectum enters the puborectalis sling at the apex of the anal sphincter complex (palpable as the anorectal ring on digital rectal examination and approximately 1–2 cm proximal to the dentate line) and ends with the squamous mucosa blending with the perianal skin, which roughly coincides with the palpable intersphincteric groove or the outermost boundary of the internal sphincter muscle. The most proximal aspect of the anal canal is lined by colorectal mucosa in which squamous metaplasia may occur. When involved by metaplasia, this zone also may be referred to as the transformation zone. Immediately proximal to the macroscopically visible dentate line, a narrow zone of transitional mucosa that is similar to urothelium is variably present. The proximal zone of the anal canal that extends from the top of the puborectalis to the dentate line measures approximately 1–2 cm. In the region of the dentate line, anal glands are subjacent to the mucosa, often penetrating through the internal sphincter into the intersphincteric plane. The distal zone of the anal canal extends from the dentate line to the mucocutaneous junction with the perianal skin and is lined by a nonkeratinizing squamous epithelium devoid of epidermal appendages (hair follicles, apocrine glands, and sweat glands).

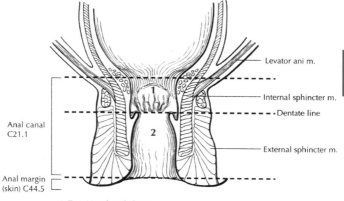

1. Transitional epithelium
2. Squamous epithelium devoid of hair and glands (not skin)

**FIGURE 15.1.** Anatomic subsites of the anal canal.

Determination of the anatomic site of origin of carcinomas that overlap the anorectal junction may be problematic. For staging purposes, such tumors should be classified as rectal cancers if their epicenter is located more than 2 cm proximal to the dentate line or proximal to the anorectal ring on digital examination and as anal canal cancers if their epicenter is 2 cm or less from the dentate line. For rectal cancers that extend beyond the dentate line, as for anal canal cancers, the superficial inguinal lymph nodes are among the regional nodal groups at risk of metastatic spread and included in cN/pN analysis (see later).

**Regional Lymph Nodes.** Lymphatic drainage and nodal involvement of anal cancers depend on the location of the primary tumor. Tumors above the dentate line spread primarily to the anorectal, perirectal, and paravertebral nodes, whereas tumors below the dentate line spread primarily to the superficial inguinal nodes.

The regional lymph nodes are as follows (Figure 15.2):

Perirctal
    Anorectal
    Perirectal
    Lateral sacral
Internal iliac (hypogastric)
Inguinal
    Superficial

All other nodal groups represent sites of distant metastasis.

**Metastatic Sites.** Cancers of the anus may metastasize to any organs, but the liver and lungs are the distal organs that are most frequently involved. Involvement of the abdominal cavity is not unusual.

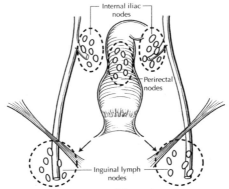

**FIGURE 15.2.** Regional lymph nodes of the anal canal.

## PROGNOSTIC FEATURES

For carcinoma of the anal canal, the 5-year observed survival rates for each of the stage groups are as follows: Stage I, $n = 637$, 69.5%; Stage II, $n = 1,711$, 61.8%; Stage IIIA, $n = 453$, 45.6%; Stage IIIB, $n = 495$, 39.6%; Stage IV, $n = 285$, 15.3%. Stage-related survival is shown in Figure 15.3.

Notably, within each stage grouping, overall 5-year survival rates for anal canal carcinomas vary significantly according to histologic type. At each stage, survival rates for patients with squamous cell carcinomas are better than that for patients with nonsquamous tumors as shown in Table 15.1.

Historically recognized histologic variants of squamous cell carcinoma, such as large cell keratinzing, large cell nonkeratinizing and basa-

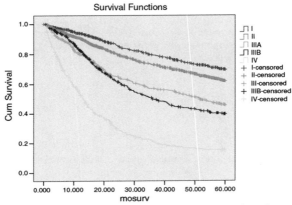

**FIGURE 15.3.** Stage-related survival for carcinoma of the anal canal.

**TABLE 15.1.** Patient outcome stratified by AJCC stage group and tumor histology (squamous vs. nonsquamous types)

| | 5-Year survival rate | | |
| Stage group | Squamous | Nonsquamous | P value |
| --- | --- | --- | --- |
| I | 71.4 | 59.1 | 0.003 |
| II | 63.5 | 52.9 | 0.001 |
| IIIA | 48.1 | 37.7 | 0.085 |
| IIIB | 43.2 | 24.4 | 0.003 |
| IV | 20.9 | 7.4 | 0.002 |

Source: National Cancer Database: Cases diagnosed 1998–1999: $n = 3,598$.

loid subtypes, have no associated prognostic differences. Therefore, the World Health Organization recommends that the generic term "squamous cell carcinoma" be used for all squamous tumors of the anal canal. Nonsquamous histologies of anal canal carcinomas include adenocarcinoma, mucinous adenocarcinoma, small cell carcinoma (high-grade neuroendocrine carcinoma), and undifferentiated carcinoma.

Human papilloma virus (HPV) may be an etiologic agent in anal carcinoma. When the data are reported, it is of value to record the HPV status in the cancer registry.

## DEFINITIONS OF TNM

### Primary Tumor (T)

TX     Primary tumor cannot be assessed
T0     No evidence of primary tumor
Tis    Carcinoma in situ (Bowen's disease, high-grade squamous intraepithelial lesion (HSIL), anal intraepithelial neoplasia II–III (AIN II–III)
T1     Tumor 2 cm or less in greatest dimension (Figure 15.4)
T2     Tumor more than 2 cm but not more than 5 cm in greatest dimension (Figure 15.5)
T3     Tumor more than 5 cm in greatest dimension (Figure 15.6)
T4     Tumor of any size invades adjacent organ(s), e.g., vagina, urethra, bladder* (Figure 15.7)

*Note: Direct invasion of the rectal wall, perirectal skin, subcutaneous tissue, or the sphincter muscle(s) is not classified as T4.

### Regional Lymph Nodes (N)

NX    Regional lymph nodes cannot be assessed
N0    No regional lymph node metastasis
N1    Metastasis in perirectal lymph node(s) (Figure 15.8)
N2    Metastasis in unilateral internal iliac and/or inguinal lymph node(s) (Figure 15.9A, B)
N3    Metastasis in perirectal and inguinal lymph nodes and/or bilateral internal iliac and/or inguinal lymph nodes (Figure 15.10A–C)

**T1**

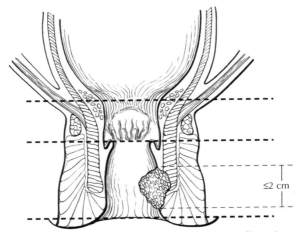

**FIGURE 15.4.** T1 is defined as tumor 2 cm or less in greatest dimension.

**T2**                              **T2**

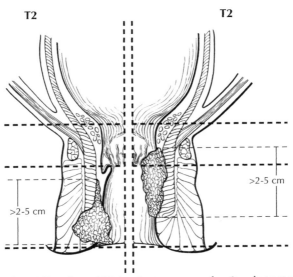

**FIGURE 15.5.** Two views of T2 showing tumor more than 2 cm but not more than 5 cm in greatest dimension. On the right side of the diagram, the tumor extends above the dentate line.

**T3**

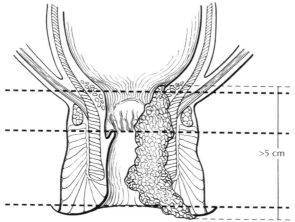

>5 cm

**FIGURE 15.6.** T3 is defined as tumor more than 5 cm in greatest dimension.

**T4**

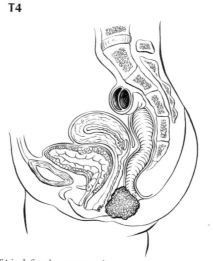

**FIGURE 15.7.** T4 is defined as tumor of any size invading adjacent organ(s), e.g., vagina (as illustrated), urethra, bladder.
*Note*: Direct invasion of the rectal wall, perirectal skin, subcutaneous tissue, or the sphincter muscle(s) is not classified as T4.

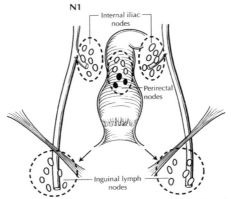

**FIGURE 15.8.** N1 is defined as metastasis in perirectal lymph node(s).

| *Distant Metastasis (M)* | | | |
|---|---|---|---|
| M0 | No distant metastasis | | |
| M1 | Distant metastasis | | |

| ANATOMIC STAGE/PROGNOSTIC GROUPS | | | |
|---|---|---|---|
| 0 | Tis | N0 | M0 |
| I | T1 | N0 | M0 |
| II | T2 | N0 | M0 |
| | T3 | N0 | M0 |
| IIIA | T1 | N1 | M0 |
| | T2 | N1 | M0 |
| | T3 | N1 | M0 |
| | T4 | N0 | M0 |
| IIIB | T4 | N1 | M0 |
| | Any T | N2 | M0 |
| | Any T | N3 | M0 |
| IV | Any T | Any N | M1 |

## PROGNOSTIC FACTORS (SITE-SPECIFIC FACTORS)
### (Recommended for Collection)

| | |
|---|---|
| Required for staging | None |
| Clinically significant | HPV Status |

## HISTOLOGIC GRADE (G)

Grade is reported in registry systems by the grade value. A two-grade, three-grade, or four-grade system may be used. If a grading system is not specified, generally the following system is used:

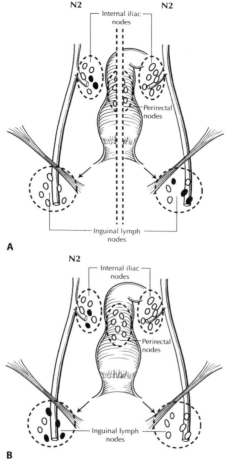

**FIGURE 15.9.** (**A**) Two views of N2, which is defined as metastasis in unilateral internal iliac (*left*) and/or inguinal lymph node(s) (*right*). (**B**) N2: metastases in unilateral internal iliac *and* inguinal lymph node(s).

| | |
|---|---|
| GX | Grade cannot be assessed |
| G1 | Well differentiated |
| G2 | Moderately differentiated |
| G3 | Poorly differentiated |
| G4 | Undifferentiated |

## HISTOPATHOLOGIC TYPE

The staging system applies to all carcinomas arising in the anal canal, including carcinomas that arise within anorectal fistulas. Melanomas, carcinoid tumors, and sarcomas are excluded from this staging system.

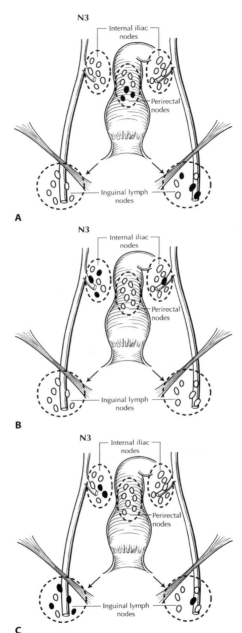

**FIGURE 15.10.** (**A**) N3 is defined as metastasis in perirectal and inguinal lymph nodes (as illustrated) and/or bilateral internal iliac and/or inguinal lymph nodes. (**B**) N3: metastases in bilateral internal iliac lymph nodes. (**C**) N3: metastases in bilateral internal iliac *and* inguinal lymph nodes.

Most carcinomas of the anal canal are squamous cell carcinomas. The WHO classification of the types and subtypes of carcinomas of the anal canal is shown later. The terms *transitional cell* and *cloacogenic carcinoma* have been abandoned, because these tumors are now recognized as nonkeratinizing types of squamous cell carcinoma.

**WHO Classification of Carcinoma of the Anal Canal***

Squamous cell carcinoma
Adenocarcinoma
> Rectal type
> Of anal glands
> Within anorectal fistula
Mucinous adenocarcinoma
Small cell carcinoma
Undifferentiated carcinoma

*The term *carcinoma*, *NOS* (not otherwise specified) is not part of the WHO classification.

Perianal skin and anal margin (junction of squamous mucosa and skin) tumor types include squamous cell carcinoma, giant condyloma (verrucous carcinoma), basal cell carcinoma, Bowen's disease, and Paget's disease. These tumors are staged as skin cancers according to the system outlined in Chap. 29.

## BIBLIOGRAPHY

Balachandra B, Marcus V, Jass JR. Poorly differentiated tumours of the anal canal: A diagnostic strategy for the surgical pathologist. Histopathology. 2007;50:163–74.

Bendell JC, Ryan DP. Current perspectives on anal cancer. Oncology. 2003;17:492–503.

Clark MA, Hartley A, Geh JI. Cancer of the anal canal. Lancet Oncol. 2004;5: 149–57.

Das P, Crane CH, Ajani JA. Current treatment for localized anal carcinoma. Curr Opin Oncol. 2007;19:396–400.

Engstrom PF, Benson AB III, Chen YJ, et al. Anal canal cancer clinical practice guidelines in oncology. J Natl Compr Canc Netw. 2005;3:510–5.

Esiashvili N, Landry J, Matthews RH. Carcinoma of the anus: strategies in management. The Oncologist. 2002;7:188–99.

Fenger C, Frisch M, Marti MC, Parc R. Tumors of the anal canal. In: Hamilton SR, Aaltonen LA, editors: World Health Organization classification of tumors. Pathology and genetics of tumors of the digestive system. Lyon: IARC; 2000. pp. 145–155.

Khatri VP, Chopra S. Clinical presentation, imaging, and staging of anal cancer. Surg Oncol Clin N Am. 2004;13:295–308.

Licitra L, Spinazze S, Doci R, et al. Cancer of the anal region. Crit Rev Oncol Hematol. 2002;43:77–92.

Moore HG, Guillem JG. Anal neoplasms. Surg Clin North Am. 2002;82:1233–51.

Sato H, Koh P-K, Bartolo DCC. Management of anal canal cancer. Dis Colon Rectum. 2005;48:1301–15.

# Gastrointestinal Stromal Tumor

## *At-A-Glance*

---

**SUMMARY OF CHANGES**

• This staging system is new for the seventh edition

---

**ANATOMIC STAGE/PROGNOSTIC GROUPS**

*Gastric GIST\**

| Group | T | N | M | Mitotic rate |
|-------|---|---|---|--------------|
| Stage IA | T1 or T2 | N0 | M0 | Low |
| Stage IB | T3 | N0 | M0 | Low |
| Stage II | T1 | N0 | M0 | High |
| | T2 | N0 | M0 | High |
| | T4 | N0 | M0 | Low |
| Stage IIIA | T3 | N0 | M0 | High |
| Stage IIIB | T4 | N0 | M0 | High |
| Stage IV | Any T | N1 | M0 | Any rate |
| | Any T | Any N | M1 | Any rate |

*Small Intestinal GIST\*\**

| Group | T | N | M | Mitotic rate |
|-------|---|---|---|--------------|
| Stage I | T1 or T2 | N0 | M0 | Low |
| Stage II | T3 | N0 | M0 | Low |
| Stage IIIA | T1 | N0 | M0 | High |
| | T4 | N0 | M0 | Low |
| Stage IIIB | T2 | N0 | M0 | High |
| | T3 | N0 | M0 | High |
| | T4 | N0 | M0 | High |
| Stage IV | Any T | N1 | M0 | Any rate |
| | Any T | Any N | M1 | Any rate |

**ICD-O-3 TOPOGRAPHY CODES**

| | |
|---|---|
| C15.0– C15.9 | Esophagus |
| C16.0– C16.9 | Stomach |
| C17.0– C17.2, C17.4– C17.9 | Small intestine |
| C18.0– C18.9 | Colon |
| C19.9 | Recto- sigmoid junction |
| C20.9 | Rectum |
| C48.1 | Specified parts of peritoneum (mesentery and omentum) |

**ICD-O-3 HISTOLOGY CODE RANGES**
8935, 8936

*\*Note*: Also to be used for omentum.

*\*\*Note*: Also to be used for esophagus, colorectal, mesentery, and peritoneum.

## INTRODUCTION

Gastrointestinal stromal tumor (GIST) is the most common mesenchymal tumor in the gastrointestinal tract. The designation of GIST refers to a specific tumor type that is generally immunohistochemically KIT-positive and is driven by KIT or PDGFRA activating mutations.

In terms of biologic potential, GISTs encompass a continuum. They include minute or small, paucicellular, mitotically inactive, obviously benign-looking tumors previously often designated as leiomyomas. At the other end of the spectrum there are larger tumors many of which contain significant mitotic activity and are histologically sarcomatous, previously often called leiomyosarcomas. In the middle, nearly all permutations of tumor size and mitotic activity occur, except that small (<2 cm) tumors with high mitotic activity are very rare. Based on the continuous biologic spectrum of GISTs, this staging scheme encompasses all GISTs. In fact, some authors maintain that most if not all GISTs should be considering having at least some potential for malignancy.

Finally, the unique management strategy for GIST needs to be considered in the staging system. In addition to a complete excision, as much as it is possible, adjuvant treatment via KIT/PDGFRA tyrosine kinase inhibitors (notably, imatinib mesylate and some second generation drugs such as sunitinib malate) are used in metastatic and unresectable GIST. Use of adjuvant therapy, especially imatinib, in GISTs deemed to be at high risk for metastasis, is being studied in clinical trials, but is currently largely experimental. This staging system attempts to assist GIST management by offering statistical probabilities of metastasis development, by tumor size and mitotic rate, the most important and most widely studied prognostic parameters in GIST.

## ANATOMY

**Primary Site.** GISTs occur throughout the gastrointestinal tract. They are most common in the stomach (60%) and small intestine (jejunum and ileum) (30%) and are relatively rare in the duodenum (5%), rectum (3%), colon (1–2%), and esophagus (<1%). In some cases, they present as disseminated tumors without a known primary site, and a small number of GISTs may be primary in the omentum or mesenteries.

**Regional Lymph Nodes.** Nodal metastasis is very rare and virtually unheard of in GIST, especially if one adheres to its rigorous histologic verification. Surgeons generally agree that nodal dissection is not indicated for GIST. In the absence of information on regional lymph node status, N0/pN0 is appropriate; NX should not be used.

**Metastastic Sites.** Metastases include intra-abdominal soft tissue, liver, and distant metastases. Presence of any of these is designated M1. Distant metastases are relatively rare in GISTs, but they are increasingly detected with sophisticated radiological studies. The most common distinct, non-abdominal metastatic sites are bone, soft tissues, and skin, whereas lung metastases are distinctly rare.

## RULES FOR CLASSIFICATION

The following staging system parallels the one used for peripheral soft tissue tumors. In addition, a numerical value for risk of metastasis is provided, based on the largest follow-up studies. Although T, N, and M definitions are identical for all GISTs, separate stage grouping schemes are provided for gastric and small intestinal tumors. Staging criteria for gastric tumors should be applied in primary, solitary omental GISTs.

Primary, solitary, mesenteric, and duodenal GISTs should be staged according to the small intestinal (jejunal-ileal) grouping. Data on GISTs in less common sites (esophagus, colon, rectum) are insufficient to allow presentation of a detailed stage grouping. It is believed that the staging criteria for small intestinal GISTs should be followed in these cases.

This staging system uses tumor size, dissemination status, and mitotic rate as the staging parameters.

**Definition of T.** *Tumor size and depth.* Because most GISTs are spherical or ovoid, the maximum tumor diameter is easy to determine. In the case of ruptured tumors, one may have to resort to estimates of the tumor size, or obtain assistance for maximum diameter measurement from radiologic studies.

The size thresholds of the greatest tumor diameter used in this staging system are 2, 5, and 10 cm. Depth of gastric or intestinal wall involved cannot be applied as practical staging criteria, because most GISTs, except the smallest ones, form transmural masses.

*Mitotic rate.* A standardized approach is needed in the determination of mitotic rate. The mitotic rate should be obtained from an area that on screening shows the highest level of mitotic activity. The mitotic rate of GIST is best expressed as the number of mitoses per 50 high-power fields using the $40\times$ magnification objective (total area 5 mm$^2$ in 50 fields). Because the counts in large prognostic studies have been obtained with "conventional" optics not employing wide field size, the number of fields needs to be adjusted. This practically means counting mitoses in 25 fields in a microscope equipped with wide field optics, to obtain a total area of 5 mm$^2$. Stringent criteria have to be followed when defining a mitosis: pyknotic or dyskaryotic nuclei must not be counted as mitoses.

For the purpose of this staging system, mitotic rates are categorized as follows:

Mitotic rates $\leq 5/50$ HPFs are considered low
Mitotic rates $> 5/50$ HPFs are considered high

**Metastases.** Intra-abdominal metastasis refers to tumor involvement in the abdominal cavity outside the main tumor mass in the peritoneum, omentum, organ serosae, and cul-de-sac, among others. Tumor multiplicity, that is, the presence of anatomically separate, multiple gastrointestinal primary tumors of various sizes, usually in the setting of neurofibromatosis type 1 or familial GIST syndrome, should not be considered intra-abdominal dissemination. Also, rare cases of multiple independent GISTs at different GI sites have been reported.

A solitary omental tumor mass should not be considered evidence of dissemination as it may represent a primary tumor. The same may be true for solitary mesenteric masses; however, experience is limited. Separation of these tumors from their gastric or intestinal origin during tumor growth is a likely explanation for primary omental and mesenteric GISTs. Furthermore, a retroperitoneal location of some segments of intestines makes a retroperitoneal location of a primary GIST also possible. However, great caution should be exercised in defining a primary extragastrointestinal GIST, so that the possibility of this being a metastasis from a gastric or intestinal origin is thoroughly excluded by clinical and radiological studies.

Liver metastasis implies the presence of tumor inside the liver parenchyma as one or more nodules. Adherence to liver capsule, even if extensive, as sometimes seen in gastric GISTs, should not be considered liver metastasis.

## PROGNOSTIC FEATURES

In some cases, patients have survived for a long time after a solitary intra-abdominal GIST metastasis. Tumors with mitotic rates in the lower end of "high mitotic rate" (6–10 mitoses/50 HPFs) may behave better than those with significantly elevated mitotic rates (>10 mitoses/50 HPFs).

There may be differences in behavior between GISTs with different types of KIT and PDGFRA mutations. Because of limitations of the universal application of mutation studies (most importantly, their limited availability), mutations are not considered in this staging system. Further research is needed to examine these and other prognostic factors in detail.

Tables 16.1 and 16.2 show the disease progression of gastric and small intestinal GISTs.

**TABLE 16.1.** Disease progression in gastric GISTs

| Stage | Tumor size (cm) | Mitotic rate | Prognostic group[a] | Observed rate of progressive disease[a] |
|---|---|---|---|---|
| Stage IA | ≤5 | Low | 1, 2 | 0–2% |
| Stage IB | >5–10 | Low | 3a | 3–4% |
| Stage II | >5–10 | High | 4 | Insufficient data |
| | >5–10 | High | 5 | 15% |
| | >10 | Low | 3b | 12% |
| Stage IIIA | >5–10 | High | 6a | 49% |
| IIIB | >10 | High | 6b | 86% |

[a]From Miettinen M, Sobin LH, Lasota J. Gastrointestinal stromal tumors of the stomach: a clinicopathologic, immunohistochemical, and molecular genetic studies of 1765 cases with long-term follow-up. Am J Surg Pathol. 2005;29:52–68, with permission from Lippincott Williams & Wilkins.

**TABLE 16.2.** Disease progression in small intestinal GIST

| Stage | Tumor size (cm) | Mitotic rate | Prognostic group[a] | Observed rate of progressive disease[a] |
|---|---|---|---|---|
| Stage IA | ≤5 | Low | 1, 2 | 0–2% |
| Stage II | >5–10 | Low | 3a | 23% |
| Stage III A | >10 | Low | 3b | 49% |
| | ≤2 | High | 4 | 50% |
| Stage IIIB | >2–5 | High | 5 | 73% |
| | >5 | High | 6a | 72% |
| | >10 | High | 6b | 89% |

[a] From Miettinen M, Makhlouf HR, Sobin LH, Lasota J. Gastrointestinal stromal tumors (GISTs) of the jejunum and ileum – a clinicopathologic, immunohistochemical and molecular genetic study of 906 cases prior to imatinib with long-term follow-up. Am J Surg Pathol. 2006;30:477–89, with permission from Lippincott Williams & Wilkins.

## DEFINITIONS OF TNM (For GISTs At All Sites)

### Primary Tumor (T)

| | |
|---|---|
| TX | Primary tumor cannot be assessed |
| T0 | No evidence for primary tumor |
| T1 | Tumor 2 cm or less |
| T2 | Tumor more than 2 cm but not more than 5 cm |
| T3 | Tumor more than 5 cm but not more than 10 cm |
| T4 | Tumor more than 10 cm in greatest dimension |

### Regional Lymph Nodes (N)

| | |
|---|---|
| NX | Regional lymph nodes cannot be assessed |
| N0 | No regional lymph node metastasis |
| N1 | Regional lymph node metastasis |

### Distant Metastasis (M)

| | |
|---|---|
| M0 | No distant metastasis |
| M1 | Distant metastasis |

## HISTOPATHOLOGIC GRADE

Grading for GISTs is dependent on mitotic rate
Low mitotic rate: 5 or fewer per 50 HPF
High mitotic rate: over 5 per 50 HPF

*Gastric GIST**

| Group | T | N | M | Mitotic rate |
|-------|---|---|---|--------------|
| Stage IA | T1 or T2 | N0 | M0 | Low |
| Stage IB | T3 | N0 | M0 | Low |
| Stage II | T1 | N0 | M0 | High |
| | T2 | N0 | M0 | High |
| | T4 | N0 | M0 | Low |
| Stage IIIA | T3 | N0 | M0 | High |
| Stage IIIB | T4 | N0 | M0 | High |
| Stage IV | Any T | N1 | M0 | Any rate |
| | Any T | Any N | M1 | Any rate |

*Small Intestinal GIST***

| Group | T | N | M | Mitotic rate |
|-------|---|---|---|--------------|
| Stage I | T1 or T2 | N0 | M0 | Low |
| Stage II | T3 | N0 | M0 | Low |
| Stage IIIA | T1 | N0 | M0 | High |
| | T4 | N0 | M0 | Low |
| Stage IIIB | T2 | N0 | M0 | High |
| | T3 | N0 | M0 | High |
| | T4 | N0 | M0 | High |
| Stage IV | Any T | N1 | M0 | Any rate |
| | Any T | Any N | M1 | Any rate |

*Note: Also to be used for omentum.

**Note: Also to be used for esophagus, colorectal, mesentery, and peritoneum.

## PROGNOSTIC FACTORS (SITE-SPECIFIC FACTORS)
### (For GISTs At All Sites)
### (Recommended for Collection)

| Required for staging | Mitotic rate |
|----------------------|--------------|
| Clinically significant | KIT immunohistochemistry |
| | Mutational status of KIT, PDGFRA |

## HISTOLOGIC GRADE (G)

Histologic grading, an ingredient in sarcoma staging, is not well suited to GISTs, because a majority of these tumors have low or relatively low mitotic rates below the thresholds used for grading of soft tissue tumors, and because GISTs often manifest aggressive features with mitotic rates below the thresholds used for soft tissue tumor grading (the lowest tier of mitotic rates for soft tissue sarcomas being 10 mitoses per 10 HPFs). In GIST staging, the grade is replaced by mitotic activity.

GX      Grade cannot be assessed
G1      Low grade; mitotic rate ≤5/50 HPF
G2      High grade, mitotic rate >5/50 HPF

## HISTOPATHOLOGIC TYPE

This staging system applies to all GISTs. The morphologic subtypes of GISTs include spindle cell (70%), epithelioid (20%), and mixed cell types. The prognostic significance of cell type remains unproven.

**16**

## BIBLIOGRAPHY

Blanke CD, Corless CL. State-of-the art therapy for gastrointestinal stromal tumors. Cancer Invest. 2005;23:274–80.

Emory TS, Sobin KH, Lukes L, Lee DH, O'Leary TJ. Prognosis of gastrointestinal smooth-muscle (stromal) tumors: dependence on anatomic site. Am J Surg Pathol. 1999;23:82–7.

Fletcher CDM, Berman JJ, Corless C, Gorstein F, Lasota J, Longley BJ, Miettinen M, O'Leary TJ, Remotti H, Rubin BP, Shmookler B, Sobin LH, Weiss SW. Diagnosis of gastrointestinal stromal tumors: a consensus approach. Hum Pathol. 2002;33:459–65; Int J Surg Pathol. 2002;10:81–9.

Lasota J, Miettinen M. KIT and PDGFRA mutations in GIST. Semin Diagn Pathol. 2006;23:91–102.

Miettinen M, Monihan JM, Sarlomo-Rikala M, Kovatich AJ, Carr NJ, Emory TS, et al. Gastrointestinal stromal tumors/smooth muscle tumors (GISTs) primary in the omentum and mesentery: clinicopathologic and immuno-histochemical study of 26 cases. Am J Surg Pathol. 1999;23:1109–18.

Miettinen M, Sarlomo-Rikala M, Sobin LH, Lasota J. Gastrointestinal stromal tumors and leiomyosarcomas in the colon: a clinicopathologic, immuno-histochemical, and molecular genetic study of 44 cases. Am J Surg Pathol. 2000;24:1339–52.

Miettinen M, Furlong M, Sarlomo-Rikala M, Burke A, Sobin LH, Lasota J. Gastro-intestinal stromal tumors, intramural leiomyomas, and leiomyosarcomas in the rectum and anus: a clinicopathologic, immunohistochemical, and molecular genetic study of 144 cases. Am J Surg Pathol. 2001;25:1121–33.

Miettinen M, El-Rifai W, Sobin LH, Lasota J. Evaluation of malignancy and progno-sis of gastrointestinal stromal tumors: a review. Hum Pathol. 2002;33:478–83.

Miettinen M, Kopczynski J, Makhlouf HR, Sarlomo-Rikala M, Gyorffy H, Burke A, et al. Gastrointestinal stromal tumors, intramural leiomyomas, and leiomyo-sarcomas in the duodenum: a clinicopathologic, immunohistochemical, and molecular genetic study of 167 cases. Am J Surg Pathol. 2003;27:625–41.

Miettinen M, Sobin LH, Lasota J. Gastrointestinal stromal tumors of the stomach: a clinicopathologic, immunohistochemical, and molecular genetic studies of 1765 cases with long-term follow-up. Am J Surg Pathol. 2005;29:52–68.

Miettinen M, Fetsch JF, Sobin LH, Lasota J. Gastrointestinal stromal tumors in patients with neurofibromatosis 1: a clinicopathologic and molecular genetic study of 45 cases. Am J Surg Pathol. 2006a;30(1):90–6.

Miettinen M, Makhlouf HR, Sobin LH, Lasota J. Gastrointestinal stromal tumors (GISTs) of the jejunum and ileum – a clinicopathologic, immuno-histochemical and molecular genetic study of 906 cases prior to imatinib with long-term follow-up. Am J Surg Pathol. 2006b;30:477–89.

# Neuroendocrine Tumors

*(Gastric, small bowel, colonic, rectal, and
ampulla of vater carcinoid tumors [well-
differentiated neuroendocrine tumors and
well-differentiated neuroendocrine carcinomas];
carcinoid tumors of the appendix [see Chap. 13]
and neuroendocrine tumors of the pancreas [see
Chap. 24] are not included.)*

## *At-A-Glance*

### SUMMARY OF CHANGES

• This staging system is new for the 7th edition

**ANATOMIC STAGE/PROGNOSTIC GROUPS**

| Stage 0 | Tis* | N0 | M0 |
|---------|------|-----|-----|
| Stage I | T1 | N0 | M0 |
| Stage IIA | T2 | N0 | M0 |
| Stage IIB | T3 | N0 | M0 |
| Stage IIIA | T4 | N0 | M0 |
| Stage IIIB | Any T | N1 | M0 |
| Stage IV | Any T | Any N | M1 |

*Note: Tis applies only to stomach.

**ICD-O-3 TOPOGRAPHY CODES**

| | |
|---|---|
| C16.0–C16.9 | Stomach |
| C17.0–C17.9 | Small intestine |
| C18.0, | Colon |
| C18.2–C18.9 | (excludes C18.1) |
| C19.9 | Recto-sigmoid junction |
| C20.9 | Rectum |
| C24.1 | Ampulla of Vater |

**ICD-O-3 HISTOLOGY CODE RANGES**
8153, 8240–8242, 8246, 8249

## INTRODUCTION

Neuroendocrine tumors (NETs) arise from the diffuse neuroendocrine system, which comprises neuroendocrine cells spread as a single cell or clusters of cells throughout the entire gastrointestinal tract, the bronchopulmonary system, and the urogenital tract. These lesions are often referred to generically using the archaic term *carcinoid* in deference to the original report of 1907 by Oberndorfer. In the past the "traditional" classification of carcinoids (1963 Sandler/Williams) was based upon their presumed embryonic origin and comprised foregut (lung, thymus, stomach, pancreas, and duodenum), midgut (from duodenum beyond the Treitz ligament to the proximal transverse colon), and hindgut carcinoids (distal colon and rectum). Although this classification is used, a tumor-based classification introduced by the World Health Organization (WHO) in 2000 has far greater scientific and clinical applicability. This classification utilizes the more generic term NET, and classification of the lesions is variously based upon size, proliferative rate, localization, differentiation, and hormone production. However, the term *carcinoid* is still in widespread use in the clinical setting and in data collected by tumor registries.

Investigation of the Surveillance Epidemiology and End Results (SEER) data base, 1973–2004, demonstrates that the incidence of gastric NETs in the US population in 2004 was 0.34/100,000, and since 1973 the annual increase in incidence has been approximately 9%. For small intestinal NETs, the annual increase in incidence since 1973 is 3.51%, and the incidence in the US population for duodenal NETs is 2.06/100,000, jejunal 0.36/100,000, and ileal 4.06/100,000 in 2004. Furthermore, NETs comprised 1.25% of all malignancies in 2004 compared to only 0.75% of all malignancies in 1994. The reason for the marked increase in incidence (prevalence) of these tumors probably represents an increased awareness by pathologists and clinicians as well as the availability of more sophisticated diagnostic tools. A connection between the introduction of potent acid suppressive medications that induce hypergastrinemia and gastric NETs has been suggested but a direct relationship remains unproven. Overall, NETs are slightly more common in women (55%); however, gastric NETs exhibit a more pronounced female predominance (64.5%). Pancreatic (66.7%) and small intestinal (53.4%) NETs are more common in men. The overall black:white ratio for GEP-NETs has increased from 1.13–1.32 since 1973. Particular sites for NETs, rather than NETs as a whole, exhibit differential incidence proclivities within the US population. As an example, duodenal NETs demonstrate an incidence propensity in black patients 3.12 times greater than what might be predicted. The lesions may also occur as a component of familial syndromes such as multiple endocrine neoplasia (MEN), von Hippel–Lindau syndrome, and neurofibromatosis and elements for the genetic basis of some associations has been suggested.

Overall the tumors exhibit a propensity for slower growth than adenocarcinomas but aggressive variants are not uncommon. In general, NETs often present a considerable diagnostic challenge especially if covert. Since the majority of small intestinal NETs (90%) are metastatic at diagnosis, a therapeutic management strategy is often complex and requires multispeciality input. A substantial number of NETs (20% of small intestinal, but <5% of gastric) exhibit disabling hormonal-induced symptomatology (flush, sweating, diarrhea, bronchospasm), which can be difficult to control. The primary tumor is usually small, may be multicentric (2% overall but as much as 33% in the small intestine) and clinical symptoms are often absent (hence diagnosis is delayed) until the tumor has metastasized to the liver. Extensive local and distant fibrosis due to production of fibroblastic growth factors is a common feature of small bowel NETs and may result in local problems (adhesive obstruction) or even cardiac valve disease.

**Primary Site.** NETs can arise from neuroendocrine cells of the entire gastroenteropancreatic system, although the small intestine is the commonest overall location (20.7%). The terminal ileal area is the most common location and lesions may be multicentric. The progenitor cell of the majority of gastro intestinal NETs is the EC cell. Gastric NETs arise from the enterochromaffin-like (ECL) cells of the fundic gastric glands. Among 12,259 GEP-NETs in the SEER database, 8.2% were gastric, 5.4% pancreatic, and 20.7% small intestinal (duodenal 19.1%, jejunal 9.2%, ileal 71.7%). The proportion of nonfunctional lesions in GEP-NETs ranges from 10 to 25% depending upon the rigorousness with which criteria of nonfunctionality are applied; some series indicate an incidence as high as 48%.

**Regional Lymph Nodes.** A rich lymphatic network surrounds the gastro-intestinal organs, and NETs exhibit an almost equal affinity for spread via the lymphatic system as well as the bloodstream.

17

### Stomach

- *Greater curvature of the stomach.* Greater curvature greater omental, gas-troduodenal, gastroepiploic, pyloric and pancreaticoduodenal nodes
- *Pancreatic and splenic areas.* Pancreaticolienal, peripancreatic, and splenic nodes
- *Lesser curvature of the stomach.* Lesser curvature, lesser omental, left gastric, cardioesophageal, common hepatic, celiac, and hepatoduode-nal nodes
- *"Distant metastasis" nodal groups.* Retropancreatic, para-aortic, portal, retroperitoneal, and mesenteric

### Small Intestine

- *Duodenum.* Duodenal, hepatic, pancreaticoduodenal, infrapyloric, gas-troduodenal, pyloric, superior mesenteric, and pericholedochal nodes
- *Ileum and jejunum.* Posterior cecal (terminal ileum only), superior mesenteric, and mesenteric NOS nodes
- *"Distant metastasis" nodal groups.* Celiac nodes

### Large Intestine

- *Cecum.* Pericolic, anterior cecal, posterior cecal, ileocolic, right colic
- *Ascending colon.* Pericolic, ileocolic, right colic, middle colic
- *Hepatic flexure.* Pericolic, middle colic, right colic
- *Transverse colon.* Pericolic, middle colic
- *Splenic flexure.* Pericolic, middle colic, left colic, inferior mesenteric
- *Descending colon.* Pericolic, left colic, inferior mesenteric, sigmoid
- *Sigmoid colon.* Pericolic, inferior mesenteric, superior rectal (hemor-rhoidal), sigmoidal, sigmoid mesenteric
- *Rectosigmoid.* Pericolic, perirectal, left colic, sigmoid mesenteric, sig-moidal, inferior mesenteric, superior rectal (hemorrhoidal), middle rectal (hemorrhoidal)

- *Rectum.* Perirectal, sigmoid mesenteric, inferior mesenteric, lateral sacral presacral, internal iliac, sacral promontory (Gerota's), internal iliac, superior rectal (hemorrhoidal), middle rectal (hemorrhoidal), inferior rectal (hemorrhoidal)

**Metastatic Sites.** The most common metastatic distribution for GEP-NETs is lymph nodes (89.8%), the liver (44.1%), lung (13.6%), peritoneum (13.6%), and pancreas (6.8%). Local spread to adjacent organs is often characterized by associated extensive fibrosis.

## RULES FOR CLASSIFICATION

**Clinical Staging.** Clinical staging depends upon the anatomic extent and hormonal activity of the primary tumor, which can be ascertained by examination before treatment. Such examination includes a medical history, physical examination, routine laboratory studies, and biochemical markers of NET disease including chromogranin A (CgA). Gastroscopy can identify lesions down to the ligament of Treitz. Endoscopic ultrasound (EUS) is a highly sensitive method for diagnostic and preoperative evaluation of NETs of the stomach, duodenum, and pancreas, since it not only identifies submucosal lesions but also facilitates staging and allows fine-needle aspiration for histology. Capsule endoscopy and enteroscopy are useful to identify small bowel lesions. Magnetic resonance imaging (MRI) and computed tomography (CT) are effective in the initial localization of NETs or their metastases with a median detection rate and sensitivity of approximately 80%. Somatostatin receptor scintigraphy (SRS) and positron emission tomography (PET) have an overall sensitivity approximately 90% to localize GI-NETs. Combinations of SRS or PET with CT or MRI imaging systems are especially effective with a high sensitivity (96–100%) for NETs detection.

**Pathologic Staging.** Pathologic staging is based on endoscopic biopsy specimens, percutaneous biopsies, fine-needle aspirates, surgical exploration, and on examination of surgically resected primary tumor, lymph nodes, and distant metastases.

## PROGNOSTIC FEATURES

Important determinants of survival in NETs are neuroendocrine cell type, nodal status, and Ki67 index. Negative predictable variables are the presence of clinical symptoms, size of primary tumor, elevated CgA and hormonally active tumor by-products, and a high mitotic index.

Gastric NETs may be subdivided into ECL cell carcinoid type I–III. Type I tumors (approximately 80–90%) originate in a hypergastrinemic milieu (rarely metastasize approximately 1–3%, 5-year survival of approximately 100%). Type II lesions are rare (5–7%), occur in the context of MEN-1 and exhibit a more aggressive neoplastic phenotype (10–30% metastasis, 5-year survival of 60–90%). Type III lesions occur in a normogastrinemic environment and constitute approximately 10–15% of tumors, behave as adenocarcinomas, are usually metastatic (50%), and have a 5-year survival

(<50%). Little biological information exists regarding the mechanisms responsible for human ECL cell transformation.

The malignancy of gastric NETs types can be further defined by elevation of levels of CCN2, metastasis associated protein 1 – MTA1, and melanoma antigen D2 – MAGE-D2, whose gene and protein expression correlates with invasion and metastatic potential.

Duodenal NETs with a tumor size greater than 2 cm, involvement of the muscularis propria, and presence of mitotic figures have a poor prognosis. The presence of regional lymph node metastases, however, cannot be predicted reliably on the basis of tumor size or depth of invasion, although EUS is of use. In a study including 89 patients with duodenal NETs, the overall 5-year survival was 60%.

Jejunoileal NETs typically present at an advanced stage and have a poor 5-year survival rate (60.5%) compared with other GI NETs. Tumor size is the most predictive factor and spread to regional lymph nodes is common at diagnosis.

Well-differentiated NETs arising in the colon are relatively rare, occuring most commonly in the cecum, although some in this location may represent extension from appendiceal carcinoids. Tumor size is probably an important prognostic indicator, but is less useful for colonic NETs because most are greater than 2 cm and involve the muscularis propria at diagnosis. Overall survival is 33–42%.

Rectal NETs have a low propensity for metastasis and have a favorable prognosis, with overall 5-year survival of 88.3%. Features predictive of poor outcome are tumor size greater than 2 cm and invasion of the muscularis propria.

Observed survival rates for 2,997 patients with GI NETs are shown in Figure 17.1.

## DEFINITIONS OF TNM

### Stomach

*Primary Tumor (T)*

| | |
|---|---|
| TX | Primary tumor cannot be assessed |
| T0 | No evidence of primary tumor |
| Tis | Carcinoma in situ/dysplasia (tumor size less than 0.5 mm), confined to mucosa |
| T1 | Tumor invades lamina propria or submucosa and 1 cm or less in size |
| T2 | Tumor invades muscularis propria or more than 1 cm in size |
| T3 | Tumor penetrates subserosa |
| T4 | Tumor invades visceral peritoneum (serosal) or other organs or adjacent structures |
| | For any T, add (m) for multiple tumors |

*Regional Lymph Nodes (N)*

| | |
|---|---|
| NX | Regional lymph nodes cannot be assessed |
| N0 | No regional lymph node metastasis |
| N1 | Regional lymph node metastasis |

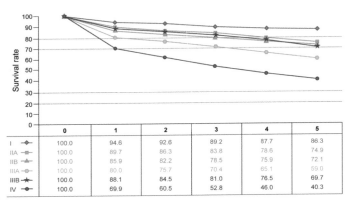

| | 0 | 1 | 2 | 3 | 4 | 5 |
|---|---|---|---|---|---|---|
| I | 100.0 | 94.6 | 92.6 | 89.2 | 87.7 | 86.3 |
| IIA | 100.0 | 89.7 | 86.3 | 83.8 | 78.6 | 74.9 |
| IIB | 100.0 | 85.9 | 82.2 | 78.5 | 75.9 | 72.1 |
| IIIA | 100.0 | 80.0 | 75.7 | 70.4 | 65.1 | 59.0 |
| IIIB | 100.0 | 88.1 | 84.5 | 81.0 | 76.5 | 69.7 |
| IV | 100.0 | 69.9 | 60.5 | 52.8 | 46.0 | 40.3 |

Years from diagnosis

**FIGURE 17.1.** Observed survival rates for 2,997 cases with GI neuroendocrine tumors. Data from the SEER 1973–2005 Public Use File diagnosed in years 1990–2000. Stage I includes 351; Stage IIA, 724; Stage IIB, 299; Stage IIIA, 115; Stage IIIB, 743; Stage IV, 765; (Stage 0 excluded due to limited numbers).

### Distant Metastases (M)

| | |
|---|---|
| M0 | No distant metastases |
| M1 | Distant metastasis |

## Duodenum/Ampulla/Jejunum/Ileum

### Primary Tumor (T)

| | |
|---|---|
| TX | Primary tumor cannot be assessed |
| T0 | No evidence of primary tumor |
| T1 | Tumor invades lamina propria or submucosa and size 1 cm or less* (small intestinal tumors); tumor 1 cm or less (ampullary tumors) |
| T2 | Tumor invades muscularis propria or size >1 cm (small intestinal tumors); tumor >1 cm (ampullary tumors) |
| T3 | Tumor invades through the muscularis propria into subserosal tissue without penetration of overlying serosa (jejunal or ileal tumors) or invades pancreas or retroperitoneum (ampullary or duodenal tumors) or into non-peritonealized tissues |
| T4 | Tumor invades visceral peritoneum (serosa) or invades other organs |
| | For any T, add (m) for multiple tumors |

*Note: Tumor limited to ampulla of Vater for ampullary gangliocytic paraganglioma.

### Regional Lymph Nodes (N)

| | |
|---|---|
| NX | Regional lymph nodes cannot be assessed |
| N0 | No regional lymph node metastasis |
| N1 | Regional lymph node metastasis |

### Distant Metastases (M)
M0    No distant metastases
M1    Distant metastasis

## Colon or Rectum

### Primary Tumor (T)
TX     Primary tumor cannot be assessed
T0     No evidence of primary tumor
T1     Tumor invades lamina propria or submucosa and size 2 cm or less
T1a    tumor size less than 1 cm in greatest dimension
T1b    tumor size 1–2 cm in greatest dimension
T2     Tumor invades muscularis propria or size more than 2 cm with invasion of lamina propria or submucosa
T3     Tumor invades through the muscularis propria into the subserosa, or into non-peritonealized pericolic or perirectal tissues
T4     Tumor invades peritoneum or other organs
       For any T, add (m) for multiple tumors

### Regional Lymph Nodes (N)
NX     Regional lymph nodes cannot be assessed
N0     No regional lymph node metastasis
N1     Regional lymph node metastasis

### Distant Metastases (M)
M0     No distant metastases
M1     Distant metastasis

### ANATOMIC STAGE/PROGNOSTIC GROUPS

| Stage 0    | Tis   | N0    | M0 |
|------------|-------|-------|----|
| Stage I    | T1    | N0    | M0 |
| Stage IIA  | T2    | N0    | M0 |
| Stage IIB  | T3    | N0    | M0 |
| Stage IIIA | T4    | N0    | M0 |
| Stage IIIB | Any T | N1    | M0 |
| Stage IV   | Any T | Any N | M1 |

### PROGNOSTIC FACTORS (SITE-SPECIFIC FACTORS)
#### (Recommended for Collection)

| | |
|---|---|
| Required for staging | None |
| Clinically significant | Preoperative plasma chromogranin A level (CgA) |
| | Urinary 5-hydroxyindolacetic acid (5-HIAA) level |
| | Mitotic count |

## HISTOLOGIC GRADE (G)

Cellular pleomorphism is not a useful feature for grading carcinoid tumors. High proliferative index has been linked with more aggressive behavior, and it has been proposed that systemic chemotherapy can be considered in the management of midgut tumors with a high mitotic count. The following grading scheme has been proposed for GI NETs:

| Grade | Mitotic count (10 HPF)* | Ki-67 index (%)** |
|-------|-------------------------|-------------------|
| G1 | <2 | ≤2 |
| G2 | 2–20 | 3–20 |
| G3 | >20 | >20 |

*Note: 10 HPF: high power field = 2 mm², at least 40 fields (at 40× magnification) evaluated in areas of highest mitotic density.

**Note: MIB1 antibody; % of 2,000 tumor cells in areas of highest nuclear labeling.

## HISTOPATHOLOGIC TYPE

This staging system applies to carcinoid tumors (well-differentiated NETs), and atypical carcinoid tumors (well-differentiated neuroendocrine carcinomas) as listed below. High-grade neuroendocrine carcinomas and mixed glandular/well-differentiated NETs are excluded and should be staged according to guidelines for staging carcinomas at that site.

Carcinoid tumor
Well-differentiated NET
Atypical carcinoid
Well-differentiated neuroendocrine carcinoma
Gangliocytic paraganglioma

## BIBLIOGRAPHY

Berge T, Linnell F. Carcinoid tumors: frequency in a defined population during a 12-year period. Acta Pathol Microbiol Scand A 1976;84:322–30.

Burke AP, Sobin LH, Federspiel BH, et al. Carcinoid tumors of the duodenum: a clinicopathologic study of 99 cases. Archives Pathol Lab Med. 1990;114:700–4.

Capella C, Solcia E, Sobin LH, et al. Endocrine tumors of the small intestine. In: Hamilton SR, Aaltonen LA, editors. World Health Organization classification of tumors. Pathology and genetics of tumours of the digestive system. Lyon: IARC Press; 2000a. p. 77–82.

Capella C, Solcia E, Sobin LH, et al. Endocrine tumours of the colon and rectum. In: Hamilton SR, Aaltonen LA, editors. World Health Organization classification of tumours. Pathology and genetics of tumours of the digestive system. Lyon: IARC Press; 2000b. p. 137–9.

Capella C, Solcia E, Sobin LH, et al. Endocrine tumours of the stomach. In: Hamilton SR, Aaltonen LA, editors. World Health Organization classification of tumours. Pathology and genetics of tumours of the digestive system. Lyon: IARC Press; 2000c. p. 53–6.

Katona TM, Jones TD, Wang M, et al. Molecular evidence for independent origin of multifocal neuroendocrine tumors of the enteropancreatic axis. Cancer Res. 2006;66:4936–42.

Kidd M, Modlin IM, Mane SM, et al. Utility of molecular genetic signatures in the delineation of gastric neoplasia. Cancer. 2006;106:1480–8.

Kloppel G, Perren A, Heitz PU. The gastroenteropancreatic neuroendocrine cell system and its tumors: the WHO classification. Annals N Y Acad Sci. 2004;1014:13–27.

Mansour JC, Chen H. Pancreatic endocrine tumors. J Surg Res. 2004:120.

Modlin IM, Kidd M, Latich I, et al. Current status of gastrointestinal carcinoids. Gastroenterology. 2005;128:1717–51.

Modlin IM, Latich I, Zikusoka M, et al. Gastrointestinal carcinoids: the evolution of diagnostic strategies. J Clin Gastroenterol. 2006;40:572–82.

Modlin IM, Lye KD, Kidd M. A 5-decade analysis of 13, 715 carcinoid tumors. Cancer. 2003;97:934–59.

Oberndorfer S. Karzinoide tumores des Dunndardms. Frankf Z Pathol 1907;426–443.

Rindi G, Kloppel G, Alhman H, et al. TNM staging of foregut (neuro)endocrine tumors: a consensus proposal including a grading system. Virchows Archiv. 2006;449:395–401.

Rindi G, Kloppel G, Couvelard A, et al. TNM staging of midgut and hindgut (neuro) endocrine tumors: a consensus proposal including a grading system. Virchows Arch. 2007;451:757–62.

Rodrigues M, Traub-Weidinger T, Li S, et al. Comparison of 111In-DOTA-DPhel-Tyr3-octreotide and 111In-DOTA-lanreotide scintigraphy and dosimetry in patients with neuroendocrine tumours. European J Nucl Med Mol Imaging. 2006;33:532–40.

Rorstad O. Prognostic indicators for carcinoid neuroendocrine tumors of the gastrointestinal tract. J Surg Oncol. 2005;89:151–60.

Seemann MD. Detection of metastases from gastrointestinal neuroendocrine tumors: prospective comparison of 18F-TOCA PET, triple-phase CT, and PET/CT. Technol Cancer Res Treat. 2007;6:213–20.

Williams ED, Sandler M. The classification of carcinoid tumors. Lancet. 1963;1:238–9.

Zar N, Garmo H, Holmberg L, et al. Long-term survival of patients with small intestinal carcinoid tumors. World J Surg. 2004;28:1163–8.

17

# Liver

*(Excluding intrahepatic bile ducts; Sarcomas and tumors metastatic to the liver are not included.)*

## *At-A-Glance*

---

### SUMMARY OF CHANGES

Intrahepatic bile ducts are no longer included in this staging chapter. The staging of liver cancer now includes only hepatocellular carcinoma

**T Category Changes**

- In the T3 category, patients with invasion of major vessels are distinguished from patients with multiple tumors, of which any are >5 cm, but lack major vessel invasion because of the markedly different prognosis of these subgroups

  - T3a includes multiple tumors, any >5 cm

  - T3b includes tumors of any size involving a major portal vein or hepatic vein

- T4 category unchanged

**N Category Changes**

- Inferior phrenic lymph nodes were reclassified to regional lymph nodes from distant lymph nodes

**Stage Grouping Changes**

- Changes in T3 classification led to changes in Stage III groupings

  - Stage IIIA now includes only T3a; patients with major vessel invasion are removed from the IIIA stage grouping

  - Stage IIIB now includes only T3b (major vessel invasion)

  - T4 is shifted to Stage IIIC

- Stage IV includes all patients with metastasis, whether nodal or distant, separated into IVA and B to permit identification of each subgroup

  - Stage IVA now includes node-positive disease (N1)

  - Stage IVB now includes distant metastasis (M1)

---

| ANATOMIC STAGE/PROGNOSTIC GROUPS | | | | ICD-O-3 TOPOGRAPHY CODES |
|---|---|---|---|---|
| Stage I | T1 | N0 | M0 | C22.0    Liver |
| Stage II | T2 | N0 | M0 | |
| Stage IIIA | T3a | N0 | M0 | ICD-O-3 HISTOLOGY CODE RANGES |
| Stage IIIB | T3b | N0 | M0 | 8170–8175 |
| Stage IIIC | T4 | N0 | M0 | |
| Stage IVA | Any T | N1 | M0 | |
| Stage IVB | Any T | Any N | M1 | |

## INTRODUCTION

Primary malignancies of the liver include tumors arising from the hepatocytes (hepatocellular carcinoma), intrahepatic bile ducts (intrahepatic cholangiocarcinoma and cystadenocarcinoma), and mesenchymal elements (primary sarcoma). Only primary hepatocellular carcinoma is included in the current staging system described here. Hepatocellular carcinoma is the most common primary cancer of the liver and is a leading cause of death from cancer worldwide. Although it is uncommon in the United States, its incidence is rising. The majority of hepatocellular carcinomas arise in a background of chronic liver disease due to viral hepatitis (B or C), ethanol-related cirrhosis, and, possibly, related steatohepatitis. Cirrhosis may dominate the clinical picture and determine the prognosis. Other important indicators of outcome in hepatocellular carcinoma are resectability for cure and the extent of vascular invasion. Previously, intrahepatic bile duct cancer was staged using the system derived for hepatocellular carcinoma, but due to the markedly different incidence, epidemiology, treatment and prognosis for these diseases, staging for bile duct cancer has been removed from this chapter. A separate staging system is included for intrahepatic bile duct (see Chap. 19).

## ANATOMY

**Primary Site.** The liver has a dual blood supply: the hepatic artery, which typically branches from the celiac artery, and the portal vein, which drains the intestine. Blood from the liver passes through the hepatic veins and enters the inferior vena cava. The liver is divided into right and left liver by a plane (Cantlie's line) projecting between the gallbladder fossa and the vena cava and defined by the middle hepatic vein. Couinaud refined knowledge about the functional anatomy of the liver and proposed division of the liver into four sectors (formerly called segments) and eight segments. In this nomenclature, the liver is divided by vertical and oblique planes or scissurae defined by the three main hepatic veins and a transverse plane or scissura that follows a line drawn through the right and left portal branches. Thus, the four traditional segments (right anterior, right posterior, left medial, and left lateral) are replaced by sectors (right anterior, right posterior, left anterior, and left posterior), and these sectors are divided into segments

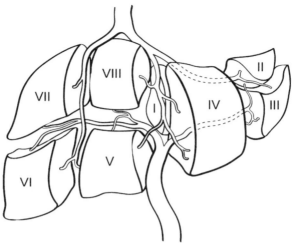

**FIGURE 18.1.** The eight segments of the liver are numbered clockwise in a frontal plane.

by the transverse scissura (Figure 18.1). The eight segments are numbered clockwise in a frontal plane. Recent advances in hepatic surgery have made possible anatomic (also called typical) resections along these planes.

Histologically, the liver is divided into lobules with central veins draining each lobule. The portal triads between the lobules contain the intrahepatic bile ducts and the blood supply, which consists of small branches of the hepatic artery and portal vein and intrahepatic lymphatic channels.

**Regional Lymph Nodes.** The regional lymph nodes are the hilar, hepatoduodenal ligament lymph nodes, inferior phrenic, and caval lymph nodes, among which the most prominent are the hepatic artery and portal vein lymph nodes. Nodal involvement should be coded as N1. Nodal involvement is now considered stage IV disease.

**Distant Metastatic Sites.** The main mode of dissemination of liver carcinomas is via the portal veins (intrahepatic) and hepatic veins. Intrahepatic venous dissemination cannot be differentiated from satellitosis or multifocal tumors and is classified as multiple tumors. The most common sites of extrahepatic dissemination are the lungs and bones. Tumors may extend through the liver capsule to adjacent organs (adrenal, diaphragm, and colon) or may rupture, causing acute hemorrhage and peritoneal metastasis.

## RULES FOR CLASSIFICATION

The T classification is based on the results of multivariate analyses of factors affecting prognosis after resection of liver carcinomas. The classification considers the presence or absence of vascular invasion (as assessed radiographically or pathologically), the number of tumor nodules (single versus multiple), and the size of the largest tumor (≤5 cm vs. >5 cm). For pathologic classification, vascular invasion includes gross as well as microscopic involvement of vessels. Major vascular invasion is defined as invasion of the branches of the main portal vein (right or left portal vein; this does not include sectoral or segmental branches) or as invasion of one or more of the three hepatic veins (right, middle, or left). Multiple tumors include satellitosis, multifocal tumors, and intrahepatic metastases. Invasion of adjacent organs other than the gallbladder or with perforation of the visceral peritoneum is considered T4.

**Validation.** Validation of T1, T2, and T3 categories of this staging system is based on multivariate analyses of outcome and survival data of single-institution and multi-institution studies of hepatic resection of hepatocellular carcinoma worldwide. The survival curves obtained from analysis of the database of the International Cooperative Study Group for Hepatocellular Carcinoma are presented in Figures 18.2 and 18.3. The system has been independently validated in several large cohorts of patients who underwent hepatic resection for hepatocellular worldwide. Recently, this system was validated in a large cohort of patients who underwent liver transplantation (Figure 18.4). As such, this is the first staging system independently validated in patients following both hepatic resection and liver transplantation.

**Clinical Staging.** Clinical staging depends on imaging procedures designed to demonstrate the size of the primary tumor and vascular invasion. Surgical exploration is not carried out if imaging shows that complete resection is not possible or if the hepatic reserve is deemed insufficient for safe resection. In the presence of cirrhosis, the Child-Pugh class and the

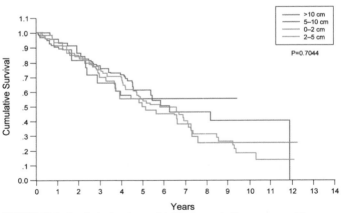

**FIGURE 18.2.** Survival of patients with T1 tumors (solitary tumor without vascular invasion), stratified by size. Size does not affect prognosis for this category (Data from Vauthey JN, Lauwers GY, Esnaola N, et al. A simplified staging for hepatocellular carcinoma. J Clin Oncol. 2002;20:1527–36).

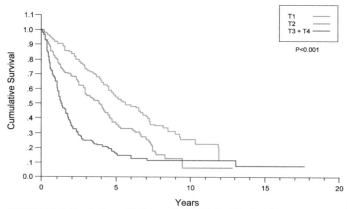

**FIGURE 18.3.** Survival stratified according to T classification (Data from Vauthey JN, Lauwers GY, Esnaola N, et al. A simplified staging for hepatocellular carcinoma. J Clin Oncol. 2002;20:1527–36).

**18**

Model of Endstage Liver Disease (MELD) score should be recorded. When advanced underlying liver disease (cirrhosis) dominates the prognosis, primary tumor factors (T classification) may become less relevant in terms of prognosis. In these instances, other clinical staging systems (Okuda staging, Cancer of the Liver Italian Program [CLIP] score, or Barcelona Clinic Liver Cancer [BCLC] staging) that combine the evaluation of liver disease and hepatocellular carcinoma may be helpful to supplement TNM staging.

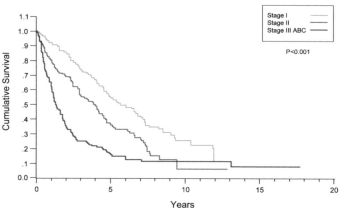

**FIGURE 18.4.** Survival stratified according to stage grouping (Data from Vauthey JN, Lauwers GY, Esnaola N, et al. A simplified staging for hepatocellular carcinoma. J Clin Oncol. 2002;20:1527–36).

**Pathologic Staging.** Complete pathologic staging consists of evaluation of the primary tumor, including histologic grade, regional lymph node status, and underlying liver disease. Regional lymph node involvement is rare (5%) except in the fibrolamellar variant of hepatocellular carcinoma. A major change from the 6th edition is that tumors with positive lymph nodes are classified as Stage IV because they carry the same prognosis as other patients with distant metastases. The grade is based on the cytopathologic study of nuclear pleomorphism as described by Edmonson and Steiner. Because of the prognostic significance of underlying liver disease in hepatocellular carcinoma, it is recommended that the results of the histopathologic analysis of the adjacent (non-tumorous) liver be reported. Severe fibrosis/cirrhosis (F1; Ishak score of 5–6) is associated with a worse prognosis than is absence of or moderate fibrosis (F0; Ishak score of 0–4). Although grade and underlying liver disease have prognostic significance, they are not included in the current staging system.

## PROGNOSTIC FEATURES

Clinical factors predictive of decreased survival duration include an elevated serum alpha-fetoprotein level and Child-Pugh class B and C liver disease. For patients who undergo tumor resection, the main predictor of poor outcome is a positive surgical margin (grossly or microscopically involved tumors indicative of incomplete resection). The effect of the extent of surgical clearance at the closest margin (<10 mm vs. >10 mm) remains controversial. Other prognostic factors associated with decreased survival include major vessel invasion and tumor size >5 cm in patients with multiple tumors.

## FIBROSIS SCORE (F)

The fibrosis score as defined by Ishak is recommended because of its prognostic value in overall survival. This scoring system uses a 0–6 scale.

F0    Fibrosis score 0–4 (none to moderate fibrosis)
F1    Fibrosis score 5–6 (severe fibrosis or cirrhosis)

## DEFINITIONS OF TNM

*Primary Tumor (T)*

| | |
|---|---|
| TX | Primary tumor cannot be assessed |
| T0 | No evidence of primary tumor |
| T1 | Solitary tumor without vascular invasion |
| T2 | Solitary tumor with vascular invasion or multiple tumors none more than 5 cm |
| T3a | Multiple tumors more than 5 cm |
| T3b | Single tumor or multiple tumors of any size involving a major branch of the portal vein or hepatic vein |
| T4 | Tumor(s) with direct invasion of adjacent organs other than the gallbladder or with perforation of visceral peritoneum |

### Regional Lymph Nodes (N)

| | |
|---|---|
| NX | Regional lymph nodes cannot be assessed |
| N0 | No regional lymph node metastasis |
| N1 | Regional lymph node metastasis |

### Distant Metastasis (M)

| | |
|---|---|
| M0 | No distant metastasis |
| M1 | Distant metastasis |

### ANATOMIC STAGE/PROGNOSTIC GROUPS

| Stage I | T1 | N0 | M0 |
|---|---|---|---|
| Stage II | T2 | N0 | M0 |
| Stage IIIA | T3a | N0 | M0 |
| Stage IIIB | T3b | N0 | M0 |
| Stage IIIC | T4 | N0 | M0 |
| Stage IVA | Any T | N1 | M0 |
| Stage IVB | Any T | Any N | M1 |

18

### PROGNOSTIC FACTORS (SITE-SPECIFIC FACTORS)
### (Recommended for Collection)

| | |
|---|---|
| Required for staging | None |
| Clinically significant | Alpha fetoprotein (AFP) |
| | Fibrosis score |
| | Hepatitis serology |
| | Creatinine (part of the Model for End Stage Liver Disease score) |
| | Bilirubin (part of the Model for End Stage Liver Disease score) |
| | Prothrombin time international normalized ratio (INR) (part of the Model for End Stage Liver Disease score) |

### HISTOLOGIC GRADE (G)

The grading scheme of Edmondson and Steiner is recommended. The system employs four grades as follows:

| | |
|---|---|
| G1 | Well differentiated |
| G2 | Moderately differentiated |
| G3 | Poorly differentiated |
| G4 | Undifferentiated |

## HISTOPATHOLOGIC TYPE

The staging system applies only to primary carcinomas of the liver. These include

Hepatocellular carcinoma
Fibrolamellar variant of hepatocellular carcinoma

Hepatocellular carcinoma is by far the more common of the two types of primary carcinoma of the liver. The staging classification does not apply to primary sarcomas or metastatic tumors, and no longer applies to tumors of the bile ducts (cholangiocarcinomas including mixed hepatocholangiocarcinoma), which are now considered in a separate, new staging system (see Chap. 19). The histologic type and subtype should be recorded, since they may provide prognostic information.

## BIBLIOGRAPHY

Bilimoria MM, Lauwers GY, Nagorney DM, et al. Underlying liver disease but not tumor factors predict long-term survival after hepatic resection of hepatocellular carcinoma. Arch Surg. 2001;136:528–35.

The Cancer of the Liver Italian Program (CLIP) investigators. Prospective validation of the CLIP score: a new prognostic system for patients with cirrhosis and hepatocellular carcinoma. Hepatology 31:840–845, 2000.

Edmondson HA, Steiner PE. Primary carcinoma of the liver: a study of 100 cases among 48,900 necropsies. Cancer. 1954;7:462–503.

Fong Y, Sun RL, Jarnagin W, et al. An analysis of 412 cases of hepatocellular carcinoma at a western center. Ann Surg. 1998;229:790–800.

Henderson JM, Sherman M, Tavill A, et al. AHPBA/AJCC consensus conference on staging of hepatocellular carcinoma: consensus statement. HPB. 2003;5:243–50.

Ikai I, Yamaoka Y, Yamamoto Y, et al. Surgical intervention for patients with stage IV-A hepatocellular carcinoma without lymph node metastasis: proposal as a standard therapy. Ann Surg. 1998;227:433–9.

Ishak K, Baptista A, Bianchi L, et al. Histological grading and staging of chronic hepatitis. J Hepatol. 1995;22:696–9.

Izumi R, Shimizu K, Ii T, Yagi M, et al. Prognostic factors of hepatocellular carcinoma in patients undergoing hepatic resection. Gastroenterology. 1994;106:720–7.

Kojiro M, Nakashima O. Histopathologic evaluation of hepatocellular carcinoma with special reference to small early stage tumor. Semin Liv Dis. 1999;19:287–96.

Lau WY, Leung KL, Leung TW, et al. Resection of hepatocellular carcinoma with diaphragmatic invasion. Br J Surg. 1995;82:264–6.

Lauwers GY, Vauthey JN. Pathological aspects of hepatocellular carcinoma: a critical review of prognostic factors. Hepatogastroenterology. 1998;45(Suppl 3):1197–202.

Lauwers GY, Terri B, Balis UJ, et al. Prognostic histologic indicators of curatively resected hepatocellular carcinomas: a multi-institutional analysis of 425 patients with definition of a histologic prognostic index. Am J Surg Pathol. 2002;26:25–34.

Lei HJ, Chau GY, Lui WY, et al. Prognostic value and clinical relevance of the 6th edition 2002 American Joint Committee on Cancer staging system in patients with resectable hepatocellular carcinoma. J Am Coll Surg. 2006;203:426–35.

Llovet JM, Bru C, Bruix J. Prognosis of hepatocellular carcinoma: the BCLC staging classification. Semin Liver Dis. 1999;19:329–38.

Nzeako UC, Goodman ZD, Ishak KG. Hepatocellular carcinoma in cirrhotic and noncirrhotic livers. A clinico-histopathologic study of 804 North American patients. Am J Clin Pathol. 1996;105:65–75.

Okuda K, Ohtsuki T, Obata H, et al. Natural history of hepatocellular carcinoma and prognosis in relation to treatment. Study of 850 patients. Cancer 1985;56:918–28.

Pawlik TM, Delman KA, Vauthey JN, et al. Tumor size predicts vascular invasion and histologic grade: implications for expanding the criteria for hepatic transplantation. Liver Transplantation. 2005;11(9):1086–92.

Pawlik TM, Poon RT, Abdalla EK, et al. Hepatectomy for hepatocellular carcinoma with major portal or hepatic vein invasion: results of a multicenter study. Surgery. 2005;137(4):403–10.

Poon RT, Fan ST, Ng IO, et al. Significance of resection margin in hepatectomy for hepatocellular carcinoma: a critical reappraisal. Ann Surg. 2000;231:544–51.

Poon RT, Fan ST. Evaluation of the new AJCC/UICC staging system for hepatocellular carcinoma after hepatic resection in Chinese patients. Surg Oncol Clin North Am. 2003;12:35–50.

Ramacciato G, Mercantini P, Cautero N, et al. Prognostic evaluation of the new American Joint Committee on Cancer/International Union Against Cancer staging system for hepatocellular carcinoma: analysis of 112 cirrhotic patients resected for hepatocellular carcinoma. Ann Surg Oncol. 2005;12:289–97.

Teh SH, Christein J, Donohue J, et al. Hepatic resection of hepatocellular carcinoma in patients with cirrhosis: Model of End-Stage Liver Disease (MELD) score predicts perioperative mortality. J Gastrointest Surg. 2005;9(9): 1207–15.

Tsai TJ, Chau GY, Lui WY, et al. Clinical significance of microscopic tumor venous invasion in patients with resectable hepatocellular carcinoma. Surgery. 2000;127:603–8.

Tung WY, Chau GY, Loong CC, et al. Surgical resection of primary hepatocellular carcinoma extending to adjacent organ(s). Eur J Surg Oncol. 1996;22: 516–20.

Varotti G, Ramacciato G, Ercolani G, et al. Comparison between the fifth and sixth editions of the AJCC/UICC TNM staging systems for hepatocellular carcinoma: multicentric study on 393 cirrhotic resected patients. Eur J Surg Oncol. 2005;31:760–7.

Vauthey JN, Klimstra D, Franceschi D, et al. Factors affecting long-term outcome after hepatic resection for hepatocellular carcinoma. Am J Surg. 1995;169:28–35.

Vauthey JN, Lauwers GY, Esnaola N, et al. A simplified staging for hepatocellular carcinoma. J Clin Oncol. 2002;20:1527–36.

Vauthey JN, Ribero D, Abdalla EK, Jonas S, Bharat A, Schumacher G, et al. Outcomes of liver transplantation in 490 patients with hepatocellular carcinoma: validation of a uniform staging after surgical treatment. J Am Coll Surg. 2007;204(5):1016–27.

Zhu LX, Wang GS, Fan ST. Spontaneous rupture of hepatocellular carcinoma. Br J Surg. 2000;83:602–7.

**18**

# Intrahepatic Bile Ducts

## *At-A-Glance*

### SUMMARY OF CHANGES

- This is a novel staging system that is independent of the staging system for hepatocellular carcinoma and independent of the staging system for extrahepatic bile duct malignancy, including hilar bile duct cancers. The rare combined hepatocellular and cholangiocarcinoma (mixed hepato-cholangio carcinomas) are included with the intrahepatic bile duct cancer staging classification

- The tumor category (T) is based on three major prognostic factors including tumor number, vascular invasion, and direct extrahepatic tumoral extension

- The nodal category (N) is a binary classification based on the presence or absence of regional lymph node metastasis

- The metastasis category (M) is a binary classification based on the presence or absence of distant disease

- Recommend collection of preoperative or pretreatment serum CA19.9

| ANATOMIC STAGE/PROGNOSTIC GROUPS | | | |
|---|---|---|---|
| Stage 0 | Tis | N0 | M0 |
| Stage I | T1 | N0 | M0 |
| Stage II | T2 | N0 | M0 |
| Stage III | T3 | N0 | M0 |
| Stage IVA | T4 | N0 | M0 |
| | Any T | N1 | M0 |
| Stage IVB | Any T | Any N | M1 |

ICD-O-3
TOPOGRAPHY
CODES
C22.1    Intrahepatic
           bile duct

ICD-O-3 HISTOLOGY
CODE RANGES
8160, 8161, 8180

## INTRODUCTION

Primary hepatobiliary malignancy includes tumors of the hepatocytes (hepatocellular carcinoma), bile ducts (cholangiocarcinoma), gallbladder, and the parenchyma of the liver (sarcoma). This TNM classification applies only to cancers arising in intrahepatic bile ducts (intrahepatic cholangio-carcinoma). Hepatocellular carcinoma, tumors of the perihilar bile duct, and gallbladder carcinomas are classified separately.

Tumors of intrahepatic bile duct origin represent 15–20% of all primary liver malignancies. The tumors of the bile ducts can be anatomically subdivided into three categories including intrahepatic, perihilar, and distal cholangiocarcinoma. The proportion of cholangiocarcinoma that is accounted for by intrahepatic tumors is approximately 20%.

Clinically, these intrahepatic tumors can be difficult to differentiate from metastatic adenocarcinomas from other primary sites. The etiologic factors that predispose to the development of intrahepatic cholangiocarcinoma include primary sclerosing cholangitis, hepatobiliary parasitosis, intrahepatic lithiasis, and chronic viral hepatitis. The overall incidence rate of intrahepatic cholangiocarcinoma is 0.7 cases per 100,000 adults in the USA. The incidence of intrahepatic cholangiocarcinoma is age-dependent, with a progressive increase in cases starting in the sixth decade of life and peaking in the ninth decade. Although less common than either hepatocellular carcinoma or hilar bile duct cancer, the incidence of intrahepatic cholangiocarcinoma is increasing.

The development of a separate staging structure for intrahepatic cholangiocarcinoma, independent of hepatocellular carcinoma, is warranted based on several differences in clinical features. Unlike hepatocellular carcinoma, multiple analyses have determined that for intrahepatic cholangiocarcinoma tumor size is not a significant prognostic factor. Additionally, intrahepatic cholangiocarcinoma differs from hepatocellular carcinoma because it has a variety of distinct growth patterns including a mass forming type, a periductal infiltrative type, and combinations of these two types.

Although it can be difficult to determine the extent of local disease on radiographic imaging, the major prognostic factors included in the staging system (tumor number, vascular invasion, perforation of the visceral peritoneum, and regional lymph node involvement) are often available from either high-resolution cross-sectional imaging/cholangiography or surgical exploration.

## ANATOMY

**Primary Site.**  At the hilar plate, the right and left hepatic bile ducts enter the liver parenchyma (Figure 19.1). Histologically these bile ducts are lined by a single layer of tall uniform columnar cells. The mucosa usually forms irregular pleats or small longitudinal folds. The walls of the bile ducts have a layer of subepithelial connective tissue and muscle fiber. However, these muscle fibers are typically sparse or absent within the hepatic parenchyma. There is a periductal neural component, which is frequently involved by cholangiocarcinomas.

The tumor growth patterns of intrahepatic cholangiocarcinoma include the mass forming type, the periductal infiltrating type, and a mixed type. Mass forming intrahepatic cholangiocarcinoma shows a radial growth pattern invading into the adjacent liver parenchyma with well-demarcated gross margins. On histopathologic examination, these are nodular sclerotic masses with distinct borders. In contrast, the periductal infiltrating type of cholangiocarcinoma demonstrates a diffuse longitudinal growth pattern along the bile duct.

The percentage of patients with the purely mass forming type is estimated to be 60% of all patients with intrahepatic cholangiocarcinoma, while the purely periductal infiltrating type represents 20% of all cases and a mixed pattern of mass forming and periductal infiltrating type represents

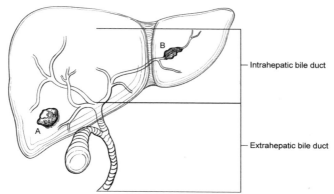

**FIGURE 19.1.** Liver diagram differentiating intrahepatic bile ducts (*open lumens*) from extrahepatic bile ducts (*across lumens*) and mass forming tumor growth pattern (**A**) from periductal infiltrating growth pattern (**B**).

the remaining 20% of cases of intrahepatic cholangiocarcinoma. Limited analyses suggest that the diffuse periductal infiltrating type is associated with a poor prognosis. However, comparison of the prognostic significance of this variable to other prognostic factors is lacking. Either histologic type may invade vascular structures, although this is less commonly observed for mass forming intrahepatic cholangiocarcinoma. Anatomically, the intrahepatic bile ducts extend from the periphery of the liver to the second order bile duct ducts (see perihilar bile duct definition).

**Regional Lymph Nodes.** Compared with primary hepatocellular carcinoma, regional lymph node metastases are more commonly associated with intrahepatic cholangiocarcinoma. The lymph node drainage patterns from the intrahepatic bile ducts demonstrate laterality. Tumors in the left lateral bi-segment (segment 2–3) of the liver may preferentially drain to lymph nodes along the lesser curvature of the stomach and subsequently to the celiac nodal basin. In contrast, intrahepatic cholangiocarcinomas of the right liver (segment 5–8) may primarily drain to hilar lymph nodes and subsequently to caval and periaortic lymph nodes.

For right liver (segment 5–8) intrahepatic cholangiocarcinomas, the regional lymph nodes include the hilar (common bile duct, hepatic artery, portal vein, and cystic duct) periduodenal and peripancreatic lymph nodes. For left liver (segment 2–4) intrahepatic cholangiocarcinomas, regional lymph nodes include hilar, and gastrohepatic lymph nodes. For intrahepatic cholangiocarcinomas, disease spread to the celiac and/or periaortic and caval lymph nodes are considered distant metastases (M1). Inferior phrenic nodes are considered regional, not distant nodes.

**Metastatic Sites.** Intrahepatic cholangiocarcinomas usually metastasize to other intrahepatic locations (classified in the T category as multiple tumors) and to the peritoneum, and subsequently, to the lungs and pleura (classified in the M category as distant metastasis).

## RULES FOR CLASSIFICATION

Intraductal papillary bile duct tumors may be identified in some patients with unilateral biliary obstruction and are classified as in situ tumors (Tis). The T classification of invasive intrahepatic cholangiocarcinoma is determined by the number of tumors present (solitary vs. multiple), the presence of vascular invasion, and the presence of visceral peritoneal perforation with or without direct involvement of local extrahepatic structures. The definition of the term "multiple tumors" includes satellitosis, multifocal tumors, and intrahepatic metastasis. Vascular invasion includes both major vessel invasion [defined as invasion of the branches of the main portal vein (right or left portal vein) or as invasion of one or more of the three hepatic veins (right, middle, or left)] and microscopic invasion of smaller intraparenchymal vascular structures identified on histopathologic examination. Direct invasion of adjacent organs, including colon, duodenum, stomach, common bile duct, portal lymph nodes, abdominal wall, and diaphragm is considered T3 disease, not as distant metastasis. Regional nodal involvement as defined above is considered N1 disease. Extraregional nodal involvement and other distant metastatic sites are classified as M1 disease.

**Validation.** Validation of T1, T2, T3, and N1 categories is based on multivariate analyses of outcome and survival data of single institution and multi-institution studies of patients with intrahepatic cholangiocarcinoma.

**Clinical Staging.** Clinical staging depends on imaging procedures designed to demonstrate the tumor growth pattern of intrahepatic cholangiocarcinoma, the number of intrahepatic masses, and the presence or absence of vascular invasion. Surgical exploration is carried out if imaging shows that a complete resection is possible and that hepatic reserve is sufficient for a safe resection. In the presence of cirrhosis, the Child-Pugh class and components of the Model for End stage Liver Disease (MELD) score should be recorded. Radiographic assessment for the presence or absence of distant metastases prior to surgical exploration is warranted.

**Pathologic Staging.** Complete pathologic staging consists of evaluation of the primary tumor, including tumor number, involvement of local regional lymph nodes, and the presence or absence of vascular invasion.

Solitary tumors with no vascular invasion and no lymph node involvement or metastasis are classified as T1. Solitary tumors with vascular invasion are classified as T2a. Multiple tumors, with or without vascular invasion, are classified as T2b. Tumors that perforate the visceral peritoneum, with or without invasion of extrahepatic structures are classified as T3. Finally, tumors with periductal invasion are classified as T4. The pathologic definition of the periductal infiltrating type is the finding of a diffuse longitudinal growth pattern along the intrahepatic bile ducts on both gross and microscopic examination. T4 includes the diffuse periductal infiltrating tumors and the mixed mass forming and periductal infiltrating tumors.

Stage I tumors are defined as T1 without regional lymph node metastasis (pN0, cN0). Stage II is defined as T2 tumors without regional lymph node involvement. Stage III is defined as T3 tumors without regional lymph node metastasis. Stage IVA is defined as either T4 or any T category with positive regional lymph nodes. Patients with distant metastasis, regardless of T and N status are considered stage IVB.

## PROGNOSTIC FEATURES

Clinical factors predictive of decreased survival include serum CA 19.9 level, the presence of underlying liver disease, and multiple tumors. For patients treated with surgical resection, the main predictors of poor outcome include regional lymph node involvement and incomplete resection. Other important prognostic factors include the finding of satellitosis or multiple intrahepatic tumors, vascular invasion, and periductal infiltrating tumor growth pattern.

Figure 19.2 shows stratification of survivals for 647 patients with confirmed intrahepatic cholangiocarcinoma based on new T category classification using SEER registry data.

## DEFINITIONS OF TNM

### *Primary Tumor (T)*

| | |
|---|---|
| TX | Primary tumor cannot be assessed |
| T0 | No evidence of primary tumor |
| Tis | Carcinoma in situ (intraductal tumor) |
| T1 | Solitary tumor without vascular invasion |
| T2a | Solitary tumor with vascular invasion |
| T2b | Multiple tumors, with or without vascular invasion |
| T3 | Tumor perforating the visceral peritoneum or involving the local extra hepatic structures by direct invasion |
| T4 | Tumor with periductal invasion |

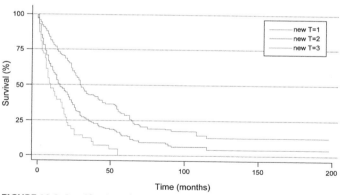

**FIGURE 19.2.** Stratification of survival for 647 patients with confirmed intrahepatic cholangiocarcinoma based on new T category classification using SEER registry data. T1: Solitary tumor without vascular invasion; T2: Solitary tumor with vascular invasion or multiple tumors; T3: Tumor perforating the visceral peritoneum or involving the local extra hepatic structures by direct invasion.

### Regional Lymph Nodes (N)

| | |
|---|---|
| NX | Regional lymph nodes cannot be assessed |
| N0 | No regional lymph node metastasis |
| N1 | Regional lymph node metastasis present |

### Distant Metastasis (M)

| | |
|---|---|
| M0 | No distant metastasis |
| M1 | Distant metastasis present |

### ANATOMIC STAGE/PROGNOSTIC GROUPS

| Stage 0 | Tis | N0 | M0 |
|---|---|---|---|
| Stage I | T1 | N0 | M0 |
| Stage II | T2 | N0 | M0 |
| Stage III | T3 | N0 | M0 |
| Stage IVA | T4 | N0 | M0 |
| | Any T | N1 | M0 |
| Stage IVB | Any T | Any N | M1 |

### PROGNOSTIC FACTORS (SITE-SPECIFIC FACTORS)
#### (Recommended for Collection)

| | |
|---|---|
| Required for staging | None |
| Clinically significant | Tumor growth pattern |
| | Primary sclerosing cholangitis |
| | CA 19-9 |

### HISTOLOGIC GRADE (G)

The histologic grade should be reported using the following scheme:

| | |
|---|---|
| G1 | Well differentiated |
| G2 | Moderately differentiated |
| G3 | Poorly differentiated |
| G4 | Undifferentiated |

### HISTOPATHOLOGIC TYPE

The staging system applies to primary carcinomas of the intrahepatic bile ducts. These include the following:

- Intrahepatic cholangiocarcinoma
  - Mass forming tumor growth pattern
  - Periductal infiltrating tumor growth pattern
  - Mixed mass forming and periductal infiltrating growth pattern
- Mixed Hepatocellular

This staging classification does not apply to primary sarcomas of the liver stroma or to liver metastases from other sites. The histopathologic subtype and, in the case of intrahepatic cholangiocarcinoma, the tumor growth pattern both should be recorded, since they may provide prognostic information.

## BIBLIOGRAPHY

Berdah SV, Delpero JR, Garcia S, Hardwigsen J, Le Treut YP. A western surgical experience of peripheral cholangiocarcinoma. Br J Surg. 1996;83(11): 1517–21.

Chen MF, Jan YY, Wang CS, Jeng LB, Hwang TL. Clinical experience in 20 hepatic resections for peripheral cholangiocarcinoma. Cancer. 1989;64(11): 2226–32.

Chou FF, Sheen-Chen SM, Chen YS, Chen MC, Chen CL. Surgical treatment of cholangiocarcinoma. Hepatogastroenterology. 1997;44(15):760–5.

Chu KM, Fan ST. Intrahepatic cholangiocarcinoma in Hong Kong. J Hepatobiliary Pancreat Surg. 1999;6(2):149–53.

El Rassi ZE, Partensky C, Scoazec JY, Henry L, Lombard-Bohas C, Maddern G. Peripheral cholangiocarcinoma: presentation, diagnosis, pathology and management. Eur J Surg Oncol. 1999;25(4):375–80.

Harrison LE, Fong Y, Klimstra DS, Zee SY, Blumgart LH. Surgical treatment of 32 patients with peripheral intrahepatic cholangiocarcinoma. Br J Surg. 1998;85(8):1068–70.

Hirohashi K, Uenishi T, Kubo S, et al. Macroscopic types of intrahepatic cholangiocarcinoma: clinicopathologic features and surgical outcomes. Hepatogastroenterology. 2002;49(44):326–9.

Isa T, Kusano T, Shimoji H, Takeshima Y, Muto Y, Furukawa M. Predictive actors for long-term survival in patients with intrahepatic cholangiocarcinoma. Am J Surg. 2001;181(6):507–11.

Kawarada Y, Yamagiwa K, Das BC. Analysis of the relationships between clinicopathologic factors and survival time in intrahepatic cholangiocarcinoma. Am J Surg. 2002;183(6):679–85.

Kim HJ, Yun SS, Jung KH, Kwun WH, Choi JH. Intrahepatic cholangiocarcinoma in Korea. J Hepatobiliary Pancreat Surg. 1999;6(2):142–8.

Lang H, Sotiropoulos GC, Fruhauf NR, et al. Extended hepatectomy for intrahepatic cholangiocellular carcinoma (ICC): when is it worthwhile? Single center experience with 27 resections in 50 patients over a 5-year period. Ann Surg. 2005;241(1):134–43.

Lieser MJ, Barry MK, Rowland C, Ilstrup DM, Nagorney DM. Surgical management of intrahepatic cholangiocarcinoma: a 31-year experience. J Hepatobiliary Pancreat Surg. 1998;5(1):41–7.

Maeda T, Adachi E, Kajiyama K, Sugimachi K, Tsuneyoshi M. Combined hepatocellular and cholangiocarcinoma: proposed criteria according to cytokeratin expression and analysis of clinicopathologic features. Hum Pathol. 1995;26(9):956–64.

McGlynn KA, Tarone RE, El-Serag HB. A comparison of trends in the incidence of hepatocellular carcinoma and intrahepatic cholangiocarcinoma in the United States. Cancer Epidemiol Biomarkers Prev. 2006;15(6):1198–203.

Nathan H, Aloia TA, Vauthey JN, et al. A proposed staging system for intrahepatic cholangiocarcinoma. Ann Surg Oncol. 2009;16:14–22.

Nozaki Y, Yamamoto M, Ikai I, et al. Reconsideration of the lymph node metastasis pattern (N factor) from intrahepatic cholangiocarcinoma using the International Union Against Cancer TNM staging system for primary liver carcinoma. Cancer. 1998;83(9):1923–9.

**19**

Ohtsuka M, Ito H, Kimura F, et al. Results of surgical treatment for intrahepatic cholangiocarcinoma and clinicopathological factors influencing survival. Br J Surg. 2002;89(12):1525–31.

Okabayashi T, Yamamoto J, Kosuge T, et al. A new staging system for mass-forming intrahepatic cholangiocarcinoma: analysis of preoperative and postoperative variables. Cancer. 2001;92(9):2374–83.

Patel T. Increasing incidence and mortality of primary intrahepatic cholangiocarcinoma in the United States. Hepatology (Baltimore). 2001;33(6):1353–7.

Pichlmayr R, Lamesch P, Weimann A, Tusch G, Ringe B. Surgical treatment of cholangiocellular carcinoma. World J Surg. 1995;19(1):83–8.

Robles R, Figueras J, Turrion VS, et al. Spanish experience in liver transplantation for hilar and peripheral cholangiocarcinoma. Ann Surg. 2004;239(2):265–71.

Shaib Y, El-Serag HB. The epidemiology of cholangiocarcinoma. Semin Liver Dis. 2004;24(2):115–25.

Shaib YH, Davila JA, McGlynn K, El-Serag HB. Rising incidence of intrahepatic cholangiocarcinoma in the United States: a true increase? J Hepatol. 2004;40(3):472–7.

Shaib YH, El-Serag HB, Nooka AK, et al. Risk factors for intrahepatic and extrahepatic cholangiocarcinoma: a hospital-based case-control study. Am J Gastroenterol. 2007;102(5):1016–21.

Shimada M, Yamashita Y, Aishima S, Shirabe K, Takenaka K, Sugimachi K. Value of lymph node dissection during resection of intrahepatic cholangiocarcinoma. Br J Surg. 2001;88(11):1463–6.

Uenishi T, Yamazaki O, Yamamoto T, et al. Serosal invasion in TNM staging of mass-forming intrahepatic cholangiocarcinoma. J Hepatobiliary Pancreat Surg. 2005;12(6):479–83.

Valverde A, Bonhomme N, Farges O, Sauvanet A, Flejou JF, Belghiti J. Resection of intrahepatic cholangiocarcinoma: a Western experience. J Hepatobiliary Pancreat Surg. 1999;6(2):122–7.

Welzel TM, McGlynn KA, Hsing AW, O'Brien TR, Pfeiffer RM. Impact of classification of hilar cholangiocarcinomas (Klatskin tumors) on the incidence of intra- and extrahepatic cholangiocarcinoma in the United States. J Natl Cancer Inst. 2006;98(12):873–5.

Yamamoto M, Takasaki K, Yoshikawa T. Extended resection for intrahepatic cholangiocarcinoma in Japan. J Hepatobiliary Pancreat Surg. 1999;6(2):117–21.

Yamasaki S. Intrahepatic cholangiocarcinoma: macroscopic type and stage classification. J Hepatobiliary Pancreat Surg. 2003;10(4):288–91.

# Gallbladder

*(Carcinoid tumors and sarcomas are not
included)*

## At-A-Glance

---

### SUMMARY OF CHANGES

- The cystic duct is now included in this classification scheme

- The N classification now distinguishes hilar nodes (N1: lymph nodes adjacent to the cystic duct, bile duct, hepatic artery, and portal vein) from other regional nodes (N2: celiac, periduodenal, and peripancreatic lymph nodes, and those along the superior mesenteric artery)

- Stage groupings have been changed to better correlate with surgical resectability and patient outcome; locally unresectable T4 tumors have been reclassified as Stage IV

- Lymph node metastasis is now classified as Stage IIIB (N1) or Stage IVB (N2)

---

**ANATOMIC STAGE/PROGNOSTIC GROUPS**

| Stage 0 | Tis | N0 | M0 |
|---|---|---|---|
| Stage I | T1 | N0 | M0 |
| Stage II | T2 | N0 | M0 |
| Stage IIIA | T3 | N0 | M0 |
| Stage IIIB | T1-3 | N1 | M0 |
| Stage IVA | T4 | N0-1 | M0 |
| Stage IVB | Any T | N2 | M0 |
| | Any T | Any N | M1 |

ICD-O-3
TOPOGRAPHY
CODES

C23.9    Gallbladder
C24.0    Cystic duct
         only

ICD-O-3 HISTOLOGY
CODE RANGES
8000–8152, 8154–8231,
8243–8245, 8250–8576,
8940–8950, 8980–8981

## INTRODUCTION

Cancers of the gallbladder are staged according to their depth of invasion into the gallbladder wall and extent of spread to surrounding structures and lymph nodes. The liver is a common site of involvement; thus, liver invasion impacts the primary tumor (T) classification. Other surrounding structures, such as the duodenum and transverse colon, are at risk of direct tumor extension. Invasion of hilar structures (common bile duct, hepatic artery, portal vein) usually renders these tumors locally unresectable. Development of jaundice suggests hilar involvement and is associated with unresectablility and poor prognosis. Cholelithiasis is associated with carcinoma of the gallbladder in the majority of cases. Many of these cancers are found incidentally following cholecystectomy, either at operation or on final histologic analysis of the specimen. Tumors encountered this way may have a better prognosis when amenable to definitive surgical resection either at the time of cholecystectomy or at a subsequent operation. As many as 50% of resected gallbladder cancers undergo definitive resection at a second operation, with the gallbladder having been removed previously for presumed benign disease. Cystic duct involvement merits consideration of formal bile duct resection at the time of the definitive operation to achieve negative margin status. Peritoneal involvement is common, and diagnostic laparoscopy at the time of surgery is usually advised. Systemic therapeutic options are limited, making prognosis for patients with unresectable disease extremely poor. Survival correlates with stage of disease.

## ANATOMY

**Primary Site.** The gallbladder is a pear-shaped saccular organ located under the liver situated in line with the physiologic division of the right and left lobes of the liver (Cantlie's line). It straddles Couinaud segments IVb and V. The organ can be divided into three parts: a fundus, a body, and a neck, which tapers into the cystic duct (Figure 20.1). The wall is considerably thinner than that of other hollow organs and lacks a submucosal layer. Its make up consists of a mucosa, a muscular layer, perimuscular connective tissue, and a serosa on one side (serosa is lacking on the side embedded in the liver). An important anatomic consideration is that the serosa along

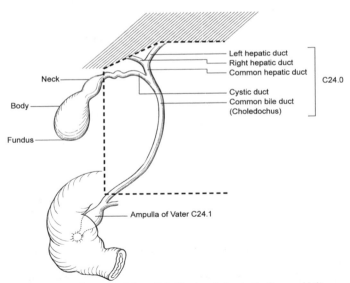

**FIGURE 20.1.** Schematic of the gallbladder in relation to the liver and biliary tract.

the liver edge is more densely adherent to the liver (cystic plate) and much of this is often left behind at the time of cholecystectomy. For this reason, partial hepatic resection incorporating portions of segments IVb and V is undertaken for some cases. Primary carcinomas of the cystic duct are included in this staging classification schema.

**Regional Lymph Nodes.** For accurate staging, all nodes removed at operation should be assessed for metastasis. Regional lymph nodes are limited to the hepatic hilus (including nodes along the common bile duct, hepatic artery, portal vein, and cystic duct). Celiac, periduodenal, peripancreatic, and superior mesenteric artery node involvement is now considered distant metastatic disease.

**Metastatic Sites.** Cancers of the gallbladder usually metastasize to the peritoneum and liver and occasionally to the lungs and pleura.

## RULES FOR CLASSIFICATION

Gallbladder cancers are staged primarily on the basis of surgical exploration or resection, but not all patients with gallbladder cancer undergo surgical resection. Many in situ and early-stage carcinomas are not recognized grossly. They are usually staged pathologically on histologic examination of the resected specimen. The T classification depends on the depth of tumor penetration into the wall of the gallbladder, on the presence or absence of tumor invasion into the liver, hepatic artery, or portal vein, and on the presence or absence of adjacent organ involvement. Direct tumor extension into the liver is not considered distant metastasis (M). Likewise, direct invasion of other adjacent organs, including colon, duodenum, stomach, common bile duct, abdominal wall, and diaphragm, is not considered distant metastasis but is classified in the T category (T3 or T4). Tumor confined to the gallbladder is classified as either T1 or T2, depending on the depth of invasion. It must be noted that because there is no serosa on the gallbladder on the side attached to the liver, a simple cholecystectomy may not completely remove a T2 tumor, even though such tumors are considered to be confined to the gallbladder.

**Validation.** Validation of stage grouping is based on multivariate analyses of outcome and survival data of the National Cancer Database (totaling 10,705 patients nationwide, Figure 20.2).

**Clinical Staging.** Clinical evaluation usually depends on the results of ultrasonography, computed tomography, and magnetic resonance cholangiopancreatography. Clinical staging may also be based on findings from surgical exploration (laparoscopic or open) when the main tumor mass is not resected.

**Pathologic Staging.** Pathologic staging is based on examination of the surgical resection specimen.

The extent of resection (R0, complete resection with grossly and microscopically negative margins of resection; R1, grossly negative but

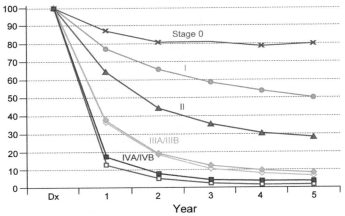

**FIGURE 20.2.** Observed survival rates for 10,705 gallbladder cancers. Data from the National Cancer Data Base (Commission on Cancer of the American College of Surgeons and the American Cancer Society) diagnosed in years 1989–1996.

microscopically positive margins of resection; R2, grossly and microscopically positive margins of resection) is a descriptor in the TNM staging system and is the most important stage-independent prognostic factor. It should be reported in all cases.

## PROGNOSTIC FEATURES

In as many as 50% of cases, gallbladder cancers are discovered at pathologic analysis after simple cholecystectomy for presumed gallstone disease. Five-year survival is 50% for patients with T1 tumors. Patients with T2 tumors have a 5-year survival rate of 29%, which appears to be improved with more radical resection. Patients with lymph node metastases (Stage IIIB or higher) or locally advanced tumors (Stage IVA or higher) rarely experience long-term survival. The site-specific prognostic factors include histologic type, histologic grade, and vascular invasion. Papillary carcinomas have the most favorable prognosis. Unfavorable histologic types include small cell carcinomas and undifferentiated carcinomas. Lymphatic and/or blood vessel invasion indicate a less favorable outcome. Histologic grade also correlates with outcome.

Patients with T2–T3 cancers discovered at pathologic analysis are usually offered a second operation for radical resection of residual tumor. This may include nonanatomic resection of the gallbladder bed (segments IVB and V of the liver) or more formal anatomic resection such as a right hepatectomy. Resection of the biliary tree is dependent on surgical decision making at the time of the definitive procedure and may be based on cystic duct margin status. Staging classification should be reported for tumors removed by either a single operation or a staged surgical procedure (cholecystectomy followed by definitive resection). In cases where the surgical procedure was staged, it should be noted whether the c... performed laparoscopically or via an open approach. ... should be made as to whether the primary tumor was loca... peritoneal or the hepatic side of the gallbladder.

## DEFINITIONS OF TNM

### *Primary Tumor (T)*

| | |
|---|---|
| TX | Primary tumor cannot be assessed |
| T0 | No evidence of primary tumor |
| Tis | Carcinoma in situ |
| T1 | Tumor invades lamina propria or muscular layer (Figure 20.3) |
| T1a | Tumor invades lamina propria |
| T1b | Tumor invades muscular layer |
| T2 | Tumor invades perimuscular connective tissue; no extension beyond serosa or into liver (Figure 20.4) |
| T3 | Tumor perforates the serosa (visceral peritoneum) and/or directly invades the liver and/or one other adjacent organ or structure, such as the stomach, duodenum, colon, pancreas, omentum, or extrahepatic bile ducts |
| T4 | Tumor invades main portal vein or hepatic artery or invades two or more extrahepatic organs or structures |

### *Regional Lymph Nodes (N)*

| | |
|---|---|
| NX | Regional lymph nodes cannot be assessed |
| N0 | No regional lymph node metastasis |
| N1 | Metastases to nodes along the cystic duct, common bile duct, hepatic artery, and/or portal vein |
| N2 | Metastases to periaortic, pericaval, superior mesenteric artery, and/or celiac artery lymph nodes |

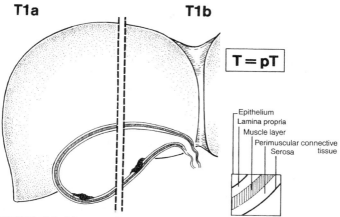

**FIGURE 20.3.** Schematic of T1, showing the tumor invading the lamina propria or muscle layer of the gallbladder.

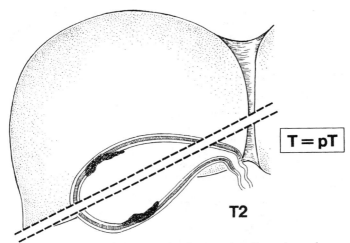

**FIGURE 20.4.** Schematic of T2, showing the tumor invading perimuscular connective tissue of the gallbladder with no extension of the tumor beyond serosa or into the liver.

| *Distant Metastasis (M)* | |
|---|---|
| M0 | No distant metastasis |
| M1 | Distant metastasis |

## ANATOMIC STAGE/PROGNOSTIC GROUPS

| Stage 0 | Tis | N0 | M0 |
|---|---|---|---|
| Stage I | T1 | N0 | M0 |
| Stage II | T2 | N0 | M0 |
| Stage IIIA | T3 | N0 | M0 |
| Stage IIIB | T1-3 | N1 | M0 |
| Stage IVA | T4 | N0-1 | M0 |
| Stage IVB | Any T | N2 | M0 |
| | Any T | Any N | M1 |

## PROGNOSTIC FACTORS (SITE-SPECIFIC FACTORS)
### (Recommended for Collection)

| Required for staging | None |
|---|---|
| Clinically significant | Tumor location |
| | Specimen type |
| | Extent of liver resection |
| | Free peritoneal side vs. hepatic side for T2 |

## HISTOLOGIC GRADE (G)

Grade is reported in registry systems by the grade value. A two-grade, three-grade, or four-grade system may be used. If a grading system is not specified, generally the following system is used:

GX     Grade cannot be assessed
G1     Well differentiated
G2     Moderately differentiated
G3     Poorly differentiated
G4     Undifferentiated

## HISTOPATHOLOGIC TYPE

The staging system applies only to primary carcinomas of the gallbladder and cystic duct. It does not apply to carcinoid tumors or to sarcoma. Adenocarcinomas are the most common histologic type. More than 98% of gallbladder cancers are carcinomas. The histologic types of carcinomas are listed below.

Carcinoma in situ
Adenocarcinoma, NOS
Papillary carcinoma
Adenocarcinoma, intestinal type
Clear cell adenocarcinoma
Mucinous carcinoma
Signet ring cell carcinoma
Squamous carcinoma
Adenosquamous carcinoma
Small cell carcinoma*
Undifferentiated carcinoma*
    Spindle and giant cell types
    Small cell types
Carcinoma, NOS
Carcinosarcoma
Other (specify)

*Grade 4 by definition

20

## BIBLIOGRAPHY

Balachandran P, Agarwal S, Krishnani N, et al. Predictors of long-term survival in patients with gallbladder cancer. J Gastrointest Surg. 2006;10(6):848–54.

Chijiiwa K, Noshiro H, Nakano K, et al. Role of surgery for gallbladder carcinoma with special reference to lymph node metastasis and stage using western and Japanese classification systems. World J Surg. 2000;24(10):1271–6.

Dixon E, Vollmer CM Jr, Sahajpal A, et al. An aggressive surgical approach leads to improved survival in patients with gallbladder cancer: a 12-year study at a North American Center. Ann Surg. 2005;241(3):385–94.

Fong Y. Treatment of T2 gallbladder cancer [comment]. Ann Surg Oncol. 2003; 10(5):490.

Fong Y, Malhotra S. Gallbladder cancer: recent advances and current guidelines for surgical therapy. Adv Surg. 2001;35:1–20.

Fong Y, Wagman L, Gonen M, et al. Evidence-based gallbladder cancer staging: changing cancer staging by analysis of data from the National Cancer Database. Ann Surg. 2006;243(6):767–71; discussion 771–4.

Hawkins WG, DeMatteo RP, Jarnagin WR, et al. Jaundice predicts advanced disease and early mortality in patients with gallbladder cancer. Ann Surg Oncol. 2004;11(3):310–5.

Kapoor VK, Sonawane RN, Haribhakti SP, et al. Gall bladder cancer: proposal for a modification of the TNM classification [see comment]. Eur J Surg Oncol. 1998;24(6):487–91.

Manfredi S, Benhamiche AM, Isambert N, et al. Trends in incidence and management of gallbladder carcinoma: a population-based study in France. Cancer. 2000;89(4):757–62.

Miller G, Jarnagin WR. Gallbladder carcinoma. EJSO. 2008;34:306–12.

Sasaki E, Nagino M, Ebata T, et al. Immunohistochemically demonstrated lymph node micrometastasis and prognosis in patients with gallbladder carcinoma. Ann Surg. 2006;244(1):99–105.

Shih SP, Schulick RD, Cameron JL, et al. Gallbladder cancer: the role of laparoscopy and radical resection. Ann Surg. 2007;245(6):893–901.

Wakabayashi H, Ishimura K, Hashimoto N, et al. Analysis of prognostic factors after surgery for stage III and IV gallbladder cancer. Eur J Surg Oncol. 2004; 30(8):842–6.

# Perihilar Bile Ducts

*(Sarcoma and carcinoid tumors are not included.)*

## *At-A-Glance*

**SUMMARY OF CHANGES**

- Extrahepatic bile duct tumors have been separated into perihilar (proximal) and distal groups and separate staging classifications defined for each

- T1 (confined to bile duct) and T2 (beyond the wall of the bile duct) have been specified histologically

- T2 includes invasion of adjacent hepatic parenchyma

- T3 is defined as unilateral vascular invasion

- T4 is defined on the basis of bilateral biliary and/or vascular invasion

- Lymph node metastasis has been reclassified as stage III (upstaged from stage II)

- The stage IV grouping defines unresectability based on local invasion (IVA) or distant disease (IVB)

**ANATOMIC STAGE/PROGNOSTIC GROUPS**

| Stage | | | |
|---|---|---|---|
| Stage 0 | Tis | N0 | M0 |
| Stage I | T1 | N0 | M0 |
| Stage II | T2a-b | N0 | M0 |
| Stage IIIA | T3 | N0 | M0 |
| Stage IIIB | T1-3 | N1 | M0 |
| Stage IVA | T4 | N0-1 | M0 |
| Stage IVB | Any T | N2 | M0 |
| | Any T | Any N | M1 |

ICD-O-3 TOPOGRAPHY CODES

C24.0    Extrahepatic bile duct (proximal or perihilar only)

ICD-O-3 HISTOLOGY CODE RANGES
8000–8152, 8154–8231, 8243–8245, 8250–8576, 8940–8950, 8980–8981

## INTRODUCTION

Proximal or perihilar cholangiocarcinomas (Klatskin tumors) involve the biliary confluence of the right or left hepatic ducts and comprise 50–70% of all cases of bile duct carcinomas (Figure 21.1). They are rare tumors, with an incidence of 1–2 per 100,000 in the USA. Early symptoms, including abdominal pain, anorexia, and weight loss, are nonspecific and occur in approximately one-third of patients. Symptoms and signs from bile duct obstruction, such as jaundice, clay-colored stools, dark urine, and pruritus, occur later in the disease.

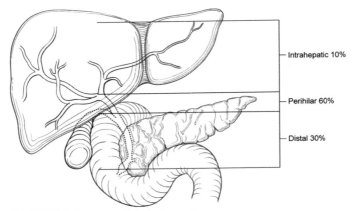

**FIGURE 21.1.** Anatomy of bile duct cancers.

Complete resection with negative histologic margins is the most robust predictor of long-term survival. However, the proximity of perihilar tumors to vital structures, including the hepatic artery, portal vein, and hepatic parenchyma, makes curative excision technically difficult. Over the past decade, improvements in imaging, perioperative care, and operative technique have allowed more patients to undergo curative resection. Recognition of the propensity of perihilar tumors for intrahepatic ductal extension, with invasion of the hepatic parenchyma in 85% of patients, has led to increased rates of extended hepatectomy (partial hepatic resection) or total hepatectomy with transplantation, with resultant increase in margin-negative resections and improved overall survival rates.

## ANATOMY

**Primary Site.** Cholangiocarcinoma can develop anywhere along the biliary tree, from proximal peripheral intrahepatic ducts to the distal intraduodenal bile duct. Extrahepatic bile duct tumors have traditionally been separated into perihilar (or proximal), middle, and distal subgroups. However, middle lesions are rare and managed either as a proximal tumor with combined hepatic and hilar resection or as a distal tumor with pancreaticoduodenectomy. In this edition of the *AJCC Cancer Staging Manual*, extrahepatic cholangiocarcinoma is divided into perihilar and distal subgroups, with middle lesions classified according to their treatment. Perihilar cholangiocarcinomas are defined anatomically as tumors located in the extrahepatic biliary tree proximal to the origin of the cystic duct. They may extend proximally into either the right hepatic duct, the left hepatic duct, or both. Laterally refers to tumor extension related to either right or left periductal regions.

The sixth edition of the *AJCC Cancer Staging Manual* classified invasion of adjacent hepatic parenchyma and unilateral vascular involvement as T3. However, patients with invasion of adjacent hepatic parenchyma have been found to have a better prognosis than patients with vascular invasion

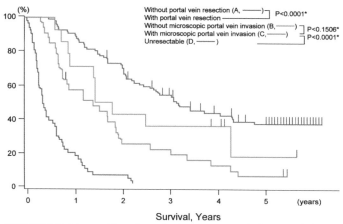

**FIGURE 21.2.** Adverse effect of vascular invasion on survival. In a study by Ebata et al. (2003), patients who underwent hepatectomy alone had a better outcome than patients who required concomitant portal vein resection, with 5-year overall survival of 37% vs. 10%, respectively.

(Figure 21.2). Thus, adjacent hepatic invasion is now classified T2, whereas unilateral vascular involvement is classified as T3.

T4 tumors are defined as those with bilateral hepatic involvement of vascular structures, bilateral tumor expansion into secondary biliary radicals, or extension to secondary biliary radicals with contralateral vascular invasion. The median survival of patients with T4 tumors is 8–13 months, and in this edition of the *AJCC Cancer Staging Manual*, T4 tumors are classified as stage IVA. However, highly selected patients with T4 tumors may be candidates for protocol-based chemoradiation followed by liver transplantation.

**Regional Lymph Nodes.** In perihilar cholangiocarcinoma, the prevalence of lymphatic metastasis increases directly with T category and ranges from 30% to 53% overall. Hilar and pericholedochal nodes in the hepatoduodenal ligament are most often involved.

**Metastatic Sites.** Perihilar cholangiocarcinoma is characterized by intrahepatic ductal extension, as well as spread along perineural and periductal lymphatic channels. While the liver is a common site of metastases, spread to other organs, especially extra-abdominal sites, is uncommon. Extrahepatic metastases have been reported in the peritoneal cavity, lung, brain, and bone.

## RULES FOR CLASSIFICATION

Most patients with perihilar cholangiocarcinoma have locoregional extension or distant metastasis that precludes resection and thus are treated without pathologic staging. A single TNM classification must apply to both clinical and pathologic staging.

**Clinical Staging.** Clinical evaluation usually depends on the results of duplex ultrasound, computed tomography, and magnetic resonance cholangiopancreatography (MRCP). The biliary extent of disease is assessed with percutaneous transhepatic cholangiography or MRCP. Clinical staging also may be based on findings from surgical exploration when the main tumor mass is not resected.

**Pathologic Staging.** Pathologic staging is based on examination of the resected specimen and/or biopsies sufficient to document the greatest extent of disease.

The extent of resection (R0, complete resection with grossly and microscopically negative margins of resection; R1, grossly negative but microscopically positive margins of resection; R2, grossly and microscopically positive margins of resection) is a descriptor in the TNM staging system and is the most important stage-independent prognostic factor and should be reported.

## PROGNOSTIC FEATURES

Patients who undergo surgical resection for localized perihilar cholangiocarcinoma have a median survival of approximately 3 years and a 5-year survival rate of 20% to 40%. In carefully selected patients with primary sclerosing cholangitis and early-stage perihilar cholangiocarcinoma, preliminary data report excellent results with neoadjuvant chemoradiation and liver transplantation. Complete resection with negative histologic margins is the major predictor of outcome, and liver resection is essential to achieve negative margins. Factors adversely associated with survival include high tumor grade, vascular invasion, lobar atrophy, and lymph node metastasis. Papillary morphology carries a more favorable prognosis than nodular or sclerosing tumors.

## DEFINITIONS OF TNM

*Primary Tumor (T)*

| | |
|---|---|
| TX | Primary tumor cannot be assessed |
| T0 | No evidence of primary tumor |
| Tis | Carcinoma in situ |
| T1 | Tumor confined to the bile duct, with extension up to the muscle layer or fibrous tissue |
| T2a | Tumor invades beyond the wall of the bile duct to surrounding adipose tissue |
| T2b | Tumor invades adjacent hepatic parenchyma |
| T3 | Tumor invades unilateral branches of the portal vein or hepatic artery |
| T4 | Tumor invades main portal vein or its branches bilaterally; or the common hepatic artery; or the second-order biliary radicals bilaterally; or unilateral second-order biliary radicals with contralateral portal vein or hepatic artery involvement |

### Regional Lymph Nodes (N)

NX    Regional lymph nodes cannot be assessed
N0    No regional lymph node metastasis
N1    Regional lymph node metastasis (including nodes along the cystic duct, common bile duct, hepatic artery, and portal vein)
N2    Metastasis to periaortic, pericaval, superior mesenteric artery, and/or celiac artery lymph nodes

### Distant Metastasis (M)

M0    No distant metastasis
M1    Distant metastasis

### ANATOMIC STAGE/PROGNOSTIC GROUPS

| Stage 0 | Tis | N0 | M0 |
|---|---|---|---|
| Stage I | T1 | N0 | M0 |
| Stage II | T2a-b | N0 | M0 |
| Stage IIIA | T3 | N0 | M0 |
| Stage IIIB | T1-3 | N1 | M0 |
| Stage IVA | T4 | N0-1 | M0 |
| Stage IVB | Any T | N2 | M0 |
| | Any T | Any N | M1 |

**21**

### PROGNOSTIC FACTORS (SITE-SPECIFIC FACTORS)
**(Recommended for Collection)**

Required for staging    None

Clinically significant    Tumor location
   Papillary variant
   Tumor growth pattern
   Primary sclerosing cholangitis
   CA 19-9

### HISTOLOGIC GRADE (G)

Grade is reported in registry systems by the grade value. A two-grade, three-grade, or four-grade system may be used. If a grading system is not specified, generally the following system is used:

GX    Grade cannot be assessed
G1    Well differentiated
G2    Moderately differentiated
G3    Poorly differentiated
G4    Undifferentiated

## HISTOPATHOLOGIC TYPE

The staging system applies to all carcinomas that arise in the perihilar extrahepatic bile ducts. Sarcomas and carcinoid tumors are excluded. Adenocarcinoma that is not further subclassified is the most common histologic type. Carcinomas account for more than 98% of cancers of the extrahepatic bile ducts. The histologic types include the following:

Carcinomas in situ
Adenocarcinoma
Adenocarcinoma, intestinal type
Clear cell adenocarcinoma
Mucinous carcinoma
Signet ring cell carcinoma
Squamous cell carcinoma
Adenosquamous carcinoma
Small cell carcinoma*
Undifferentiated carcinoma*
    Spindle and giant cell types
    Small cell types
Papillomatosis
Papillary carcinoma, noninvasive
Papillary carcinoma, invasive
Carcinoma, NOS
Other (specify)

*Grade 4 by definition.

## BIBLIOGRAPHY

Abdalla EK, Vauthey JN. Biliary tract cancer. Curr Opin Gastroenterol. 2001;17: 450–7.

Baton O, Azoulay D, Adam DV, et al. Major hepatectomy for hilar cholangiocarcinoma type 3 and 4: prognostic factors and longterm outcomes. J Am Coll Surg. 2007;204:250–60.

De Groen PC, Gores GJ, LaRusso NF, et al. Biliary tract cancers. N Engl J Med. 1999;341:1368–78.

DeOliveira ML, Cunningham SC, Cameron JL, et al. Cholangiocarcinoma: thirty-one-year experience with 564 patients at a single institution. Ann Surg. 2007;245:755–62.

Ebata T, Nagino M, Kamiya J, et al. Hepatectomy with portal vein resection for hilar cholangiocarcinoma: audit of 52 consecutive cases. Ann Surg. 2003;238:720–7.

Hemming AW, Reed AI, Fujita S, et al. Surgical management of hilar cholangiocarcinoma. Ann Surg. 2005;241:693–702.

Hong SM, Kim MJ, Pi DY, et al. Analysis of extrahepatic bile duct carcinomas according to the New American Joint Committee on cancer staging system focused on tumor classification problems in 222 patients. Cancer. 2005;104: 802–10.

Jarnagin WR, Fong Y, DeMatteo RP, et al. Staging, resectability, and outcome in 225 patients with hilar cholangiocarcinoma. Ann Surg. 2001;234:507–17.

Jarnagin WR, Bowne W, Klimstra DS, et al. Papillary phenotype confers improved survival after resection of hilar cholangiocarcinoma. Ann Surg. 2005;241:703–12.

Khan AZ, Makuuchi M. Trends in the surgical management of Klatskin tumors. Br J Surg. 2007;94:393–4.

Kitagawa Y, Nagino M, Kamiya J, et al. Lymph node metastasis from hilar cholangiocarcinoma: audit of 110 patients who underwent regional and paraaortic node dissection. Ann Surg. 2001;233:385–92.

Nagino M, Kamiya J, Nishio H, et al. Two hundred forty consecutive portal vein embolizations before extended hepatectomy for biliary cancer: surgical outcome and long-term follow-up. Ann Surg. 2006;243:364–72.

Nagorney DM, Kendrick ML. Hepatic resection in the treatment of hilar cholangiocarcinoma. Adv Surg. 2006;40:159–71.

Nakeeb A, Pitt HA, Sohn TA, et al. Cholangiocarcinoma. A spectrum of intrahepatic, perihilar, and distal tumors. Ann Surg. 1996;224:463–75.

Neuhaus P, Jonas S, Bechstein WO, et al. Extended resections for hilar cholangiocarcinoma. Ann Surg. 1999;230:808–19.

Nishio H, Nagino M, Oda K, et al. TNM classification for perihilar cholangiocarcinoma: comparison between 5th and 6th editions of the AJCC/UICC staging system. Langenbecks Arch Surg. 2005;390:319–27.

Rea DJ, Heimbach JK, Rosen CB, et al. Liver transplantation with neoadjuvant chemoradiation is more effective than resection for hilar cholangiocarcinoma. Ann Surg. 2005;242:451–61.

Seyama Y, Kubota K, Sano K, et al. Long-term outcome of extended hemihepatectomy for hilar bile duct cancer with no mortality and high survival rate. Ann Surg. 2003;238:73–83.

Vauthey JN, Blumgart LH. Recent advances in the management of cholangiocarcinomas. Semin Liver Dis. 1994;14:109–14.

21

# 22

# Distal Bile Duct

*(Sarcoma and carcinoid tumors are not included.)*

## *At-A-Glance*

### SUMMARY OF CHANGES

- Extrahepatic bile duct was a single chapter in the sixth edition, this has been divided into two chapters for the seventh edition [Perihilar Bile Ducts (see Chap. 21) and Distal Bile Duct]

- Two site-specific prognostic factors, preoperative or pretreatment serum carcinoembryonic antigen and CA19.9, are recommended for collection

| ANATOMIC STAGE/PROGNOSTIC GROUPS | | | |
|---|---|---|---|
| Stage 0 | Tis | N0 | M0 |
| Stage IA | T1 | N0 | M0 |
| Stage IB | T2 | N0 | M0 |
| Stage IIA | T3 | N0 | M0 |
| Stage IIB | T1 | N1 | M0 |
| | T2 | N1 | M0 |
| | T3 | N1 | M0 |
| Stage III | T4 | Any N | M0 |
| Stage IV | Any T | Any N | M1 |

ICD-O-3 TOPOGRAPHY CODES

C24.0 Distal bile duct only

ICD-O-3 HISTOLOGY CODE RANGES

8000–8152, 8154–8231, 8243–8245, 8250–8576, 8940–8950, 8980–8981

## INTRODUCTION

Malignant tumors can develop anywhere along the extrahepatic bile ducts. Of these tumors, 70–80% involve the confluence of the right and left hepatic ducts (perihilar carcinomas), and about 20–30% arise more distally. Diffuse involvement of the ducts is rare, occurring in only about 2% of cases. As a result of differences in anatomy of the bile duct and consideration of local factors that relate to resectability, extrahepatic bile duct carcinomas have been divided into perihilar and distal bile duct cancers. All malignant tumors of the extrahepatic bile ducts inevitably cause partial or complete ductal obstruction. Because the bile ducts have a small diameter, the signs and symptoms of obstruction usually occur while tumors are relatively small. Distal bile duct tumors are classified as those lesions

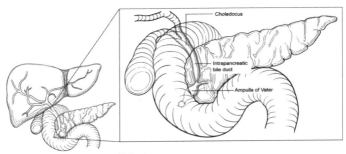

**FIGURE 22.1.** Anatomy of bile duct cancers.

arising between the junction of the cystic duct–bile duct and the ampulla of Vater. This TNM classification applies only to cancers arising in the extrahepatic bile ducts above the ampulla of Vater (Figure 22.1). It includes malignant tumors that develop in congenital choledochal cysts and tumors that arise in the intrapancreatic portion of the common bile duct. Patients with advanced (metastatic) disease and a primary tumor in the intrapancreatic portion of the common bile duct may be misclassified as having pancreatic cancer if surgical resection is not performed. In such cases, it is often impossible to determine (from radiographic images or endoscopy) whether a tumor arises from the intrapancreatic portion of the bile duct, the ampulla of Vater, or the pancreas. Tumors of the pancreas and ampulla of Vater are staged separately.

## ANATOMY

**Primary Site.** The cystic duct connects to the gallbladder and joins the common hepatic duct to form the common bile duct, which passes posterior to the first part of the duodenum, traverses the head of the pancreas, and then enters the second part of the duodenum through the ampulla of Vater. Histologically, the bile ducts are lined by a single layer of tall, uniform columnar cells. The mucosa usually forms irregular pleats or small longitudinal folds. The walls of the bile ducts have a layer of subepithelial connective tissue and muscle fibers. It should be noted that the muscle fibers are most prominent in the distal segment of the common bile duct. The extrahepatic ducts lack a serosa but are surrounded by varying amounts of adventitial adipose tissue. Adipose tissue surrounding the fibromuscular wall is not considered part of the bile duct mural anatomy. Invasion of the perimural adventitial adipose tissue is considered extension beyond the bile duct wall.

**Regional Lymph Nodes.** Accurate tumor staging requires that all lymph nodes that are removed be analyzed. Optimal histologic examination of a pancreaticoduodenectomy specimen should include analysis of a minimum of 12 lymph nodes. If the resected lymph node is negative but this number examined is not met, pN0 should still be assigned. The regional lymph nodes are the same as those resected for cancers of the head of the pancreas; i.e., nodes along the common bile duct, hepatic artery, and back toward the celiac trunk, the posterior and anterior pancreaticoduodenal nodes, and the nodes along the superior mesenteric vein and the right lateral wall of the superior mesenteric artery. Anatomic division of regional lymph nodes is not necessary; however, separately submitted lymph nodes should be reported as submitted.

**Metastatic Sites.** Carcinomas that arise in the distal segment of the common bile duct can spread to the pancreas, duodenum, stomach, colon, or omentum. Distant metastases usually occur late in the course of the disease and are most often found in the liver, lungs, and peritoneum.

## RULES FOR CLASSIFICATION

Most often, patients are staged following surgery and pathologic examination. In a third to a half of cases, surgical resection is not attempted because of local/regional extension, and patients are treated without pathologic staging. A single TNM classification applies to both clinical and pathologic staging. With advances in imaging, integrated radiologic and pathologic staging of patients can be satisfactorily achieved.

**Clinical Staging.** Clinical evaluation usually depends on the results of ultrasonography, contrast-enhanced multidetector computerized tomography (CT), or magnetic resonance cholangiopancreatography (MRCP), including arterial and portal venous phases, with thin sections whenever possible. Clinical staging may also be based on findings from surgical exploration when the main tumor mass is not resected.

**Pathologic Staging.** Pathologic staging depends on surgical resection and pathologic examination of the specimen and associated lymph nodes.

The extent of resection (R0, complete resection with grossly and microscopically negative margins of resection; R1, grossly negative but microscopically positive margins of resection; R2, grossly and microscopically positive margins of resection) is a descriptor in the TNM staging system and is the most important stage-independent prognostic factor and should be reported.

## PROGNOSTIC FEATURES

Patients who undergo surgical resection for localized bile duct adenocarcinoma have a median survival of approximately 2 years and a 5-year survival of 20–40% based on extent of disease at the time of surgery. Several adverse prognostic factors based on the pathologic characteristics of the primary tumor have been reported for carcinomas of the extrahepatic bile ducts. These include histologic type, histologic grade, and vascular, lymphatic, and perineural invasion. Papillary carcinomas have a more favorable outcome than other types of carcinoma. High-grade tumors (grades 3–4) have a less favorable outcome than low-grade tumors (grades 1–2). Positive surgical margins have emerged as a very important prognostic factor. Residual tumor classification (R0, R1, R2) should be reported if the margins are involved.

Patients who undergo pancreaticoduodenectomy for localized periampullary adenocarcinoma of nonpancreatic origin have a superior survival duration compared with similarly treated patients who have adenocarcinoma of pancreatic origin (median survival 3–4 years compared with 18–24 months; 5-year survival 35–45% compared with 10–20%). However, as is true of the natural history of pancreatic adenocarcinoma, extent of disease and the histologic characteristics of the primary tumor predict survival duration. Even in patients who undergo a potentially curative resection, the presence of lymph node metastasis, poorly differentiated histology, positive margins of resection, and tumor invasion into the pancreas are associated with a less favorable outcome. Histologic evidence of tumor extension from the ampulla into the pancreatic parenchyma appears to reflect the extent of both local and regional disease. Perineural invasion, ulceration, and high histopathologic grade are also adverse prognostic factors. Although tumor size is not part of the TNM classification, it has prognostic significance.

Preoperative or pretreatment level of two serum markers, carcinoembryonic antigen and CA19-9, may have prognostic significance and their collection is recommended.

## DEFINITIONS OF TNM

### Primary Tumor (T)

| | |
|---|---|
| TX | Primary tumor cannot be assessed |
| T0 | No evidence of primary tumor |
| Tis | Carcinoma in situ |
| T1 | Tumor confined to the bile duct histologically |
| T2 | Tumor invades beyond the wall of the bile duct |
| T3 | Tumor invades the gallbladder, pancreas, duodenum, or other adjacent organs without involvement of the celiac axis, or the superior mesenteric artery |
| T4 | Tumor involves the celiac axis, or the superior mesenteric artery |

### Regional Lymph Nodes (N)

| | |
|---|---|
| NX | Regional lymph nodes cannot be assessed |
| N0 | No regional lymph node metastasis |
| N1 | Regional lymph node metastasis |

### Distant Metastasis (M)

| | |
|---|---|
| M0 | No distant metastasis |
| M1 | Distant metastasis |

## ANATOMIC STAGE/PROGNOSTIC GROUPS

| Stage 0 | Tis | N0 | M0 |
|---|---|---|---|
| Stage IA | T1 | N0 | M0 |
| Stage IB | T2 | N0 | M0 |
| Stage IIA | T3 | N0 | M0 |
| Stage IIB | T1 | N1 | M0 |
| | T2 | N1 | M0 |
| | T3 | N1 | M0 |
| Stage III | T4 | Any N | M0 |
| Stage IV | Any T | Any N | M1 |

## PROGNOSTIC FACTORS (SITE-SPECIFIC FACTORS)
### (Recommended for Collection)

| Required for staging | None |
|---|---|
| Clinically significant | Tumor location |
| | Carcinoembryonic antigen (CEA) |
| | CA 19-9 |

## HISTOLOGIC GRADE (G)

Grade is reported in registry systems by the grade value. A two-grade, three-grade, or four-grade system may be used. If a grading system is not specified, generally the following system is used:

GX Grade cannot be assessed
G1 Well differentiated
G2 Moderately differentiated
G3 Poorly differentiated
G4 Undifferentiated

## HISTOPATHOLOGIC TYPE

The staging system applies to all carcinomas that arise in the distal extrahepatic bile ducts. Sarcomas and carcinoid tumors are excluded. Adenocarcinoma without specific subtype features is the most common histologic type. Carcinomas account for more than 98% of cancers of the distal extrahepatic bile ducts. The histologic types include:

Carcinomas in situ
Adenocarcinoma
Adenocarcinoma, intestinal type
Clear cell adenocarcinoma
Mucinous carcinoma
Signet ring cell carcinoma
Squamous cell carcinoma
Adenosquamous carcinoma

Small cell carcinoma
Undifferentiated carcinoma
    Spindle and giant cell types
    Small cell types
Papillary carcinoma, noninvasive
Papillary carcinoma, invasive
Carcinoma, NOS
Other (specify)

## BIBLIOGRAPHY

DeOliveira ML, Cunningham SC, Cameron JL, et al. Cholangiocarcinoma: thirty-one-year experience with 564 patients at a single institution. Ann Surg. 2007;245(5):755–62.

Fong Y, Blumgart LH, Lin E, Fortner JG, Brennan MF. Outcome of treatment for distal bile duct cancer. Br J Surg. 1996;83(12):1712–5.

He P, Shi JS, Chen WK, Wang ZR, Ren H, Li H. Multivariate statistical analysis of clinicopathologic factors influencing survival of patients with bile duct carcinoma. World J Gastroenterol. 2002;8(5):943–6.

Hong SM, Cho H, Lee OJ, Ro JY. The number of metastatic lymph nodes in extrahepatic bile duct carcinoma as a prognostic factor. Am J Surg Pathol. 2005;29(9):1177–83.

Hong SM, Kim MJ, Pi DY, Jo D, Cho HJ, Yu E, et al. Analysis of extrahepatic bile duct carcinomas according to the New American Joint Committee on Cancer staging system focused on tumor classification problems in 222 patients. Cancer. 2005;104(4):802–10.

Hong SM, Kim MJ, Cho H, Pi DY, Jo D, Yu E, et al. Superficial vs deep pancreatic parenchymal invasion in the extrahepatic bile duct carcinomas: a significant prognostic factor. Mod Pathol. 2005;18(7):969–75.

Hong SM, Cho H, Moskaluk CA, Yu E. Measurement of the invasion depth of extrahepatic bile duct carcinoma: an alternative method overcoming the current T classification problems of the AJCC staging system. Am J Surg Pathol. 2007;31(2):199–206.

Kayahara M, Nagakawa T, Ohta T, Kitagawa H, Tajima H, Miwa K. Role of nodal involvement and the periductal soft-tissue margin in middle and distal bile duct cancer. Ann Surg. 1999;229(1):76–83.

Murakami Y, Uemura K, Hayashidani Y, Sudo T, Hashimoto Y, Ohge H, et al. Prognostic significance of lymph node metastasis and surgical margin status for distal cholangiocarcinoma. J Surg Oncol. 2007;95(3):207–12.

Murakami Y, Uemura K, Hayashidani Y, Sudo T, Ohge H, Sueda T. Pancreatoduodenectomy for distal cholangiocarcinoma: prognostic impact of lymph node metastasis. World J Surg. 2007;31(2):337–42.

Riall TS, Cameron JL, Lillemoe KD, Winter JM, Campbell KA, Hruban RH, et al. Resected periampullary adenocarcinoma: 5-year survivors and their 6- to 10-year follow-up. Surgery. 2006;140(5):764–72.

Sasaki R, Takahashi M, Funato O, Nitta H, Murakami M, Kawamura H, et al. Prognostic significance of lymph node involvement in middle and distal bile duct cancer. Surgery. 2001;129(6):677–83.

Yoshida T, Matsumoto T, Sasaki A, Morii Y, Aramaki M, Kitano S. Prognostic factors after pancreatoduodenectomy with extended lymphadenectomy for distal bile duct cancer. Arch Surg. 2002;137(1):69–73.

# Ampulla of Vater

## *At-A-Glance*

> **SUMMARY OF CHANGES**
> • The definitions of TNM and the Stage Grouping for this chapter have not changed from the Sixth Edition

| ANATOMIC STAGE/PROGNOSTIC GROUPS | | | |
|---|---|---|---|
| Stage 0 | Tis | N0 | M0 |
| Stage 1A | T1 | N0 | M0 |
| Stage IB | T2 | N0 | M0 |
| Stage IIA | T3 | N0 | M0 |
| Stage IIB | T1 | N1 | M0 |
| | T2 | N1 | M0 |
| | T3 | N1 | M0 |
| Stage III | T4 | Any N | M0 |
| Stage IV | Any T | Any N | M1 |

ICD-O-3 TOPOGRAPHY CODES

C24.1    Ampulla of Vater

ICD-O-3 HISTOLOGY CODE RANGES

8000–8152, 8154–8231, 8243–8245, 8250–8576, 8940–8950, 8980–8981

## INTRODUCTION

The ampulla of Vater is strategically located at the confluence of the pancreatic and common bile ducts (Figure 23.1). Most tumors that arise in this small structure obstruct the common bile duct, causing jaundice, abdominal pain, occasionally pancreatitis, and bleeding. Clinically and pathologically, carcinomas of the ampulla may be difficult to differentiate from those arising in the head of the pancreas or in the distal segment of the common bile duct. Primary cancers of the ampulla are not common, accounting for roughly 15–25% of neoplasms arising in the periampullary region, although they constitute a high proportion of malignant tumors occurring in the duodenum. Tumors of the ampulla must be differentiated from those arising in the second part of the duodenum and invading the ampulla. Carcinomas of the ampulla and periampullary region are often associated with familial adenomatous polyposis coli.

## ANATOMY

**Primary Site.** The ampulla is a small dilated duct less than 1.5-cm long, formed in most individuals by the union of the terminal segments of the pancreatic and common bile ducts. In 42% of individuals, however,

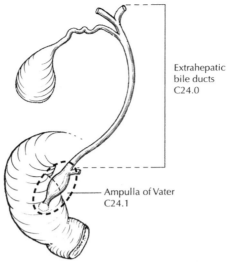

Extrahepatic
bile ducts
C24.0

Ampulla of Vater
C24.1

**FIGURE 23.1.** Anatomy of the ampulla of Vater, strategically located at the confluence of the pancreatic and common bile ducts.

the ampulla is the termination of the common duct only, the pancreatic duct having its own entrance into the duodenum adjacent to the ampulla. In these individuals, the ampulla may be difficult to locate or even nonexistent. The ampulla opens into the duodenum, usually on the posterior-medial wall, through a small mucosal elevation, the duodenal papilla, which is also called the papilla of Vater. Although carcinomas can arise either in the ampulla or on the papilla, they most commonly arise near the junction of the mucosa of the ampulla with that of the papilla. It may not be possible to determine the exact site of origin for large tumors. Nearly all cancers that arise in this area are well-differentiated adenocarcinomas.

**Regional Lymph Nodes.** A rich lymphatic network surrounds the pancreas and periampullary region, and accurate tumor staging requires that all lymph nodes that are removed be analyzed. The regional lymph nodes are the peripancreatic lymph nodes, which also include the lymph nodes along the hepatic artery and portal vein. Anatomic division of regional lymph nodes is not necessary. However, separately submitted lymph nodes should be reported as submitted. Optimal histologic examination of a pancreaticoduodenectomy specimen should include analysis of a minimum of 12 lymph nodes. If the resected lymph nodes are negative, but this number examined is not met, pN0 should still be assigned. The number of lymph nodes sampled and the number of involved lymph nodes should be recorded.

**Metastatic Sites.** Tumors of the ampulla may infiltrate adjacent structures, such as the wall of the duodenum, the head of the pancreas, and extrahepatic bile ducts. Metastatic disease is most commonly found in the liver and peritoneum and is less commonly seen in the lungs and pleura.

---

## RULES FOR CLASSIFICATION

Most patients are staged pathologically after examination of the resected specimen. Classification is based primarily on local extension. The T classification depends on extension of the primary tumor through the ampulla of Vater or the sphincter of Oddi into the duodenal wall or beyond into the head of the pancreas or contiguous soft tissue. The designation T4 most commonly refers to local soft tissue invasion, but even T4 tumors are usually locally resectable.

**Clinical Staging.** Endoscopic ultrasonography and computed tomography are effective in preoperative staging and in evaluating resectability of ampullary carcinomas. Magnetic resonance imaging with magnetic resonance cholangiopancreatography may be helpful, especially in the setting of complete obstruction of the pancreatic duct. Fluorodeoxyglucose positron emission tomography (FDG-PET) has not emerged as useful in the initial evaluation of ampullary neoplasms, although it may be useful in detection of metastatic disease. Laparoscopy is occasionally performed for patients who are believed to have localized, potentially resectable tumors to exclude peritoneal metastases and small metastases on the surface of the liver.

**Pathologic Staging.** Pathologic staging depends on surgical resection and pathologic examination of the specimen and associated lymph nodes. The finding of positive regional lymph nodes has a significant negative impact on survival, with 5-year overall survival rates in one study falling from 63% for node negative patients to 40% for patients with one positive regional lymph node and 0% for those with four or more positive nodes. The completeness of resection (R0, complete resection with no residual tumor; R1, microscopic residual tumor; R2, macroscopic residual tumor) is not part of the TNM staging system but is prognostically of great significance.

## PROGNOSTIC FEATURES

Patients who undergo pancreaticoduodenectomy for localized periampullary adenocarcinoma of non-pancreatic origin have a superior survival duration compared with similarly treated patients who have adenocarcinoma of pancreatic origin (median survival 3–4 years compared with 18–24 months; 5-year survival 35–45% compared with 10–20%). However, as is true of the natural history of pancreatic adenocarcinoma, extent of disease and the histologic characteristics of the primary tumor predict survival duration. Even in patients who undergo a potentially curative resection, the presence of lymph node metastases, poorly differentiated histology, positive margins of resection, and tumor invasion into the pancreas are associated with a less favorable outcome. Histologic evidence of tumor extension from the ampulla into the pancreatic parenchyma appears to reflect the extent of both local and regional disease. Perineural invasion, ulceration, and high histopathologic grade are also adverse prognostic factors.

Although tumor size is not part of the TNM classification, it has prognostic significance. Tumor involvement (positivity) of resection margins repeatedly has been demonstrated to be an adverse prognostic factor. The residual tumor classification (R1, or R2) should be reported if the margins are involved.

Lymph node metastasis in patients with adenocarcinoma of the ampulla of Vater is consistently reported to be a predictor of poor outcome, although it does not appear to be as powerful a predictor of disease recurrence or short survival duration as for pancreatic carcinoma. The actuarial 5-year survival following potentially curative surgery in node-positive patients with pancreatic adenocarcinoma is 0–5%; in those with ampullary adenocarcinoma it is 15–30%. Extended retroperitoneal lymphadenectomy has not been shown to improve survival. Tumors with papillary histology have a better outcome than non-papillary tumors. Two serum markers may have prognostic significance and should be routinely collected before surgery or treatment begins and may be useful to assess treatment response. These are carcinoembryonic antigen (CEA) and CA19-9.

## DEFINITIONS OF TNM

### Primary Tumor (T)

| | |
|---|---|
| TX | Primary tumor cannot be assessed |
| T0 | No evidence of primary tumor |
| Tis | Carcinoma in situ |
| T1 | Tumor limited to ampulla of Vater or sphincter of Oddi |
| T2 | Tumor invades duodenal wall |
| T3 | Tumor invades pancreas |
| T4 | Tumor invades peripancreatic soft tissues or other adjacent organs or structures other than pancreas |

### Regional Lymph Nodes (N)

| | |
|---|---|
| NX | Regional lymph nodes cannot be assessed |
| N0 | No regional lymph node metastasis |
| N1 | Regional lymph node metastasis |

### Distant Metastasis (M)

| | |
|---|---|
| M0 | No distant metastasis |
| M1 | Distant metastasis |

### ANATOMIC STAGE/PROGNOSTIC GROUPS

| Stage 0 | Tis | N0 | M0 |
|---|---|---|---|
| Stage IA | T1 | N0 | M0 |
| Stage IB | T2 | N0 | M0 |
| Stage IIA | T3 | N0 | M0 |
| Stage IIB | T1 | N1 | M0 |
| | T2 | N1 | M0 |
| | T3 | N1 | M0 |
| Stage III | T4 | Any N | M0 |
| Stage IV | Any T | Any N | M1 |

## PROGNOSTIC FACTORS (SITE-SPECIFIC FACTORS)
### (Recommended for Collection)

| | |
|---|---|
| Required for staging | None |
| Clinically significant | Preoperative or pretreatment carcinoembryonic antigen (CEA) |
| | Preoperative or pretreatment CA 19-9 |

## HISTOLOGIC GRADE (G)

Grade is reported in registry systems by the grade value. A two-grade, three-grade, or four-grade system may be used. If a grading system is not specified, generally the following system is used:

GX     Grade cannot be assessed
G1     Well differentiated
G2     Moderately differentiated
G3     Poorly differentiated
G4     Undifferentiated

## HISTOPATHOLOGIC TYPE

The staging system applies to all primary carcinomas that arise in the ampulla or on the duodenal papilla. Adenocarcinomas are the most common histologic type. The classification does not apply to carcinoid tumors or to other neuroendocrine tumors. The following histologic types are included:

Carcinoma in situ
Adenocarcinoma
Adenocarcinoma, intestinal type
Clear cell adenocarcinoma
Mucinous carcinoma
Signet ring cell carcinoma
Squamous cell carcinoma
Adenosquamous carcinoma
Small cell carcinoma*
Undifferentiated carcinoma*
    Spindle and giant cell types
Papillary carcinoma, noninvasive
Papillary carcinoma, invasive
Carcinoma
Other (specify)

*Grade 4 by definition

## OUTCOMES RESULTS

Observed survival rates for 4,328 cases with carcinoma of the ampulla of Vater from 1998 to 2002 are shown in Figure 23.2.

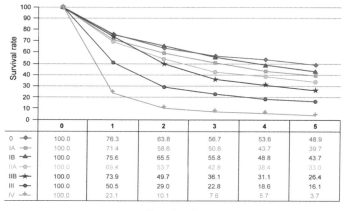

| | 0 | 1 | 2 | 3 | 4 | 5 |
|---|---|---|---|---|---|---|
| 0 | 100.0 | 76.3 | 63.8 | 56.7 | 53.6 | 48.9 |
| IA | 100.0 | 71.4 | 58.6 | 50.6 | 43.7 | 39.7 |
| IB | 100.0 | 75.6 | 65.5 | 55.8 | 48.8 | 43.7 |
| IIA | 100.0 | 69.4 | 53.7 | 42.8 | 38.4 | 33.0 |
| IIB | 100.0 | 73.9 | 49.7 | 36.1 | 31.1 | 26.4 |
| III | 100.0 | 50.5 | 29.0 | 22.8 | 18.6 | 16.1 |
| IV | 100.0 | 23.1 | 10.1 | 7.6 | 5.7 | 3.7 |

Years from diagnosis

**FIGURE 23.2.** Observed survival rates for 4,328 cases with carcinoma of the ampulla of Vater. Data from the National Cancer Data Base (Commission on Cancer of the American College of Surgeons and the American Cancer Society) diagnosed in years 1998–2002. Stage 0 includes 118 patients; Stage IA, 892; Stage IB, 807; Stage IIA 554; Stage IIB, 1,206; Stage III, 546; and Stage IV, 205.

## BIBLIOGRAPHY

Abrams RA, Yeo CJ. Combined modality adjuvant therapy for resected periampullary pancreatic and nonpancreatic adenocarcinoma: a review of studies and experience at The Johns Hopkins Hospital, 1991–2003. Surg Oncol Clin North Am. 2004;13:621–38.

Bakkevold KE, Kambestad B. Staging of carcinoma of the pancreas and ampulla of Vater: tumor (T), lymph node (N), and distant metastasis (M) as prognostic factors. Int J Pancreatol. 1995;17:249–59.

Bettschart V, Rahman MQ, Engelken FJ, et al. Presentation, treatment, and outcome in patients with ampullary tumors. Br J Surg. 2004;91:1600–7.

De Castro SMM, van Heek NT, Kuhlmann KFD, et al. Surgical management of neoplasms of the ampulla of Vater: local resection or pancreatoduodenectomy and prognostic factors for survival. Surgery. 2004;136:994–1002.

Howe JR, Klimstra DS, Moccia RD, et al. Factors predictive of survival in ampullary carcinoma. Ann Surg. 1998;228:87–94.

Hsu HP, Yang TM, Hsieh YH, et al. Predictors for patterns of failure after pancreaticoduodenectomy in ampullary cancer. Ann Surg Oncol. 2007;14:50–60.

Katz MH, Bouvet M, Al-Refaie W, et al. Non-pancreatic periampullary adenocarcinomas: an explanation for favorable prognosis. Hepato-Gastroenterology. 2004;51:842–6.

Kennedy EP, Yeo CJ. Pancreaticoduodenectomy with extended retroperitoneal lymphadenectomy for periampullary carcinoma. Surg Oncol Clin North Am. 2007;16:157–76.

Kim RD, Kundhal PS, McGilvray ID, Cattral MS, Taylor B, et al. Predictors of failure after pancreaticoduodenectomy for ampullary carcinoma. J Am Coll Surg. 2006;202:112–9.

Qiao QL, Zhao YG, Ye ML, et al. Carcinoma of the ampulla of Vater: factors influencing long-term survival of 127 patients with resection. World J Surg. 2007;31:137–43.

Riall TS, Cameron JL, Lillemoe KD, et al. Resected periampullary adenocarcinoma: 5-year survivors and their 6- to 10-year follow-up. Surgery.
2006;140:764–72.

Sakata J, Shirai Y, Wakai T, et al. Number of positive lymph nodes independently
affects long-term survival after resection in patients with ampullary carcinoma. Eur J Surgical Oncol. 2007;33:346–51.

Todoroki T, Koike N, Morishita Y, et al. Patterns and predictors of failure after
curative resections of carcinoma of the ampulla of Vater. Ann Surg Oncol.
2003;10:1176–83.

Walsh RM, Connelly M, Baker M. Imaging for the diagnosis and staging of periampullary carcinomas. Surg Endosc. 2003;17:1514–20.

23

# Exocrine and Endocrine Pancreas

## *At-A-Glance*

---

### SUMMARY OF CHANGES

- Pancreatic neuroendocrine tumors (including carcinoid tumors) are now staged by a single pancreatic staging system

- Survival tables and figures have been added for adenocarcinoma and neuroendocrine tumors

- The definition of TNM and the Anatomic Stage/Prognostic Groupings for this chapter have not changed from the sixth edition for exocrine tumors

---

| ANATOMIC STAGE/PROGNOSTIC GROUPS | | | |
|---|---|---|---|
| Stage 0 | Tis | N0 | M0 |
| Stage IA | T1 | N0 | M0 |
| Stage IB | T2 | N0 | M0 |
| Stage IIA | T3 | N0 | M0 |
| Stage IIB | T1 | N1 | M0 |
| | T2 | N1 | M0 |
| | T3 | N1 | M0 |
| Stage III | T4 | Any N | M0 |
| Stage IV | Any T | Any N | M1 |

ICD-O-3 TOPOGRAPHY CODES

C25.0    Head of pancreas

C25.1    Body of pancreas

C25.2    Tail of pancreas

C25.3    Pancreatic duct

C25.4    Islets of Langerhans (endocrine pancreas)

C25.7    Other specified parts of pancreas

C25.8    Overlapping lesion of pancreas

C25.9    Pancreas, NOS

ICD-O-3 HISTOLOGY CODE RANGES
8000–8576, 8940–8950, 8980–8981

# INTRODUCTION

In the USA, pancreatic cancer is the second most common malignant tumor of the gastrointestinal tract and the fourth leading cause of cancer-related death in adults. The disease is difficult to diagnose, especially in its early stages, and pessimism regarding pancreatic cancer has resulted in underutilization of surgery for resectable patients. Most pancreatic cancers arise in the head of the pancreas, often causing bile duct obstruction that results in clinically evident jaundice. Cancers that arise in either the body or the tail of the pancreas are insidious in their development and often far advanced when first detected. Most pancreatic cancers are adenocarcinomas, which originate from the pancreatic duct cells. Pancreatic neuroendocrine carcinomas also arising from pancreatic duct cells capable of neuroendocrine differentiation comprise 3–5% of pancreatic malignancies. Surgical resection remains the only potentially curative approach, although multimodality therapy consisting of systemic agents, and often radiation, may improve survival. Staging of pancreatic cancers depends on the size and extent of the primary tumor.

# ANATOMY

**Primary Site.** The pancreas is a long, coarsely lobulated gland that lies transversely across the posterior abdomen and extends from the duodenum to the splenic hilum. The organ is divided into a head with a small uncinate process, a neck, a body, and a tail. The anterior aspect of the body of the pancreas is in direct contact with the posterior wall of the stomach; posteriorly, the pancreas extends to the inferior vena cava, superior mesenteric vein, splenic vein, and left kidney

**Regional Lymph Nodes.** A rich lymphatic network surrounds the pancreas, and accurate tumor staging requires that all lymph nodes that are removed be analyzed. Optimal histologic examination of a pancreaticoduodenectomy specimen should include analysis of a minimum of 12 lymph nodes. The standard regional lymph node basins and soft tissues resected for tumors located in the head and neck of the pancreas include lymph nodes along the common bile duct, common hepatic artery, portal vein, posterior and anterior pancreaticoduodenal arcades, and along the superior mesenteric vein and right lateral wall of the superior mesenteric artery. For cancers located in body and tail, regional lymph node basins include lymph nodes along the common hepatic artery, celiac axis, splenic artery, and splenic hilum. Anatomic division of regional lymph nodes is not necessary. However, separately submitted lymph nodes should be reported as labeled by the surgeon.

**Metastatic Sites.** Distant spread is common on presentation and typically involves the liver, peritoneal cavity, and lungs. Metastases to other sites are uncommon.

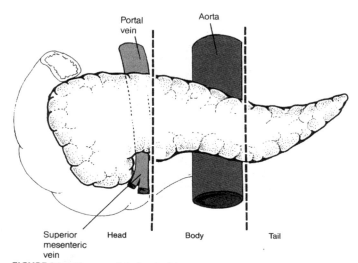

**FIGURE 24.1.** Tumors of the head of the pancreas are those arising to the right of the superior mesenteric–portal vein confluence.

## DEFINITION OF LOCATION

Tumors of the head of the pancreas are those arising to the right of the superior mesenteric–portal vein confluence (Figure 24.1). The uncinate process is part of the pancreatic head. Tumors of the body of the pancreas are defined as those arising between the left edge of the superior mesenteric–portal vein confluence and the left edge of the aorta. Tumors of the tail of the pancreas are those arising to the left of the left edge of the aorta.

## RULES FOR CLASSIFICATION

Because only a minority of patients with pancreatic cancer undergo surgical resection of the pancreas (and adjacent lymph nodes), a single TNM classification must apply to both clinical and pathologic staging.

### Changes from the Sixth Edition

1. Pancreatic neuroendocrine tumors and carcinoid tumors were specifically excluded in prior editions of the AJCC *Cancer Staging Manual.* Pancreatic neuroendocrine tumors typically have a better prognosis than adenocarcinoma. However, neuroendocrine tumors can be staged by the exocrine cancer staging system. Although tumor size and the presence of lymph node metastases are of questionable importance, the survival discrimination seen likely stems from T and N stage serving as proxy for other prognostic factors that have been shown to be significant for neuroendocrine tumors such as tumor differentiation and functional status. Inclusion of these tumors in the staging system will improve data collection to facilitate investigation of prognostic factors.

**24**

2. Survival tables have been added for pancreatic adenocarcinoma and neuroendocrine tumors. These data from the National Cancer Data Base (NCDB) offer prognostic information for patients, provide detailed information for treatment decisions, and improve for stratification in clinical trials.

**Clinical Staging.** Information necessary for the clinical staging of pancreatic cancer can be obtained from physical examination and three-dimensional radiographic imaging studies, which include triphasic, contrast-enhanced multislice computed tomography or magnetic resonance imaging (MRI). On the basis of the interpretation of CT images and chest radiographs, patients can be classified as having localized resectable (Stage I or II), locally advanced (Stage III), or metastatic (Stage IV) pancreatic cancer. Endoscopic ultrasonography (when done by experienced gastroenterologists) also provides information helpful for clinical staging and is the procedure of choice for performing fine-needle aspiration biopsy of the pancreas. Tumor involvement of the superior mesenteric or portal veins will usually be classified as T3 in the current AJCC T classification. Such tumors are considered resectable in some centers and there are limited data on the prognostic significance of venous invasion. The distinction between T3 and T4 reflects the difference between potentially resectable (T3) and locally advanced (T4) primary pancreatic tumors, both of which demonstrate radiographic or pathologic evidence of extrapancreatic tumor extension. The standard radiographic assessment of resectability includes evaluation for peritoneal or hepatic metastases; the patency of the superior mesenteric vein and portal vein and the relationship of these vessels and their tributaries to the tumor; and the relationship of the tumor to the superior mesenteric artery, celiac axis, and hepatic artery.

Laparoscopy may be performed on patients believed to have localized, potentially resectable tumors to exclude peritoneal metastases and small metastases on the surface of the liver. Laparoscopy will reveal tiny (<1 cm) peritoneal or liver metastases and upstage (to Stage IV) approximately 10% of patients with tumors in the pancreatic head, and probably a greater percentage of patients with tumors in the body and tail. The necessity of obtaining peritoneal cytology from washings during laparoscopy remains controversial. At present, positive peritoneal cytology is considered M1 disease.

**Pathologic Staging.** The College of American Pathologists (CAP) Checklist for Endocrine or Exocrine Pancreatic Tumors is recommended as a guideline for the pathologic evaluation of these pancreatic resection specimens (http://www.cap.org/apps/cap.portal?_nfpb=true&_pageLabel=reference). Partial resection (pancreaticoduodenectomy or distal pancreatectomy) or complete resection of the pancreas, including the tumor and associated regional lymph nodes, provides the information necessary for pathologic staging. In pancreaticoduodenectomy specimens, the bile duct, pancreatic duct, and superior mesenteric artery margins should be evaluated grossly and microscopically. The superior mesenteric artery margin has also been termed the retroperitoneal, mesopancreatic, and unicate margin. In total pancreatectomy specimens, the bile duct and retroperitoneal margins should be

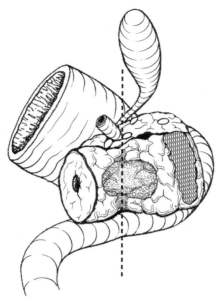

**FIGURE 24.2.** The retroperitoneal pancreatic margin (hatched area; also referred to as the mesenteric or uncinate) consists of soft tissue that often contains perineural tissue adjacent to the superior mesenteric artery.

assessed. Duodenal (with pylorus-preserving pancreaticoduodenectomy) and gastric (with standard pancreaticoduodenectomy) margins are rarely involved, but their status should be included in the surgical pathology report. Reporting of margins may be facilitated by ensuring documentation of the pertinent margins: (1) Common bile (hepatic) duct, (2) pancreatic neck, (3) superior mesenteric artery margin, (4) other soft tissue margins (i.e., posterior pancreatic), duodenum, and stomach.

Particular attention should be paid to the superior mesenteric artery margin (soft tissue that often contains perineural tissue adjacent to the right lateral wall of the superior mesenteric artery; see Figure 24.2) because most local recurrences arise in the pancreatic bed along this critical margin. The soft tissue between the anterior surface of the inferior vena cava and the posterior aspect of the pancreatic head and duodenum is best referred to as the posterior pancreatic margin (not the retroperitoneal margin). The superior mesenteric artery margin (retroperitoneal or uncinate margin) should be inked as part of the gross evaluation of the specimen; the specimen is then cut perpendicular to the inked margin for histologic analysis. The closest microscopic approach of the tumor to the margin should be recorded in millimeters.

Seeding of the peritoneum (even if limited to the lesser sac region) is considered M1. Similarly, peritoneal fluid that contains cytologic (microscopic) evidence of carcinoma is considered M1. In patients without ascites, the implications of positive peritoneal cytology are not clear at this time, although the available data suggest that this finding predicts a short survival. Therefore, positive peritoneal cytology is also considered M1.

## PROGNOSTIC FEATURES

**Adenocarcinoma.** Patients who undergo surgical resection for localized nonmetastatic adenocarcinoma of the pancreas have a long-term survival rate of approximately 20% and a median survival of 12–20 months (Table 24.1). Patients with locally advanced, non-metastatic disease have a median survival of 6–10 months (Table 24.2). Patients with metastatic disease have a short survival (3–6 months), the length of which depends on the extent of disease, performance status, and response to systemic therapy.

A number of investigators have examined pathologic factors of the resected tumor (in patients with apparently localized, resectable pancreatic cancer) in an effort to establish reliable prognostic variables associated with decreased survival duration. Metastatic disease in regional lymph nodes, poorly differentiated histology, and increased size of the primary tumor have been associated with decreased survival duration. Perineural invasion, lymphovascular invasion, and elevated CA 19-9 levels are also associated with a poor prognosis. Another prognostic factor of importance in patients who undergo pancreaticoduodenectomy is incomplete resection. Therefore, margin assessment is of major importance in the gross and microscopic evaluation of the pancreaticoduodenectomy specimen. It is important to note that the extent of resection (R0, complete resection with grossly and microscopically negative margins of resection; R1, grossly negative but microscopically positive margins of resection; R2, grossly and microscopically positive margins of resection) is not part of the TNM staging system but is prognostically significant. Retrospective pathologic analysis of archival material does not allow accurate assessment of the margins of resection or of the number of lymph nodes retrieved; this information must be obtained when the specimen is removed and examined in the surgical pathology laboratory. The margin of resection most likely to be positive is the superior mesenteric artery margin along the right lateral border of the superior mesenteric artery. This margin is defined as the soft tissue margin directly adjacent to the proximal 3–4 cm of the superior mesenteric artery and is inked for evaluation of margin status on permanent-section histologic evaluation (see the "Pathologic Staging" section). Incomplete resection resulting in a grossly positive retroperitoneal margin provides no survival advantage from surgical resection (compared with those who receive chemoradiation and no surgery).

**Neuroendocrine Tumors.** Patients who undergo surgical resection for localized neuroendocrine carcinoma of the pancreas have a 5-year overall survival rate of approximately 55.4%, significantly better than patients with pancreatic adenocarcinoma (Table 24.3). Those who do not undergo resection have 5-year survival of approximately 15.6%. The natural history of these tumors is poorly understood due to their relative rarity, but demonstrated prognostic factors include patient age, distant metastases, tumor functional status, and degree of differentiation. Including these tumors in

**TABLE 24.1.** Five-year overall survival for pancreatic adenocarcinoma from the National Cancer Data Base: surgical

| | Surgical patients | | Observed survival | | | | | | Median survival (months) |
|---|---|---|---|---|---|---|---|---|---|
| | Number of patients | (%) | 1-Year (%) | 2-Year (%) | 3-Year (%) | 4-Year (%) | 5-Year (%) | | |
| Stage IA | 1886 | 8.8 | 71.3 | 50.2 | 40.7 | 34.7 | 31.4 | | 24.1 |
| Stage IB | 2364 | 11.0 | 67.3 | 45.4 | 35.3 | 29.6 | 27.2 | | 20.6 |
| Stage IIA | 3846 | 17.9 | 60.7 | 34.9 | 23.8 | 18.4 | 15.7 | | 15.4 |
| Stage IIB | 7828 | 36.4 | 52.7 | 23.8 | 14.4 | 10.2 | 7.7 | | 12.7 |
| Stage III | 2850 | 13.2 | 44.5 | 19.3 | 11.0 | 8.1 | 6.8 | | 10.6 |
| Stage IV | 2738 | 12.7 | 19.2 | 8.4 | 5.3 | 3.7 | 2.8 | | 4.5 |
| Total | 21,512 | | | | | | | | 12.6 |

From Bilimoria KY, Bentrem DJ, Ko CY, et al. Validation of the 6th edition AJCC Pancreatic Cancer Staging System: report from the National Cancer Database. Cancer. 2007;110(4):738–44, with permission of Wiley.

24

**TABLE 24.2.** Five-year overall survival for pancreatic adenocarcinoma from the National Cancer Data Base: no surgery

| | Nonsurgical patients | | Observed survival | | | | | Median survival (months) |
|---|---|---|---|---|---|---|---|---|
| | Number of patients | (%) | 1-Year (%) | 2-Year (%) | 3-Year (%) | 4-Year (%) | 5-Year (%) | |
| Stage IA | 3,412 | 4.4 | 29.2 | 10.5 | 6.2 | 4.6 | 3.8 | 6.8 |
| Stage IB | 4,298 | 5.4 | 26.0 | 9.4 | 5.7 | 4.0 | 3.4 | 6.1 |
| Stage IIA | 8,486 | 10.1 | 25.0 | 7.7 | 4.1 | 2.8 | 2.4 | 6.2 |
| Stage IIB | 6,570 | 11.8 | 26.9 | 7.7 | 3.8 | 2.6 | 2.0 | 6.7 |
| Stage III | 12,981 | 13.0 | 27.0 | 7.3 | 3.4 | 2.4 | 1.8 | 7.2 |
| Stage IV | 64,454 | 55.2 | 8.3 | 2.3 | 1.2 | 0.8 | 0.6 | 2.5 |
| Total | 100,201 | | | | | | | 3.5 |

From Bilimoria KY, Bentrem DJ, Ko CY, et al. Validation of the 6th edition AJCC Pancreatic Cancer Staging System: report from the National Cancer Database. Cancer. 2007;110(4):738–44, with permission of Wiley.

**TABLE 24.3.** Five and ten-year survival rates for patients who underwent resection of pancreatic neuroendocrine tumors

| | Observed survival[a] | | Relative survival[b] | | |
|---|---|---|---|---|---|
| | 5-Year (%) | 10-Year (%) | 5-Year (%) | 10-Year (%) | Median survival |
| Stage I | 61.0 | 46.0 | 75.6 | 71.1 | 112 months |
| Stage II | 52.0 | 28.8 | 64.3 | 45.8 | 63 months |
| Stage III | 41.4 | 18.5 | 60.5 | 33.1 | 46 months |
| Stage IV | 15.5 | 5.1 | 19.9 | 8.9 | 14 months |

From Bilimoria KY, Bentrem DJ, Merkow RP, et al: Application of the pancreatic adenocarcinoma staging system to pancreatic neuroendocrine tumors. J Am Coll Surg. 2007; 205(4):558–63.

[a] Comparisons between each stage group are significant to $P < 0.0001$.

[b] Survival adjusted for patient age by matching against 1990 United States Census Bureau data.

the pancreatic cancer staging system will allow for improved data collection and subsequent identification of potential prognostic factors. Importantly, the classification of these tumors as "benign" or "malignant" is not consistent, thus all pancreatic neuroendocrine tumors irrespective of being classified as benign or malignant should be staged by this system and reported to cancer registries.

## DEFINITIONS OF TNM

### Primary Tumor (T)

TX      Primary tumor cannot be assessed
T0      No evidence of primary tumor
Tis     Carcinoma in situ*
T1      Tumor limited to the pancreas, 2 cm or less in greatest dimension
T2      Tumor limited to the pancreas, more than 2 cm in greatest dimension
T3      Tumor extends beyond the pancreas but without involvement of the celiac axis or the superior mesenteric artery
T4      Tumor involves the celiac axis or the superior mesenteric artery (unresectable primary tumor)

*This also includes the "PanInIII" classification.

### Regional Lymph Nodes (N)

NX     Regional lymph nodes cannot be assessed
N0     No regional lymph node metastasis
N1     Regional lymph node metastasis

### Distant Metastasis (M)

M0     No distant metastasis
M1     Distant metastasis

24

## ANATOMIC STAGE/PROGNOSTIC GROUPS

| Stage 0 | Tis | N0 | M0 |
|---------|-----|-----|-----|
| Stage IA | T1 | N0 | M0 |
| Stage IB | T2 | N0 | M0 |
| Stage IIA | T3 | N0 | M0 |
| Stage IIB | T1 | N1 | M0 |
| | T2 | N1 | M0 |
| | T3 | N1 | M0 |
| Stage III | T4 | Any N | M0 |
| Stage IV | Any T | Any N | M1 |

## PROGNOSTIC FACTORS (SITE-SPECIFIC FACTORS)
### (Recommended for Collection)

| | |
|---|---|
| Required for staging | None |
| Clinically significant | Preoperative CA 19-9 |
| | Preoperative carcinoembryonic antigen (CEA) |
| | Preoperative plasma chromogranin A level (CgA) (endocrine pancreas) |
| | Mitotic count (endocrine pancreas) |

## HISTOLOGIC GRADE (G)

Grade is reported in registry systems by the grade value. A two-grade, three-grade, or four-grade system may be used. If a grading system is not specified, generally the following system is used:

| | |
|-----|-----|
| GX | Grade cannot be assessed |
| G1 | Well differentiated |
| G2 | Moderately differentiated |
| G3 | Poorly differentiated |
| G4 | Undifferentiated |

## HISTOPATHOLOGIC TYPE

The staging system applies to all arise in the pancreas. Neuroendocrine tumors have a distinctly different tumor biology and better long-term survival; however, the TNM system provides reasonable stage discrimination. The following tumors are included:

Severe ductal dysplasia/carcinoma in situ (PanIn III; pancreatic intraepithelial neoplasia)
Ductal adenocarcinoma
Mucinous noncystic carcinoma
Signet ring cell carcinoma
Adenosquamous carcinoma

Undifferentiated carcinoma
    Spindle and giant cell types
    Small cell types
Mixed ductal-endocrine carcinoma
Osteoclast-like giant cell tumor
Serous cystadenocarcinoma
Mucinous cystadenocarcinoma
Intraductal papillary mucinous carcinoma with or without invasion
    (IPMN)
Acinar cell carcinoma
Acinar cell cystadenocarcinoma
Mixed acinar-endocrine carcinoma
Pancreaticoblastoma
Solid pseudopapillary carcinoma
Borderline (uncertain malignant potential) tumors
    Mucinous cystic tumor with moderate dysplasia
    Intraductal papillary-mucinous tumor with moderate dysplasia
    Solid pseudopapillary tumor
Composite carcinoid (combined with adenocarcinoma)
Adenocarcinoid tumor
Mixed islet cell and exocrine adenocarcinoma
Islet cell carcinoma
Insulinoma
Glucagonoma
Gastrinoma
Vipoma
Somatostatinoma
Enteroglucagonoma
Carcinoid tumor, NOS
Atypical carcinoid tumor
Neuroendocrine carcinoma, NOS

## BIBLIOGRAPHY

Albores-Saavedra J, Heffess C, Hruban RH, et al. Recommendations for the
    reporting of pancreatic specimens containing malignant tumors. Am J Clin
    Pathol. 1999;111:304–7.
Bilimoria KY, Bentrem DJ, Merkow RP, et al. Application of the pancreatic ade-
    nocarcinoma staging system to pancreatic neuroendocrine tumors. J Am
    Coll Surg. 2007a;205(4):558–63.
Bilimoria KY, Bentrem DJ, Ko CY, et al. Validation of the 6th edition AJCC Pan-
    creatic Cancer Staging System: report from the National Cancer Database.
    Cancer. 2007b;110(4):738–44.
Bilimoria KY, Talamonti MD, Tomlinson JS, et al. Prognostic score predicting
    survival after resection of pancreatic neuroendocrine tumors: analysis of
    3851 patients. Ann Surg. 2008;247(3):490–500.
Birkmeyer JD, Finlayson SR, Tosteson AN, et al. Effect of hospital volume on in-
    hospital mortality with pancreaticoduodenectomy. Surgery. 1999a;125:250–6.
Birkmeyer JD, Warshaw AL, Finlayson SR, et al. Relationship between hospi-
    tal volume and late survival after pancreaticoduodenectomy. Surgery.
    1999b;126:178–83.

**24**

Bold RJ, Charnsangavej C, Cleary KR, et al. Major vascular resection as part of pancreaticoduodenectomy for cancer: radiologic, intraoperative, and pathologic analysis. J Gastrointest Surg. 1999;3:233–43.

Brennan MF, Kattan MW, Klimstra D, Conlon K. Prognostic nomogram for patients undergoing resection for adenocarcinoma of the pancreas. Ann Surg. 2004;240(2):293–8.

Cameron JL, Riall TS, Coleman J, Belcher KA. One thousand consecutive pancreaticoduodenectomies. Ann Surg. 2006;244(1):10–5.

Conlon KC, Klimstra DS, Brennan MF. Long-term survival after curative resection for pancreatic ductal adenocarcinoma: clinicopathologic analysis of 5-year survivors. Ann Surg. 1996;223:273–9.

Evans DB, Abbruzzese JL, Willett CG. Cancer of the pancreas. In: DeVita VT, Hellman S, Rosenberg SA, editors. Cancer, principles and practice of oncology. 6th ed. Philadelphia, PA: J.B. Lippincott; 2002.

Fuhrman GM, Charnsangavej C, Abbruzzese JL, et al. Thin-section contrast-enhanced computed tomography accurately predicts resectability of malignant pancreatic neoplasms. Am J Surg. 1994;167:104–111.

Geer RJ, Brennan MF. Prognostic indicators for survival after resection of pancreatic adenocarcinoma. Am J Surg. 1993;165:68–72.

Gold EB, Goldin SB. Epidemiology of and risk factors for pancreatic cancer. Surg Oncol Clin N Am. 1998;7:67–91.

Millikan KW, Deziel DJ, Silverstein JC, et al. Prognostic factors associated with resectable adenocarcinoma of the head of the pancreas. Am Surg. 1999;65:618–24.

Nitecki SS, Sarr MG, Colby TV, et al. Long-term survival after resection for ductal adenocarcinoma of the pancreas: is it really improving? Ann Surg. 1995;221:59–66.

Sohn TA, Yeo CJ, Cameron JL, et al. Resected adenocarcinoma of the pancreas–616 patients: results, outcomes, and prognostic indicators. J Gastrointest Surg. 2000;4:567–79.

Staley C, Cleary K, Abbruzzese J, et al. Need for standardized pathologic staging of pancreaticoduodenectomy specimens. Pancreas. 1996;12:373–80.

Suits J, Frazee R, Erickson RA. Endoscopic ultrasound and fine needle aspiration for the valuation of pancreatic masses. Arch Surg. 1999;134:639–43.

Tomlinson JS, Jain S, Bentrem DJ, et al. Accuracy of staging node negative pancreas cancer: a potential quality measure. Arch Surg. 2007;142:767–74.

Traverso LW, Longmire WP Jr. Preservation of the pylorus in pancreaticoduodenectomy. Surg Gynecol Obstet. 1978;146:959–62.

van Eeden S, Offerhaus GJA. Historical, current and future perspectives on gastrointestinal and pancreatic endocrine tumors. Virchows Arch. 2006;448:1–6.

Whipple AO, Parsons WW, Mullin CR. Treatment of carcinoma of the ampulla of Vater. Ann Surg. 1935;102:263–9.

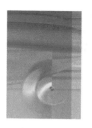

# PART IV
# Thorax

# Lung

*(Carcinoid tumors are included. Sarcomas and
other rare tumors are not included.)*

## *At-A-Glance*

### SUMMARY OF CHANGES

* This staging system is now recommended for the classification of both non-small cell and small cell lung carcinomas and for carcinoid tumors of the lung

* The T classifications have been redefined:

  * T1 has been subclassified into T1a (≤2 cm in size) and T1b (>2–3 cm in size)

  * T2 has been subclassified into T2a (>3–5 cm in size) and T2b (>5–7 cm in size)

  * T2 (>7 cm in size) has been reclassified as T3

  * Multiple tumor nodules in the same lobe have been reclassified from T4 to T3

  * Multiple tumor nodules in the same lung but a different lobe have been reclassified from M1 to T4

* No changes have been made to the N classification. However, a new international lymph node map defining the anatomical boundaries for lymph node stations has been developed

* The M classifications have been redefined:

  * M1 has been subdivided into M1a and M1b

  * Malignant pleural and pericardial effusions have been reclassified from T4 to M1a

  * Separate tumor nodules in the contralateral lung are considered M1a

  * M1b designates distant metastases

| ANATOMIC STAGE/PROGNOSTIC GROUPS | | | |
|---|---|---|---|
| **Occult Carcinoma** | TX | N0 | M0 |
| Stage 0 | Tis | N0 | M0 |
| Stage IA | T1a | N0 | M0 |
|  | T1b | N0 | M0 |
| Stage IB | T2a | N0 | M0 |
| Stage IIA | T2b | N0 | M0 |
|  | T1a | N1 | M0 |
|  | T1b | N1 | M0 |
|  | T2a | N1 | M0 |

**ICD-O-3
TOPOGRAPHY
CODES**

| | |
|---|---|
| C34.0 | Main bronchus |
| C34.1 | Upper lobe, lung |
| C34.2 | Middle lobe, lung |
| C34.3 | Lower lobe, lung |

**25**

| Stage IIB | T2b | N1 | M0 |
|---|---|---|---|
| | T3 | N0 | M0 |
| Stage IIIA | T1a | N2 | M0 |
| | T1b | N2 | M0 |
| | T2a | N2 | M0 |
| | T2b | N2 | M0 |
| | T3 | N1 | M0 |
| | T3 | N2 | M0 |
| | T4 | N0 | M0 |
| | T4 | N1 | M0 |
| Stage IIIB | T1a | N3 | M0 |
| | T1b | N3 | M0 |
| | T2a | N3 | M0 |
| | T2b | N3 | M0 |
| | T3 | N3 | M0 |
| | T4 | N2 | M0 |
| | T4 | N3 | M0 |
| Stage IV | Any T | Any N | M1a |
| | Any T | Any N | M1b |

C34.8    Overlapping lesion of lung

C34.9    Lung, NOS

ICD-O-3 HISTOLOGY CODE RANGES
8000–8576, 8940–8950, 8980–8981

# INTRODUCTION

Lung cancer is among the most common malignancies in the Western world and is the leading cause of cancer deaths in both men and women. The primary etiology of lung cancer is exposure to tobacco smoke. Other less common factors, such as asbestos exposure, may contribute to the development of lung cancer. In recent years, the level of tobacco exposure, generally expressed as the number of cigarette pack-years of smoking, has been correlated with the biology and clinical behavior of this malignancy. Lung cancer is usually diagnosed at an advanced stage and consequently the overall 5-year survival for patients is approximately 15%. However, patients diagnosed when the primary tumor is resectable experience 5-year survivals ranging from 20 to 80%. Clinical and pathologic staging is critical to selecting patients appropriately for surgery and multimodality therapy.

# ANATOMY

**Primary Site.** Carcinomas of the lung arise either from the alveolar lining cells of the pulmonary parenchyma or from the mucosa of the tracheo-bronchial tree. The trachea, which lies in the middle mediastinum, divides into the right and left main bronchi, which extend into the right and left lungs, respectively. The bronchi then subdivide into the lobar bronchi in the upper, middle, and lower lobes on the right and the upper and lower lobes on the left. The lungs are encased in membranes called the visceral pleura. The inside of the chest cavity is lined by a similar membrane called the parietal pleura. The potential space between these two membranes is the pleural space. The mediastinum contains structures in between the lungs, including the heart, thymus, great vessels, lymph nodes, and esophagus.

The great vessels include:

Aorta
Superior vena cava
Inferior vena cava
Main pulmonary artery
Intrapericardial segments of the trunk of the right and left pulmonary artery
Intrapericardial segments of the superior and inferior right and left pulmonary veins

**Regional Lymph Nodes.** The regional lymph nodes extend from the supraclavicular region to the diaphragm. During the past three decades, two different lymph node maps have been used to describe the regional lymph nodes potentially involved by lung cancers. The first such map, proposed by Naruke (Figure 25.1) and officially endorsed by the Japan Lung Cancer Society, is used primarily in Japan. The second, the Mountain-Dresler modification of the American Thoracic Society (MD-ATS) lymph node map (Figure 25.2), is used in North America and Europe. The nomenclature for the anatomical locations of lymph nodes differs between these two maps especially with respect to nodes located in the

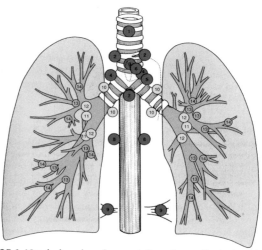

**FIGURE 25.1.** Naruke lymph node map. 1, Superior mediastinal or highest mediastinal; 2, paratracheal; 3, pretracheal; 3a, anterior mediastinal; 3p, retrotracheal or posterior mediastinal; 4, tracheobronchial; 5, subaortic or Botallo's; 6, paraaortic (ascending aorta); 7, subcarinal; 8, paraesophageal (below carina); 9, pulmonary ligament; 10, hilar; 11, interlobar; 12, lobar: upper lobe, middle lobe, and lower lobe; 13, segmental; 14, subsegmental. (From The Japan Lung Cancer Society. Classification of Lung Cancer. First English Edition. Tokyo: Kanehara & Co., 2000, used with permission.)

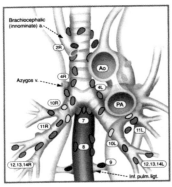

**Superior Mediastinal Nodes**

- 1 Highest Mediastinal
- 2 Upper Paratracheal
- 3 Pre-vascular and Retrotracheal
- 4 Lower Paratracheal
  (including Azygos Nodes)

  $N_2$ = single digit, ipsilateral
  $N_3$ = single digit, contralateral or supraclavicular

**Aortic Nodes**

- 5 Subaortic (A-P window)
- 6 Para-aortic (ascending aorta or phrenic)

**Inferior Mediastinal Nodes**

- 7 Subcarinal
- 8 Paraesophageal (below carina)
- 9 Pulmonary Ligament

**N₁ Nodes**

- ○ 10 Hilar
- 11 Interlobar
- 12 Lobar
- 13 Segmental
- 14 Subsegmental

**FIGURE 25.2.** Mountain/Dresler lymph node map. (From Mountain CF, Dresler CM. Regional lymph node classification for lung cancer staging. Chest 1997;111:1718–1723, used with permission.)

paratracheal, tracheobronchial angle, and subcarinal areas. Recently, the International Association for the Study of Lung Cancer (IASLC) proposed a lymph node map (Figure 25.3) that reconciles the discrepancies between these two previous maps, considers other published proposals, and provides more detailed nomenclature for the anatomical boundaries of lymph nodes stations. Table 25.1 shows the definition for lymph node stations in all three maps. The IASLC lymph node map is now the recommended means of describing regional lymph node involvement for lung cancers. Analyses of a large international lung cancer database suggest that for purposes of prognostic classification, it may be appropriate to amalgamate lymph node stations into "zones" (Figure 25.3). However, the use of lymph node "zones" for N staging remains investigational and needs to be confirmed by future prospective studies.

There are no evidence-based guidelines regarding the *number* of lymph nodes to be removed at surgery for adequate staging. However, adequate N staging is generally considered to include sampling or dissection of lymph nodes from stations 2R, 4R, 7, 10R, and 11R for right-sided tumors, and stations 5, 6, 7, 10 L, and 11 L for left-sided tumors. Station 9 lymph nodes

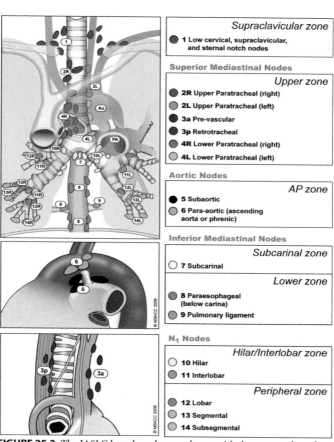

Supraclavicular zone

● 1 Low cervical, supraclavicular, and sternal notch nodes

**Superior Mediastinal Nodes**

Upper zone

● 2R Upper Paratracheal (right)
◐ 2L Upper Paratracheal (left)
● 3a Pre-vascular
● 3p Retrotracheal
● 4R Lower Paratracheal (right)
○ 4L Lower Paratracheal (left)

**Aortic Nodes**

AP zone

● 5 Subaortic
◐ 6 Para-aortic (ascending aorta or phrenic)

**Inferior Mediastinal Nodes**

Subcarinal zone

○ 7 Subcarinal

Lower zone

● 8 Paraesophageal (below carina)
◐ 9 Pulmonary ligament

**N₁ Nodes**

Hilar/Interlobar zone

○ 10 Hilar
◐ 11 Interlobar

Peripheral zone

◐ 12 Lobar
○ 13 Segmental
○ 14 Subsegmental

**FIGURE 25.3.** The IASLC lymph node map shown with the proposed amalgamation of lymph node levels into *zones*. (© Memorial Sloan-Kettering Cancer Center, 2009.)

should also be evaluated for lower lobe tumors. The more peripheral lymph nodes at stations 12–14 are usually evaluated by the pathologist in lobectomy or pneumonectomy specimens but may be separately removed when sublobar resections (e.g., segmentectomy) are performed. There is evidence to support the recommendation that histological examination of hilar and mediastinal lymphenectomy specimen(s) will ordinarily include 6 or more lymph nodes/stations. Three of these nodes/stations should be mediastinal, including the sub-carinal nodes and three from N1 nodes/stations.

25

**Distant Metastatic Sites.** The most common metastatic sites are the brain, bones, adrenal glands, contralateral lung, liver, pericardium, kidneys, and subcutaneous tissues. However, virtually any organ can be a site of metastatic disease.

**TABLE 25.1.** Definition for lymph node stations in Japan Lung Cancer Society Map, MD-ATS Map, and IASLC Map

| Japan Lung Cancer Society map | MD-ATS map | IASLC map |
|---|---|---|
| *1 Low cervical, supraclavicular and sternal notch nodes* | | |
| Located in the area of the upper 1/3 of the intrathoracic trachea. Boundary level from the upper margin of the subclavian artery or the apex to the crossing point of the upper margin of the left brachiocephalic vein and the midline of the trachea | Nodes lying above a horizontal line at the upper rim of the brachiocephalic (left innominate) vein where it ascends to the left, crossing in front of the trachea at its midline | Upper border: lower margin of cricoid cartilage<br><br>Lower border: clavicles bilaterally and, in the midline, the upper border of the manubrium, 1R designates right-sided nodes, 1L, left-sided nodes in this region<br><br>For lymph node station 1, the midline of the trachea serves as the border between 1R and 1L |
| *2 Paratracheal lymph nodes* | *2 Upper paratracheal nodes* | |
| Located in the area between the superior mediastinal lymph nodes (1) and the tracheobronchial lymph nodes (4). Paratracheal lymph nodes with primary tumor can be defined as ipsilateral lymph nodes; paratracheal lymph nodes without primary tumor can be defined as contralateral lymph nodes | Nodes lying above a horizontal line drawn tangential to the upper margin of the aortic arch and below the inferior boundary of No. 1 nodes | 2R: Upper border: apex of the right lung and pleural space, and in the midline, the upper border of the manubrium<br><br>Lower border: intersection of caudal margin of innominate vein with the trachea<br><br>As for lymph node station 4R, 2R includes nodes extending to the left lateral border of the trachea<br><br>2L: Upper border: apex of the left lung and pleural space, and in the midline, the upper border of the manubrium<br><br>Lower border: superior border of the aortic arch |

| 3 Pretracheal lymph nodes | 3 Pre-vascular and retrotracheal nodes | |
|---|---|---|
| Located in the area anterior to the trachea and inferior to the superior mediastinal lymph nodes (1). On the right side, the boundary is limited to the posterior wall of the superior vena cava. On the left side, the boundary is limited to the posterior wall of the brachiocephalic vein | Prevascular and retrotracheal nodes may be designated 3A and 3P; midline nodes are considered to be ipsilateral | 3a: Prevascular |
| | | On the right: |
| | | Upper border: apex of chest |
| | | Lower border: level of carina |
| | | Anterior border: posterior aspect of sternum |
| | | Posterior border: anterior border of superior vena cava |
| 3a Anterior mediastinal lymph nodes | | On the left: |
| On the right side, located in the area anterior to the superior vena cava. On the left side, the boundary is limited to the line connecting the left bracheocephalic vein and the ascending aorta | | Upper border: apex of chest |
| | | Lower border: level of carina |
| | | Anterior border: posterior aspect of sternum |
| | | Posterior border: left carotid artery |
| 3p Retrotracheal mediastinal lymph nodes/ Posterior mediastinal lymph nodes | | 3p: Retrotracheal |
| Located in the retrotracheal or posterior area of the trachea | | Upper border: apex of chest |
| | | Lower border: carina |

continued

25

**TABLE 25.1.** Definition for lymph node stations in Japan Lung Cancer Society Map, MD-ATS Map, and IASLC Map (continued)

| Japan Lung Cancer Society map | MD-ATS map | IASLC map |
|---|---|---|
| *4 Tracheobronchial lymph nodes* | *4 Lower paratracheal nodes* | |
| Located in the area superior to the carina. On the right side, located medial to the azygos vein. On the left side, located in the area surrounded by the medial wall of the aortic arch | The lower paratracheal nodes on the right lie to the right of the midline of the trachea between a horizontal line drawn tangential to the upper margin of the aortic arch and a line extending across the right main bronchus at the upper margin of the upper lobe bronchus, and contained within the mediastinal pleural envelope; the lower paratracheal nodes on the left lie to the left of the midline of the trachea between a horizontal line drawn tangential to the upper margin of the aortic arch and a line extending across the left main bronchus at the level of the upper margin of the left upper lobe bronchus, medial to the ligamentum arteriosum and contained within the mediastinal pleural envelope. Researchers may wish to designate the lower paratracheal nodes as No. 4s (superior) and No. 4i (inferior) subsets for study purposes; the No. 4s nodes may be defined by a horizontal line extending across the trachea and drawn tangential to the cephalic border of the azygos vein; the No. 4i nodes may be defined by the lower boundary of No. 4s and the lower boundary of no. 4, as described above | 4R: includes right paratracheal nodes, and pretracheal nodes extending to the left lateral border of trachea<br><br>Upper border: intersection of caudal margin of innominate vein with the trachea<br><br>Lower border: lower border of azygos vein<br><br>4L: includes nodes to the left of the left lateral border of the trachea, medial to the ligamentum arteriosum<br><br>Upper border: upper margin of the aortic arch<br><br>Lower border: upper rim of the left main pulmonary artery |

| 5 Subaortic lymph nodes/Botallo's lymph nodes | | 5 Subaortic (aorto-pulmonary window) | |
|---|---|---|---|
| Located in the area adjacent to the ligamentum arteriosum (Botallo's ligament). The boundary extends from the aortic arch to the left main pulmonary artery | Subaortic nodes are lateral to the ligamentum arteriosum or the aorta or left pulmonary artery and proximal to the first branch of the left pulmonary artery and lie within the mediastinal pleural envelope | Subaortic lymph nodes lateral to the ligamentum arteriosum | |
| | | Upper border: the lower border of the aortic arch | |
| | | Lower border: upper rim of the left main pulmonary artery | |
| 6 Para-aortic nodes (ascending aorta or phrenic) | | | |
| Located along the ascending aorta, and in the area of the lateral wall of the aortic arch. Posterior boundary limited to the site of the vagal nerve | Nodes lying anterior and lateral to the ascending aorta and the aortic arch or the innominate artery, beneath a line tangential the upper margin of the aortic arch | Lymph nodes anterior and lateral to the ascending aorta and aortic arch | |
| | | Upper border: a line tangential to the upper border of the aortic arch | |
| | | Lower border: the lower border of the aortic arch | |
| 7 Subcarinal nodes | | | |
| Located in the area below the carina, where the trachea bifurcates to the two main bronchi | Nodes lying caudal to the carina of the trachea, but not associated with the lower lobe bronchi or arteries within the lung | Upper border: the carina of the trachea | |
| | | Lower border: the upper border of the lower lobe bronchus on the left; the lower border of the bronchus intermedius on the right | |

continued

25

**TABLE 25.1.** Definition for lymph node stations in Japan Lung Cancer Society Map, MD-ATS Map, and IASLC Map (continued)

| Japan Lung Cancer Society map | MD-ATS map | IASLC map |
|---|---|---|
| *8 Para-esophageal nodes (below carina)* | | |
| Located below the subcarinal lymph nodes, and along the esophagus | Nodes lying adjacent to the wall of the esophagus and to the right or left of the midline, excluding subcarinal nodes | Nodes lying adjacent to the wall of the esophagus and to the right or left of the midline, excluding subcarinal nodes |
| | | Upper border: the upper border of the lower lobe bronchus on the left; the lower border of the bronchus intermedius on the right |
| | | Lower border: the diaphragm |
| *9 Pulmonary ligament nodes* | | |
| Located in the area of the posterior and the lower edge of the inferior pulmonary vein | Nodes lying within the pulmonary ligament, including those in the posterior wall, and lower part of the inferior pulmonary vein | Nodes lying within the pulmonary ligament |
| | | Upper border: the inferior pulmonary vein |
| | | Lower border: the diaphragm |
| *10 Hilar nodes* | | |
| Located around the right and left main bronchi | The proximal lobar nodes, distal to the mediastinal pleural reflection and the nodes adjacent to the bronchus intermedius on the right; radiographically, the hilar shadow may be created by enlargement of both hilar and interlobar nodes | Includes nodes immediately adjacent to the mainstem bronchus and hilar vessels including the proximal portions of the pulmonary veins and main pulmonary artery |
| | | Upper border: the lower rim of the azygos vein on the right; upper rim of the pulmonary artery on the left |
| | | Lower border: interlobar region bilaterally |

| *11 Interlobar nodes* | | |
|---|---|---|
| Located between the lobar bronchi. On the right side, subclassified into two groups: | Nodes lying between the lobar bronchi | Between the origin of the lobar bronchi |
| 11s: Superior interlobar nodes: located at the bifurcation of the upper and middle lobar bronchi | | 11s: between the upper lobe bronchus and bronchus intermedius on the right |
| 11i: Inferior interlobar nodes: located at the bifurcation of the middle and lower lobar bronchi | | 11i: between the middle and lower lobe bronchi on the right |
| *12 Lobar nodes* | | |
| Located in the area around the lobar branches, which are subclassified into three groups: | Nodes adjacent to the distal lobar bronchi | Adjacent to the lobar bronchi |
| 12u: Upper lobar lymph nodes | | |
| 12m: Middle lobar lymph nodes | | |
| 12l: Lower lobar lymph nodes | | |
| *13 Segmental nodes* | | |
| Located along the segmental branches | Nodes adjacent to the segmental bronchi | Adjacent to the segmental bronchi |
| *14 Subsegmental nodes* | | |
| Located along the subsegmental branches | Nodes around the subsegmental bronchi | Adjacent to the subsegmental bronchi |

25

## RULES FOR CLASSIFICATION

Lung cancers are broadly classified as either non-small cell (approximately 85% of tumors) or small cell carcinomas (15% of tumors). This general histological distinction reflects the clinical and biological behavior of these two tumor types. Approximately half of all non-small cell lung cancers (NSCLC) are either localized or locally advanced at the time of diagnosis and are treated by resection alone, or by combined modality therapy with or without resection. By contrast, small cell lung cancers (SCLC) are metastatic in 80% of cases at diagnosis. The 20% of SCLC that are initially localized to the hemithorax are usually locally advanced tumors managed by combination chemotherapy and radiotherapy. Less than 10% of SCLC are detected at a very early stage when they can be treated by resection and adjuvant chemotherapy.

The TNM staging system has traditionally been used for NSCLC. Although it is supposed to be applied also to SCLC, in practice these tumors have been classified as "limited" or "extensive" disease, a staging system introduced in the 1950s by the Veterans' Administration Lung Study Group for use in their clinical trials. Limited disease (LD) was characterized by tumors confined to one hemithorax, although local extension and ipsilateral supraclavicular nodes could also be present if they could be encompassed in the same radiation portal as the primary tumor. No extrathoracic metastases could be present. All other patients were classified as extensive disease (ED). In 1989, a consensus report from the IASLC recommended that LD be defined as tumors limited to one hemithorax with regional lymph node metastases including hilar, ipsilateral and contralateral mediastinal and ipsilateral and contralateral supraclavicular nodes. This report also recommends that patients with ipsilateral pleural effusion regardless of whether cytology positive or negative should be considered to have LD if no extrathoracic metastases were detected. More recently, analysis of an international database developed by the IASLC that includes 8088 SCLC patients showed that the TNM staging system is applicable to SCLC. Therefore, the staging system being presented in this edition of the staging manual should now be applied to both NSCLC and SCLC.

Bronchopulmonary carcinoid tumors are also frequently classified according to the TNM staging system for NSCLC, even though they are not officially included in the AJCC or UICC staging manuals. Recent analysis of both the SEER and the IASLC international lung tumor databases indicates that the TNM staging system for NSCLC is also applicable to bronchopulmonary carcinoid tumors. Therefore, typical carcinoid and atypical carcinoid tumors should also now be routinely classified according to the TNM system used for NSCLC and SCLC.

**Clinical Staging.** Clinical classification (cTNM) is based on the evidence acquired before treatment, including physical examination, imaging studies (e.g., computed and positron emission tomography), laboratory tests, and staging procedures such as bronchoscopy or esophagoscopy with ultrasound directed biopsies (EBUS, EUS), mediastinoscopy, mediastinotomy, thoracentesis, and thoracoscopy (VATS) as well as exploratory thoracotomy.

**Pathologic Staging.** Pathological classification uses the evidence acquired before treatment, supplemented or modified by the additional evidence acquired during and after surgery, particularly from pathologic examination. The pathologic stage provides additional precise data used for estimating prognosis and calculating end results.

- The pathologic assessment of the primary tumor (pT) entails resection of the primary tumor sufficient to evaluate the highest pT category.
- The complete pathologic assessment of the regional lymph nodes (pN) ideally entails removal of a sufficient number of lymph nodes to evaluate the highest pN category.
- If pathologic assessment of lymph nodes reveals negative nodes but the number of lymph node stations examined are fewer than suggested above, classify the N category as pN0.
- Isolated tumor cells (ITC) are single tumor cells or small clusters of cells not more than 0.2 mm in greatest dimension that are usually detected by immunohistochemistry or molecular methods. Cases with ITC in lymph nodes or at distant sites should be classified as N0 or M0, respectively. The same applies to cases with findings suggestive of tumor cells or their components by non-morphologic techniques such as flow cytometry or DNA analysis.
- The following classification of ITC may be used:

| | |
|---|---|
| pN0 | No regional lymph node metastasis histologically, no examination for ITC |
| pN0(i−) | No regional lymph node metastasis histologically, negative morphological findings for ITC |
| pN0(i+) | No regional lymph node metastasis histologically, positive morphological findings for ITC |
| pN0(mol−) | No regional lymph node metastasis histologically, negative non-morphological findings for ITC |
| pN0(mol+) | No regional lymph node metastasis histologically, positive non-morphological findings for ITC |

- The pathologic assessment of metastases may be either clinical or pathologic when the T and/or N categories meet the criteria for pathologic staging (pT, pN, cM, or pM).

Pathologic staging depends on the proven anatomic extent of disease, whether or not the primary lesion has been completely removed. If a biopsied primary tumor technically cannot be removed, or when it is unreasonable to remove it, and if the highest T and N categories or the M1 category of the tumor can be confirmed microscopically, the criteria for pathologic classification and staging have been satisfied without total removal of the primary cancer.

**Basis for Current Revisions to the Lung Cancer Staging System.** The 6th edition of the *AJCC Cancer Staging Manual*, introduced in 2002, made no changes to the previous edition with regards to lung cancer. The proposals for lung cancer staging in the 5th edition, published in 1997, were based on a relatively small database of 5,319 cases of NSCLC accumulated since 1975 by Dr. Clifton Mountain at the MD Anderson Cancer Center (Houston, TX, USA). During this time, there had been many refinements

**25**

to the techniques available for clinical staging, principally the routine use of computed tomography and more recently, an increasing use of positron emission tomography. The database was largely from a single institution, containing cases predominantly treated surgically. Repeated iterations of the TNM staging system had seen recommendations for lung cancer staging evolve with little internal validation and no external validation of the descriptors or the stage groupings. Increasingly reports from other databases challenged some of the descriptors and stage groupings. In preparation for this 7th edition of the staging manual, the IASLC established a Lung Cancer Staging Project in 1998 to bring together the large databases available worldwide to inform recommendations for revision that would be intensively validated. The results of this project were accepted by the International Union Against Cancer (UICC) and the AJCC as the primary source for revisions of the lung cancer staging system in the 7th editions of their staging manuals.

The IASLC lung cancer database includes cases from 46 sources in more than 19 countries, diagnosed between 1990 and 2000 and treated by all modalities of care. A total of 100,869 cases were submitted to the data center at Cancer Research and Biostatistics (Seattle, WA, USA). After an initial sift to exclude cases outside the study period, those for whom cell type was not known, cases not newly diagnosed at the point of entry, and those with inadequate information on stage, treatment, or follow-up, 81,015 cases remained for analysis. Of these, 67,725 were NSCLC and 13,290 were SCLC. The analyses of the T, N, and M descriptors and the subsequent analysis of TNM subsets and stage groupings were derived from the cases of NSCLC and subsequently validated also in the SCLC cases and carcinoids. Survival was measured from the date of entry (date of diagnosis for registries, date of registration for protocols) for clinically staged data and the date of surgery for pathologically staged data and was calculated by the Kaplan–Meier method. Prognostic groups were assessed by Cox regression analysis.

Where the analyses showed descriptors to have a prognosis that differed from the other descriptors in any T or M category, two alternative strategies were considered: (1) Retain that descriptor in the existing category, identified by alphabetical subscripts. For example, additional pulmonary nodules in the lobe of the primary, considered to be T4 in the 6th edition, would become T4a, whereas additional pulmonary nodules in other ipsilateral lobes, designed as M1 in the 6th edition, would become M1a. (2) Allow descriptors to move between categories, to a category containing other descriptors with a similar prognosis, e.g., additional pulmonary nodules in the lobe of the primary would move from T4 to T3, and additional pulmonary nodules in other ipsilateral lobes would move from M1 to T4. The first strategy had the advantage of allowing, to a large extent, retrograde compatibility with existing databases. Unfortunately, this generated a large number of descriptors (approximately 20) and an impractically large number of TNM subsets (>180). For this reason, backward compatibility was compromised and strategy (2) was preferred for its clinical utility. A small number of candidate stage grouping schemes were developed initially using a recursive partitioning and amalgamation algorithm. The analysis grouped cases based on best stage (pathologic, if available, otherwise clinical) after determination of best-split points based on overall

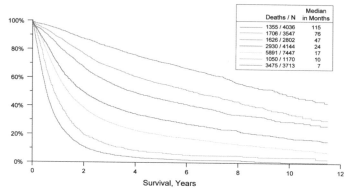

**FIGURE 25.4.** Survival in all NSCLC by TNM stage (according to "best" based on a combination of clinical and pathologic staging.

survival on indicator variables for the newly presented TM categories and an ordered variable for N category, excluding NX cases (Figures 25.4 and 25.5). The analysis was performed on a randomly selected training set comprising two-thirds of the available data that met the requirements for conversion to newly presented T and M categories, reserving the other one-third of cases for later validation. The random selection process was stratified by type of database submission and time period of case entry (1990–1994 vs. 1995–2000).

Selection of a final stage grouping proposal from among the candidate schemes was done based on its statistical properties in the training set and its relevance to clinical practice and by consensus.

Table 25.2 shows a comparison of the 6th edition and 7th edition TNM for lung cancer to assure clarity for the user. The final 7th edition TNM is described in the "Definitions of TNM" section that follows.

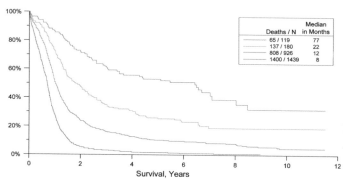

**FIGURE 25.5.** Survival in all SCLC by TNM stage (according to "best" stage based on a combination of clinical and pathologic staging in the IASLC lung database).

**TABLE 25.2.** Stage grouping comparisons: 6th edition vs. 7th edition descriptors, T and M categories, and stage groupings

| Sixth edition T/M descriptor | 7th edition T/M | N0 | N1 | N2 | N3 |
|---|---|---|---|---|---|
| T1 (≤2 cm) | T1a | IA | IIA | IIIA | IIIB |
| T1 (>2–3 cm) | T1b | IA | IIA | IIIA | IIIB |
| T2 (≤5 cm) | T2a | IB | **IIA** | IIIA | IIIB |
| T2 (>5–7 cm) | T2b | **IIA** | IIB | IIIA | IIIB |
| T2 (>7 cm) | T3 | **IIB** | **IIIA** | IIIA | IIIB |
| T3 invasion | | IIB | IIIA | IIIA | IIIB |
| T4 (same lobe nodules) | | **IIB** | **IIIA** | **IIIA** | IIIB |
| T4 (extension) | T4 | **IIIA** | **IIIA** | IIIB | IIIB |
| M1 (ipsilateral lung) | | **IIIA** | **IIIA** | **IIIB** | **IIIB** |
| M1 (pleural effusion) | M1a | **IV** | **IV** | **IV** | **IV** |
| M1 (contralateral lung) | | IV | IV | IV | IV |
| M1 (distant) | M1b | IV | IV | IV | IV |

Cells in bold indicate a change from the 6th edition for a particular TNM category.

From Goldstraw P, Crowley J, Chansky K et al: The IASLC Lung Cancer Staging Project: Proposals for the revision of the TNM stage groupings in the forthcoming (seventh) edition of the TNM classification of malignant tumours. J Thorac Oncol 2:706–714, 2007, with permission.

## PROGNOSTIC FEATURES

The IASLC lung cancer database, although retrospective, provides the largest published analyses of prognostic factors in both NSCLC and SCLC. Potentially useful prognostic variables for lung cancer survival that were considered included: TNM stage, tumor histology, patient age, sex, and performance status, various laboratory values and molecular markers.

**Clinical Factors.** Analyses of the IASLC lung cancer database revealed that in addition to clinical stage, performance status and patient age and sex (male gender being associated with a worse survival) were important prognostic factors for both NSCLC and SCLC. In NSCLC, squamous cell carcinoma was associated with a better prognosis for patients with Stage III disease but not in other tumor stages. In advanced NSCLC (Stages IIIB/IV), some laboratory tests (principally white blood cells and hypercalcemia) were also important prognostic variables. In SCLC, albumin was an independent biological factor. Analyses that incorporate these factors along with overall TNM stage stratify both NSCLC and SCLC patients into 4 groups that have distinctly different overall survivals. In addition to these, a recent study of 455 patients with completely resected pathologic Stage I NSCLC suggests that high preoperative serum carcinoembryonic antigen (CEA) levels identify patients who have a poor prognosis, especially if those levels also remain elevated postoperatively. Other retrospective studies report that the intensity of hypermetabolism on FDG-PET scan is correlated with outcome in NSCLC patients managed surgically. Additional prospective studies are needed to validate these findings and to determine whether FDG-PET is prognostic across all lung cancer stages and histologies.

In the lung, arterioles are frequently invaded by cancers. For this reason, the V classification is applicable to indicate vascular invasion, whether venous or arteriolar.

**Biological Factors.** In recent years, multiple biological and molecular markers have been found to have prognostic value for survival in lung cancer, particularly NSCLC. These are summarized in Table 25.3. Although some molecular abnormalities, for example EGFR and K-ras mutations, are now being used to stratify patients for treatment, none is yet routinely used for lung cancer staging.

## DEFINITIONS OF TNM

*Primary Tumor (T)*

TX     Primary tumor cannot be assessed, or tumor proven by the presence of malignant cells in sputum or bronchial washings but not visualized by imaging or bronchoscopy

T0     No evidence of primary tumor

Tis     Carcinoma in situ

T1     Tumor 3 cm or less in greatest dimension, surrounded by lung or visceral pleura, without bronchoscopic evidence of invasion more proximal than the lobar bronchus (i.e., not in the main bronchus)*

T1a     Tumor 2 cm or less in greatest dimension

T1b     Tumor more than 2 cm but 3 cm or less in greatest dimension

**25**

### Primary Tumor (T) (continued)

**T2**  Tumor more than 3 cm but 7 cm or less or tumor with any of the following features (T2 tumors with these features are classified T2a if 5 cm or less); Involves main bronchus, 2 cm or more distal to the carina; Invades visceral pleura (PL1 or PL2); Associated with atelectasis or obstructive pneumonitis that extends to the hilar region but does not involve the entire lung

**T2a**  Tumor more than 3 cm but 5 cm or less in greatest dimension

**T2b**  Tumor more than 5 cm but 7 cm or less in greatest dimension

**T3**  Tumor more than 7 cm or one that directly invades any of the following: parietal pleural (PL3) chest wall (including superior sulcus tumors), diaphragm, phrenic nerve, mediastinal pleura, parietal pericardium; or tumor in the main bronchus (less than 2 cm distal to the carina* but without involvement of the carina; or associated atelectasis or obstructive pneumonitis of the entire lung or separate tumor nodule(s) in the same lobe

**T4**  Tumor of any size that invades any of the following: mediastinum, heart, great vessels, trachea, recurrent laryngeal nerve, esophagus, vertebral body, carina, separate tumor nodule(s) in a different ipsilateral lobe

*The uncommon superficial spreading tumor of any size with its invasive component limited to the bronchial wall, which may extend proximally to the main bronchus, is also classified as T1a.

**TABLE 25.3.** Metaanalyses published on the prognostic value of biological or genetic markers for survival in lung cancer

| Biological variable | Prognostic factor | Reference |
| --- | --- | --- |
| bcl-2 | Favorable | Martin et al. 2003 |
| TTF1 | Adverse | Berghmans et al. 2006 |
| Cox2 | Adverse | Mascaux et al. 2006 |
| EGFR overexpression | Adverse | Nakamura et al. 2006 |
| | | Meert et al. 2002 |
| EGFR mutation | Favorable | Marks et al. 2007 |
| ras | Adverse | Mascaux et al. 2006 |
| | | Huncharek et al. 1999 |
| Ki67 | Adverse | Martin et al. 2004 |
| HER2 | Adverse | Meert et al. 2003 |
| | | Nakamura et al. 2005 |
| VEGF | Adverse | Delmotte et al. 2002 |
| Microvascular density | Adverse | Meert et al. 2002 |
| p53 | Adverse | Steels et al. 2001 |
| | | Mitsudomi et al. 2000 |
| | | Huncharek et al. 2000 |
| Aneuploidy | Adverse | Choma et al. 2001 |

Adapted from Sculier JP et al. The IASLC Lung Cancer Staging Project: The impact of additional prognostic factors on survival and their relationship with the anatomical extent of disease expressed by the 6th edition of the TNM classification of malignant tumours and the proposals for the 7th edition, *J Thorac Oncol* 3(4):457–466, 2008, with permission.

### Regional Lymph Nodes (N)

NX     Regional lymph nodes cannot be assessed
N0     No regional lymph node metastases
N1     Metastasis in ipsilateral peribronchial and/or ipsilateral hilar lymph nodes and intrapulmonary nodes, including involvement by direct extension
N2     Metastasis in ipsilateral mediastinal and/or subcarinal lymph node(s)
N3     Metastasis in contralateral mediastinal, contralateral hilar, ipsilateral or contralateral scalene, or supraclavicular lymph node(s)

### Distant Metastasis (M)

M0     No distant metastasis
M1     Distant metastasis
M1a    Separate tumor nodule(s) in a contralateral lobe tumor with pleural nodules or malignant pleural (or pericardial) effusion*
M1b    Distant metastasis

From Goldstraw P, Crowley J, Chansky K, et al.: The IASLC Lung Cancer Staging Project: Proposals for the revision of the TNM stage groupings in the forthcoming (seventh) edition of the TNM classification of malignant tumours. *J Thorac Oncol* 2:706–714, 2007, with permission.

*Most pleural (and pericardial) effusions with lung cancer are due to tumor. In a few patients, however, multiple cytopathologic examinations of pleural (pericardial) fluid are negative for tumor, and the fluid is nonbloody and is not an exudate. Where these elements and clinical judgment dictate that the effusion is not related to the tumor, the effusion should be excluded as a staging element and the patient should be classified as M0.

### ANATOMIC STAGE/PROGNOSTIC GROUPS

| Occult carcinoma | TX | N0 | M0 |
|---|---|---|---|
| Stage 0 | Tis | N0 | M0 |
| Stage IA | T1a | N0 | M0 |
| | T1b | N0 | M0 |
| Stage IB | T2a | N0 | M0 |
| Stage IIA | T2b | N0 | M0 |
| | T1a | N1 | M0 |
| | T1b | N1 | M0 |
| | T2a | N1 | M0 |
| Stage IIB | T2b | N1 | M0 |
| | T3 | N0 | M0 |
| Stage IIIA | T1a | N2 | M0 |
| | T1b | N2 | M0 |
| | T2a | N2 | M0 |
| | T2b | N2 | M0 |
| | T3 | N1 | M0 |

**25**

|            | T3    | N2    | M0  |
|------------|-------|-------|-----|
|            | T4    | N0    | M0  |
|            | T4    | N1    | M0  |
| Stage IIIB | T1a   | N3    | M0  |
|            | T1b   | N3    | M0  |
|            | T2a   | N3    | M0  |
|            | T2b   | N3    | M0  |
|            | T3    | N3    | M0  |
|            | T4    | N2    | M0  |
|            | T4    | N3    | M0  |
| Stage IV   | Any T | Any N | M1a |
|            | Any T | Any N | M1b |

## PROGNOSTIC FACTORS (SITE-SPECIFIC FACTORS)
### (Recommended for Collection)

| | |
|---|---|
| Required for staging | None |
| Clinically significant | Pleural/elastic layer invasion (based on H&E and elastic stains) |
| | Separate tumor nodules |
| | Vascular invasion – V classification (venous or arteriolar) |

## HISTOPATHOLOGIC GRADE (G)

| | |
|---|---|
| GX | Grade cannot be assessed |
| G1 | Well differentiated |
| G2 | Moderately differentiated |
| G3 | Poorly differentiated |
| G4 | Undifferentiated |

## ADDITIONAL NOTES REGARDING TNM DESCRIPTORS

The T category is defined by the size and extent of the primary tumor. Definitions have changed from the prior edition of TNM. For the T2 category, visceral pleural invasion is defined as invasion to the surface of the visceral pleura or invasion beyond the elastic layer. On the basis of a review of published literature, the IASLC Staging Committee recommends that elastic stains can be used in cases where it is difficult to identify invasion of the elastic layer by hematoxylin and eosin (H&E) stains. A tumor that falls short of completely traversing the elastic layer is defined as PL0. A tumor that extends through the elastic layer is defined as PL1 and one that extends to the surface of the visceral pleural as PL2. Either PL1 or PL2 status allows classification of the primary tumor as T2. Extension of the tumor to the parietal pleura is defined as PL3 and categorizes the primary tumor as T3.

Direct tumor invasion into an adjacent ipsilateral lobe (i.e., invasion across a fissure) is classified as T2a. These definitions are illustrated in a report by Travis et al., referenced in the bibliography of this chapter.

Multiple tumors may be considered to be synchronous primaries if they are of different histological cell types. When multiple tumors are of the same cell type, they should only be considered to be synchronous primary tumors if in the opinion of the pathologist, based on features such as associated carcinoma in situ or differences in morphology, immunohistochemistry, and/or molecular studies, they represent differing subtypes of the same histopathological cell type, and also have no evidence of mediastinal nodal metastases or of nodal metastases within a common nodal drainage. Synchronous primary tumors are most commonly encountered when dealing with either bronchioloalveolar carcinomas or adenocarcinomas of mixed subtype with a bronchioloalveolar component. Multiple synchronous primary tumors should be staged separately. The highest T category and stage of disease should be assigned and the multiplicity or the number of tumors should be indicated in parenthesis, e.g., T2(m) or T2(5).

Vocal cord paralysis (resulting from involvement of the recurrent branch of the vagus nerve), superior vena caval obstruction, or compression of the trachea or esophagus may be related to direct extension of the primary tumor or to lymph node involvement. The treatment options and prognosis associated with this direct extension of the primary tumor fall within the T4N0-1 (Stage IIIA) category; therefore, a classification of T4 is recommended. If the primary tumor is peripheral, vocal cord paralysis is usually related to the presence of N2 disease and should be classified as such.

The designation of "Pancoast" tumors relates to the symptom complex or syndrome caused by a tumor arising in the superior sulcus of the lung that involves the inferior branches of the brachial plexus (C8 and/or T1) and, in some cases, the stellate ganglion. Some superior sulcus tumors are more anteriorly located and cause fewer neurological symptoms but encase the subclavian vessels. The extent of disease varies in these tumors, and they should be classified according to the established rules. If there is evidence of invasion of the vertebral body or spinal canal, encasement of the subclavian vessels, or unequivocal involvement of the superior branches of the brachial plexus (C8 or above), the tumor is then classified as T4. If no criteria for T4 disease pertain, the tumor is classified as T3.

Tumors directly invading the diaphragm in the absence of other signs of locally advanced disease are rare, constituting less than 1% of all cases of potentially resectable NSCLC. These tumors are considered to be T3, but appear to have a poor prognosis, even after complete resection and in the absence of N2 disease. The classification of such tumors may need to be reevaluated in the future as more survival data become available.

The term "satellite nodules" was included in the 6th edition of the *AJCC Cancer Staging Manual.* It was defined as additional small nodules in the same lobe as the primary tumor but anatomically distinct from it that could be recognized grossly. Additional small nodules that could be identified only microscopically were not included in this definition. The term "satellite nodules" is being deleted from this edition of the *Staging Manual* because it is confusing, has no scientific basis, and is at variance with the

25

UICC Staging Manual. The term "additional tumor nodules" should be used to describe grossly recognizable multiple carcinomas in the same lobe. Such nodules are classified as T3. This definition does not apply to one grossly detected tumor associated with multiple separate microscopic foci.

## HISTOPATHOLOGIC TYPE

The World Health Organization histologic classification of tumors of the lung, 2004, is shown in Table 25.4.

**TABLE 25.4.** World Health Organization histologic classification of tumors of the lung, 2004

| Malignant epithelial tumors | ICD |
|---|---|
| Squamous cell carcinoma | 8070/3 |
|   Papillary | 8052/3 |
|   Clear cell | 8084/3 |
|   Small cell | 8073/3 |
|   Basaloid | 8083/3 |
| Small cell carcinoma | 8041/3 |
|   Combined small cell carcinoma | 8045/3 |
| Adenocarcinoma | 8140/3 |
|   Adenocarcinoma, mixed subtype | 8255/3 |
|   Acinar adenocarcinoma | 8550/3 |
|   Papillary adenocarcinoma | 8260/3 |
|   Bronchioloalveolar carcinoma | 8250/3 |
|     Nonmucinous | 8252/3 |
|     Mucinous | 8253/3 |
|     Mixed nonmucinous and mucinous or indeterminate | 8254/3 |
|   Solid adenocarcinoma with mucin production | 8230/3 |
|   Fetal adenocarcinoma | 8333/3 |
|   Mucinous ("colloid") carcinoma | 8480/3 |
|   Mucinous cystadenocarcinoma | 8470/3 |
|   Signet ring adenocarcinoma | 8490/3 |
|   Clear cell adenocarcinoma | 8310/3 |
| Large cell carcinoma | 8012/3 |
|   Large cell neuroendocrine carcinoma | 8013/3 |
|     Combined large cell neuroendocrine carcinoma | 8013/3 |
|   Basaloid carcinoma | 8123/3 |
|   Lymphoepithelioma-like carcinoma | 8082/3 |
|   Clear cell carcinoma | 8310/3 |
|   Large cell carcinoma with rhabdoid phenotype | 8014/3 |
| Adenosquamous carcinoma | 8560/3 |

*continued*

**TABLE 25.4.** World Health Organization histologic classification of tumors of the lung, 2004 (continued)

| Malignant epithelial tumors | ICD |
|---|---|
| Sarcomatoid carcinoma | 8033/3 |
| Pleomorphic carcinoma | 8022/3 |
| Spindle cell carcinoma | 8032/3 |
| Giant cell carcinoma | 8031/3 |
| Carcinosarcoma | 8980/3 |
| Pulmonary blastoma | 8972/3 |
| Carcinoid tumor | 8240/3 |
| Typical carcinoid | 8240/3 |
| Atypical carcinoid | 8249/3 |
| Salivary gland tumors | |
| Mucoepidermoid carcinoma | 8430/3 |
| Adenoid cystic carcinoma | 8200/2 |
| Epithelial-myoepithelial carcinoma | 8562/3 |

Morphology code of the International Classification of Diseases for Oncology (ICD-0) and the Systematized Nomenclature of Medicine (http://snowmed.org). Behavior is coded /0 for benign tumors, /3 for malignant tumors, and /1 for borderline or uncertain behavior.

From Travis WD, et al., eds. Tumours of the Lung, Pleura, Thymus and Heart. World Health Organization Classification of Tumours. Lyon: IARC Press, 2004, p. 10, with permission of IARC Press.

## BIBLIOGRAPHY

Berghmans T, Paesmans M, Mascaux C, et al. Thyroid transcription factor 1 – a new prognostic factor in lung cancer: A meta-analysis. Ann Oncol. 2006;17: 1673–6.

Delmotte P, Martin B, Paesmans M, et al. VEGF et survie des patients atteints d'un cancer pulmonaire. Rev Mal Respir. 2002;19(5 Pt 1):577–84.

Goldstraw P, Crowley JJ. The International Association for the Study of Lung Cancer international staging project on lung cancer. J Thorac Oncol. 2006;1: 281–6.

Goldstraw P, Crowley J, Chansky K, et al. The IASLC Lung Cancer Staging Project: Proposals for the revision of the TNM stage groupings in the forthcoming (seventh) edition of the TNM classification of malignant tumours. J Thorac Oncol. 2007;2:706–14.

Groome PA, Bolejack V, Crowley JJ, et al. The IASLC Lung Cancer Staging Project: Validation of the proposals for revision of the T, N, and M descriptors and consequent stage groupings in the forthcoming (seventh) edition of the TNM classification of malignant tumours. J Thorac Oncol. 2007;2:694–705.

Huncharek M, Muscat J, Geschwind JF. K-ras oncogene mutation as a prognostic marker in non-small cell lung cancer: A combined analysis of 881 cases. Carcinogenesis. 1999;20:1507–10.

Huncharek M, Kupelnick B, Geschwind JF, et al. Prognostic significance of p53 mutations in non-small cell lung cancer: A meta-analysis of 829 cases from eight published studies. Cancer Let. 2000;153:219–26.

Kato H, Kawate N, Kobayashi K et al, editors. The Japan Lung Cancer Society: Classification of lung cancer (ed First English Edition). Tokyo: Kanehara & Co., 2000.

Marks JL, Broderick S, Zhou Q, et al. Prognostic implications of EGFR and KRAS mutations in resected lung adenocarcinoma. J Thorac Oncol. 2008;3:111–6.

**25**

Martin B, Paesmans M, Berghmans T, et al. Role of bcl-2 as a prognostic factor for survival in lung cancer: A systematic review of the literature with meta-analysis. Br J Cancer. 2003;89:55–64.

Martin B, Paesmans M, Mascaux C, et al. Ki-67 expression and patients survival in lung cancer: Systematic review of the literature with meta-analysis. Br J Cancer. 2004;9:2018–25.

Martini N, Melamed MR. Multiple primary lung cancers. J Thorac Cardiovasc Surg. 1975;70:606–12.

Mascaux C, Iannino N, Martin B, et al. The role of RAS oncogene in survival of patients with lung cancer: A systematic review of the literature with meta-analysis. Br J Cancer. 2005;92:131–9.

Mascaux C, Martin B, Paesmans M, et al. Has Cox-2 a prognostic role in non-small cell lung cancer? A systematic review of the literature with meta-analysis of the survival results. Br J Cancer. 2006;95:139–45.

Matsuguma H, Nakahara R, Igarashi S, et al. Pathologic stage I non-small cell lung cancer with high levels of preoperative serum carcinoembryonic antigen: Clinicopathologic characteristics and prognosis. J Thorac Cardiovasc Surg. 2008;135:44–9.

Meert AP, Martin B, Delmotte P, et al. The role of EGF-R expression on patient survival in lung cancer: A systematic review with meta-analysis. Eur Respir J. 2002;20:975–81.

Meert AP, Paesmans M, Martin B, et al. The role of microvessel density on the survival of patients with lung cancer: A systematic review of the literature with meta-anslysis. Br J Cancer. 2002;87:694–701.

Meert AP, Martin B, Paesmans M, et al. The role of HER-2/neu expression on the survival of patients with lung cancer: A systematic review of the literature. Br J Cancer. 2003;89:959–65.

Mitsudomi T, Hamajima N, Ogawa M, et al. Prognostic significance of p53 alterations in patients with non-small cell lung cancer: A meta-analysis. Clin Cancer Res. 2000;6:4055–63.

Mountain CF, Dresler CM. Regional lymph node classification for lung cancer staging. Chest. 1997;111:1718–23.

Nakamura H, Kawasaki N, Taguchi M, et al. Association of HER-2 overexpression with prognosis in nonsmall cell lung carcinoma: A meta-analysis. Cancer. 2005;103:1865–73.

Nakamura H, Kawasaki N, Taguchi M, et al. Survival impact of epidermal growth factor receptor overexpression in patients with non-small cell lung cancer: A meta-analysis. Thorax. 2006;61:140–5.

Postmus PE, Brambilla E, Chansky K, et al. The IASLC Lung Cancer Staging Project: Proposals for revision of the M descriptors in the forthcoming (seventh) edition of the TNM classification of lung cancer. J Thorac Oncol. 2007;2:686–93.

Rami-Porta R, Ball D, Crowley J, et al. The IASLC Lung Cancer Staging Project: Proposals for the revision of the T descriptors in the forthcoming (seventh) edition of the TNM classification for lung cancer. J Thorac Oncol. 2007;2:593–602.

Rusch VW, Crowley J, Giroux DJ, et al. The IASLC Lung Cancer Staging Project: Proposals for the revision of the N descriptors in the forthcoming seventh edition of the TNM classification for lung cancer. J Thorac Oncol. 2007;2:603–12.

Sculier J-P, Chansky K, Crowley JJ, et al. The IASLC Lung Cancer Staging Project: The impact of additional prognostic factors on survival and their relationship with the anatomical extent of disease expressed by the 6th edition of the TNM Classification of Malignant Tumours and the proposals for the 7th edition. J Thorac Oncol. 2008;3(5):457–66.

Shepherd FA, Crowley J, Van Houtte P, et al. The IASLC Lung Cancer Staging Project: Proposals regarding the clinical staging of small cell lung cancer in the forthcoming (seventh) edition of the TNM classification for lung cancer. J Thorac Oncol. 2007;2(12):1067–77.

Steels E, Paesmans M, Berghmans T, et al. Role of p53 as a prognostic factor for survival in lung cancer: A systematic review of the literature with a meta-analysis. Eur Respir J. 2001;18:705–19.

Travis WD, Brambilla E, Müller-Hermelink HK, et al., editors. World Health Organization Classification of tumours: Pathology and genetics of tumours of the lung, pleura, thymus and heart. Lyon, France: IARC Press, 2004.

Travis WD, Brambilla E, Rami-Porta R, et al. Visceral pleural invasion: Pathologic criteria and use of elastic stains: Proposal for the 7th edition of the TNM classification for lung cancer. J Thorac Oncol. 2008;3:1384–90.

Travis WD, Giroux DJ, Chansky K, et al. The IASLC Lung Cancer Staging Project: Proposals for the inclusion of carcinoid tumors in the forthcoming (seventh) edition of the TNM classification for lung cancer. J Thorac Oncol. 2008;3:1213–23.

Wittekind C, Greene FL, Henson DE, et al., editors. UICC International Union Against Cancer: TNM supplement: A commentary on uniform use. New York: Wiley-Liss, 2003.

Zielinski M, Rami-Porta R. Proposals for changes in the Mountain and Dresler mediastinal and pulmonary lymph node map. J Thorac Oncol. 2007;2:3–6.

25

# Pleural Mesothelioma

## *At-A-Glance*

**SUMMARY OF CHANGES**

• Peridiaphragmatic lymph nodes have been added to the N2 category

| ANATOMIC STAGE/PROGNOSTIC GROUPS | | | |
|---|---|---|---|
| Stage I | T1 | N0 | M0 |
| Stage IA | T1a | N0 | M0 |
| Stage IB | T1b | N0 | M0 |
| Stage II | T2 | N0 | M0 |
| Stage III | T1, T2 | N1 | M0 |
| | T1, T2 | N2 | M0 |
| | T3 | N0, N1, N2 | M0 |
| Stage IV | T4 | Any N | M0 |
| | Any T | N3 | M0 |
| | Any T | Any N | M1 |

ICD-O-3
TOPOGRAPHY
CODES
C38.4     Pleura, NOS

ICD-O-3 HISTOLOGY
CODE RANGES
9050–9053

## INTRODUCTION

Malignant mesotheliomas are relatively rare tumors that arise from the mesothelium lining the pleural, pericardial, and peritoneal cavities. They represent less than 2% of all cancers. The most common risk factor for malignant mesotheliomas is previous exposure to asbestos. The latency period between the asbestos exposure and the development of malignant mesothelioma is generally 20 years or more. Although peritoneal mesotheliomas are thought to occur in individuals who have had more extensive exposure than those with pleural mesothelioma, there is no clearly documented relationship between the amount of asbestos exposure and the subsequent development of this neoplasm. Malignant mesotheliomas were previously thought to be virulent tumors. However, this impression was probably related to the fact that most mesotheliomas are diagnosed when they are already at an advanced stage. Recent data indicate that the clinical and biological behavior of mesotheliomas is variable and that most mesotheliomas grow relatively slowly.

All mesotheliomas are fundamentally epithelial tumors. However, their morphology ranges from a pure epithelial appearance to an entirely sarcomatoid or even desmoplastic one. Distinguishing the pleomorphic histology

26

of mesotheliomas from that of other neoplasms can be difficult, especially for the pure epithelial mesotheliomas that may closely resemble metastatic adenocarcinoma. Therefore, confirmation of the histological diagnosis by immunohistochemistry and/or electron microscopy is essential.

During the past 30 years, many staging systems have been proposed for malignant pleural mesothelioma. The first staging system for this disease published by the American Joint Committee on Cancer (AJCC) and simultaneously accepted by the International Union Against Cancer appeared in the fifth edition of the *AJCC Staging Manual*. The staging system described here represents an adoption of the one proposed in 1995 by the International Mesothelioma Interest Group (IMIG), which was based on updated information about the relationships between tumor T and N status and overall survival. This system has been validated by several surgical reports, but will likely require revision in the future as further data in larger numbers of patients become available. This staging system applies only to tumors arising in the pleura. Peritoneal and pericardial mesotheliomas are rare and do not lend themselves easily to a TNM staging system.

## ANATOMY

**Primary Site.** The mesothelium covers the external surface of the lungs and the inside of the chest wall. It is usually composed of flat tightly connected cells no more than one layer thick.

**Regional Lymph Nodes.** The regional lymph nodes include:

Intrathoracic
Scalene
Supraclavicular
Internal mammary
Peridiaphragmatic

The regional lymph node map and nomenclature adopted for the mesothelioma staging system is identical to that used for lung cancer. See Chap. 25 for a detailed list of intrathoracic lymph nodes. For pN, histologic examination of a mediastinal lymphadenectomy or lymph node sampling specimen will ordinarily include regional nodes taken from the ipsilateral N1 and N2 nodal stations. In addition, mesotheliomas often metastasize to lymph nodes not involved by lung cancers, most commonly the internal mammary and peridiaphragmatic nodes. These latter two regions also are classified as N2 nodal stations. Contralateral mediastinal and supraclavicular nodes may be available if a mediastinoscopy or node biopsy is also performed. If involved by metastatic disease these would be staged as N3.

**Distant Metastatic Sites.** Advanced malignant pleural mesotheliomas often metastasize widely to uncommon sites, including retroperitoneal lymph nodes, the brain, and spine, or even to organs such as the thyroid or prostate. However, the most frequent sites of metastatic disease are the peritoneum, contralateral pleura, and lung.

## RULES FOR CLASSIFICATION

This staging system serves both clinical and pathologic staging. Clinical staging depends on imaging; most frequently computed tomography (CT) and more recently FDG positron emission tomography (FDG-PET) scanning. Pathologic staging is based on surgical resection. The extent of disease before and after resection should be carefully documented. In some cases, complete N classification may not be possible, especially if technical unresectable tumor (T4) is found at thoracotomy which prevents access to both N1 and N2 lymph nodes. In this situation, the pN stage should be based on the histological findings in whichever lymph nodes were removed or should be designated as pNX if no lymph nodes could be removed.

## PROGNOSTIC FEATURES

Several factors are reported to have prognostic significance in patients with malignant pleural mesothelioma. Histological subtype and patient performance status are consistently reported as prognostically significant. Patient age, gender, symptoms (absence or presence of chest pain), and history of asbestos exposure are also cited in various studies as potential prognostic factors. The intensity of primary tumor hypermetabolism on FDG-PET scan as measured by the standardized uptake value (SUV) has also been reported to correlate with overall survival, with tumor SUV greater than 10 being associated with a worse outcome. Further analysis of these various factors in a large multicenter database is needed to determine their true prognostic validity.

## DEFINITIONS OF TNM

### IMIG Staging System for Diffuse Malignant Pleural Mesothelioma

*Primary Tumor (T)*

| | |
|---|---|
| TX | Primary tumor cannot be assessed |
| T0 | No evidence of primary tumor |
| T1 | Tumor limited to the ipsilateral parietal pleura with or without mediastinal pleura and with or without diaphragmatic pleural involvement |
| T1a | No involvement of the visceral pleura |
| T1b | Tumor also involving the visceral pleura |
| T2 | Tumor involving each of the ipsilateral pleural surfaces (parietal, mediastinal, diaphragmatic, and visceral pleura) with at least one of the following: |
| |     Involvement of diaphragmatic muscle |
| |     Extension of tumor from visceral pleura into the underlying pulmonary parenchyma |

**26**

### Primary Tumor (T) (continued)

T3   Locally advanced but potentially resectable tumor
     Tumor involving all of the ipsilateral pleural surfaces (parietal, mediastinal, diaphragmatic, and visceral pleura) with at least one of the following:

>   Involvement of the endothoracic fascia
>   Extension into the mediastinal fat
>   Solitary, completely resectable focus of tumor extending into the soft tissues of the chest wall
>   Nontransmural involvement of the pericardium

T4   Locally advanced technically unresectable tumor
     Tumor involving all of the ipsilateral pleural surfaces (parietal, mediastinal, diaphragmatic, and visceral pleura) with at least one of the following:

>   Diffuse extension or multifocal masses of tumor in the chest wall, with or without associated rib destruction
>   Direct transdiaphragmatic extension of tumor to the peritoneum
>   Direct extension of tumor to the contralateral pleura
>   Direct extension of tumor to mediastinal organs
>   Direct extension of tumor into the spine
>   Tumor extending through to the internal surface of the pericardium with or without a pericardial effusion or tumor involving the myocardium

### Regional Lymph Nodes (N)

NX   Regional lymph nodes cannot be assessed
N0   No regional lymph node metastases
N1   Metastases in the ipsilateral bronchopulmonary or hilar lymph nodes
N2   Metastases in the subcarinal or the ipsilateral mediastinal lymph nodes including the ipsilateral internal mammary and peridiaphragmatic nodes
N3   Metastases in the contralateral mediastinal, contralateral internal mammary, ipsilateral or contralateral supraclavicular lymph nodes

### Distant Metastasis (M)

M0   No distant metastasis
M1   Distant metastasis present

## ANATOMIC STAGE/PROGNOSTIC GROUPS

| | | | |
|---|---|---|---|
| Stage I | T1 | N0 | M0 |
| Stage IA | T1a | N0 | M0 |
| Stage IB | T1b | N0 | M0 |
| Stage II | T2 | N0 | M0 |
| Stage III | T1, T2 | N1 | M0 |
| | T1, T2 | N2 | M0 |
| | T3 | N0, N1, N2 | M0 |
| Stage IV | T4 | Any N | M0 |
| | Any T | N3 | M0 |
| | Any T | Any N | M1 |

## PROGNOSTIC FACTORS (SITE-SPECIFIC FACTORS)
### (Recommended for Collection)

| | |
|---|---|
| Required for staging | None |
| Clinically significant | Histological subtype (epithelioid, mixed or biphasic, sarcomatoid, desmoplastic) |
| | History of asbestos exposure |
| | Presence or absence of chest pain |
| | FDG-PET SUV |

## HISTOLOGIC GRADE (G)

Grade is reported in registry systems by the grade value. A two-grade, three-grade, or four-grade system may be used. If a grading system is not specified, generally the following system is used:

| | |
|---|---|
| GX | Grade cannot be assessed |
| G1 | Well differentiated |
| G2 | Moderately differentiated |
| G3 | Poorly differentiated |
| G4 | Undifferentiated |

## HISTOPATHOLOGIC TYPE

There are four types of malignant pleural mesothelioma, which are listed here in descending order of frequency:

1. Epithelioid
2. Biphasic (at least 10% of both epithelioid and sarcomatoid components)
3. Sarcomatoid
4. Desmoplastic

26

In general, the pure epithelioid tumors are associated with a better prognosis than the biphasic or sarcomatoid tumors. Despite their bland histological appearance, desmoplastic tumors appear to have the worst prognosis. The biology underlying these differences is not yet understood.

## BIBLIOGRAPHY

Bottomley A, Coens C, Efficace F, et al. Symptoms and patient-reported well being: Do they predict survival in malignant pleural mesothelioma? A prognostic factor analysis of EORTC-NCIC 08983: Randomized phase III study of cisplatin with or without raltitrexed in patients with malignant pleural mesothelioma. J Clin Oncol. 2007;25:5770–6.

Boutin C, Rey F, Gouvernet J, et al. Thoracoscopy in pleural malignant mesothelioma: a prospective study of 188 consecutive patients. Part 2: Prognosis and staging. Cancer. 1993;72:394–404.

Edwards JG, Stewart DJ, Martin-Ucar A, et al. The pattern of lymph node involvement influences outcome after extrapleural pneumonectomy for malignant mesothelioma. J Thorac Cardiovasc Surg. 2006;131:981–7.

Fennell DA, Parmar A, Shamash J, et al. Statistical validation of the EORTC prognostic model for malignant pleural mesothelioma based on three consecutive phase II trials. J Clin Oncol. 2005;23:184–9.

Flores RM, Akhurst T, Gonen M, et al. Positron emission tomography (PET) predicts survival in malignant pleural mesothelioma (MPM). J Thorac Cardiovasc Surg. 2006;132:763–8.

Flores RM, Zakowski M, Venkatraman E, et al. Prognostic factors in the treatment of malignant pleural mesothelioma at a large tertiary referral center. J Thorac Oncol. 2007;2:957–65.

Flores RM, Routledge T, Seshan VE, et al. The impact of lymph node station on survival in 348 patients with surgically resected malignant pleural mesothelioma: Implications for revision of the American Joint Committee on Cancer staging system. J Thorac Cardiovasc Surg. 2008;136(3):605–10.

Ruffie P, Feld R, Minkin S, et al. Diffuse malignant mesothelioma of the pleura in Ontario and Quebec: a retrospective study of 332 patients. J Clin Oncol. 1989;7:1157–68.

Rusch VW. The International Mesothelioma Interest Group: a proposed new international TNM staging system for malignant pleural mesothelioma. Chest. 1995;108:1122–8.

Rusch VW, Venkatraman E. The importance of surgical staging in the treatment of malignant pleural mesothelioma. J Thorac Cardiovasc Surg. 1996;111:815–26.

Rusch VW, Venkatraman ES. Important prognostic factors in patients with malignant pleural mesothelioma, managed surgically. Ann Thorac Surg. 1999;68:1799–804.

Sugarbaker DJ, Strauss GM, Lynch TJ, et al. Node status has prognostic significance in the multimodality therapy of diffuse, malignant mesothelioma. J Clin Oncol. 1993;11(6):1172–8.

Sugarbaker DJ, Flores RM, Jaklitsch MT, et al. Resection margins, extrapleural nodal status, and cell type determine postoperative long-term survival in trimodality therapy of malignant pleural mesothelioma: results of 183 patients. J Thorac Cardiovasc Surg. 1999;117:54–65.

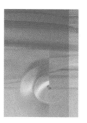

# PART V
# Musculoskeletal Sites

# Bone

*(Primary malignant lymphoma and multiple myeloma are not included.)*

## At-A-Glance

| SUMMARY OF CHANGES |
|---|
| • Stage III is reserved for G3, G4 |

| ANATOMIC STAGE/PROGNOSTIC GROUPS | | | | |
|---|---|---|---|---|
| Stage IA | T1 | N0 | M0 | G1,2 Low grade, GX |
| Stage IB | T2 | N0 | M0 | G1,2 Low grade, GX |
| | T3 | N0 | M0 | G1,2 Low grade, GX |
| Stage IIA | T1 | N0 | M0 | G3, 4 High grade |
| Stage IIB | T2 | N0 | M0 | G3, 4 High grade |
| Stage III | T3 | N0 | M0 | G3, 4 |
| Stage IVA | Any T | N0 | M1a | Any G |
| Stage IVB | Any T | N1 | Any M | Any G |
| | Any T | Any N | M1b | Any G |

**ICD-O-3 TOPOGRAPHY CODES**

C40.0   Long bones of upper limb, scapula, and associated joints

C40.1   Short bones of upper limb and associated joints

C40.2   Long bones of lower limb and associated joints

C40.3   Short bones of lower limb and associated joints

C40.8   Overlapping lesion of bones, joints, and articular cartilage of limbs

C40.9   Bone of limb, NOS

C41.0   Bones of skull and face and associated joints

C41.1   Mandible

C41.2   Vertebral column

C41.3   Rib, sternum, clavicle, and associated joints

C41.4   Pelvic bones, sacrum, coccyx, and associated joints

C41.8   Overlapping lesion of bones, joints, and articular cartilage

C41.9   Bone, NOS

**ICD-O-3 HISTOLOGY CODE RANGES**
8800–9136, 9142–9582

## INTRODUCTION

This classification is used for all primary malignant tumors of bone except primary malignant lymphoma and multiple myeloma. These tumors are relatively rare, representing less than 0.2% of all malignancies. Osteosarcoma (35%), chondrosarcoma (30%), and Ewing's sarcoma (16%) are the three most common forms of primary bone cancer. Osteosarcoma and Ewing's sarcoma develop mainly in children and young adults, whereas chondrosarcoma is usually found in middle aged and older adults. Data from these three histologies analyzed at multiple institutions, predominantly influence this staging system. Staging of bone sarcomas is the process whereby patients are evaluated with regard to histology, as well as the local and distant extent of disease. Bone sarcomas are staged based on grade, size, and the presence and location of metastases. The system is designed to help stratify patients according to known risk factors.

## ANATOMY

**Primary Site.**  All bones of the skeleton are included in this system. The current staging system does not take into account anatomic site. However, anatomic site is known to influence outcome, and therefore outcome data should be reported specifying site.

Site groups for bone sarcoma:

- Extremity
- Pelvis
- Spine

**Regional Lymph Nodes.**  Regional lymph metastases from bone tumors are extremely rare.

**Metastatic Sites.**  A metastatic site includes any site beyond the regional lymph nodes of the primary site. Pulmonary metastases are the most frequent site for all bone sarcomas. Extra pulmonary metastases occur infrequently, and may include secondary bone metastases, for example.

## RULES FOR CLASSIFICATION

**Clinical Staging.**  Clinical staging includes all relevant data prior to primary definitive therapy, including physical examination, imaging, and biopsy. It is dependent on the T, N, M characteristics of the identified tumor. T is divided into lesions of maximum dimension 8 cm or less (T1), and lesions greater than 8 cm (T2). T3 has been redefined to include only high-grade tumors, discontinuous, within the same bone. Metastatic disease should be evaluated for and described. In general, the minimum clinical staging workup of a bone sarcoma should include axial imaging using MRI and/or CT, CT scan of the chest, and technetium scintigraphy of the entire skeleton.

The radiograph remains the mainstay in determining whether a lesion of bone requires staging and usually is the modality that permits reliable prediction of the probable histology of a lesion of bone.

Local staging of all bone sarcomas is most accurately achieved by magnetic resonance (MR) imaging. Axial imaging, complemented by either coronal or sagittal imaging planes using T1- and T2-weighted SPIN-echo sequences, most often provides accurate depiction of intra- and extraosseous tumor. To improve conspicuity in locations such as the pelvis or vertebrae, these sequences could be augmented by fat-suppressed pulse sequences. The maximum dimension of the tumor must be measured prior to any treatment. The decision to use intravenous contrast should be based upon medical appropriateness.

Computerized tomography (CT) has a limited role in local staging of tumors. In those situations, where characterization of a lesion by radiography may be incomplete or difficult because of inadequate visualization of the matrix of a lesion, CT may be preferred to MR imaging. The role of CT in these circumstances is to characterize the lesion and determine whether it is potentially malignant or not, and the obtained CT images may suffice for local staging. CT remains the examination of choice for evaluating the presence or absence of pulmonary metastases.

Technetium scintigraphy is the examination of choice for evaluating the entire skeleton to determine whether there are multiple bony lesions. The role of positron emission tomography (PET) in the evaluation and staging of bone sarcomas remains incompletely defined. Reports indicate usefulness in detecting extrapulmonary metastases, evaluating response to chemotherapy, and determining local recurrence adjacent to prosthetic implants.

**Biopsy.** Biopsy of the tumor completes the staging process, and the location of the biopsy must be carefully planned to allow for eventual en bloc resection of the entire biopsy tract together with a malignant neoplasm. Staging of the lesion should precede biopsy. Imaging the tumor after biopsy may compromise the accuracy of the staging process.

**Pathologic Staging.** The pathologic diagnosis is based on the microscopic examination of tissue, correlated with imaging studies. Pathologic staging pTNM includes pathologic data obtained from examination of a resected specimen sufficient to evaluate the highest T category, histopathologic type and grade, regional lymph nodes as appropriate, or distant metastasis. Because regional lymph node involvement from bone tumors is rare, the pathologic stage grouping includes any of the following combinations: pT pG pN pM, or pT pG cN cM, or cT cN pM. Grade should be assigned to all bone sarcomas. Based upon published outcomes data, the current staging system accommodates a two-tiered (low vs. high grade) for recording stage.

**Restaging of Recurrent Tumors.** The same staging should be used when a patient requires restaging of sarcoma recurrence. Such reports should specify whether patients have primary lesions or lesions that were previously treated and have subsequently recurred. The identification and reporting of etiologic factors such as radiation exposure and inherited or genetic syndromes are encouraged.

## PROGNOSTIC FEATURES

Known prognostic factors for malignant bone tumors are as follows. (1) T1 tumors have a better prognosis than T2 tumors. (2) Histopathologic low grade (G1, G2) has a better prognosis than high grade (G3, G4). (3) Location of the primary tumor is a prognostic factor. Patients who have an anatomically resectable primary tumor have a better prognosis than those with a non-resectable tumor, and tumors of the spine and pelvis tend to have a poorer prognosis. (4) The size of the primary tumor is a prognostic factor for osteosarcoma and Ewing's sarcoma. Ewing's sarcoma patients with a tumor 8 cm or less in greatest dimension have a better prognosis than those with a tumor greater than 8 cm. Osteosarcoma patients with a tumor 9 cm or less in greatest dimension have a better prognosis than those with a tumor greater than 9 cm. (5) Patients who have a localized primary tumor have a better prognosis than those with metastases. (6) Certain metastatic sites are associated with a poorer prognosis than other sites: bony and hepatic metastases convey a much worse prognosis than do lung metastases, and patients with solitary lung metastases have a better prognosis than those with multiple lung lesions. (7) Histologic response of the primary tumor to chemotherapy is a prognostic factor for osteosarcoma and Ewing's sarcoma. Those patients with a "good" response, >90% tumor necrosis, have a better prognosis than those with less necrosis. (8) Patients with osteosarcoma who experience pathologic fractures may have a poorer prognosis, particularly if their fracture does not heal during chemotherapy. (9) Recent studies have shown that the biologic behavior of osteosarcoma and Ewing's sarcoma is related to specific molecular abnormalities identified in these neoplasms. As with soft tissue sarcomas, investigation has been undertaken to identify molecular markers that are useful both as prognostic tools as well as in directing treatment. The results of this investigation have shown that the biologic behavior of osteosarcoma and Ewing's sarcoma can be related to specific molecular abnormalities. For practical purposes, prognostically relevant molecular aberrations are considered in terms of gene translocations, expression of multidrug resistance genes, expression of growth factor receptors, and mutations in cell cycle regulators.

Investigation as to whether the type of fusion gene detected in Ewing's sarcoma has prognostic significance has been met with mixed results. Initial studies suggested that the EWS-FLI1 type 1 fusion gene was associated with longer relapse-free survival in patients with localized disease and have been confirmed with a subsequent study which found an association between type 1 EWS-FLI1 and overall survival by multivariate analysis. In contrast, a study concluded that no prognostic value was attributed to different fusion genes when evaluated for event-free and overall survival by univariate analysis.

P-glycoprotein, the product of the multidrug resistance 1 gene (MDR1), functions to remove certain chemotherapeutic drugs, such as doxorubicin, from tumor cells. In osteosarcoma, P-glycoprotein status has been noted to be an independent predictor of clinical outcome and to be associated with a ninefold increase in the odds of death and a fivefold increase in the odds of metastases in patients with Stage IIB osteosarcoma. Further investigation showed that P-glycoprotein-positivity at diagnosis emerged as the single factor significantly associated with an unfavorable outcome from survival and multivariate analyses and this association was strong enough to be useful in stratifying patients in whom alternative treatments were being considered.

Also in osteosarcoma, investigation of human epidermal growth factor receptor 2 (HER2)/erbB-2 has led to differing results between investigators as well. Gorlick et al. identified a significant percentage (42.6%) of initial biopsies with high levels of HER2/erbB-2 expression. They noted that there was a correlation with histologic response to neoadjuvant chemotherapy and event-free survival. Zhou et al. noted an association between HER2/erbB-2 expression with an increased risk of metastasis. Scotlandi also confirmed an advantage in event-free survival with HER2 overexpression. Subsequent analysis by Scotlandi has failed to show HER2 amplification/overexpression by immunohistochemistry/CISH and FISH, respectively.

In Ewing's sarcoma, the status of several cell cycle regulators has been shown to correlate with outcome. Aberrant P53, p16INK4A, and p14ARF expression has been shown by several investigators to identify a subset of patients whose tumors will exhibit aggressive behavior and a poor response to chemotherapy. Additional studies revealed that loss of INK4 expression correlated with metastatic disease at presentation and also showed a trend toward shortened survival. Suppression of the cyclin-dependant kinase inhibitor p27(kip1) by EWS-FLI1 has been associated with poor event-free survival in univariate analysis and the expression level of p27 correlates significantly with patient survival. Overall event-free survival has been correlated to P53 alteration in osteosarcoma as well.

A variety of other markers have been described as relevant to the prognosis of osteosarcoma. This includes KI-67, a proliferative marker which has been suggested as a marker for the development of pulmonary metastasis. Heat shock proteins (HSP) have been shown to aid in the growth and development of tumors and overexpression of HSP27 specifically has been shown to carry negative prognostic value. Overexpression of parathyroid hormone Type 1 has been shown to confer an aggressive phenotype in osteosarcoma. Platelet-derived growth factor-AA expression was found to be an independent predictor of tumor progression in osteosarcoma. Nuclear survivin expression/localization has been associated with prolonged survival. Vascular endothelial growth factor expression in untreated osteosarcoma is predictive of pulmonary metastasis and poor prognosis. HLA class I expression has been shown to be associated with significantly better overall and event-free survival than patients lacking HLA class I expression in osteosarcoma. Finally, telomerase expression in osteosarcoma is associated with decreased progression free survival and overall survival.

Investigation to identify molecular markers in chondrosarcoma has progressed at a slower pace. Rozeman et al. investigated a variety of markers, none of which had prognostic importance independent of histologic grade. Decreased Indian Hedgehog signaling and loss of INK4A/p16 has been found to be important in the progression of peripheral chondrosarcoma and enchondroma, respectively.

## DEFINITIONS OF TNM

### Primary Tumor (T)

| | |
|---|---|
| TX | Primary tumor cannot be assessed |
| T0 | No evidence of primary tumor |
| T1 | Tumor 8 cm or less in greatest dimension |
| T2 | Tumor more than 8 cm in greatest dimension |
| T3 | Discontinuous tumors in the primary bone site |

### Regional Lymph Nodes (N)

| | |
|---|---|
| NX | Regional lymph nodes cannot be assessed |
| N0 | No regional lymph node metastasis |
| N1 | Regional lymph node metastasis |

*Note*: Because of the rarity of lymph node involvement in bone sarcomas, the designation NX may not be appropriate and cases should be considered N0 unless clinical node involvement is clearly evident.

### Distant Metastasis (M)

| | |
|---|---|
| M0 | No distant metastasis |
| M1 | Distant metastasis |
| M1a | Lung |
| M1b | Other distant sites |

### ANATOMIC STAGE/PROGNOSTIC GROUPS

| | | | | |
|---|---|---|---|---|
| Stage IA | T1 | N0 | M0 | G1,2 Low grade, GX |
| Stage IB | T2 | N0 | M0 | G1,2 Low grade, GX |
| | T3 | N0 | M0 | G1,2 Low grade, GX |
| Stage IIA | T1 | N0 | M0 | G3, 4 High grade |
| Stage IIB | T2 | N0 | M0 | G3, 4 High grade |
| Stage III | T3 | N0 | M0 | G3, 4 |
| Stage IVA | Any T | N0 | M1a | Any G |
| Stage IVB | Any T | N1 | Any M | Any G |
| | Any T | Any N | M1b | Any G |

## PROGNOSTIC FACTORS (SITE-SPECIFIC FACTORS)
### (Recommended for Collection)

| | |
|---|---|
| Required for staging | Grade |
| Clinically significant | Three dimensions of tumor size |
| | Percentage necrosis post neoadjuvant systemic therapy from pathology report |
| | Number of resected pulmonary metastases from pathology report |

## HISTOLOGIC GRADE (G)

27

Grade is reported in registry systems by the grade value. A two-grade, three-grade, or four-grade system may be used. If a grading system is not specified, generally the following system is used:

GX     Grade cannot be assessed
G1     Well differentiated – low grade
G2     Moderately differentiated – low grade
G3     Poorly differentiated
G4     Undifferentiated

*Note*: Ewing's sarcoma is classified as G4.

## HISTOPATHOLOGIC TYPE

### Classification of Primary Malignant Bone Tumors

1. Osteosarcoma
   a. Intramedullary high grade
      • Osteoblastic
      • Chondroblastic
      • Fibroblastic
      • Mixed
      • Small cell
      • Other (telangiectatic, epithelioid, chondromyxoid fibroma-like, chondroblastoma-like, osteoblastoma-like, giant cell rich)
   b. Intramedullary low grade
   c. Juxtacortical high grade (high grade surface osteosarcoma)
   d. Juxtacortical intermediate grade chondroblastic (periosteal osteosarcoma)
   e. Juxtacortical low grade (parosteal osteosarcoma)
2. Chondrosarcoma
   a. Intramedullary
      • Conventional (hyaline/myxoid)
      • Clear cell
      • Dedifferentiated
      • Mesenchymal
   b. Juxtacortical
3. Primitive neuroectodermal tumor/Ewing's sarcoma
4. Angiosarcoma
   a. Conventional
   b. Epithelioid hemangioendothelioma
5. Fibrosarcoma/malignant fibrous histiocytoma
6. Chordoma
   a. Conventional
   b. Dedifferentiated
7. Adamantinoma
   a. Conventional
   b. Well differentiated – osteofibrous dysplasia-like

8. Other
   a. Liposarcoma
   b. Leiomyosarcoma
   c. Malignant peripheral nerve sheath tumor
   d. Rhabdomyosarcoma
   e. Malignant mesenchymoma
   f. Malignant hemangiopericytoma

## BIBLIOGRAPHY

Aigner T, Muller S, Neureiter D, Illstrup DM, Kirchner T, Bjornsson J. Prognostic relevance of cell biologic and biochemical features in conventional chondrosarcomas. Cancer. 2002;94(8):2273–81.

Bacci G, Ferrari S, Longhi A, Donati D, Manfrini M, Giacomini S, et al. Nonmetastatic osteosarcoma of the extremity with pathologic fracture at presentation: local and systemic control by amputation or limb salvage after preoperative chemotherapy. Acta Orthop Scand. 2003;74(4): 449–54.

Baldini N, Scotlandi K, Barbanti-Brodano G, Manara MC, Maurici D, Bacci G, et al. Expression of P-glycoprotein in high-grade osteosarcomas in relation to clinical outcome. N Engl J Med. 1995;333(21):1380–5.

Barri G, Ferrari S, Bertoni F, et al. Prognostic factors in non-metastatic Ewings' sarcoma of bone treated with adjuvant chemotherapy: analysis of 359 patients at the Istituto Ortopedico Rizzoli. J Clin Oncol. 2000;18: 4–11.

Biermann JS, Adkins D, Benjamin R, Brigman B, Chow W, Conrad EU, et al. Bone cancer: clinical practice guidelines in oncology. J Natl Compr Cancer Netw. 2007;5(4):420–37.

Brenner W, Conrad EU, Eary JF. FDG PET imaging for grading and prediction of outcome in chondrosarcoma patients. Eur J Nucl Med Mol Imaging. 2004;31(2):189–95.

Cotterill SJ, Ahrens S, Paulussen M, Jurgens HF, Voute PA, Gadner H, et al. Prognostic factors in Ewing's tumor of bone: analysis of 975 patients form the European integral group cooperative Ewing's sarcoma study group. J Clin Oncol. 2000;18:3108–14.

Damron TA, Ward WG, Stewart A. Osteosarcoma, chondrosarcoma, and Ewing's sarcoma: a national cancer data base report. Clin Ortho Relat Res. 2007;459: 40–7.

Davis A, Bell R, Goodwin P. Prognostic factors in osteosarcoma: a critical review. J Clin Oncol. 1994;12(2):423–31.

de Alava E, Kawai A, Healey JH, Fligman I, Meyers PA, Huvos AG, et al. EWS-FLI1 fusion transcript structure is an independent determinant of prognosis in Ewing's sarcoma. J Clin Oncol. 1998;16(4):1248–55.

de Alava E, Antonescu CR, Panizo A, Leung D, Meyers PA, Huvos AG, et al. Prognostic impact of P53 status in Ewing's sarcoma. Cancer. 2000;89(4): 783–92.

Enneking WF, Spanier S, Goodman M. A system for the surgical staging of musculoskeletal sarcoma. Clin Orthop Relat Res. 1980;153:106–20.

Fiorenza F, Abudu A, Grimer RJ, et al. Risk factors for survival and local control in chondrosarcoma of bone. J Bone Joint Surg. 2002;84B:93–9.

Folpe AL, Lyles RH, Sprouse JT, Conrad EU, Eary JF. (F-18) Fluorodeoxyglucose positron emission tomography as a predictor of pathologic grade and other prognostic variables in bone and soft tissue sarcoma. Clin Cancer Res. 2000;6(4):1279–87.

Foukas AF, Deshmukh NS, Grimer RJ, Mangham DC, Mangos EG, Taylor S. Stage-IIB osteosarcomas around the knee. a study of MMP-9 in surviving tumour cells. J Bone Joint Surg. 2002;84B(5):706–11.

Fuchs B, Valenzuela RG, Sim FH. Pathologic fracture as a complication in the treatment of Ewing's sarcoma. Clin Orthop Relat Res. 2003;415:25–30.

Ginsberg JP, de Alava E, Ladanyi M, Wexler LH, Kovar H, Paulussen M, et al. EWS-FLI1 and EWS-ERG gene fusions are associated with similar clinical phenotypes in Ewing's sarcoma. J Clin Oncol. 1999;17(6):1809–14.

Gorlick R, Huvos AG, Heller G, Aledo A, Beardsley GP, Healey JH, et al. Expression of HER2/erbB-2 correlates with survival in osteosarcoma. J Clin Oncol. 1999;17(9):2781–8.

Ham SJ, Kroon HM, Koops HS, Hoekstra HJ. Osteosarcoma of the pelvis: oncologist results of 40 patients registered by The Netherlands committee on bone tumours. Eur J Surg Oncol. 2000;26(1):53–60.

Hameetman L, Rozeman LB, Lombaerts M, Oosting J, Taminiau AH, Cleton-Jansen AM, et al. Peripheral chondrosarcoma progression is accompanied by decreased Indian hedgehog signaling. J Pathol. 2006;209(4):501–11.

Hayden JB, Hoang BH. Osteosarcoma: basic science and clinical implications. Orthop Clin North Am. 2006;37(1):1–7.

Heck RK, Stacy GS, Flaherty MJ, Montag AG, Peabody TD, Simon MA. A comparison study of staging systems for bone sarcomas. Clin Orthop Relat Res. 2003;415:64–71.

Heck RK, Peabody TD, Simon MA. Staging of primary malignancies of bone. CA Cancer J Clin. 2006;56(6):366–75.

Hernandez-Rodriguez NA, Correa E, Sotelo R, Contreras-Paredes A, Gomez-Ruiz C, Green L, et al. Ki-67: a proliferative marker that may predict pulmonary metastases and mortality of primary osteosarcoma. Cancer Detect Prev. 2001;25(2):210–5.

Hornicek FJ, Gebhardt MC, Wolfe MW, Kharrazi FD, Takeshita H, Parekh SG, et al. P-glycoprotein levels predict poor outcome in patients with osteosarcoma. Clin Orthop Relat Res. 2000;373:11–7.

Huang HY, Illei PB, Zhao Z, Mazumdar M, Huvos AG, Healey JH, et al. Ewing sarcomas with p53 mutation or p16/p14ARF homozygous deletion: a highly lethal subset associated with poor chemoresponse. J Clin Oncol. 2005;23(3):548–58.

Jadvar H, Gamie S, Ramanna L, Conti PS. Musculoskeleta system. Semin Nucl Med. 2004;34(4):254–61.

Kager L, Zoubek A, Potschger U, et al. Primary metastatic osteosarcoma: presentation and outcome of patients treated on neoadjuvant cooperative osteosarcoma study group protocols. J Clin Oncol. 2003;21:2011–8.

Kaya M, Wada T, Akatsuka T, Kawaguchi S, Nagoya S, Shindoh M, et al. Vascular endothelial growth factor expression in untreated osteosarcoma is predictive of pulmonary metastasis and poor prognosis. Clin Cancer Res. 2000;6(2):572–7.

Kim MS, Cho WH, Song WS, Lee SY, Jeon DC. Time dependency of prognostic factors in patients with stage II osteosarcomas. Clin Orthop Relat Res. 2007;463:157–65.

Kneisl JS, Patt JC, Johnson JC, Zuger JH. Is PET useful in detecting occult non-pulmonary metastases in pediatric bone sarcomas? Clin Orthop Relat Res. 2006;450:101–4.

Leerapun T, Hugate RR, Inwards CY, Scully SP, Sim FH. Surgical management of conventional grade I chondrosarcoma of long bones. Clin Orthop Relat Res. 2007;463:166–72.

Lewis DR, Ries LA. Cancer of the bone and joint (chapter 10). In: Gloeckler Ries LA, Young JL, Keel GE, Eisner MP, Lin YD, Horner M-J, editors. Cancer survival among adults: US seer program, 1988–2001 (patient and tumor characteristics, National Cancer Institute). Bethesda, MD: NIH Publication No. 07-6215; 2007. p. 81–8.

Lin PP, Jaffe N, Herzog CE, Costelloe CM, Deavers MT, Kelly JS, et al. Chemotherapy response in an important predictor of local recurrence in Ewing sarcoma. Cancer. 2007;109(3):603–11.

Maitra A, Roberts H, Weinberg AG, Geradts J. Aberrant expression of tumor suppressor proteins in the Ewing family of tumors. Arch Pathol Lab Med. 2001;125(9):1207–12.

Mankin HJ, Hornicek FJ, Rosenberg AE, Harmon DC. Survival data for 648 patients with osteosarcoma treated at one institution. Clin Orthop Relat Res. 2004;429:286–91.

Matsunobu T, Tanaka K, Matsumoto Y, Nakatani F, Sakimura R, Hanada M, et al. The prognostic and therapeutic relevance of p27kip1 in Ewing's family tumors. Clin Cancer Res. 2004;10(3):1003–12.

Miller SL, Hoffer FA, Reddick WE, Wu S, Glasso JO, Gronemeyer SA, et al. Tumor volume or dynamic contrast-enhanced MRI for prediction of clinical outcome of Ewing sarcoma family of tumors. Pediatr Radiol. 2001;31(7): 518–23.

O'Sullivan B, Catton CN. Soft tissue sarcomas (chapter 23). In: Gospodarowicz MK, O'Sullivan B, Sobin LH, editors. Prognostic factors in cancer (third edition). New York: Wiley; 2006. p. 181–6.

Ozaki T, Flege S, Liljenqvist U, et al. Osteosarcoma of the spine: experience of the cooperative osteosarcoma study group. Cancer (Phila). 2002;94: 1069–77.

Paulussen M, Ahrens S, Dunst J, Winkelmann W, Exner GU, Kotz R, et al. Localized Ewing tumor of bone: final results of the cooperative Ewing's sarcoma study CESS 86. J Clin Oncol. 2001;19(6):1818–29.

Peabody TD, Gibbs CP, Simon MA. Evaluation and staging of musculoskeletal neoplasms. J Bone Joint Surg. 1998;80A:1204–18.

Pring ME, Weber KL, Unni KK, et al. Chondrosarcoma of the pelvis. A review of sixty-four cases. J Bone Joint Surg. 2001;83A:1630–42.

Reith JD, Horodyski MB, Scarborough MT. Grade 2 chondrosarcoma: stage i or stage ii tumor? Clin Orthop. 2003;415:45–51.

Rodriguez-Galindo C, Shah N, McCarville MB, Billups CA, Neel MN, Rao BN, et al. Outcome after local recurrence of osteosarcoma: The St. Jude Children's Research Hospital Experience (1970–2000). Cancer. 2004;100(9): 1928–35.

Rosier RN, Bukata SV. Sarcomas of bone (chapter 57). In: Chang AE, Ganz PA, Hayes DF, Kinsella TJ, Pass HI, Schiller JH, Stone RM, Strecher VJ, editors. Oncology: an evidence-based approach. New York: Springer; 2006. p. 1025–38.

Rougraff BT, Simon MA, Kneisl JS, Greenberg DB, Mankin, HJ. Limb salvage compared with amputation for osteosarcoma of the distal end of the femur: a long-term oncological, functional, and quality-of-life study. J Bone Joint Surg. 1994;76A:649–56.

Rozeman LB, Hogendoorn PC, Bovee JV. Diagnosis and prognosis of chondrosarcoma of bone. Expert Rev Mol Diagn. 2002;2(5):461–72.

Saifuddin A. The accuracy of imaging in the local staging of appendicular osteosarcoma. Skeletal Radiol. 2002;31(4):191–201.

Sanders RP, Drissi R, Billups CA, Daw NC, Valentine MB, Dome JS. Telomerase expression predicts unfavorable outcome in osteosarcoma. J Clin Oncol. 2004;22(18):3790–7.

Scully SP, Ghert MA, Zurakowski D, Thompson RC, Gebhardt MC. Pathologic fracture in osteosarcoma: prognostic importance and treatment implications. J Bone Joint Surg. 2002;84:49–57.

Serra M, Scotland K, Reverter-Branchat G, Ferrari S, Manara MC, Benini S, et al. Value of P-glycoprotein and clinicopathologic factors as the basis for new treatment strategies in high-grade osteosarcoma of the extremities. J Clin Oncol. 2003;21(3):536–42.

Serra M, Pasello M, Manara MC, Scotlandi K, Ferrari S, Bertoni F, et al. May P-glycoprotein status be used to stratify high-grade osteosarcoma patients? Results from the Italian/Scandinavian sarcoma group 1 treatment protocol. Int J Oncol. 2006;29(6):1459–68.

Smeland S, Muller C, Alvegard TA, et al. Scandanavian sarcoma group osteosarcoma study SSG VIII: prognostic factors for outcome and the role of replacement salvage chemotherapy for poor histological responders. Eur J Cancer. 2003;39:488–94.

Soderstrom M, Ekfors TO, Bohling TO, et al. No improvement in the overall survival of 194 patients with chondrosarcoma in Finland in 1971–1990. Acta Orthop Scand. 2003;74:344–50.

Somers GR, Ho M, Zielenska M, Squire JA, Thorner PS. HER2 amplification and overexpression is not present in pediatric osteosarcoma: a tissue microarray study. Pediatr Dev Pathol. 2005;8(5):525–32.

Sucato DJ, Rougraff B, McGrath BE, Sizinski J, Davis M, Papandonatos G, Green D, Szarzanowicz T. Ewing's sarcoma of the pelvis. Long-term survival and functional outcome. Clin Orthop Relat Res. 2000;373:193–201.

Sulzbacher I, Birner P, Trieb K, Traxler M, Lang S, Chott A. Expression of platelet-derived growth factor-AA is associated with tumor progression in osteosarcoma. Mod Pathol. 2003;16(1):66–71.

Talac R, Yaszemski MJ, Currier BL, et al. Relationship between surgical margins and local recurrence in sarcomas of the spine. Clin Orthop. 2002;397: 127–32.

Trieb K, Lehner R, Stulnig T, Sulzbacher I, Shroyer KR. Survivin expression in human osteosarcoma is a marker for survival. Eur J Surg Oncol. 2003;29(4): 379–82.

Tsuchiya T, Sekine K, Hinohara S, Namiki T, Nobori T, Kaneko Y. Analysis of the p16INK4, p14ARF, p15, TP53, and MDM2 genes and their prognostic implications in osteosarcoma and Ewing sarcoma. Cancer Genet Cytogenet. 2000;120(2):91–8.

Tsukahara T, Kawaguchi S, Torigoe T, Asanuma H, Nakazawa E, Shimozawa K, et al. Prognostic significance of HLA class I expression in osteosarcoma defined by anti-pan HLA class I monoclonal antibody, EMR8–5. Cancer Sci. 2006;97(12):1374–80.

Uozaki H, Ishida T, Kakiuchi C, Horiuchi H, Gotoh T, Iijima T, Imamura T, Machinami R. Expression of heat shock proteins in osteosarcoma and its relationship to prognosis. Pathol Res Pract. 2000;196(10):665–73.

van Beerendonk HM, Rozeman LB, Taminiau AH, Sciot R, Bovee JV, Cleton-Jansen AM, et al. Molecular analysis of the INK4A/INK4A-arf gene locus in conventional (central) chondrosarcomas and enchondromas: indication of an important gene for tumour progression. J Pathol. 2004;202(3): 359–66.

Willmore-Payne C, Holden JA, Zhou H, Gupta D, Hirschowitz S, Wittwer CT, et al. Evaluation of Her-2/neu gene status in osteosarcoma by fluorescence in situ hybridization and multiplex and monoplex polymerase chain reactions. Arch Pathol Lab Med. 2006;130(5):691–8.

Wuisman P, Enneking WF. Prognosis for patients who have osteosarcoma with skip metastasis. J Bone Joint Surg. 1990;72A(1):60–8.

Yang R, Hoang BH, Kubo T, Kawano H, Chou A, Sowers R, et al. Over-expression of parathyroid hormone type 1 receptor confers an aggressive phenotype in osteosarcoma. Int J Cancer. 2007;121(5):943–54.

---

Zhou H, Randall RL, Brothman AR, Maxwell T, Coffin CM, Goldsby RE. Her-2/neu expression in osteosarcoma increases risk of lung metastasis and can be associated with gene amplification. J Pediatr Hematol Oncol. 2003;25(1):27–32.

Zoubek A, Dockhorn-Dworniczak B, Delattre O, Christiansen H, Niggli F, Gatterer-Menz I, et al. Does expression of different EWS chimeric transcripts define clinically distinct risk groups of ewing tumor patients. J Clin Oncol. 1996;14(4):1245–51.

# Soft Tissue Sarcoma

*(Kaposi's sarcoma, fibromatosis [desmoid tumor], and sarcoma arising from the dura mater, brain, parenchymatous organs, or hollow viscera are not included.)*

## *At-A-Glance*

### SUMMARY OF CHANGES

- Gastrointestinal stromal tumor (GIST) is now included in Chap. 16; fibromatosis (desmoid tumor), Kaposi's sarcoma, and infantile fibrosarcoma are no longer included in the histological types for this site

- Angiosarcoma, extraskeletal Ewing's sarcoma, and dermatofibrosarcoma protuberans have been added to the list of histologic types for this site

- N1 disease has been reclassified as Stage III rather than Stage IV disease

- Grading has been reformatted from a four grade to a three-grade system as per the criteria recommended by the College of American Pathologists

### ANATOMIC STAGE/PROGNOSTIC GROUPS

| Stage | T | N | M | G |
|---|---|---|---|---|
| Stage IA | T1a | N0 | M0 | G1, GX |
| | T1b | N0 | M0 | G1, GX |
| Stage IB | T2a | N0 | M0 | G1, GX |
| | T2b | N0 | M0 | G1, GX |
| Stage IIA | T1a | N0 | M0 | G2, G3 |
| | T1b | N0 | M0 | G2, G3 |
| Stage IIB | T2a | N0 | M0 | G2 |
| | T2b | N0 | M0 | G2 |
| Stage III | T2a, T2b | N0 | M0 | G3 |
| | Any T | N1 | M0 | Any G |
| Stage IV | Any T | Any N | M1 | Any G |

**ICD-O-3 TOPOGRAPHY CODES**

| | |
|---|---|
| C38.0 | Heart |
| C38.1 | Anterior mediastinum |
| C38.2 | Posterior mediastinum |
| C38.3 | Mediastinum, NOS |
| C38.8 | Overlapping lesion of heart, mediastinum, and pleura |
| C47.0 | Peripheral nerves and autonomic nervous system of head, face, and neck |
| C47.1 | Peripheral nerves and autonomic nervous system of upper limb and shoulder |
| C47.2 | Peripheral nerves and autonomic nervous system of lower limb and hip |

| C47.3 | Peripheral nerves and autonomic nervous system of thorax | C48.0 | Retro-peritoneum | | soft tissues of thorax |
|---|---|---|---|---|---|
| | | C48.1 | Specified parts of peritoneum | C49.4 | Connective, subcutane-ous, and other soft tissues of abdomen |
| C47.4 | Peripheral nerves and autonomic nervous system of abdomen | C48.2 | Peritoneum, NOS | | |
| | | C48.8 | Overlapping lesion of retro-peritoneum and peritoneum | C49.5 | Connective, subcutaneous, and other soft tissues of pelvis |
| C47.5 | Peripheral nerves and autonomic nervous system of pelvis | C49.0 | Connective, subcutaneous, and other soft tissues of head, face, and neck | C49.6 | Connective, subcutane-ous, and other soft tissues of trunk, NOS |
| C47.6 | Peripheral nerves and autonomic nervous system of trunk, NOS | C49.1 | Connective, subcutane-ous, and other soft tissues of upper limb and shoulder | C49.8 | Overlapping lesion of con-nective, subcuta-neous, and other soft tissues |
| C47.8 | Overlap-ping lesion of peripheral nerves and autonomic nervous system | C49.2 | Connective, subcutaneous, and other soft tissues of lower limb and hip | C49.9 | Connective, subcutaneous, and other soft tissues, NOS |
| C47.9 | Autonomic nervous sys-tem, NOS | C49.3 | Connective, subcutane-ous, and other | ICD-O-3 HISTOLOGY CODE RANGES 8800–8820, 8823–8935, 8940–9136, 9142–9582 | |

## INTRODUCTION

The staging system applies to all soft tissue sarcomas except Kaposi's sarcoma, gastrointestinal stromal tumors, fibromatosis (desmoid tumor), and infantile fibrosarcoma. In addition, sarcomas arising within the confines of the dura mater, including the brain, and sarcomas arising in parenchymatous organs and from hollow viscera are not optimally staged by this system.

Data to support this staging system are based on current analyses from multiple institutions and represent the recommendations of an AJCC task force on soft tissue sarcoma. In the era of cytoreductive neoadjuvant treatments, clinical and pathologic staging may be altered in the future. Because pathologic staging drives adjuvant therapy decisions, patients should be restaged after neoadjuvant therapies have been administered.

Histologic type, grade, and tumor size and depth are essential for staging. Histologic grade of a sarcoma is one of the most important param-eters of the staging system. Grade is based on analysis of various pathologic features of a tumor, such as histologic subtype, degree of differentiation, mitotic activity, and necrosis. Accurate grading requires an adequate sample of well-fixed tissue for evaluation. Accurate grading is not always possible on the basis of needle biopsies or in tumors that have been previously irradiated or treated with chemotherapy. The current staging system does not take into account anatomic site. However, anatomic site is known to influence outcome, and therefore outcome data should be reported specifying site. This is particularly applicable in sites such as head and neck and retroperitoneum, where grade (head and neck) or size (retroperitoneum) may disproportionately drive prognosis relative to other staging criteria in comparison with sarcomas arising elsewhere in the body. Primary sarcomas of the breast are another special situation in which the tumor should be staged and managed as would any comparably staged sarcoma located elsewhere in the body (e.g., staged and treated in a manner analogous to an extremity sarcoma). Generic grouping of site is accepted. The following site groups can be used for reports that include sarcomas arising in tissues other than soft tissues (such as parenchymal organs). Extremity and superficial trunk can be combined; viscera, including all the intra-abdominal viscera, can also be combined. Where enough numbers exist, these can be reported by subdivision into the various components of the gastrointestinal tract. Lung, gastrointestinal, genitourinary, and gynecologic sarcomas should be grouped separately.

**Site Groups for Soft Tissue Sarcoma**

Head and neck
Extremity and superficial trunk
Gastrointestinal
Genitourinary
Visceral retroperitoneal
Gynecologic
Breast
Lung, pleura, mediastinum
Other

## ANATOMY

### Staging of Soft Tissue Sarcoma

**Inclusions.** The present staging system applies to soft tissue sarcomas. Primary sarcomas can arise from a variety of soft tissues. These tissues include fibrous connective tissue, fat, smooth or striated muscle, vascular tissue, peripheral neural tissue, and visceral tissue.

**Regional Lymph Nodes.** Involvement of regional lymph nodes by soft tissue sarcomas is uncommon in adults.

**Metastatic Sites.** Metastatic sites for soft tissue sarcoma are often dependent on the original site of the primary lesion. For example, the most common site of metastatic disease for patients with extremity sarcoma is the lung, whereas retroperitoneal and gastrointestinal sarcomas often have liver as the first site of metastasis.

# RULES FOR CLASSIFICATION

**Clinical Staging.** Clinical staging is dependent on characteristics of T, N, and M. T is divided into lesions of maximum dimension 5 cm or less and lesions of more than 5 cm in greatest dimension. Tumor size can be measured clinically or radiologically. Metastatic disease should be described according to the most likely sites of metastasis. In general, the minimal clinical staging workup of soft tissue sarcoma is accomplished by axial imaging of the involved site using MRI or CT scan and by imaging of the lungs, the most likely site for occult metastatic disease, using chest CT scans.

**Pathologic Staging.** Pathologic (pTNM) staging consists of the removal and pathologic evaluation of the primary tumor and clinical/radiologic evaluation for regional and distant metastases. In circumstances where it is not possible to obtain accurate measurements of the excised primary sarcoma specimen, it is acceptable to use radiologic assessment to assign a pT stage using the dimensions of the sarcoma. In examining the primary tumor, the pathologist should subclassify the lesion and assign a histopathologic grade. Occasionally, immunohistochemistry or cytogenetics may be necessary for accurate assignment of subtype. Assignment of grade can be affected by prior administration of chemotherapy and/or radiotherapy. Lesions initially assigned a high-grade status, after response to presurgical treatments, may have a less ominous appearance on microscopic examination and therefore may be assigned a lower grade than the initial designation; occasionally, the reverse situation is observed due to either sampling error or presurgical treatment elimination of lower grade cells in these typically heterogeneous tumors.

**Definition of T.** Although size is currently designated as ≤5 cm or >5 cm, particular emphasis should be placed on providing size measurements (or even volume determinants) in sites other than the extremity or superficial trunk. Size should be regarded as a continuous variable, with 5 cm as merely an arbitrary division that makes it possible to dichotomize patient populations.

**Depth.** Depth is evaluated relative to the investing fascia of the extremity and trunk. *Superficial* is defined as lack of any involvement of the superficial investing muscular fascia in extremity or trunk lesions. For staging, nonsuperficial head and neck, intrathoracic, intra-abdominal, retroperitoneal, and visceral lesions are considered to be deep lesions.

Depth is also an independent variable and is defined as follows:

1. Superficial – located entirely in the subcutaneous tissues without any degree of extension through the muscular fascia or into underlying muscle. In these cases, pretreatment imaging studies demonstrate a subcutaneous tumor without involvement of muscle, and excisional pathology reports demonstrate a tumor located within the subcutaneous tissues without extension into underlying muscle.

2. Deep – located partly or completely within one or more muscle groups within the extremity. Deep tumors may extend through the muscular fascia into the subcutaneous tissues or even to the skin but the critical criterion is location of any portion of the tumor within the muscular compartments of the extremity. In these cases, pretreatment imaging studies demonstrate a tumor located completely or in part within the muscular compartments of the extremity.

3. Depth is evaluated in relation to tumor size (T):
   a. Tumor $\leq 5$ cm: T1a = superficial, T1b = deep
   b. Tumor $> 5$ cm: T2a = superficial, T2b = deep

**Nodal Disease.** Nodal involvement is rare in adult soft tissue sarcomas. In the assigning of stage group, patients whose nodal status is not determined to be positive for tumor, either clinically or pathologically, should be designated as N0.

**Grade.** Grade should be assigned to all sarcomas. Historically the AJCC soft tissue staging system has used a four-grade system, but within the soft tissue sarcoma staging groups this effectively functioned as a two-stage system by combining G1/G2 (low) and G3/G4 (high). The traditional AJCC grading system based on differentiation (well, moderate, poor, and undifferentiated) is poorly suited to soft tissue sarcoma. Comprehensive grading of soft tissue sarcomas is strongly correlated with disease-specific survival and incorporates differentiation (histology-specific), mitotic rate, and extent of necrosis. The two most widely employed grading systems, French (FNCLCC) and NIH, are three-grade systems. In accordance with the College of American Pathologists (CAP) recommendations (see Rubin et al. below), the French system (see Guillou et al. below) is preferred over the NIH system for reasons of ease of use/reproducibility and perhaps slightly superior performance. This revision of the AJCC staging system incorporates a three-tiered grading system. Applying histologic grading to core needle biopsies is problematic when neoadjuvant chemotherapy or radiation has been administered. However, given the importance of grade to staging and treatment, efforts to separate sarcomas on needle biopsies into at least two tiers (i.e., low and high grade) as described above are encouraged. In many instances the type of sarcoma will readily permit this distinction (i.e., Ewing sarcoma/PNET, malignant fibrous histiocytoma), whereas in less obvious instances the difficulty of assigning grade should be noted. In general, multiple core needle biopsies disclosing a high-grade sarcoma can be regarded as high grade since the probability of subsequent downgrading is remote, but limited cores biopsies of low-grade sarcoma carry a risk of subsequent upgrading.

**FNCLCC Grading.** The FNCLCC grade is determined by three parameters: differentiation (histology specific), mitotic activity, and extent of necrosis. Each parameter is scored: differentiation (1–3), mitotic activity (1–3), and necrosis (0–2). The scores are summed to designate grade.

Grade 1    2 or 3
Grade 2    4 or 5
Grade 3    6–8

**TABLE 28.1.** Histology-specific tumor differentiation score

| Histologic type | Score |
|---|---|
| Atypical lipomatous tumor/well-differentiated liposarcoma | 1 |
| Myxoid liposarcoma | 2 |
| Round cell liposarcoma | 3 |
| Pleomorphic liposarcoma | 3 |
| Dedifferentiated liposarcoma | 3 |
| Fibrosarcoma | 2 |
| Myxofibrosarcoma [myxoid malignant fibrous histiocytoma (MFH)] | 2 |
| Typical storiform MFH (sarcoma, NOS) | 2 |
| MFH, pleomorphic type (patternless pleomorphic sarcoma) | 3 |
| Giant cell and inflammatory MFH (pleomorphic sarcoma, NOS with giant cells or inflammatory cells) | 3 |
| Well-differentiated leiomyosarcoma | 1 |
| Conventional leiomyosarcoma | 2 |
| Poorly differentiated/pleomorphic/epithelioid leiomyosarcoma | 3 |
| Biphasic/monophasic synovial sarcoma | 3 |
| Poorly differentiated synovial sarcoma | 3 |
| Pleomorphic rhabdomyosarcoma | 3 |
| Mesenchymal chondrosarcoma | 3 |
| Extraskeletal osteosarcoma | 3 |
| Ewing sarcoma/primitive neuroectodermal tumor | 3 |
| Malignant rhabdoid tumor | 3 |
| Undifferentiated sarcoma | 3 |

*Note*: Grading of malignant peripheral nerve sheath tumor, embryonal and alveolar rhabdomyosarcoma, angiosarcoma, extraskeletal myxoid chondrosarcoma, alveolar soft part sarcoma, clear cell sarcoma, and epithelioid sarcoma is not recommended under this system.

Modified from Guillou L, Coindre JM, Bonichon F, et al. Comparative study of the National Cancer Institute and French Federation of Cancer Centers Sarcoma Group grading systems in a population of 410 adult patients with soft tissue sarcoma. J Clin Oncol. 1997;15:350–62, with permission.

***Differentiation.*** Tumor differentiation is histology specific and is generally scored as follows:

Score 1    Sarcomas closely resembling normal, mature mesenchymal tissue
Score 2    Sarcomas of definite histologic type
Score 3    Synovial sarcomas, embryonal sarcomas, undifferentiated sarcomas, and sarcomas of unknown/doubtful tumor type

Tumor differentiation score is the most subjective aspect of the FNCLCC system (Table 28.1). In addition, it is not validated for every subtype of sarcoma and inapplicable to certain subtypes as noted below. However, this score is critical given its proportional weight such that any sarcoma assigned a differentiation score of 3 will be at least intermediate to high grade.

***Mitotic Count.*** In the most mitotically active area of the sarcoma, ten successive high-power fields (HPFs) (one HPF at 400× magnification = 0.1734 mm$^2$) are assessed using a 40× objective.

Score 1    0–9 mitoses per 10 HPFs
Score 2    10–19 mitoses per 10 HPFs
Score 3    20 or more mitoses per 10 HPFs

*Tumor Necrosis.* Evaluated on gross examination and validated with histologic sections.

Score 0    No tumor necrosis
Score 1    Less than or equal to 50% tumor necrosis
Score 2    More than 50% tumor necrosis

**Restaging of Recurrent Tumors.** The same staging should be used when a patient requires restaging of sarcoma recurrence. Such reports should specify whether patients have primary lesions or lesions that were previously treated and have subsequently recurred. The identification and reporting of etiologic factors such as radiation exposure and inherited or genetic syndromes are encouraged. Appropriate workup for recurrent sarcoma should include cross-sectional imaging (CT scan or MRI scan) of the tumor, a CT scan of the chest, and a tissue biopsy to confirm diagnosis prior to initiation of therapy.

## PROGNOSTIC FEATURES

**Neurovascular and Bone Invasion.** In earlier staging systems, neurovascular and bone invasion by soft tissue sarcomas had been included as a determinant of stage. It is not included in the current staging system, and no plans are proposed to add it at the present time. Nevertheless, neurovascular and bone invasion should always be reported where possible, and further studies are needed to determine whether or not such invasion is an independent prognostic factor.

**Molecular Markers.** Molecular markers and genetic abnormalities are being evaluated as determinants of outcome. At the present time, however, insufficient data exist to include specific molecular markers in the staging system.

    For the present time, molecular and genetic markers should be considered as important information to aid in histopathologic diagnosis, rather than as determinants of stage.

**Validation.** The current staging system has the capacity to discriminate the overall survival of patients with soft tissue sarcoma. Patients with Stage I lesions are at low risk for disease-related mortality, whereas Stages II and III entail progressively greater risk.

## DEFINITION OF TNM

### Primary Tumor (T)

| | |
|---|---|
| TX | Primary tumor cannot be assessed |
| T0 | No evidence of primary tumor |
| T1 | Tumor 5 cm or less in greatest dimension* |
| T1a | Superficial tumor |
| T1b | Deep tumor |
| T2 | Tumor more than 5 cm in greatest dimension* |
| T2a | Superficial tumor |
| T2b | Deep tumor |

*Note: Superficial tumor is located exclusively above the superficial fascia without invasion of the fascia; deep tumor is located either exclusively beneath the superficial fascia, superficial to the fascia with invasion of or through the fascia, or both superficial yet beneath the fascia.

### Regional Lymph Nodes (N)

| | |
|---|---|
| NX | Regional lymph nodes cannot be assessed |
| N0 | No regional lymph node metastasis |
| N1* | Regional lymph node metastasis |

*Note: Presence of positive nodes (N1) in M0 tumors is considered Stage III.

### Distant Metastasis (M)

| | |
|---|---|
| M0 | No distant metastasis |
| M1 | Distant metastasis |

### ANATOMIC STAGE/PROGNOSTIC GROUPS

| Stage IA | T1a | N0 | M0 | G1, GX |
|---|---|---|---|---|
| | T1b | N0 | M0 | G1, GX |
| Stage IB | T2a | N0 | M0 | G1, GX |
| | T2b | N0 | M0 | G1, GX |
| Stage IIA | T1a | N0 | M0 | G2, G3 |
| | T1b | N0 | M0 | G2, G3 |
| Stage IIB | T2a | N0 | M0 | G2 |
| | T2b | N0 | M0 | G2 |
| Stage III | T2a, T2b | N0 | M0 | G3 |
| | Any T | N1 | M0 | Any G |
| Stage IV | Any T | Any N | M1 | Any G |

### PROGNOSTIC FACTORS (SITE-SPECIFIC FACTORS)
### (Recommended for Collection)

| | |
|---|---|
| Required for staging | Grade |
| Clinically significant | Neurovascular invasion as determined by pathology |
| | Bone invasion as determined by imaging |
| | If pM1, source of pathologic metastatic specimen |

**TABLE 28.2.** Five-year survival rates in extremity soft tissue sarcoma

| Stage | N | Freedom from local recurrence (%) | Disease-free survival (%) | Overall survival (%) |
|-------|-----|-------|-------|-------|
| I | 137 | 88.04 | 86.13 | 90.00 |
| II | 491 | 81.97 | 71.68 | 80.89 |
| III | 469 | 83.44 | 51.77 | 56.29 |

Local recurrence, disease-free survival, and overall survival by stage.

Source: Data from Memorial Sloan-Kettering Cancer Center (MSKCC) for the time period of July 1, 1982 to June 30, 2000.

Table 28.2 presents the 5-year survival rates in extremity soft tissue sarcomas.

## HISTOLOGIC GRADE (G)

(FNCLCC System Preferred)

| | |
|-----|-----|
| GX | Grade cannot be assessed |
| G1 | Grade 1 |
| G2 | Grade 2 |
| G3 | Grade 3 |

## HISTOPATHOLOGIC TYPE

Tumors included in the soft tissue category are listed below as per the 2002 World Health Organization classification of tumors:

Adipocytic Tumors
> Dedifferentiated liposarcoma*
> Myxoid/round cell liposarcoma
> Pleomorphic liposarcoma

Fibroblastic/Myofibroblastic Tumors
> Fibrosarcoma**
> Myxofibrosarcoma, low grade
> Low-grade fibromyxoid sarcoma
> Sclerosing epithelioid fibrosarcoma

So-called Fibrohistiocytic Tumors
> Undifferentiated pleomorphic sarcoma/malignant fibrous histiocytoma (MFH) (including pleomorphic, giant cell, myxoid/high-grade myxofibrosarcoma and inflammatory forms)

Smooth Muscle Tumors
> Leiomyosarcoma

Skeletal Muscle Tumors
> Rhabdomyosarcoma (embryonal, alveolar, and pleomorphic forms)

Vascular Tumors
> Epithelioid hemangioendothelioma
> Angiosarcoma, deep***

Tumors of Peripheral Nerves
> Malignant peripheral nerve sheath tumor

Chondro-osseous Tumors
    Extraskeletal chondrosarcoma
      (mesenchymal and other variants)
    Extraskeletal osteosarcoma
Tumors of Uncertain Differentiation
    Synovial sarcoma
    Epithelioid sarcoma
    Alveolar soft part sarcoma
    Clear cell sarcoma of soft tissue
    Extraskeletal myxoid chondrosarcoma
    Primitive neuroectodermal tumor (PNET)/extraskeletal Ewing
      tumor
    Desmoplastic small round cell tumor
    Extrarenal rhabdoid tumor
    Undifferentiated sarcoma; sarcoma, not otherwise specified
    (NOS)

*Notes*: *It is recognized that dedifferentiated liposarcoma primarily arises in the context of deep atypical lipomatous tumor/well-differentiated liposarcoma, a sarcoma of intermediate malignancy due to lack of metastatic capacity.

**The category of fibrosarcoma can be considered to be inclusive of fibrosarcomatous differentiation in dermatofibrosarcoma protuberans.

***Cutaneous angiosarcoma may be difficult to stage using the AJCC system. Gastrointestinal stromal tumor (GIST) is addressed in Chap. 16.)

The following histologic types are *not* included: inflammatory myofibroblastic tumor, fibromatosis (desmoid tumor), mesothelioma, sarcomas arising in tissues apart from soft tissue (e.g., parenchymal organs).

## BIBLIOGRAPHY

Behranwala KA, A'Hern R, Omar AM, et al. Prognosis of lymph node metastasis in soft tissue sarcoma. Ann Surg Oncol. 2004;11:714–9.

Billingsley KG, Burt ME, Jara E, Ginsberg RJ, Woodruff JM, Leung DHY, et al. Pulmonary metastases from soft tissue sarcoma: analysis of patterns of disease and postmetastasis survival. Ann Surg. 1999;229(5):602–10.

Brennan MF. Staging of soft tissue sarcomas. Ann Surg Oncol. 1999;6:8–9.

Brennan MF, Kattan MW, Klimstra D, et al. Prognostic nomogram for patients undergoing resection for adenocarcinoma of the pancreas. Ann Surg. 2004; 240:293–8.

Coindre JM. Pathology and grading of soft tissue sarcomas. Cancer Treat Res. 1993;67:1–22.

Coindre JM, Terrier P, Bui NB, Bonichon F, Collin CF, Le Doussal V, et al. Prognostic factors in adult patients with locally controlled soft tissue sarcoma: a study of 546 patients from the French Federation of Cancer Centers Sarcoma Group. J Clin Oncol. 1996;14(3):869–77.

Dalal KM, Kattan MW, Antonescu CR, et al. Subtype specific prognostic nomogram for patients with primary liposarcoma of the retroperitoneum, extremity, or trunk. Ann Surg. 2006;244:381–91.

Fleming JB, Berman R, Cheng S, Chen NP, Hunt K, Feig BW, et al. Long-term outcome of patients with American Joint Committee on Cancer Stage IIB extremity soft tissue sarcoma. J Clin Oncol. 1999;17(9):2772–80.

Guillou L, Coindre JM, Bonichon F, Bui NB, Terrier P, Collin CF, et al. Comparative study of the National Cancer Institute and French Federation of Cancer Centers Sarcoma Group grading systems in a population of 410 adult patients with soft tissue sarcoma. J Clin Oncol. 1997;15:350–62.

Heslin MJ, Lewis JJ, Nadler E, Newman E, Woodruff JM, Casper ES, et al. Prognostic factors associated with long-term survival for retroperitoneal sarcoma: implications for management. J Clin Oncol. 1997;15(8):2832–9.

Kattan MW, Leung DH, Brennan MF. Postoperative nomogram for 12-year sarcoma-specific death. J Clin Oncol. 2002;20:791–6.

Kattan MW, Heller G, Brennan MF. A competing-risks nomogram for sarcoma-specific death following local recurrence. Stat Med. 2003;22:3515–25.

Kotilingam D, Lev DC, Lazar AJ, Pollock RE. Staging soft tissue sarcoma: evolution and change. CA Cancer J Clin. 2006;56:282–91.

Pisters PWT, Pollock RE. Prognostic factors in soft tissue sarcoma. In: Gospodarowicz M, O'Sullivan B, editors. UICC: prognostic factors in cancer. New York: Wiley; 2006.

Pisters PWT, Leung DHY, Woodruff JM, Shi W, Brennan MF. Analysis of prognostic factors in 1041 patients with localized soft tissue sarcomas of the extremities. J Clin Oncol. 1996;14:1679–89.

Riad S, Griffin AM, Liberman B, et al. Lymph node metastasis in soft tissue sarcoma in an extremity. Clin Orthop Relat Res. 2004;426:129–34.

Rubin, BP, Fletcher CDM, Inwards C, et al. Protocol for the examination of specimens from patients with soft tissue tumors of intermediate malignant potential, malignant soft tissue tumors, and borderline/locally aggressive and malignant bone tumors. Arch Pathol Lab Med. 2006;130(11):1616–29.

Van Glabbeke M, van Oosterom AT, Oosterhuis JW, Mouridsen H, Crowther D, Somers R, et al. Prognostic factors for the outcome of chemotherapy in advanced soft tissue sarcoma: an analysis of 2185 patients treated with anthracycline-containing first-line regimens – European Organization for Research and Treatment of Cancer Soft Tissue and Bone Sarcoma Group study. J Clin Oncol. 1999;17(1):150–7.

Weiss SW, Goldblum JR. Enzinger and Weiss's soft tissue tumor, 4th ed. Philadelphia, PA: Mosby-Harcourt Brace; 2001.

World Health Organization classification of tumours. Pathology and genetics. Tumours of soft tissue and bone. Lyon: IARC; 2002.

**28**

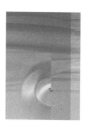

# PART VI
# Skin

# Cutaneous Squamous Cell Carcinoma and Other Cutaneous Carcinomas

## At-A-Glance

### SUMMARY OF CHANGES

- The previous edition chapter, entitled "Carcinoma of the Skin," has been eliminated and two chapters have been created in its place:

  - Merkel Cell Carcinoma: An entirely new chapter specifically for Merkel cell carcinoma (MCC) has been designed (see Chap. 30)

  - This chapter has been renamed "Cutaneous Squamous Cell Carcinoma and Other Cutaneous Carcinomas" and is an entirely new staging system that, for the first time, reflects a multidisciplinary effort to provide a mechanism for staging nonmelanoma skin cancers according to evidence-based medicine. In total, seven board-certified disciplines collaborated to develop this chapter: Dermatology, Otolaryngology-Head and Neck Surgery, Surgical Oncology, Dermatopathology, Oncology, Plastic Surgery, and Oral and Maxillofacial Surgery. The title of this chapter reflects the basis of the data, which is focused on cutaneous squamous cell carcinoma (cSCC). All other nonmelanoma skin carcinomas (except Merkel cell carcinoma) will be staged according to the cSCC staging system

- Anatomic site of the eyelid is not included – staged by Ophthalmic Carcinoma of the Eyelid (see Chap. 48)

- The T staging has eliminated the 5-cm-size breakpoint and invasion of extradermal structures for T4. Two cm continues to differentiate T1 and 2, however, a list of clinical and histologic "high-risk features" has been created that can increase the T staging, independent of tumor size

- Grade has been included as one of the "high-risk features" within the T category and now contributes toward the final stage grouping. Other "high-risk features" include primary anatomic site ear or hair-bearing lip, >2 mm depth, Clark level ≥IV, or perineural invasion

- Advanced T stage is reserved for bony extension or involvement (e.g., maxilla, mandible, orbit, temporal bone, or perineural invasion of skull base or axial skeleton for T3 and T4, respectively)

- Nodal (N) staging has been completely revised to reflect published evidence-based data demonstrating that survival decreases with increasing nodal size and number of nodes involved

- Because the majority of cSCC tumors occur on the head and neck, the seventh edition staging system for cSCC and other cutaneous carcinomas was made congruent with the AJCC Head and Neck staging system

| ANATOMIC STAGE/PROGNOSTIC GROUPS | | | |
|---|---|---|---|
| Stage 0 | Tis | N0 | M0 |
| Stage I | T1 | N0 | M0 |
| Stage II | T2 | N0 | M0 |
| Stage III | T3 | N0 | M0 |
| | T1 | N1 | M0 |
| | T2 | N1 | M0 |
| | T3 | N1 | M0 |
| Stage IV | T1 | N2 | M0 |
| | T2 | N2 | M0 |
| | T3 | N2 | M0 |
| | T Any | N3 | M0 |
| | T4 | N Any | M0 |
| | T Any | N Any | M1 |

**ICD-O-3 TOPOGRAPHY CODES**

| | |
|---|---|
| C44.0 | Skin of lip, NOS |
| C44.2 | External ear |
| C44.3 | Skin of other and unspecified parts of the face |
| C44.4 | Skin of scalp and neck |
| C44.5 | Skin of trunk |
| C44.6 | Skin of upper limb and shoulder |
| C44.7 | Skin of lower limb and hip |
| C44.8 | Overlapping lesion of skin |
| C44.9 | Skin, NOS |
| C63.2 | Scrotum, NOS |

**ICD-O-3 HISTOLOGY CODE RANGES**
8000–8246, 8248–8576, 8940–8950, 8980–8981

## INTRODUCTION

The term nonmelanoma skin carcinoma (NMSC) includes approximately 82 types of skin malignancies with wide variability in prognosis, ranging from those that generally portend a poor prognosis, such as Merkel cell carcinoma (MCC), to the far more frequent and clinically favorable basal cell carcinoma (BCC) and cutaneous squamous cell carcinoma (cSCC). Because of important differences in natural behavior of MCC and other NMSC, the previous chapter entitled "Carcinoma of the Skin," has been split in this seventh edition into two separate chapters entitled "Merkel Cell Carcinoma" (see Chap. 30) and the current chapter, which has been renamed as "Cutaneous Squamous Cell Carcinoma (cSCC) and Other Cutaneous Carcinomas." Although the primary focus of the discussion in this chapter is on cSCC, the staging system applies to all NMSC except MCC. Recently published data regarding prognostic factors has been utilized as the basis for this new and revised staging system.

The incidence of cSCC and other carcinomas of the skin varies globally, but is thought to be increasing overall since the 1960s at a rate of 3–8% per year.[1] In the United States, NMSC is the most frequent cancer.[2] Although the vast majority of these tumors present at Stage I and II, cSCC is responsible for the majority of NMSC deaths[3] and accounts for a approximately 20% of all skin cancer-related deaths.[4] The high incidence of cSCC and BCC is thought to be mostly the result of sun exposure and mutagenic effects of ultraviolet (UV) light.[5] BCC and cSCC tumors are far more common in fair skinned patients and typically located on anatomic areas exposed to the sun, such as the head, neck, or extremities. Incidence varies with geographic latitude as well as ozone depletion, with a high incidence in areas such as Australia and New Zealand.[1,6-13] Other risk factors for developing NMSC include advanced age and induced or acquired immunosuppression, seen after solid organ transplantation[14-16] or in patients diagnosed and treated for leukemia or lymphoma. Male gender is a well-described risk factor for the development of cSCC.[5]

A completely revised staging system is described herein, along with operational definitions. This new staging system was designed based on published evidence-based data demonstrating significant mortality associated with specific clinical and histologic features. This revised version of cSCC staging more accurately reflects the prognosis and natural history of cSCC and therefore will be more applicable to treatment planning and design of clinical trials for carcinomas of the skin. Because a significant number of NMSC primaries occur on the head and neck, concordance with the head and neck staging system was planned and achieved. The major differences between the new chapter entitled "Cutaneous Squamous Cell Carcinoma and Other Cutaneous Carcinomas" and the chapter found in the sixth edition AJCC manual entitled "Carcinoma of the Skin" are summarized below. The chapter summary outlines the major revisions while more details about the staging system revision rationale and interpretation are forthcoming in separate manuscripts (in preparation).

Cutaneous SCC of the eyelid is relatively common. In developing the staging system for this edition of the *AJCC Cancer Staging Manual*, both the Ophthalmic Task Force and the cSCC Task Force developed staging systems for cSCC of the eyelid. The cSCC Task Force used the system reported herein for all cSCC and the Ophthalmic Task Force used a different system to be applied to all eyelid tumors (Table 29.1). The final decision of the Editorial Board was to assign eyelid cSCC staging to the Ophthalmic eyelid staging system, and to recommend collection for eyelid cSCC of the prognostic and high-risk factors defined below for all cSCC so that future staging revisions will be based on as high-level evidence as possible (see Carcinoma of the Eyelid, Chap. 48).

## ANATOMY

**Primary Site.** Cutaneous squamous cell and other carcinomas can occur anywhere on the skin. Cutaneous SCC and BCC most commonly arise on anatomic sites that have been exposed to sunlight.[5] Cutaneous SCC can also arise in skin that was previously scarred or ulcerated – that is, at sites of burns and chronic ulcers (chronic inflammation). All of the components of the skin (epidermis, dermis, and adnexal structures) can give rise to malignant neoplasms.

**TABLE 29.1.** Comparison of sixth edition and seventh editions

| Factor | 6th Edition | 7th Edition | Comments |
|---|---|---|---|
| Tumor types included | All NMSC were included | Merkel Cell Carcinoma placed in a separate chapter, current chapter covers Squamous Cell Carcinoma and other Cutaneous Carcinomas | Merkel Cell Carcinoma natural history differs significantly from other NMSC |
| Anatomic sites | Excluded eyelid | cSCC of the eyelid are to be staged using the system defined in chapter 48, Carcinoma of the Eyelid | Ophthalmic staging system will stage NMSC tumors and eyelid is not included within this new cSCC chapter. The NMSC task force will continue to collect and analyze prognostic factors for cSCC and the 8th edition AJCC NMSC task force will analyze their data which includes eyelid |
| Tumor size threshold | T1: ≤2 cm<br>T2: 2–5 cm<br>T3: >5 cm | T1: ≤2 cm<br>T2: >2 cm | Lack of evidence to support 5-cm threshold |
| Histopathologic grade | Not included in the final stage grouping | Included as part of the T staging and therefore contributes to final staging | Degree of differentiation has been reported as a risk factor for cSCC |
| High-risk features | Not used for T or final staging | "High-risk features" can upgrade T staging and include: histologic grade, anatomic site ear or hair-bearing lip, >2-mm depth, Clark level ≥IV, or perineural invasion | Many different histologic or clinical determinants have been reported to predict cSCC recurrence or metastasis |
| Histologic extradermal invasion | Used to determine T4 | Eliminated | Lack of data demonstrating uniform prognostic effect |

| | | | |
|---|---|---|---|
| Anatomic sites | Not used for T or final staging | Added as high-risk features | Specific anatomic sites confer worse prognosis |
| Cranial or facial bone involvement | Included as T4, invasion of extradermal structure | Invasion of maxilla, mandible, orbit, or temporal bone defined as T3 | Correlates with head and neck cancer staging |
| Invasion of skull base or axial skeleton | Included as T4, invasion of extradermal structure | T4 is redefined as tumor involvement of skull base or axial skeleton | Correlates with head and neck cancer staging and recently published data |
| N staging | Based on presence (N1) or absence (N0) of nodal disease | N0–N3 disease has been established based on size and number of nodal metastases | (1) Congruence with head and neck staging is achieved and (2) published data shows decreasing survival with increased size or number of metastatic nodal involvement |
| M staging | Based on presence (M1) or absence (M0) of distant metastasis | No change | M remains the only unchanged staging determinant |

Nonaggressive NMSC, such as BCC, usually grow solely by local extension, both horizontally and vertically. Continued local extension may result in growth into deep structures, including adipose tissue, cartilage, muscle, and bone. Perineural extension is a particularly insidious form of local extension, as this is often clinically occult. If neglected for an extended length of time, nodal metastasis can occur with nonaggressive NMSC.

Aggressive NMSC, including cSCC and some types of sebaceous and eccrine neoplasms, also grow by local lateral and vertical extension early in their natural history. Once deeper extension occurs, growth may become discontinuous, resulting in deeper local extension, in transit metastasis, and nodal metastasis. In more advanced cases, cSCC and other tumors can extend along cranial foramina through the skull base into the cranial vault. Uncommon types of NMSC vary considerably in their propensity for metastasis.

**Regional Lymph Nodes.**  When deep invasion and eventual metastasis occurs, local and regional lymph nodes are the most common sites of metastasis. Nodal metastasis usually occurs in an orderly manner, initially in a single node, which expands in size. Eventually, multiple nodes become involved with metastasis. Metastatic disease may spread to secondary nodal basins, including contralateral nodes when advanced. Uncommonly, nodal metastases may bypass a primary nodal basin.

**Metastatic Sites.**  Nonaggressive NMSC more often involves deep tissue by direct extension than by metastasis. After metastasizing to nodes, cSCC may spread to visceral sites, including lung.

## RULES FOR CLASSIFICATION

The clinical and pathologic classifications are identical. However, pathologic staging uses the symbol p as a prefix.

**Clinical Staging.**  The clinical staging of skin cancer is based on inspection and palpation of the involved area and the regional lymph nodes. Imaging studies may be important to stage cSCC for which there is clinical suspicion for nodal metastasis or bone invasion.

**Pathologic Staging.**  Complete resection of the primary tumor site is required for accurate pathologic staging and for cure. Surgical resection of lymph node tissue is necessary when involvement is suspected. Pathologists should comment on histologic characteristics of the tumor, particularly depth, grade, and perineural invasion. Low-grade tumors show considerable cell differentiation, uniform cell size, infrequent cellular mitoses and nuclear irregularity, and intact intercellular bridges. High-grade tumors show poor differentiation, spindle cell characteristics, necrosis, high mitotic activity, and deep invasion. Depth of cSCC invasion, as measured by Breslow depth, correlates with metastatic potential.

## PROGNOSTIC FEATURES

Most studies that analyze early stage cSCC are retrospective in nature and do not rely on multivariate analysis. The revision of the staging system for Stage I and II cSCC was primarily based on consensus opinion of the NMSC Task Force. Poor prognosis for recurrence and metastasis has been correlated with multiple factors such as anatomic site, tumor diameter, poor differentiation, perineural invasion, as well extension >2 mm depth. These prognostic factors are discussed in detail below. They apply primarily to cSCC and an aggressive subset of NMSC, but rarely to BCC. The following rationale determined the multiple factors used for the T staging:

**Tumor Diameter.**  Tumor size refers to the maximum clinical diameter of the cSCC lesion. In the sixth edition AJCC staging system, 2- and 5-cm tumor size thresholds were used to define the primary tumor (T) and were the sole criteria for T1, T2, and T3. Multiple studies corroborate a correlation between tumor size and more biologically aggressive disease, including local recurrence and metastasis in univariate analysis.[4,17–19] Tumor size remains a significant variable on multivariate analysis in some reports. Several published studies point toward 2 cm as a threshold beyond which tumors are more likely to metastasize to lymph nodes. A 3.8-fold risk of recurrence and metastasis for tumors >2 cm was noted by Mullen[18] when reviewing M.D. Anderson Cancer Center's database of 149 cSCC on the trunk and extremities. In a large review of all published literature on the prognosis of SCC occurring on the skin and lip since 1940, Rowe et al.[4] found that among tumors that exceeded 2 cm in diameter, the local recurrence rate was double (15 vs. 7%) and metastatic rates were triple (30 vs. 9%) the rates when the primary was ≤2 cm.

After considering all of this published data, the AJCC cSCC Task Force decided to continue 2 cm as one of the key delineating features between T1 and T2 cSCC staging in the seventh edition AJCC Manual (Table 29.1). This threshold was decided based on the existing published data that ≥2 cm clinical diameter is associated with a poor prognosis. In addition, this breakpoint allowed congruence between cSCC and Head and Neck Staging. Prognostically relevant breakpoints beyond 2 cm are difficult to establish. A limited number of studies suggest 4 cm as significant thresholds,[20] while others show other factors to be important.[17] Therefore, there is a lack of sufficient evidence to support the 5-cm break point featured in the previous NMSC staging system. Thus, a 5-cm breakpoint has been removed from the seventh edition AJCC T staging definitions for cSCC.

**High-Risk Tumor Features.**  Although 2 cm is recognized by many to be an important size cutoff, the metastatic potential of tumors smaller than 2 cm cannot be ignored, as they too can metastasize. In a prospective study of 266 patients with head and neck cSCC metastatic to lymph nodes, the majority of patients had tumors <2 cm in size, leading the investigators to conclude that size alone is a poor predictor of outcome.[12] A review of 915 cSCC in Netherlands' national registry over a 10-year period (comparing nonmetastatic and metastatic lesions matched for gender, location, and other clinicopathologic variables) suggested that the risk of metastasis significantly increased with tumors >1.5 cm.[21] In conceptualizing how to integrate the multiple other clinicopathologic tumor characteristics into the overall staging system, the NMSC Task Force felt that the independent prognostic validity of the multiple other features was insufficient to accurately place them into stage-specific locations. Instead, the Task Force approved a group of "high-risk" features which are combined with diameter to classify tumors as T1 or T2 (Table 29.1).

Additionally, because of data suggesting that immunosuppression correlates with worse prognosis as described in Lee et al. (in preparation), strong consideration was given toward including immunosuppression as a risk factor. However, because strict TNM criteria preclude inclusion of clinical risk factors in the staging system, this factor should be collected by tumor registries as a site-specific factor rather than incorporated in the final staging system. For centers collecting such data and performing studies, immunosuppressed status may be designated with an "I" after the staging designation.

*Depth of Tumor.* Recent studies show that both tumor thickness and the depth of invasion are important variables for the prognosis of cSCC. Prospective studies showed that increasing tumor thickness[22,23] as well as anatomic depth[17] of invasion correlate with an increased risk of metastases. In an initial study, no metastases were associated with primary tumors less than 2 mm in depth (tumor thickness), but a metastatic rate of 15% was noted with tumors greater than 6 mm in depth.[17] This study also reported increasing metastatic rates as tumor invasion progressed from dermis to subcutaneous adipose tissue, to muscle, or bone.[17] Based on the prospective and multivariate data, the seventh edition AJCC cSCC staging system incorporates >2 mm Breslow depth as one of the high-risk features in the T classification. Clark's level ≥IV is included as an additional high-risk feature. Differentiation between the prognostic contributions of Breslow thickness vs. Clark level will depend on future studies.

*Anatomic Site.* Specific anatomic locations on the hair-bearing lip and ear appear to have an increased local recurrence and metastatic potential and thus have been categorized as high risk in the seventh edition system (Table 29.1).

*Perineural Invasion.* Goepfert et al., in their review of 520 patients with 967 cSCC of the face, found an increased incidence of cervical lymphadenopathy and distant metastasis, as well as significantly reduced survival in patients with tumors that showed perineural invasion.[24] Several univariate studies, all retrospective, have also confirmed that perineural invasion has a negative prognostic impact in cSCC.[25-27]

*Histopathologic Grade or Differentiation.* Early studies recognized that the histological grade or degree of differentiation of a cSCC affects prognosis: the more well-differentiated, the less aggressive the clinical course.[28] In 1978, Mohs, in his review of "microscopically controlled surgery," reported significant differences in cure rates for well-differentiated tumors (99.4%)

compared with poorly differentiated tumors (42.1%).[29] A multivariate analysis has also confirmed that histopathologic grade correlates with recurrence.[30] The sixth edition staging system used a separate G classification system to denote histopathologic grade, however, grade did not contribute toward overall stage grouping (Table 29.1). For the seventh edition AJCC cSCC staging, histopathologic grade includes poorly differentiated tumors as one of the several high-risk features.

**Extension to Bony Structures.** In the sixth edition T staging system, the T4 designation was used for tumors that "invaded extradermal structures." The most common and important instances of deep anatomic extension for cSCC involve extension to bone of the head and neck and perineural extension to bony structures vs. the skull base. Based on these considerations, in the seventh edition cSCC staging system, T3 designation denotes direct invasion of cSCC into cranial bone structures. The T4 designation is reserved for direct or perineural invasion of the skull base independent of tumor thickness or depth (Table 29.1) consistent with data from several head and neck studies suggesting that cSCC extending to skull base is associated to poor prognosis similar to advanced lymph node disease.[8–11,31,32] While published studies include facial nerve involvement in nodal staging,[8–11,31,32] the NMSC Task Force decided to separate this factor from nodal status and include it in the T staging in order to understand its unique contribution to prognosis. The NMSC Task Force reached consensus that, similarly, extension of cSCC to axial skeleton should also merit a T4 designation.

**Evidence-Based Medicine and Nodal Disease.** Since the sixth edition AJCC manual, four studies have examined the outcomes in patients with cSCC and regional lymph node metastasis. Approximately 761 patients from ten centers and three countries (Table 29.2) have been studied suggesting the number nodes involved and size of lymph node metastasis correlates with poor prognosis.

In 2002, O'Brien et al.[8] conducted a prospective study with multivariate analysis and therein proposed a new clinical staging system for cSCC. He used a new staging system in which he separated the parotid gland involvement from the cervical node metastasis and applied this new P (parotid) N (neck) system to 87 patients with parotid and cervical cSCC metastasis to analyze the influence of clinical stage, extent of surgery, and pathologic findings on outcome by applying this new staging system The multivariate analysis showed that increasing P stage, positive margins, and a failure to have postoperative radiotherapy independently predicted decrease in local control. It also demonstrated that positive surgical margins and the advanced (N2) clinical and pathologic neck disease were independent risk factors for survival. The results from this study concluded that patients with metastatic cSCC in both the parotid gland and neck have significantly worse prognosis than those in the parotid gland only. O'Brien et al. recommended that a new clinical staging system for cSCC of the head and neck should separate parotid (P) and neck disease (N) nodal involvement.[8]

In 2003, Palme et al.[9] in a retrospective, multicenter study, independently tested this new PN staging system on 126 patients with metastatic

**TABLE 29.2.** Published data on advanced cSCC tumors

| | Number of patients | Type of study | Major statistically significant conclusions | Number of centers | Number of countries |
|---|---|---|---|---|---|
| O'Brien et al.[8] | 87 | Prospective, multivariate analysis | Advanced nodal disease associated with (a/w) poor prognosis | 1 | 1 |
| Palme et al.[9] | 126 | Retrospective, multivariate | Immunosuppression, single modality treatment, advanced parotid disease a/w poor prognosis | 1 | 1 |
| Audet et al.[31] | 56 | Retrospective, multivariate | Facial nerve involvement, advanced parotid disease a/w poor prognosis | 1 | 1 |
| Andruchow et al.[11] | 322 | Retrospective, multivariate | Advanced parotid and pathologic cervical lymph node disease a/w poor prognosis | 6 | 3 |
| Ch'ng et al.[32] | 170 | Prospective, multivariate | Advanced disease a/w poor prognosis | 1 | 1 |
| Total patients | 761 | | | | |

Included in the nodal analysis were studies where prospective or retrospective data and multivariate analysis were performed. Survival was based on overall survival[8,11] or disease-specific survival.[9,31,32] Follow-up varied from at least 1 year,[31] 18 months,[32] 2 years,[8,11] or 5 years.[9] Total numbers of patients may be 649; however, the real number of patients is likely to be less than 600 since some analyses likely have overlapping patients.[8,9,11,31]

cSCCs involving the parotid and/or neck. The multivariate analysis showed that advanced P staging (P2 and P3) were independent risk factors for a decrease in local control rate, and the pathologic involvement of neck nodes did not worsen survival of patients with parotid disease. Overall, this analysis concluded that single-modality therapy, P3 stage, and presence of immunosuppression independently predicted a decrease in survival. This study confirmed that the extent of metastatic disease in the parotid gland significantly influences outcome and that separating the parotid from the neck metastasis may be useful.[9]

In 2004, Audet et al.,[31] in their retrospective study on 56 patients with previously untreated metastatic head and neck cSCC involving the parotid gland, confirmed that metastatic cSCC to the parotid gland is an aggressive neoplasm that requires combination therapy. They also reported that the presence of a lesion in excess of 6 cm or with facial nerve involvement is associated with a poor prognosis.[31]

In 2006, a larger cohort, multicenter, retrospective study was conducted by Andruchow et al.[11] on 322 patients from six independent institutions to further clarify the clinical behavior of metastatic cSCC and to determine whether or not the proposed changes to the clinical staging system could be validated. In this study, 322 patients with parotid and/or neck metastatic cSCC were restaged with the O'Brien P and N staging system and were followed up for at least 2 years. Both univariate and multivariate analysis confirmed that survival was significantly worse for patients with advanced P stage, suggesting a revised classification of nodal status.[11] This concept of increasing nodal disease correlating with decreased survival was confirmed in a separate prospective analysis of 67 patients with metastatic disease.[32]

Patient survival from the published studies is shown in Figure 29.1. Based on this data, the NMSC Task Force decided that there is sufficient evidence to stage patients according to increasing nodal disease. While preliminary data exists to suggest that cervical disease may portend a worse prognosis than similar disease in the parotid, there is insufficient data to support this separation at this time. Separating out facial nerve involvement or involvement of the skull base (now T4) from extensive parotid disease will further clarify the prognosis of these patients.

**Immunosuppression and Advanced Disease.**   It is well known that immunosuppressed patients are at risk for developing malignancies, especially cSCCs. Organ transplant recipients develop squamous cell carcinoma 65 times more frequently than in age-matched controls.[33,34] The cSCCs in immunocompromised patients are more aggressive: they are numerous, tend to recur, and metastasize at a higher rate.[14,15,35–41] It has been reported that immunocompromised patients have a 7.2 times increased risk of local recurrence and a 5.3 times increased risk of any recurrence of disease.[42] Mortality is also increased with skin cancer, the fourth most common cause of death in a renal transplant cohort.[43] In transplant recipients, cSCC develops 10–30 years earlier than in immunocompetent hosts.[3,4]

Histopathology of cSCC in an immunocompromised host show more acantholytic changes, early dermal invasion, infiltrative growth pattern, Bowen's disease with carcinoma, and increased depth of the primary.[44] Tumors in immunocompromised patients can range widely in size from

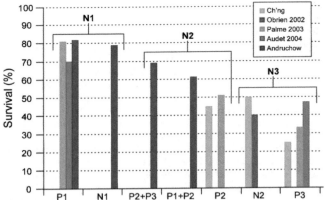

**FIGURE 29.1.** Published survival rates for advanced cSCC disease. Published studies for advanced cSCC disease have described survival according to O'Brien[8] using the P and N system proposed therein (X-axis). Reported overall or disease-specific survival is represented by the Y-axis. To achieve concordance with the Head and Neck AJCC staging, the NMSC Task Force recommended a three-stage system (*brackets*) to include both parotid and nodal disease together until future studies determine their individual contributions to prognosis.

6 to 75 mm; however, Lindelof and colleagues[45] report that most lethal cSCCs in their study were 5–19 mm in diameter. They also point out that focusing on tumor size may be misleading in immunocompromised populations because small tumors can behave very aggressively. For centers prospectively studying cSCC, recording of presence and type of immunosuppression is recommended.

## CONCLUSIONS

The seventh edition of the AJCC Staging Manual features MCC as a separate chapter and cSCC is staged in this chapter entitled "Cutaneous Squamous cell and Other Carcinomas." The remainder of NMSC tumors (such as appendageal tumors and BCC) will also be included within the cSCC chapter since those tumors can rarely be advanced and are occasionally described to undergo metastasis. As the first published staging system devoted specifically to cSCC prognosis, this represents an important step for better understanding and studying the prognosis of this potentially metastatic tumor. Additionally, since many cSCC tumors occur on the head and neck, the seventh edition cSCC staging system is congruent with Head and Neck Cancer staging system. Furthermore, the new T staging definitions for the seventh edition for cSCC now capture additional features believed to correlate with high-risk cSCC in order to more meaningfully stratify patients based on prospective systematic data. Certainly there is still a need for multivariate data analysis, particularly to determine the relative contributions of the various described T factors influencing cSCC prognosis.

Finally, the new N staging definitions are congruent with Head and Neck staging and reflect recent data that suggests that prognosis is inversely correlated with increasing nodal disease.

## DEFINITIONS OF TNM

Definitions for clinical (cTNM) and pathologic (pTNM) classifications are the same. Patients with cSCC in situ are categorized as Tis. Carcinomas that are indeterminate or cannot be staged should be category TX. Carcinomas 2 cm or less in diameter are T1, if they have fewer than two high-risk features. Clinical high-risk features include primary site on ear or hair-bearing lip. Histologic high-risk features include depth >2 mm, Clark level ≥IV/V, poor differentiation, and the presence of perineural invasion. Tumors greater than 2 cm in diameter are classified as T2. Tumors 2 cm or less in diameter are classified as T2 if the tumor has two or more high-risk features. Invasion into facial bones is classified as T3, while invasion to base of skull or axial skeleton is classified as T4.

Local and regional metastases most commonly present in the regional lymph nodes. The actual status of nodal metastases identified by clinical inspection or imaging and the status and number of positive and total nodes by pathologic analysis must be reported for staging purposes. In instances where lymph node status is not recorded, a designation of NX is used. A solitary parotid or regional lymph node metastasis measuring 3 cm or less in size is given a N1 designation. Several different lymph node states are classified as N2: N2a represents a single ipsilateral lymph node, more than 3 cm but not more than 6 cm in greatest dimension; N2b is defined by multiple ipsilateral lymph nodes, none more than 6 cm in greatest dimension; N2c includes bilateral or contralateral lymph nodes, none more than 6 cm in greatest dimension. Nodal metastases more than 6 cm in greatest dimension are classified as N3.

Distant metastases are staged primarily by the presence (M1) or absence (M0) of metastases in distant organs or sites outside of the regional lymph nodes.

| *Primary Tumor (T)** | |
|---|---|
| TX | Primary tumor cannot be assessed |
| T0 | No evidence of primary tumor |
| Tis | Carcinoma in situ |
| T1 | Tumor 2 cm or less in greatest dimension with less than two high-risk features** |
| T2 | Tumor greater than 2 cm in greatest dimension *or* Tumor any size with two or more high-risk features* |
| T3 | Tumor with invasion of maxilla, mandible, orbit, or temporal bone |
| T4 | Tumor with invasion of skeleton (axial or appendicular) or perineural invasion of skull base |

*Excludes cSCC of the eyelid (see Chap. 48).

**High-risk features for the primary tumor (T) staging

| Depth/invasion | >2 mm thickness |
| | Clark level $\geq$ IV |
| | Perineural invasion |
| Anatomic location | Primary site ear |
| | Primary site non-hair-bearing lip |
| Differentiation | Poorly differentiated or undifferentiated |

### Regional Lymph Nodes (N)

| | |
|---|---|
| NX | Regional lymph nodes cannot be assessed |
| N0 | No regional lymph node metastases |
| N1 | Metastasis in a single ipsilateral lymph node, 3 cm or less in greatest dimension |
| N2 | Metastasis in a single ipsilateral lymph node, more than 3 cm but not more than 6 cm in greatest dimension; or in multiple ipsilateral lymph nodes, none more than 6 cm in greatest dimension; or in bilateral or contralateral lymph nodes, none more than 6 cm in greatest dimension |
| N2a | Metastasis in a single ipsilateral lymph node, more than 3 cm but not more than 6 cm in greatest dimension |
| N2b | Metastasis in multiple ipsilateral lymph nodes, none more than 6 cm in greatest dimension |
| N2c | Metastasis in bilateral or contralateral lymph nodes, none more than 6 cm in greatest dimension |
| N3 | Metastasis in a lymph node, more than 6 cm in greatest dimension |

### Distant Metastasis (M)

| | |
|---|---|
| M0 | No distant metastases |
| M1 | Distant metastases |

## ANATOMIC STAGE/PROGNOSTIC GROUPS

Patients with primary cSCC or other cutaneous carcinomas with no evidence (clinical, radiologic, or pathologic) of regional or distant metastases are divided into two stages: Stage I for tumors measuring $\leq$2 cm in size and Stage II for those that are greater than 2 cm in size. In instances where there is clinical concern for extension of tumor into bone and radiologic evaluation has been performed (and is negative), these data may be included to support the Stage I vs. II designation. Tumors that are $\leq$2 cm in size can be upstaged to Stage II if they contain two or more high-risk features. Stage III patients are those with (1) clinical, histologic, or radiologic evidence of one solitary node measuring $\leq$3 cm in size or (2) Tumor extension into bone: maxilla, mandible, orbit, or temporal bone. Stage IV patients are those with (1) tumor with direct or perineural invasion of skull base or axial skeleton, (2) $\geq$2 lymph nodes or (3) single or multiple lymph nodes measuring >3 cm in size or (4) distant metastasis.

| Stage | T | N | M |
|-------|---|---|---|
| Stage 0 | Tis | N0 | M0 |
| Stage I | T1 | N0 | M0 |
| Stage II | T2 | N0 | M0 |
| Stage III | T3 | N0 | M0 |
| | T1 | N1 | M0 |
| | T2 | N1 | M0 |
| | T3 | N1 | M0 |
| Stage IV | T1 | N2 | M0 |
| | T2 | N2 | M0 |
| | T3 | N2 | M0 |
| | T Any | N3 | M0 |
| | T4 | N Any | M0 |
| | T Any | N Any | M1 |

**29**

## PROGNOSTIC FACTORS (SITE-SPECIFIC FACTORS)
### (Recommended for Collection)

| | |
|---|---|
| Required for staging | Tumor thickness (in mm) |
| | Clark's level |
| | Presence/absence of perineural invasion |
| | Primary site location on ear or hair-bearing lip |
| | Histologic grade |
| | Size of largest lymph node metastasis |
| Clinically significant | No additional factors |

## HISTOLOGIC GRADE (G)

Grade is reported in registry systems by the grade value. A two-grade, three-grade, or four-grade system may be used. If a grading system is not specified, generally the following system is used:

| | |
|---|---|
| GX | Grade cannot be assessed |
| G1 | Well differentiated |
| G2 | Moderately differentiated |
| G3 | Poorly differentiated |
| G4 | Undifferentiated |

## HISTOPATHOLOGIC TYPE

The classification applies only to carcinomas of the skin, primarily cSCC and other carcinomas. It also applies to the adenocarcinomas that develop from eccrine or sebaceous glands and to the spindle cell variant of cSCC. Microscopic verification is necessary to group by histologic type. A form of in situ cSCC or intraepidermal cSCC is often referred to as Bowen's disease. This lesion should be coded as Tis.

# BIBLIOGRAPHY

1. Diepgen TL, Mahler V. The epidemiology of skin cancer. Br J Dermatol. 2002;146 Suppl 61:1–6.
2. Housman TS, Feldman SR, Williford PM, et al. Skin cancer is among the most costly of all cancers to treat for the Medicare population. J Am Acad Dermatol. 2003;48:425–9.
3. Alam M, Ratner D. Cutaneous squamous-cell carcinoma. N Engl J Med. 2001;344:975–83.
4. Rowe DE, Carroll RJ, Day CL Jr. Prognostic factors for local recurrence, metastasis, and survival rates in squamous cell carcinoma of the skin, ear, and lip. Implications for treatment modality selection. J Am Acad Dermatol. 1992;26:976–90.
5. Preston DS, Stern RS. Nonmelanoma cancers of the skin. N Engl J Med. 1992;327:1649–62.
6. Zak-Prelich M, Narbutt J, Sysa-Jedrzejowska A. Environmental risk factors predisposing to the development of basal cell carcinoma. Dermatol Surg. 2004;30:248–52.
7. Nolan RC, Chan MT, Heenan PJ. A clinicopathologic review of lethal non-melanoma skin cancers in Western Australia. J Am Acad Dermatol. 2005;52:101–8.
8. O'Brien CJ, McNeil EB, McMahon JD, et al. Significance of clinical stage, extent of surgery, and pathologic findings in metastatic cutaneous squamous carcinoma of the parotid gland. Head Neck. 2002;24:417–22.
9. Palme CE, O'Brien CJ, Veness MJ, et al. Extent of parotid disease influences outcome in patients with metastatic cutaneous squamous cell carcinoma. Arch Otolaryngol Head Neck Surg. 2003;129:750–3.
10. Veness MJ, Palme CE, Smith M, et al. Cutaneous head and neck squamous cell carcinoma metastatic to cervical lymph nodes (nonparotid): a better outcome with surgery and adjuvant radiotherapy. Laryngoscope. 2003;113:1827–33.
11. Andruchow JL, Veness MJ, Morgan GJ, et al. Implications for clinical staging of metastatic cutaneous squamous carcinoma of the head and neck based on a multicenter study of treatment outcomes. Cancer. 2006;106:1078–83.
12. Veness MJ, Palme CE, Morgan GJ. High-risk cutaneous squamous cell carcinoma of the head and neck: results from 266 treated patients with metastatic lymph node disease. Cancer. 2006;106:2389–96.
13. Veness MJ, Ong C, Cakir B, et al. Squamous cell carcinoma of the lip. Patterns of relapse and outcome: reporting the Westmead Hospital experience, 1980–1997. Australas Radiol. 2001;45:195–9.
14. Ulrich C, Schmook T, Sachse MM, et al. Comparative epidemiology and pathogenic factors for nonmelanoma skin cancer in organ transplant patients. Dermatol Surg. 2004;30:622–7.
15. Ramsay HM, Fryer AA, Hawley CM, et al. Factors associated with nonmelanoma skin cancer following renal transplantation in Queensland, Australia. J Am Acad Dermatol. 2003;49:397–406.
16. Veness MJ, Quinn DI, Ong CS, et al. Aggressive cutaneous malignancies following cardiothoracic transplantation: the Australian experience. Cancer. 1999;85:1758–64.
17. Breuninger H, Black B, Rassner G. Microstaging of squamous cell carcinomas. Am J Clin Pathol. 1990;94:624–7.
18. Mullen JT, Feng L, Xing Y, et al. Invasive squamous cell carcinoma of the skin: defining a high-risk group. Ann Surg Oncol. 2006;13:902–9.
19. Dinehart SM, Pollack SV. Metastases from squamous cell carcinoma of the skin and lip. An analysis of twenty-seven cases. J Am Acad Dermatol. 1989;21:241–8.

20. Moore BA, Weber RS, Prieto V, et al. Lymph node metastases from cutaneous squamous cell carcinoma of the head and neck. Laryngoscope. 2005;115: 1561–7.
21. Quaedvlieg PJ, Creytens DH, Epping GG, et al. Histopathological characteristics of metastasizing squamous cell carcinoma of the skin and lips. Histopathology. 2006;49:256–64.
22. Breuninger H, Schaumburg-Lever G, Holzschuh J, et al. Desmoplastic squamous cell carcinoma of skin and vermilion surface: a highly malignant subtype of skin cancer. Cancer. 1997;79:915–9.
23. Brantsch KD, Meisner C, Schonfisch B, et al. Analysis of risk factors determining prognosis of cutaneous squamous-cell carcinoma: a prospective study. Lancet Oncol. 2008;9:713–20.
24. Goepfert H, Dichtel WJ, Medina JE, et al. Perineural invasion in squamous cell skin cancer of the head and neck. Am J Surg. 1984;148:542–7.
25. Fagan JJ, Collins B, Barnes L, et al. Perineural invasion in squamous cell carcinoma of the head and neck. Arch Otolaryngol Head Neck Surg. 1998;124:637–40.
26. Garcia-Serra A, Hinerman RW, Mendenhall WM, et al. Carcinoma of the skin with perineural invasion. Head Neck. 2003;25:1027–33.
27. Lawrence N, Cottel WI. Squamous cell carcinoma of skin with perineural invasion. J Am Acad Dermatol. 1994;31:30–3.
28. Broders AC. Squamous-cell epithelioma of the skin: a study of 256 cases. Ann Surg. 1921;73:141–60.
29. Mohs F. Chemosurgery: microscopically controlled surgery for skin cancer. Springfield IL: Charles C. Thomas; 1978.
30. Eroglu A, Berberoglu U, Berreroglu S. Risk factors related to locoregional recurrence in squamous cell carcinoma of the skin. J Surg Oncol. 1996;61:124–30.
31. Audet N, Palme CE, Gullane PJ, et al. Cutaneous metastatic squamous cell carcinoma to the parotid gland: analysis and outcome. Head Neck. 2004;26:727–32.
32. Ch'ng S, Maitra A, Allison RS, et al. Parotid and cervical nodal status predict prognosis for patients with head and neck metastatic cutaneous squamous cell carcinoma. J Surg Oncol. 2008;98:101–5.
33. Jensen P, Hansen S, Moller B, et al. Are renal transplant recipients on CsA-based immunosuppressive regimens more likely to develop skin cancer than those on azathioprine and prednisolone? Transplant Proc. 1999;31:1120.
34. Jensen P, Hansen S, Moller B, et al. Skin cancer in kidney and heart transplant recipients and different long-term immunosuppressive therapy regimens. J Am Acad Dermatol. 1999;40:177–86.
35. Jemec GB, Holm EA. Nonmelanoma skin cancer in organ transplant patients. Transplantation. 2003;75:253–7.
36. Herrero JI, Espana A, Quiroga J, et al. Nonmelanoma skin cancer after liver transplantation. Study of risk factors. Liver Transplant. 2005;11:1100–6.
37. Berg D, Otley CC. Skin cancer in organ transplant recipients: epidemiology, pathogenesis, and management. J Am Acad Dermatol. 2002;47:1–17; quiz 18–20.
38. Bordea C, Wojnarowska F, Millard PR, et al. Skin cancers in renal-transplant recipients occur more frequently than previously recognized in a temperate climate. Transplantation. 2004;77:574–9.
39. Fortina AB, Piaserico S, Caforio AL, et al. Immunosuppressive level and other risk factors for basal cell carcinoma and squamous cell carcinoma in heart transplant recipients. Arch Dermatol. 2004;140:1079–85.
40. Patel MJ, Liégeois NJ. Skin cancer and the solid organ transplant recipient. Curr Treat Options Oncol. 2008;9:251–8.

41. Moloney FJ, Comber H, O'Lorcain P, et al. A population-based study of skin cancer incidence and prevalence in renal transplant recipients. Br J Dermatol. 2006;154:498–504.

42. Southwell KE, Chaplin JM, Eisenberg RL, et al. Effect of immunocompromise on metastatic cutaneous squamous cell carcinoma in the parotid and neck. Head Neck. 2006;28:244–8.

43. Marcen R, Pascual J, Tato AM, et al. Influence of immunosuppression on the prevalence of cancer after kidney transplantation. Transplant Proc 2003;35: 1714–6.

44. Smith KJ, Hamza S, Skelton H. Histologic features in primary cutaneous squamous cell carcinomas in immunocompromised patients focusing on organ transplant patients. Dermatol Surg. 2004;30:634–41.

45. Boffetta P, Gridley G, Lindelof B. Cancer risk in a population-based cohort of patients hospitalized for psoriasis in Sweden. J Invest Dermatol. 2001;117: 1531–7.

# Merkel Cell Carcinoma

*(Staging for Merkel Cell of the eyelid [C44.1]*
*is not included in this chapter – see Chap. 48,*
*"Carcinoma of the Eyelid")*

## *At-A-Glance*

### SUMMARY OF CHANGES

• This is the first staging chapter specific for Merkel cell carcinoma. Merkel cell carcinoma was previously included in the "Carcinoma of the Skin" chapter

**30**

### ANATOMIC STAGE/PROGNOSTIC GROUPS

Patients with primary Merkel cell carcinoma with no evidence of regional or distant metastases (either clinically or pathologically) are divided into two stages: Stage I for primary tumors ≤2 cm in size and Stage II for primary tumors >2 cm in size. Stages I and II are further divided into A and B substages based on method of nodal evaluation. Patients who have pathologically proven node negative disease (by microscopic evaluation of their draining lymph nodes) have improved survival (substaged as A) compared with those who are only evaluated clinically (substaged as B). Stage II has an additional substage (IIC) for tumors with extracutaneous invasion (T4) and negative node status regardless of whether the negative node status was established microscopically or clinically. Stage III is also divided into A and B categories for patients with microscopically positive and clinically occult nodes (IIIA) and macroscopic nodes (IIIB). There are no subgroups of Stage IV Merkel cell carcinoma.

| Stage 0 | Tis | N0 | M0 |
|---------|------|-----|-----|
| Stage IA | T1 | pN0 | M0 |
| Stage IB | T1 | cN0 | M0 |
| Stage IIA | T2/T3 | pN0 | M0 |
| Stage IIB | T2/T3 | cN0 | M0 |
| Stage IIC | T4 | N0 | M0 |

### ICD-O-3 TOPOGRAPHY CODES

| | |
|------|------|
| C44.0 | Skin of lip, NOS |
| C44.2 | External ear |
| C44.3 | Skin of other and unspecified parts of face |
| C44.4 | Skin of scalp and neck |
| C44.5 | Skin of trunk |
| C44.6 | Skin of upper limb and shoulder |
| C44.7 | Skin of lower limb and hip |
| C44.8 | Overlapping lesion of skin |
| C44.9 | Skin, NOS |
| C51.0 | Labium majus |
| C51.1 | Labium minus |
| C51.2 | Clitoris |
| C51.8 | Overlapping lesion of vulva |
| C51.9 | Vulva, NOS |
| C60.0 | Prepuce |
| C60.1 | Glans penis |
| C60.2 | Body of penis |
| C60.8 | Overlapping lesion of penis |
| C60.9 | Penis, NOS |
| C63.2 | Scrotum, NOS |

## INTRODUCTION

Merkel cell carcinoma (MCC) is a relatively rare, potentially aggressive primary cutaneous neuroendocrine carcinoma, originally described by Tang and Toker in 1972 as trabecular carcinoma.[1] The mortality rate is twice that observed in melanoma (33% vs. 15%). Although the molecular pathogenesis remains largely unknown, ultraviolet radiation and immune suppression are likely significant predisposing factors. The identification of a novel polyomavirus termed *Merkel cell polyomavirus* in the majority of MCC tumors suggests a viral component in many cases.[2] Merkel cell carcinoma occurs most commonly on sun-exposed skin in fair-skinned individuals older than 50 years with a slight male predominance.[3,4] An increased incidence is also observed in patients with HIV infection, leukemias, and organ transplantation.[4-6] Merkel cell carcinoma is increasing in frequency, rising from 0.15 cases per 100,000 in 1986 to 0.44 cases per 100,000 in 2001. Much of this increase in reported frequency is likely due to increased recognition and improved techniques for diagnosis.[7] Currently in the United States, approximately 1,500 cases of MCC are diagnosed annually.[8] As the US population ages and improved transplantation regimens prolong the lives of organ transplant recipients, the incidence of MCC will likely continue to rise.

Merkel cell carcinoma has a nonspecific clinical presentation, though rapid growth of a firm, red to violaceous, nontender papule or nodule is often noted.[4] Diagnosis is made via biopsy, almost invariably with the aid of immunohistochemistry, classically demonstrating a peri-nuclear dot pattern of cytokeratin-20 staining. The majority of patients present with clinically localized disease. However, the disease can rapidly spread to regional and distant sites. The regional draining nodal basin is the most common site for recurrence.[9] The natural history of the disease is variable but heavily dependent on the stage at time of diagnosis.

Five different staging systems for Merkel cell carcinoma have been described in the literature and all are currently in use.[10-14] Depending on the system used, Stage III MCC could represent local, nodal, or metastatic disease. This situation impedes effective patient–physician communication, data comparison, and outcomes analysis. Therefore, development of a standardized, data-driven staging system is important for improving clinical care and research in this disease. Moreover, a separate staging system for MCC is appropriate given its unique behavior compared with other malignancies that will remain in the "Cutaneous Squamous Cell Carcinoma and other Cutaneous Carcinomas" staging chapter (see Chap. 29). This new staging system is based on an analysis of over 4,700 patients using the National Cancer Database as well as extensive review of the literature.

**Primary Sites.** Merkel cell carcinoma is postulated to arise from the Merkel cell, a neuroendocrine cell of the skin.[1] MCC can occur anywhere on the skin but arises most often in sun-exposed areas. It occurs most commonly on the head and neck, followed by the extremities. In 14% of cases, the primary site remains unknown with MCC presentation in nodal or visceral sites.[4]

**Regional Lymph Nodes.** The draining regional lymph nodes are the most common site of metastasis. Regional lymph node metastasis occurs relatively frequently and early, even in the absence of deep local extension or large primary tumor size. Thirty-two percent of clinically negative draining lymph node basins were in fact positive for microscopic metastases as revealed by sentinel or elective lymphadenectomy.[15] Intralymphatic "in transit" regional metastases also occur but are uncommon. For MCC, an in transit metastasis is defined as a tumor distinct from the primary lesion and located either (1) between the primary lesion and the draining regional lymph nodes or (2) distal to the primary lesion. In contrast to melanoma, for MCC there is no separate subclassification of in transit metastases based on distance from the primary (i.e., no *satellite* metastasis classification). By convention, the term "regional nodal metastases" refers to disease confined to one nodal basin or two contiguous nodal basins, as in patients with nodal disease in combinations of femoral/iliac, axillary/supraclavicular, or cervical/supraclavicular metastases or in primary truncal disease with axillary/femoral, bilateral axillary, or bilateral femoral metastases.

**Metastatic Sites.** Merkel cell carcinoma can metastasize to virtually any organ site. Metastases occur most commonly to distant lymph nodes, followed by the liver, lung, bone, and brain.[16]

## RULES FOR CLASSIFICATION

The primary difference between the definitions of clinical and pathologic nodal staging is whether the regional lymph nodes were staged by clinical/radiologic exam only or by pathologic exam (after partial or complete lymphadenectomy).

**Clinical Staging.** Clinical staging is defined as regional lymph nodes that are staged by clinical inspection and palpation of the involved area and the regional lymph nodes and/or by radiologic studies. For cases without documentation of abnormal regional nodes on physical exam, patients should be considered to not have macroscopic nodal disease.

**Pathologic Staging.** Pathologic staging is defined as regional lymph nodes that are staged by focused (sentinel lymph node biopsy), therapeutic, or complete lymphadenectomy. With regard to Merkel cell carcinoma, the distinction between clinical vs. pathologic staging is highly significant. The natural history of MCC is variable and dependent on the pathologic stage at time of presentation. Sentinel lymph node biopsy should be performed routinely on MCC patients, as approximately 32% of patients without palpable lymph nodes will have positive sentinel lymph node biopsies.[15] Pathologic staging with negative sentinel lymph node biopsy at time of diagnosis is a predictor of improved survival.[12] Despite these issues, approximately two-thirds of MCC patients captured in the National Cancer Database did not have pathologic staging of the regional nodes.

## PROGNOSTIC FEATURES AND SURVIVAL RESULTS

Survival in Merkel cell carcinoma is based on stage at presentation (Figure 30.1). Overall survival relative to an age- and sex-matched population was determined using 4,700 Merkel cell carcinoma patients in the National Cancer Database registry (manuscript in preparation). Tumor size is a continuous variable with increasing tumor size correlating with modestly poorer prognosis (Figure 30.2). True lymph node negativity by pathologic evaluation portends a better prognosis compared with patients whose lymph nodes are only evaluated by clinical or radiographic examination (Figure 30.3). This is in large part likely due to the high rate (33%) of false negative nodal determination by clinical exam alone.[15] Thus, patients should have pathologic evaluation of the draining nodal basin to most accurately predict survival and guide optimal therapy. Percent relative survival based on stage is shown in Figure 30.4.

Profound immune suppression, such as in HIV/AIDS, chronic lymphocytic leukemia, or solid organ transplantation have all been associated with worse survival in MCC.[6,17] Further, immunosuppressed patients frequently present with more advanced disease.[4]

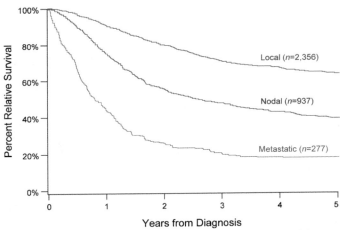

**FIGURE 30.1.** Relative survival for Merkel cell carcinoma by extent of disease at time of diagnosis. Percent relative survival was calculated for cases in the National Cancer Database using age- and sex-matched control data from the Centers for Disease Control and Prevention.

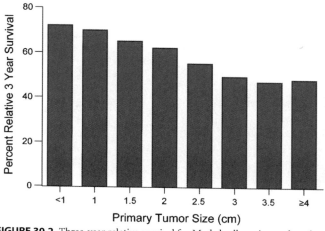

**FIGURE 30.2.** Three-year relative survival for Merkel cell carcinoma based on primary tumor dimension. While increased tumor dimension is associated with worse prognosis, these differences were modest, suggesting that tumor size alone is a poor predictor of survival. Total number of patients was 3,297, and individual groups were as follows: <1 cm = 517, 1 cm = 641, 1.5 cm = 519, 2 cm = 432, 2.5 cm = 288, 3 cm = 291, 3.5 cm = 123, ≥4 cm = 486.

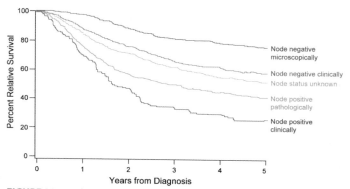

**FIGURE 30.3.** Relative survival among 4,426 Merkel cell carcinoma patients by node status. Percent relative survival was calculated for cases in the National Cancer Database using age- and sex-matched control data from the Centers for Disease Control and Prevention. Relative survival curves shown are divided into node negative patients (*top two lines*), nodes status unknown (*middle line*), and node positive patients (*bottom two lines*). The *curve* indicated by "Node positive pathologically" includes pathologic node positive patients with clinical node status negative or unknown. Total number of patients was 4,426, and individual groupings were as follows: node negative microscopically = 630, node negative clinically = 1,726, node status unknown = 1,134, node positive pathologically = 794, node positive clinically = 143.

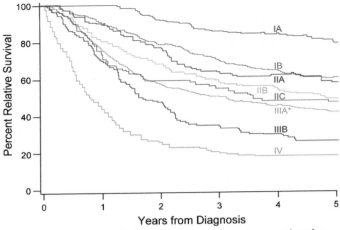

**FIGURE 30.4.** Relative survival for 2,856 Merkel cell carcinoma patients by stage. Percent relative survival was calculated for cases in the National Cancer Database using age- and sex-matched control data from the Centers for Disease Control and Prevention. Stages are as indicated in the figure except for Stage IIIA which could not be derived using this dataset. The *curve* marked "IIIA*" represents pathologically node positive patients, with the clinical node status unknown or negative. It is anticipated that true Stage IIIA patients (clinical node status negative) have better survival than the line marked with "IIIA*." Total number of patients was 2,856, and individual substages were as follows: IA = 266, IB = 754, IIA = 124, IIB = 414, IIC = 84, IIIA* = 794, IIIB = 143, IV = 277.

## DEFINITIONS OF TNM

Those patients with MCC presentations where the primary tumor cannot be assessed should be categorized as TX. Patients with Merkel cell carcinoma in situ are categorized as Tis. The T category of MCC is classified primarily by measuring the maximum dimension of the tumor: 2 cm or less (T1), greater than 2 cm but not more than 5 cm (T2), and greater than 5 cm (T3). Extracutaneous invasion by the primary tumor into bone, muscle, fascia, or cartilage is classified as T4. Inclusion of 2 cm MCC tumors as T1 is consistent with the prior AJCC staging system but differs from other frequently used MCC staging systems[12,14] that categorize 2 cm tumors as T2. The breakdown of T category is conserved from the prior version of AJCC staging for "Carcinoma of the Skin."

Regional metastases most commonly present in the regional lymph nodes. A second staging definition is related to nodal tumor burden: microscopic vs. macroscopic. Therefore, patients without clinical or radiologic evidence of lymph node metastases but who have pathologically documented nodal metastases are defined by convention as exhibiting "microscopic" or "clinically occult" nodal metastases. In contrast, MCC patients with both clinical evidence of nodal metastases *and* pathologic examination confirming nodal metastases are defined by convention as having "macroscopic" or "clinically apparent" nodal metastases. Nodes clinically positive by exam and negative by pathology would be classified as pN0. Clinically positive nodes in the draining nodal basin that are assumed to be involved with Merkel cell carcinoma but are without pathologic confirmation (no pathology performed) should be classified as N1b and the pathologic classification would be NX. Then in determining the stage grouping, it would be Stage IIIB defaulting to the higher N category.

Distant metastases are defined as metastases that have spread beyond the draining lymph node basin, including cutaneous, nodal, and visceral sites.

### Primary Tumor (T)

| | |
|-----|-----|
| TX | Primary tumor cannot be assessed |
| T0 | No evidence of primary tumor (e.g., nodal/metastatic presentation without associated primary) |
| Tis | In situ primary tumor |
| T1 | Less than or equal to 2 cm maximum tumor dimension |
| T2 | Greater than 2 cm but not more than 5 cm maximum tumor dimension |
| T3 | Over 5 cm maximum tumor dimension |
| T4 | Primary tumor invades bone, muscle, fascia, or cartilage |

### Regional Lymph Nodes (N)

| | |
|-----|-----|
| NX | Regional lymph nodes cannot be assessed |
| N0 | No regional lymph node metastasis |
| cN0 | Nodes negative by clinical exam* (no pathologic node exam performed) |
| pN0 | Nodes negative by pathologic exam |
| N1 | Metastasis in regional lymph node(s) |
| N1a | Micrometastasis** |
| N1b | Macrometastasis*** |
| N2 | In transit metastasis**** |

*Clinical detection of nodal disease may be via inspection, palpation, and/ or imaging.

**Micrometastases are diagnosed after sentinel or elective lymphadenectomy.

***Macrometastases are defined as clinically detectable nodal metastases confirmed by therapeutic lymphadenectomy or needle biopsy.

****In transit metastasis: a tumor distinct from the primary lesion and located either (1) between the primary lesion and the draining regional lymph nodes or (2) distal to the primary lesion.

---

### Distant Metastasis (M)

| | |
|---|---|
| M0 | No distant metastasis |
| M1 | Metastasis beyond regional lymph nodes |
| M1a | Metastasis to skin, subcutaneous tissues or distant lymph nodes |
| M1b | Metastasis to lung |
| M1c | Metastasis to all other visceral sites |

## ANATOMIC STAGE/PROGNOSTIC GROUPS

Patients with primary Merkel cell carcinoma with no evidence of regional or distant metastases (either clinically or pathologically) are divided into two stages: Stage I for primary tumors ≤2 cm in size and Stage II for primary tumors >2 cm in size. Stages I and II are further divided into A and B substages based on method of nodal evaluation. Patients who have pathologically proven node negative disease (by microscopic evaluation of their draining lymph nodes) have improved survival (substaged as A) compared to those who are only evaluated clinically (substaged as B). Stage II has an additional substage (IIC) for tumors with extracutaneous invasion (T4) and negative node status regardless of whether the negative node status was established microscopically or clinically. Stage III is also divided into A and B categories for patients with microscopically positive and clinically occult nodes (IIIA) and macroscopic nodes (IIIB). There are no subgroups of Stage IV Merkel cell carcinoma.

| Stage 0 | Tis | N0 | M0 |
|---|---|---|---|
| Stage IA | T1 | pN0 | M0 |
| Stage IB | T1 | cN0 | M0 |
| Stage IIA | T2/T3 | pN0 | M0 |
| Stage IIB | T2/T3 | cN0 | M0 |
| Stage IIC | T4 | N0 | M0 |
| Stage IIIA | Any T | N1a | M0 |
| Stage IIIB | Any T | N1b/N2 | M0 |
| Stage IV | Any T | Any N | M1 |

## PROGNOSTIC FACTORS (SITE-SPECIFIC FACTORS)
### (Recommended for Collection)

| | |
|---|---|
| Required for staging | None |
| Clinically significant | Measured thickness (depth) |
| | Tumor base transection status |
| | Profound immune suppression |
| | Tumor infiltrating lymphocytes in the primary tumor (TIL) |
| | Growth pattern of primary tumor |
| | Size of tumor nests in regional lymph nodes |

Clinical status of regional lymph nodes
Regional lymph nodes pathological extracapsular extension
Isolated tumor cells in regional lymph node(s)

## HISTOLOGIC GRADE (G)

Histologic grade is not used in the staging of Merkel cell carcinoma.

## HISTOPATHOLOGIC TYPE

While several distinct morphologic patterns have been described for MCC, these have not been reproducibly found to be of prognostic significance. These histologic subtypes include: intermediate type (most common), small cell type (second most common), and trabecular type (least common but most characteristic pattern of MCC).

**30**

## REFERENCES

1. Tang CK, Toker C. Trabecular carcinoma of the skin: an ultrastructural study. Cancer. 1978;42(5):2311–21.
2. Feng H, Shuda M, Chang Y, Moore PS. Clonal integration of a polyomavirus in human merkel cell carcinoma. Science. 2008;319:1096–100.
3. Agelli M, Clegg LX. Epidemiology of primary Merkel cell carcinoma in the United States. J Am Acad Dermatol. 2003;49(5):832–41.
4. Heath ML, Jaimes N, Lemos B, et al. Clinical characteristics of Merkel cell carcinoma at diagnosis in 195 patients: the AEIOU features. J Am Acad Dermatol. 2008;58(3):375–81.
5. Kanitakis J, Euvrard S, Chouvet B, Butnaru AC, Claudy A. Merkel cell carcinoma in organ-transplant recipients: report of two cases with unusual histological features and literature review. J Cutan Pathol. 2006;33(10):686–94.
6. Penn I, First MR. Merkel's cell carcinoma in organ recipients: report of 41 cases. Transplantation. 1999;68(11):1717–21.
7. Hodgson NC. Merkel cell carcinoma: changing incidence trends. J Surg Oncol. 2005;89(1):1–4.
8. Lemos B, Nghiem P. Merkel cell carcinoma: more deaths but still no pathway to blame. J Invest Dermatol. 2007;127(9):2100–3.
9. Medina-Franco H, Urist MM, Fiveash J, Heslin MJ, Bland KI, Beenken SW. Multimodality treatment of Merkel cell carcinoma: case series and literature review of 1024 cases. Ann Surg Oncol. 2001;8(3):204–8.
10. Allen PJ, Zhang ZF, Coit DG. Surgical management of Merkel cell carcinoma. Ann Surg. 1999;229(1):97–105.
11. AJCC cancer staging manual. 6th ed. Chicago, IL: Springer; 2002.
12. Allen PJ, Bowne WB, Jaques DP, Brennan MF, Busam K, Coit DG. Merkel cell carcinoma: prognosis and treatment of patients from a single institution. J Clin Oncol. 2005;23(10):2300–9.
13. Clark JR, Veness MJ, Gilbert R, O'Brien CJ, Gullane PJ. Merkel cell carcinoma of the head and neck: Is adjuvant radiotherapy necessary? Head Neck. 2007;29(3):249–57.
14. Yiengpruksawan A, Coit DG, Thaler HT, Urmacher C, Knapper WK. Merkel cell carcinoma. Prognosis and management. Arch Surg. 1991;126(12):1514–9.

15. Gupta SG, Wang LC, Penas PF, Gellenthin M, Lee SJ, Nghiem P. Sentinel lymph node biopsy for evaluation and treatment of patients with Merkel cell carcinoma: the Dana-Farber experience and meta-analysis of the literature. Arch Dermatol. 2006;142(6):685–90.

16. Voog E, Biron P, Martin JP, Blay JY. Chemotherapy for patients with locally advanced or metastatic Merkel cell carcinoma. Cancer. 1999;85(12):2589–95.

17. Buell JF, Trofe J, Hanaway MJ, et al. Immunosuppression and Merkel cell cancer. Transplant Proc. 2002;34(5):1780–1.

# Melanoma of the Skin

## *At-A-Glance*

---

### SUMMARY OF CHANGES

- Mitotic rate (histologically defined as mitoses/mm², not mitoses/10 HPF) is an important primary tumor prognostic factor. A mitotic rate equal to or greater than 1/mm² denotes a melanoma at higher risk for metastasis. It should now be used as one defining criteria of T1b melanomas

- Melanoma thickness and tumor ulceration continue to be used in defining strata in the T category. For T1 melanomas, in addition to tumor ulceration, mitotic rate replaces level of invasion as a primary criterion for defining the subcategory of T1b

- The presence of nodal micrometastases can be defined using either H&E or immunohistochemical staining (previously, only the H&E could be used)

- There is no lower threshold of tumor burden defining the presence of regional nodal metastasis. Specifically, nodal tumor deposits less than 0.2 mm in diameter (previously used as the threshold for defining nodal metastasis) are included in the staging of nodal disease as a result of the consensus that smaller volumes of metastatic tumor are still clinically significant. A lower threshold of clinically insignificant nodal metastases has not been defined based on evidence

- The site of distant metastases [nonvisceral (i.e., skin/soft tissue/distant nodal) vs. lung vs. all other visceral metastatic sites] continues to represent the primary component of categorizing the M category

- An elevated serum lactic dehydrogenase (LDH) level remains a powerful predictor of survival and is also to be used in defining the M category

- Survival estimates for patients with intralymphatic regional metastases (i.e., satellites and in transit metastasis) are somewhat better than for the remaining cohort of Stage IIIB patients. Nevertheless, Stage IIIB still represents the closest statistical fit for this group, so the current staging definition for intralymphatic regional metastasis has been retained

- The prognostic significance of microsatellites has been established less broadly. The Melanoma Task Force recommended that this uncommon feature be retained in the N2c category, largely because the published literature is insufficient to substantiate revision of the definitions used in the Sixth Edition *Staging Manual*

- The staging definition of metastatic melanoma from an unknown primary site was clarified, such that isolated metastases arising in lymph nodes, skin, and subcutaneous tissues are to be categorized as Stage III rather than Stage IV

- The definitions of tumor ulceration, mitotic rate and microsatellites were clarified

- Lymphoscintigraphy followed by lymphatic mapping and sentinel lymph node biopsy (sentinel lymphadenectomy) remain important components of melanoma staging and should be used (or discussed with the patient) in defining occult Stage III disease among patients who present with clinical Stage IB or II melanoma

---

## ANATOMIC STAGE/PROGNOSTIC GROUPS

| Clinical Staging* | | | | Pathologic Staging** | | | |
|---|---|---|---|---|---|---|---|
| Stage 0 | Tis | N0 | M0 | 0 | Tis | N0 | M0 |
| Stage IA | T1a | N0 | M0 | IA | T1a | N0 | M0 |
| Stage IB | T1b | N0 | M0 | IB | T1b | N0 | M0 |
| | T2a | N0 | M0 | | T2a | N0 | M0 |
| Stage IIA | T2b | N0 | M0 | IIA | T2b | N0 | M0 |
| | T3a | N0 | M0 | | T3a | N0 | M0 |
| Stage IIB | T3b | N0 | M0 | IIB | T3b | N0 | M0 |
| | T4a | N0 | M0 | | T4a | N0 | M0 |
| Stage IIC | T4b | N0 | M0 | IIC | T4b | N0 | M0 |
| Stage III | Any T | ≥N1 | M0 | IIIA | T1–4a | N1a | M0 |
| | | | | | T1–4a | N2a | M0 |
| | | | | IIIB | T1–4b | N1a | M0 |
| | | | | | T1–4b | N2a | M0 |
| | | | | | T1–4a | N1b | M0 |
| | | | | | T1–4a | N2b | M0 |
| | | | | | T1–4a | N2c | M0 |
| | | | | IIIC | T1–4b | N1b | M0 |
| | | | | | T1–4b | N2b | M0 |
| | | | | | T1–4b | N2c | M0 |
| | | | | | Any T | N3 | M0 |
| Stage IV | Any T | Any N | M1 | IV | Any T | Any N | M1 |

*Clinical staging includes microstaging of the primary melanoma and clinical/radiologic evaluation for metastases. By convention, it should be used after complete excision of the primary melanoma with clinical assessment for regional and distant metastases.

**Pathologic staging includes microstaging of the primary melanoma and pathologic information about the regional lymph nodes after partial or complete lymphadenectomy. Pathologic Stage 0 or Stage IA patients are the exception; they do not require pathologic evaluation of their lymph nodes.

## ICD-O-3 TOPOGRAPHY CODES

| | |
|---|---|
| C44.0 | Skin of lip, NOS |
| C44.1 | Eyelid |
| C44.2 | External ear |
| C44.3 | Skin of other and unspecified parts of face |
| C44.4 | Skin of scalp and neck |
| C44.5 | Skin of trunk |
| C44.6 | Skin of upper limb and shoulder |
| C44.7 | Skin of lower limb and hip |
| C44.8 | Overlapping lesion of skin |
| C44.9 | Skin, NOS |
| C51.0 | Labium majus |
| C51.1 | Labium minus |
| C51.2 | Clitoris |
| C51.8 | Overlapping lesion of vulva |
| C51.9 | Vulva, NOS |
| C60.0 | Prepuce |
| C60.1 | Glans penis |
| C60.2 | Body of penis |
| C60.8 | Overlapping lesion of penis |
| C60.9 | Penis, NOS |
| C63.2 | Scrotum, NOS |

ICD-O-3 HISTOLOGY CODE RANGES
8720–8790

## INTRODUCTION

The sixth edition of the AJCC staging system for cutaneous melanoma has been widely adopted over the past 5 years and few major changes are recommended for the seventh edition. The AJCC Melanoma Staging Database represents a collaborative, international effort developed over several decades. An analysis of prognostic factors involving almost 60,000 patients from these 14 cancer centers and organizations was performed to validate

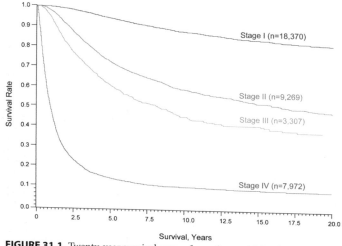

**FIGURE 31.1.** Twenty-year survival curves for patients with localized melanoma (Stages I and II), regional metastases (Stage III), and distant metastases (Stage IV). The *numbers* in *parentheses* are the numbers of patients from the AJCC Melanoma Staging Database used to calculate the survival rates. The differences between the *curves* are highly significant ($p < 0.0001$).

the staging categories and groupings for the seventh edition. The TNM categories and the stage groupings are defined in the following chapter. Twenty-year survival rates for patients with Stages I–IV melanoma are shown in Figure 31.1. Differences between the sixth edition version and the seventh edition version of the melanoma staging system are listed in Table 31.1. Within each stage grouping and subgroups, there is a uniform risk for survival (Figure 31.1).

## ANATOMY

**Primary Sites.** Cutaneous melanoma can occur anywhere on the skin. It occurs most commonly on the extremities in female subjects and on the trunk in male subjects.

**Regional Lymph Nodes.** The regional lymph nodes are the most common site of metastases. The widespread use of cutaneous lymphoscintigraphy followed by lymphatic mapping and sentinel lymph node biopsy has greatly enhanced the ability to identify nodal micrometastases and to define the stage of clinically node-negative melanoma patients. Indeed, the distribution of Stage III patients has changed dramatically since the last melanoma staging review; those patients presenting with clinically occult nodal metastases (Stage IIIA) comprise the majority of the Stage III patients, and the number of patients with clinically detectable metastases (Stage IIIB and IIIC) has declined considerably.

**TABLE 31.1.** Changes in the melanoma staging system comparing the sixth edition (2002) version with the current version (2009)

| Factor | 6th Edition criteria | 7th Edition criteria | Comments |
|---|---|---|---|
| Thickness | Primary determinant of T staging; thresholds of 1.0, 2.0, 4.0 mm | Same | Correlation of metastatic risk is a continuous variable |
| Level of invasion | Used only for defining T1 melanomas | No longer used | Clark's levels $\geq$IV or V may be used in rare instances as a criterion for defining T1b melanoma *only* if mitotic rate cannot be determined in a nonulcerated T1 melanoma |
| Ulceration | Included as a second determinant of T and N staging | Same | Signifies a locally advanced lesion; dominant prognostic factor for grouping Stage I, II, and III |
| Mitotic rate per $mm^2$ | Not Used | Used for categorizing T1 melanoma | Mitosis $\geq$1/$mm^2$ used as a primary determinant for defining T1b melanoma |
| Satellite metastases | In N category | Same | Merged with in transit lesions |
| Immunohistochemical detection of nodal metastases | Not allowed | Allowed | Must include at least one melanoma-specific marker (e.g., HMB-45, Melan-A, MART 1) |
| 0.2-mm threshold of defined node-positive | Implied | No lower threshold of staging node-positive disease | |
| Number of nodal metastases | Dominant determinant of N staging | Same | Thresholds of 1 vs. 2–3 vs. $\geq$4 nodes |
| Metastatic "volume" | Included as a second determinant of N staging | Same | Clinically occult ("microscopic") vs. clinically apparent ("macroscopic") nodal volume |
| Lung metastases | Separate category as M1b | Same | Has a somewhat better prognosis than other visceral metastases |
| Elevated serum LDH | Included as a second determinant of M staging | Same | Recommend a second confirmatory LDH if elevated |
| Clinical vs. pathologic staging | Sentinel node results incorporated into definition of pathologic staging | | Large variability in outcome between clinical and pathologic staging; Sentinel node staging encouraged for standard patient care and should be required prior to entry into clinical trials |

Intralymphatic local and regional metastases may also become clinically manifest as (1) *satellite* metastases (defined arbitrarily as grossly visible cutaneous and/or subcutaneous metastases occurring within 2 cm of the primary melanoma); (2) *microsatellites* – microscopic and discontinuous cutaneous and/or subcutaneous metastases found on pathologic examination adjacent to a primary melanoma; or (3) *in transit* metastases (defined arbitrarily as clinically evident cutaneous and/or subcutaneous metastases identified at a distance greater than 2 cm from the primary melanoma in the region between the primary and the first echelon of regional lymph nodes). These manifestations of melanoma constitute a small but clinically significant and distinctive category of patients, with considerable risk of both additional locoregional and distant metastases.

**Metastatic Sites.** Melanoma can metastasize to virtually any organ site. Distant metastases most commonly occur in the skin or soft tissues, the lung, liver, brain, bone, or gastrointestinal tract.

## RULES FOR CLASSIFICATION

31

The definitions of clinical vs. pathologic stage grouping differ according to whether the regional lymph nodes are staged by clinical/radiographic exam or by pathologic evaluation of the nodal status.

**Clinical Staging.** Clinical Stages I and II are confined to those patients who have no evidence of metastases, either at regional or distant sites based upon clinical, radiographic, and/or laboratory evaluation. Stage III melanoma patients are those with clinical or radiographic evidence of regional metastases, either in the regional lymph nodes or intralymphatic metastases manifesting as either satellite or in transit metastases. Clinical Stage III groupings rely on clinical and/or radiographic assessment of the regional lymph nodes, which is inherently difficult, especially with respect to assessing both the presence and the number of metastatic nodes. The Melanoma Task Force therefore made no subgroup definitions of clinically staged patients with nodal or intralymphatic regional metastases. They are all categorized as clinical Stage III disease. Clinical Stage IV melanoma patients have metastases at a distant site(s) and are not substaged.

**Pathologic Staging.** In contrast to clinical staging, there is greater accuracy (both qualitatively and quantitatively) in defining distinctive prognostic subgroups when combining pathologic information from the primary melanoma and from pathologic examination of the regional lymph nodes after sentinel or complete lymphadenectomy.

Pathologic Stages I and II melanoma comprise those patients who have no evidence of regional or distant metastases, when clinically appropriate use of sentinel lymph node biopsy demonstrates the absence of nodal metastases after careful pathologic examination and routine clinical and radiographic examination demonstrate the absence of distant metastases. Pathologic Stage III melanoma patients have pathologic evidence of regional metastases, either in the regional lymph nodes or at intralymphatic sites. The quantitative classification for pathologic nodal status requires

**TABLE 31.2.** Five-year survival rates of pathologically staged patients (from the 2008 AJCC Melanoma Staging Database)

| | IA | IB | IIA | IIB | IIC | IIIA | IIIB | IIIC |
|---|---|---|---|---|---|---|---|---|
| Ta: nonulcerated | T1a | T2a | T3a | T4a | | N1a | N1b | N3 |
| | 97% | 91% | 79% | 71% | | N2a | N2b | 47% |
| | | | | | | 78% | 48% | |
| Tb: ulcerated[a] | | T1b | T2b | T3b | T4b | | N1a | N1b N2b |
| | | 94% | 82% | 68% | 53% | | N2a | N3 |
| | | | | | | | 55% | 38% |

Note that the stage groupings involve upstaging to account for melanoma ulceration, where thinner melanomas with ulceration are grouped with the next greatest T substage for nonulcerated melanomas.

[a] The presence of tumor ulceration of a primary melanoma (designated Tb) causes upstaging by one substage compared to a nonulcerated melanoma (designated Ta).

careful pathologic examination of the surgically resected nodal basin and documentation of number of lymph nodes examined and the number of nodes that contain metastases. Pathologic Stage IV melanoma patients have histological documentation of metastases at one or more distant sites.

With the widespread use of sentinel lymph node biopsy, it is clear that there is considerable stage migration of patients previously staged as "node negative," but who in fact have undetected nodal metastases. These previously understaged Stage III patients have revealed an extraordinary heterogeneity of metastatic risk within Stage III melanoma. Thus, the range of survival rates among various subgroups of pathologically defined Stage III patients is quite large, ranging from 38 to 78% 5-year survival (Table 31.2).[1,2]

**Clinical vs. Pathologic Staging.** The AJCC Melanoma Task Force recommends that sentinel lymph node biopsy be performed as a staging procedure in patients for whom the information will be useful in planning subsequent treatment and follow-up regimens. Specifically, the procedure should be recommended for (or at least discussed with) patients who have T1b, T2, T3, or T4 melanomas, and clinically or radiographically uninvolved regional lymph nodes. In all prospective studies performed to date involving such patients, sentinel node status was one of the most powerful independent prognostic factors examined.[3–17]

The AJCC Melanoma Task Force also strongly recommends that sentinel lymph node biopsy be required as an entry criterion for all melanoma patients presenting with clinical Stage IB or II disease (including T1a patients with melanoma = 1.00 mm) before entry into clinical trials involving new surgical techniques or adjuvant therapy.

By convention, clinical staging should be performed after complete excision of the primary melanoma (including microstaging) with *clinical* assessment of regional lymph nodes. Pathologic staging will use information gained from *both* microstaging of the primary melanoma and pathologic evaluation of the nodal status after sentinel lymph node biopsy and/ or complete regional lymphadenectomy.

In some centers, ultrasound examination of the regional lymph nodes and fine needle aspiration (FNA) of abnormal lymph nodes has been used to detect small nodal metastases.[18–22] The sensitivity, specificity, and yield of this diagnostic approach have been variable and its use should not replace sentinel lymph node biopsy in clinical Stage IB and II patients when the ultrasound examination and needle biopsy are negative or inconclusive.[20,21] In contrast, when the cytologic examination after a needle biopsy demonstrates the presence of melanoma, a sentinel lymph node biopsy is superfluous in that nodal basin and the final staging is determined after complete or formal regional lymphadenectomy, when the number of metastatic lymph nodes can be pathologically assessed.[23]

Significant differences in survival rates have been identified for melanoma patients who were clinically staged compared with those whose nodal disease was staged pathologically.[1,24,25] These survival differences between clinically and pathologically staged patients were statistically significant among all T categories except for T4b.[1,24] The differences were most striking in patients with clinical T2b – T4a T categories; 10-year survival rates for the same T category of clinically vs. pathologically staged patients varied significantly with diminished survival ranging from 12 to 29% in absolute numbers among clinically vs. pathologically staged patients.[1,24] These results highlight the compelling prognostic value of knowing the nodal status as identified by lymphatic mapping and sentinel lymph node biopsy.

## PROGNOSTIC FEATURES

**Primary Tumor.** Twenty-year survival rates for each of the T categories in clinically staged patients are shown in Table 31.2 and Figure 31.2.

*Melanoma Thickness.* The T category of melanoma is classified primarily by measuring the thickness of the melanoma as defined by Dr. Alexander Breslow.[26,27] In the seventh edition staging version, the T category thresholds of melanoma thickness are still defined in even integers (1.0, 2.0, and 4.0 mm). Although these are arbitrary thresholds for staging purposes, they were previously determined to represent both a statistical "best fit" for the (N0) patient population and the thresholds most compatible with contemporary clinical decision making.[1,24]

The AJCC Melanoma Staging Database includes prospectively accumulated data on over 27,000 melanoma patients with clinically or pathologically localized melanoma (Stage I and II) for whom tumor thickness and follow-up information is available. As tumor thickness increased, there was a highly significant decline in 5- and 10-year survival ($p < 0.001$). Among the 5,296 patients with 0.01–0.5-mm thick melanomas, the 10-year survival was 96%, while it was 89% in the 6,545 patients with 0.51–1.00 mm thick, 80% in the 8,046 patients with 1.01–2.00 mm thick, 65% in 3,539 patients with 2.01–3.00 mm thick, 57% in the 1,752 patients with 3.01–4.00 mm thick, and 54% in the 1,464 patients with 4.01–6.00-mm thick melanomas. For patients with tumor thickness greater than 6.00 mm, the 10-year survival rate was 42%.

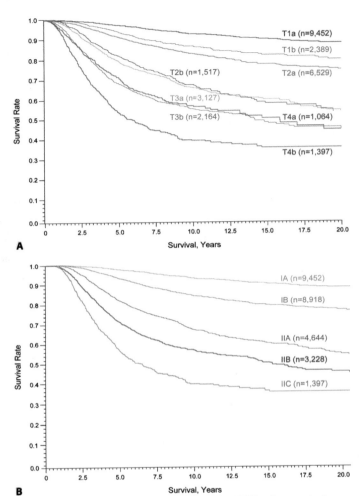

**FIGURE 31.2.** Twenty-year survival rates from the AJCC melanoma staging database comparing the different T categories (**A**) and the stage groupings (**B**) for stages I and II melanoma.

*Melanoma Ulceration.* The second criterion for determining T category is primary tumor ulceration, i.e., the presence or absence of a completely intact epidermis above the primary melanoma based upon a histopathologic examination. Melanoma ulceration is defined as the combination of the following features: full-thickness epidermal defect (including absence of stratum corneum and basement membrane), evidence of reactive changes (i.e., fibrin deposition and neutrophils), and thinning, effacement, or reactive hyperplasia of the surrounding epidermis in the absence of trauma or a recent surgical procedure.[28-32]

**TABLE 31.3.** 2008 AJCC Melanoma Staging Database: Stage I/II survival by current T classification

| T classification | $N^a$ | Survival rate ± SE | |
|---|---|---|---|
| | | 5-Year | 10-Year |
| T1a | 9,452 | 0.972 ± 0.002 | 0.927 ± 0.005 |
| T1b | 2,389 | 0.936 ± 0.007 | 0.865 ± 0.011 |
| T2a | 6,529 | 0.913 ± 0.004 | 0.829 ± 0.007 |
| T2b | 1,517 | 0.818 ± 0.012 | 0.673 ± 0.019 |
| T3a | 3,127 | 0.790 ± 0.009 | 0.661 ± 0.012 |
| T3b | 2,164 | 0.678 ± 0.013 | 0.553 ± 0.015 |
| T4a | 1,064 | 0.709 ± 0.018 | 0.569 ± 0.023 |
| T4b | 1,397 | 0.533 ± 0.018 | 0.394 ± 0.021 |

[a] The number of patients listed are those for whom all the T classification data was available and with sufficient follow-up.

Survival rates for patients with an ulcerated melanoma are proportionately lower than those of patients with a nonulcerated melanoma of equivalent T category, but are remarkably similar to those of patients with a nonulcerated melanoma of the next highest T category (Figure 31.2 and Tables 31.2 and 31.3).

**Melanoma Mitotic Rate.** Primary tumor mitotic rate has been introduced as a required element for the seventh edition melanoma staging system. Data from the AJCC Melanoma Staging Database demonstrated a highly significant correlation with increasing mitotic rate and declining survival rates (Tables 31.4 and 31.5), especially within thin melanoma subgroups. In a multifactorial analysis of 10,233 patients with clinically localized melanoma, mitotic rate was the second most powerful predictor of survival outcome, after tumor thickness (Table 31.6). Single institutions have also identified mitotic rate as an adverse prognostic factor.[33–37]

Mitotic rate should be assessed on all primary melanomas. The recommended approach to enumerating mitoses is to first find the areas in the dermis containing the most mitotic figures, the so-called hot spot. After counting the mitoses in the hot spot, the count is extended to adjacent fields until an area

**TABLE 31.4.** Data from the 2008 AJCC Melanoma Staging Database demonstrating a highly significant correlation between increasing mitotic rate and declining survival in patients with localized melanoma (stages I and II)

| Number of mitoses/mm² | n | Survival rate ± SE | |
|---|---|---|---|
| | | 5-Year | 10-Year |
| 0–0.99 | 3,312 | 0.973 ± 0.004 | 0.927 ± 0.007 |
| 1.00–1.99 | 2,117 | 0.920 ± 0.007 | 0.842 ± 0.012 |
| 2.00–4.99 | 3,254 | 0.869 ± 0.007 | 0.754 ± 0.012 |
| 5.00–10.99 | 2,049 | 0.781 ± 0.011 | 0.680 ± 0.018 |
| 11.00–19.99 | 673 | 0.695 ± 0.022 | 0.576 ± 0.027 |
| ≥20.0 | 259 | 0.594 ± 0.039 | 0.476 ± 0.050 |
| Total | 11,664[a] | | |

[a] Includes patients with mitosis, tumor thickness, and follow-up information available.

**TABLE 31.5.** Survival rates for 4861 T1 melanoma patients (1.00 mm or less) subgrouped by thickness and mitotic rate of the primary melanoma

| Thickness (mm) | Mitosis | N | Survival rate ± SE | |
| | | | 5-Year | 10-Year |
|---|---|---|---|---|
| 0.01–0.50 | <1.0 | 1,194 | 0.991 ± 0.004 | 0.974 ± 0.086 |
| 0.01–0.50 | ≥1.0 | 327 | 0.970 ± 0.012 | 0.952 ± 0.017 |
| 0.51–1.00 | <1.0 | 1,472 | 0.977 ± 0.005 | 0.930 ± 0.010 |
| 0.51–1.00 | ≥1.0 | 1,868 | 0.935 ± 0.006 | 0.871 ± 0.012 |

corresponding to 1 mm$^2$ is assessed. If no hot spot can be found and mitoses are sparse and randomly scattered throughout the lesion, then a representative mitosis is chosen and beginning with that field the count is then extended to adjacent fields until an area corresponding to 1 mm$^2$ is assessed. The count then is expressed as the number of mitoses/mm$^2$ (i.e., an area corresponding to approximately four high power fields at 400× in most microscopes). To obtain accurate measurement, calibration of individual microscopes is recommended. For classifying thin (≤1 mm) melanomas, the threshold for a nonulcerated melanoma to be defined as T1b is ≥1 mitoses/mm$^2$.

When the invasive component of tumor is <1 mm$^2$ (in area), the number of mitoses present in 1 mm$^2$ of dermal tissue that includes the tumor should be enumerated and recorded as a number per millimeter squared. Alternatively, in tumors where the invasive component is <1 mm$^2$ in area, the simple presence or absence of a mitosis can be designated as *at least* 1/mm$^2$ (i.e., "mitogenic") or 0/mm$^2$ (i.e., "nonmitogenic"), respectively. At some institutions, when mitotic figures are not found after numerous fields are examined, the mitotic count has been described as "<1/mm$^2$." For most tumor registries, the designation "<1/mm$^2$" equals 0 as has been customarily used in the past. This practice may be continued for historical data. For the future, we urge pathologists to list 0 or 1 or more, and this practice should also be demanded by clinicians.

It is common and appropriate practice with small, thin melanomas to have the technician place multiple sections cut from the block on a single slide. As a guide, we suggest that no more than two slides with such multiple sections be evaluated so that exhaustive evaluation of the lesion is not performed. Excellent interobserver reproducibility among specialist, general, and trainee pathologists for their assessment of mitotic rate as defined above has been previously described.[37a]

*Level of Invasion.* The level of invasion, as defined by Dr. Wallace Clark,[38] has been used for over 40 years for various staging systems of melanomas. Although Clark's levels of invasion have prognostic significance in univariate analysis, numerous publications have shown that the level of invasion is less reproducible among pathologists and does not reflect prognosis as accurately as tumor thickness.[26,29,39–42] In the sixth edition of the *Cancer Staging Manual,* level of invasion was used in defining the specific subgroup of thin (T1) melanomas.[24,43–49] However, newer information has demonstrated that while level of invasion is an independent prognostic factor, it has the lowest statistical correlation with survival rates compared with the other six independent prognostic variables (Table 31.6).

**TABLE 31.6.** Multivariate Cox regression analysis of prognostic factors in 10,233 patients with localized cutaneous melanoma (Stage I and II)

| Variable | Chi-square values (1 d.f.) | P | HR | 95% CI |
|---|---|---|---|---|
| Tumor thickness | 84.6 | <0.0001 | 1.25 | 1.19–1.31 |
| Mitotic rate | 79.1 | <0.0001 | 1.26 | 1.20–1.32 |
| Ulceration | 47.2 | <0.0001 | 1.56 | 1.38–1.78 |
| Age | 40.8 | <0.0001 | 1.16 | 1.11–1.22 |
| Gender | 32.4 | <0.0001 | 0.70 | 0.62–0.79 |
| Site | 29.1 | <0.0001 | 1.38 | 1.23–1.54 |
| Clark's level | 8.2 | 0.0041 | 1.15 | 1.04–1.26 |

**Defining T1 Melanomas.** In the T1 cohort of melanomas, the assignment of T1a is restricted to melanomas with three criteria (1) ≤1.0 mm thick, (2) absence of ulceration, and (3) mitotic rate of *less than* 1/mm². Thus, T1b melanomas are now defined as those whose tumor thickness is ≤1.0 mm *and* have *at least* 1 mitosis/mm² or tumor ulceration. This is a major change from the sixth edition Cancer Staging Manual where the level of invasion was used to define T1b melanomas. In the rare circumstances where the mitotic rate cannot be accurately determined, a level invasion of either IV or V as defined by Clark can be used to categorize patients into the T1b classification.

These recommendations were made after reviewing the statistical information involving 4,861 T1 melanomas from the updated AJCC Melanoma Staging Database demonstrating that mitotic rate was the most powerful predictor of survival outcome for T1 melanoma patients, and conversely, that the level of invasion was no longer statistically significant when mitotic rate and ulceration were included (data not shown). Ten-year survival rates ranged from 97% for T1 melanomas of 0.01–0.50 mm in thickness and <1 mitosis/mm² to 87% for 0.51–1.00 mm melanomas with ≥1 mitosis/mm² (Table 31.5). In the latter group, the 10-year survival rates dropped to 85% if the melanoma was also ulcerated.

**TABLE 31.7.** Multivariate Cox regression analysis of prognostic factors in 1,338 patients with regional lymph node metastases (Stage III)

| Variable | Chi-square values (1 d.f.) | | |
|---|---|---|---|
| | All patient with stage III (n = 1,338) | Patient with micro-metastasis (n = 1,070) | Patients with macro-metastasis (n = 268) |
| No. of positive nodes | 27.4 | 27.8 | 5.0 |
| Ulceration | 17.5 | 13.5 | 2.1 |
| Tumor thickness | 9.1 | 9.4 | 1.1 |
| Tumor burden (micro vs. macro) | 4.7 | – | – |
| Mitotic rate | 4.4 | 12.7 | 0.2 |
| Age | 24.8 | 15.8 | 7.1 |
| Site | 4.3 | 4.7 | 0.4 |
| Gender | 0.5 | 0.4 | 0.2 |
| Clark's level | 0.1 | 0.0 | 0.2 |

*Sentinel Nodal Staging in T1b Melanoma.* In the sixth edition of the AJCC *Staging Manual* it was recommended that sentinel node staging be considered in patients presenting with T1bN0M0 or thicker melanomas, based upon the secondary features of either tumor ulceration or Clark's level IV depth of invasion, which were associated with an approximately 10% yield of occult nodal metastases. The use of mitotic rate for the purpose of classifying thin melanomas as T1b in the seventh edition was based on a survival analysis. The AJCC Melanoma Staging Database did not contain sufficient data for precisely estimating risk for occult nodal micrometastases in this population. However, preliminary evidence from several other large studies would suggest that T1b melanomas (as defined in the new system) of ≥0.76 mm in thickness are associated with an approximately 10% risk of occult nodal metastases. Conversely, T1a melanomas with <1 mitoses/mm$^2$, or T1b melanomas <0.5 mm in thickness have a very low risk of nodal micrometastases. These data may be helpful when discussing the indications for sentinel lymph node biopsy for staging with individual patients with T1b melanoma.

*Melanoma In Situ, Indeterminate Melanomas, Multiple Primary Melanomas.* Patients with melanoma in situ are categorized as Tis. Those patients with melanoma presentations that are indeterminate or cannot be microstaged should be categorized as TX. However, when the pathology of the initial biopsy finds that the tumor was transected at the base, the maximal thickness should be recorded without the addition of any residual tumor found in the re-excision. If the total thickness found in the re-excision is greater than the thickness of the original biopsy, then only the maximal thickness in the re-excision should be recorded. When patients present with multiple primary melanomas, the T category staging is based upon the melanoma with the worst prognostic features.

*Melanoma Growth Patterns.* The data used to derive the TNM categories were largely based on melanomas with superficial spreading and nodular growth patterns. There is some evidence that melanomas of other growth patterns, namely lentigo maligna, acral lentiginous, and desmoplastic melanomas, have a different etiology and natural history.[50–55] At present, the same staging criteria should be used for melanomas with all growth patterns, even though their prognosis may differ somewhat from the more commonly occurring growth patterns.

**Regional Lymph Nodes.** The 2008 AJCC Staging Melanoma Database contains over 3,400 Stage III patients, the vast majority of whom presented with micrometastases after a sentinel lymph node biopsy and completion lymphadenectomy. A multivariate Cox regression analysis of the database demonstrated that the number of tumor-bearing nodes, tumor burden at the time of staging (i.e., microscopic vs. macroscopic), and presence or absence of ulceration of the primary melanoma were the most predictive independent factors for survival in these patients (Table 31.7). These characteristics were incorporated into the stage grouping criteria. For example, the presence of tumor ulceration was used as a criterion for a higher assigned substage due to lower observed survival rates, such that,

**TABLE 31.8.** 2008 AJCC melanoma staging database: Five- and ten-year survival rates for stage III melanoma substages

| Stage | N | Survival rate ± SE | |
| --- | --- | --- | --- |
| | | 5-Year | 10-Year |
| IIIA | 1,196 | 0.78 ± 0.02 | 0.68 ± 0.02 |
| IIIB[a] (including N2c) | 1,391 | 0.59 ± 0.02 | 0.43 ± 0.02 |
| IIIB (excluding N2c) | 992 | 0.54 ± 0.02 | 0.38 ± 0.03 |
| IIIC | 720 | 0.40 ± 0.02 | 0.24 ± 0.03 |

[a] 399 N2c patients (intralymphatic metastases) had 5- and 10-year survival rates of 69% and 52%.

there was a uniform 5-year survival probability within each of the Stage III subgroups (see Table 31.2).

***Number of Metastatic Nodes.*** This factor is the primary criterion for defining the N category, because the number of metastatic nodes correlated best with 10-year survival outcomes in all substages of Stage III in the AJCC analysis (see Table 31.7).[24] Thus, patients with one node involved by metastasis are categorized as N1, those with 2–3 metastatic nodes as N2 and those with ≥4 metastatic nodes involved (or matted nodes) are defined as N3. Survival rates for these N subgroups are shown in Figure 31.3.

***Micrometastases vs. Macrometastases.*** Another significant prognostic feature for patients with nodal metastases is the tumor burden of nodal metastases (Table 31.7). This terminology is defined operationally, not by actual measurements. Thus, those patients without clinical or radiographic evidence of lymph node metastases but who have pathologically documented

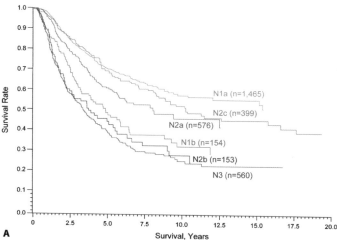

**FIGURE 31.3.** Twenty-year survival rates from the AJCC melanoma staging database comparing the different N categories (**A**) and the stage groupings (**B**) for stage III melanoma. (**C**) This figure shows the more favorable survival for the subgroup of stage III patients with satellites or in transit lesions.

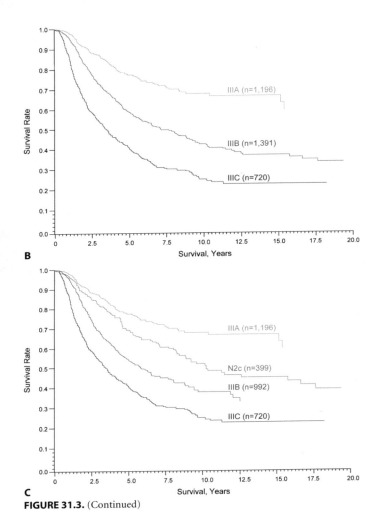

**B**

**C**

**FIGURE 31.3.** (Continued)

nodal metastases are defined by convention as "microscopic" or "clinically occult" nodal metastases. It is recognized that such nodal metastases may vary in dimensions (especially for deep-seated nodes or in obese patients), but such a delineation can be identified in the medical record, based upon the preoperative clinical exam and the operative notation about the intent of the lymphadenectomy (i.e., whether it is a completion lymphadenectomy after sentinel lymph node biopsy for clinically occult disease or a "therapeutic" lymphadenectomy for clinically detected disease). Survival rates for these two patient groups are significantly different.[24,39,56]

*Immunohistochemical Detection of Micrometastases.* Immunohistology should always be adjunctive to good quality hematoxylin and eosin (H&E) stained sections. That being said, for the purposes of staging for nodal metastases, it is no longer mandatory for histopathologic confirmation using standard H&E staining, although this is highly recommended. With the availability of immunohistochemical (IHC) staining, it is now possible to detect nodal metastases as small as <0.1-mm or even aggregates of a few cells.[57,58] The availability of immunohistochemical methods to detect melanoma-associated antigens is sufficiently available worldwide, that the AJCC Melanoma Task Force considers it acceptable to classify node-positive metastases based solely on immunohistochemical staining of melanoma-associated markers. In the sixth edition of the *Cancer Staging Manual*, micrometastases were only defined when they were detected by standard H&E staining.

Since some IHC markers are sensitive, but not specific, for staining melanoma cells (e.g., S100, tyrosinase), the definitive diagnosis must include detection with at least one melanoma-associated marker (e.g., HMB-45, Melan-A/MART-1) if cellular morphology is not otherwise diagnostic.[59] These "specific" melanoma markers are of limited sensitivity and may not stain up to 15% of melanomas. In several studies, however, the combination of permanent H&E sections with multiple levels and S-100, Melan-A, and/or HMB-45 IHC increased the overall diagnostic sensitivity of sentinel lymph node biopsy.[60–62]

The reverse transcriptase polymerase chain reaction (RT-PCR) technique may detect metastases not identifiable by the light microscope. Such sophisticated detection procedures may be incorporated into future staging criteria, but at the present time are associated with conflicting results in the literature and are therefore not sufficiently standardized to warrant their inclusion at this time.

*Node Positive Threshold for Defining Nodal Micrometastases.* There is no definitive evidence that defines a lower threshol of microscopically identifiable tumor burden that should not be used to define node positive disease for staging purposes. Evidence published in the melanoma literature demonstrates that even small volumes of metastatic tumor (e.g., those of 0.1 mm or less in diameter) are associated with a worse prognosis than pathologically negative nodes over time.[57,58] The concept that isolated tumor cells in the lymph nodes (especially in subcapsular sinuses) are of no adverse biological significance cannot be substantiated for melanoma at this time, and a lower threshold of clinically insignificant nodal metastases has not been defined based on any evidence known to the AJCC Melanoma Task Force membership. These findings are in contrast to the findings often cited from breast cancer where micrometastases of <0.2 mm are defined as "not clinically relevant" and therefore not used as a criterion for staging node positive breast cancer.[63]

*Intralymphatic Metastases.* The third criterion for defining the N category is the presence or absence of satellites or in transit metastases, regardless of the number of lesions. The available data show no substantial difference in survival outcome for these two anatomically defined entities.[40] The clinical or microscopic presence of satellites around a primary melanoma or of in transit metastases between the primary melanoma site and the regional lymph node basin represent intralymphatic metastases that portend a relatively poor prognosis.[40,64-70]

The sixth edition staging manual classification of Stage III melanoma included those patients with regional lymph node metastases or with metastases within the lymphatics manifesting as either satellite (including microsatellites) or in transit metastases. The latter situation would be designated as "N2c" without nodal metastases or "N3" with synchronous nodal metastasis. The identification of satellite or in transit metastases is associated with a poorer survival rate comparable to that of patients with Stage IIIB melanoma (without concomitant nodal metastases) or IIIC melanoma (with nodal metastases or arising from an ulcerated primary melanoma). The 2008 AJCC Melanoma Staging Database contained new information about patients with intralymphatic metastases (N2c). The 5- and 10-year survival rates were 69% and 52%, respectively (see Figure 31.3). These are somewhat more favorable than that previously reported in the literature and higher than the remaining cohort of Stage IIIB patients (Table 31.8).[40] Nonetheless, the AJCC Melanoma Task Force noted that the category of Stage IIIB was presently the closest fit and recommended that the sixth edition staging definition be retained.

The data for microsatellites is less robust, but the more limited evidence shows that the survival outcome is comparable to that of patients with clinically detectable satellite metastases. Microscopic satellites are defined as any discontinuous nest of intralymphatic metastatic cells >0.05 mm in diameter that are clearly separated by normal dermis (not fibrosis or inflammation) from the main invasive component of melanoma by a distance of at least 0.3 mm. The significance of the microscopic satellites relates to their being highly predictive of recurrent locoregional involvement and lower survival rates in patients with otherwise uninvolved lymph nodes.

In the past, the definition of microsatellites has varied and this may account for some of the differences in results regarding their prognostic significance. As a result, the level of evidence regarding the prognostic significance of microsatellites is not as robust, but the available data indicates that this finding is an adverse finding associated with an increased risk of regional recurrences and a decreased disease-free survival rate similar to that of clinically detectable satellites.[65-67,70-72] Whether microsatellites represent an independent predictor of survival outcome is less clear but at present the preponderance of evidence suggests that this feature represents an adverse prognostic factor for survival.[70-72] Accordingly, the AJCC Melanoma Task Force has recommended that this feature of early lymphatic metastases, as defined above, be retained in the category of N2c melanoma.

***Contiguous or Multiple Nodal Basins and Staging.*** By convention, the term regional nodal metastases refers to disease confined to one nodal basin or two contiguous nodal basins, such as patients with nodal disease involving combinations of femoral/iliac, axillary/supraclavicular, cervical/supraclavicular, axillary/femoral or bilateral axillary/femoral metastases. All such patients would be categorized as having Stage III melanoma.

**Distant Metastasis.** In patients with distant metastases, the site(s) of metastases and elevated serum levels of lactate dehydrogenase (LDH) are used to delineate the M categories into three groups: M1a, M1b, and M1c, with 1-year survival rates ranging from 40 to 60% (Figures 31.4 and 31.5).

*Site(s) of Distant Metastases.* Patients with distant metastasis in the skin, subcutaneous tissue, or distant lymph nodes are categorized as M1a provided the LDH level is normal; they have a relatively better prognosis compared with those patients with metastases located in any other anatomic site.[24,54,73–76] Patients with metastasis to the lung and a normal LDH level are categorized as M1b and have an "intermediate" prognosis when comparing survival rates. Those patients with metastases to any other visceral sites or with an elevated LDH level have a relatively worse prognosis and are designated as M1c (Figure 31.4).

*Elevated Serum Lactate Dehydrogenase.* Although it is uncommon in staging classifications to include serum factors, an exception was made for elevated levels of serum LDH. The updated AJCC Melanoma Staging Database clearly demonstrates that this is an independent and highly significant predictor of survival outcome among patients who present with or develop Stage IV disease (Figure 31.5). The mechanism(s) or source(s) of elevated LDH isoenzymes are unknown, and generally the elevations have a nonspecific pattern of elevation among the various LDH isoenzymes. Nevertheless, the clinical results that have emerged from the assessment of total LDH values in relation to outcome are striking in that survival rates are significantly reduced in those patients with an elevated serum LDH at the time of initial Stage IV diagnosis. Thus 1- and 2-year overall survival

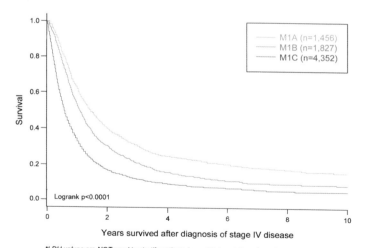

M1A (n=1,456)
M1B (n=1,827)
M1C (n=4,352)

Logrank p<0.0001

Survival

Years survived after diagnosis of stage IV disease

*LDH values are NOT used to stratify patients here–this is only based on site of metastasis

**FIGURE 31.4.** Survival curves of 7,635 patients with metastatic melanomas at distant sites (stage IV) subgrouped by M category site of disease (LDH levels not included in stratification). The number of patients is shown in *parentheses.*

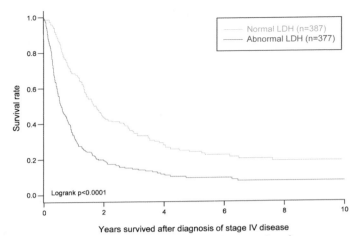

**FIGURE 31.5.** Survival curves of 764 patients with metastatic melanomas at distant sites (stage IV) subgrouped by normal and abnormal serum LDH levels. The number of patients is shown in *parentheses*.

rates for those Stage IV patients in the 2008 AJCC Melanoma Staging Database with a normal serum LDH were 65% and 40%, respectively, compared with 32% and 18%, respectively, when the serum LDH was elevated at the time of staging. Furthermore, this factor was among the most predictive independent factors of diminished survival in all published studies when it was analyzed in a multivariate analysis, even after accounting for site and number of metastases.[77–80] Therefore, when the serum LDH is elevated above the upper limits of normal at the time of staging, such patients with distant metastases are assigned to M1c regardless of the site of their distant metastases. To confirm the elevated serum LDH for staging purposes, it is recommended to obtain two or more determinations obtained more than 24 h apart, since an elevated serum LDH on a single determination can be falsely positive due to hemolysis or other factors unrelated to melanoma metastases.

*Number of Metastases.* The number of metastases at distant sites has previously been documented as an important prognostic factor.[54,73,75,76] This was also confirmed by preliminary multivariate analyses using the AJCC Melanoma Staging Database. However, this feature was not incorporated into this version of the staging system due to the significant variability in the deployment of diagnostic tests to comprehensively search for distant metastases. These may range from a chest x-ray in some centers to high-resolution double-contrast CT, PET/CT, and MRI in others. Until the indications and types of tests used are better standardized, the number of metastases cannot reliably or reproducibly be used for staging purposes.

*Metastatic Melanoma from an Unknown Primary Site.* In general, the staging criteria for unknown primary metastatic melanoma should be the same as those for known primary melanomas. Potential sources could be primary cutaneous melanomas that have been previously biopsied or which have regressed, or from mucosal or ocular primary sites. When patients have an initial presentation of metastases in the lymph nodes, these should be presumed to be regional (Stage III instead of Stage IV) if an appropriate staging workup does not reveal any other sites of metastases. These patients have a prognosis and natural history that is similar to, if not more favorable than, patients with the same staging characteristics from a known primary cutaneous melanoma.[81],[82] A careful history should be obtained and a close examination of the skin from which lymphatics drain to that nodal basin should be made for previous biopsy scars or areas of depigmentation. If there have been previous biopsies, the pathology should be reviewed to determine if, in retrospect, any of these may have been a primary melanoma.

When there are localized metastases to the skin or subcutaneous tissues, these should also be presumed to be regional (i.e., Stage III instead of Stage IV) if an appropriate staging workup does not reveal any other sites of metastases. In patients with presumed skin metastases from an unknown primary site, pathology review by an experienced pathologist or dermatopathologist is appropriate to confirm that the lesion is not a variant of a primary melanoma, particularly a melanoma with a regressed junctional component. In some patients, examination of the skin with a Wood's light (Black or UV light) reveals skin changes of a regressed primary melanoma that can be confirmed pathologically.[83]

All other circumstances (i.e., metastases to a visceral site and no known primary melanoma) should be categorized as Stage IV melanoma, using the M1 classification criteria described above reflecting metastatic site and serum LDH status.

**Stage Groups**

*Localized Melanoma (Stages I and II).* Patients with primary melanomas with no evidence of regional or distant metastases (either clinically or pathologically) are divided into two stages: Stage I for early-stage patients with relatively "low risk" for metastases and melanoma-specific mortality and Stage II for those with "intermediate risk" for metastases and melanoma-specific mortality. Within each stage, the presence of melanoma ulceration heralds an increased relative risk for metastases compared to patients with melanomas of equivalent thickness without ulceration. Therefore, Stage I patients are subdivided into two subgroups (1) Stage IA are T1 melanomas with mitotic rate of $<1/mm^2$ and without ulceration (T1aN0M0 melanomas) and (2) Stage IB are either T1 melanomas with mitotic rate of at least $1/mm^2$ or histopathologic evidence of ulceration (T1bN0M0) or those T2 melanomas without ulceration regardless of mitotic rate (T2aN0M0). Stage II patients constitute three subgroups (1) Stage IIA are T2 melanomas with ulceration (T2bN0M0) or T3 melanomas without ulceration (T3aN0M0); (2) Stage IIB are either T3 melanomas with ulceration (T3bN0M0) or T4 melanomas without ulceration (T4aN0M0); and (3) Stage IIC are T4 melanomas with ulceration (T4bN0M0). Survival rates for these stage groupings are shown in Figure 31.2.

***Regional Metastases (Stage III).*** There are no substages assigned for clinical Stage III melanoma. The major determinants of outcome for pathologic Stage III melanoma are (1) the number of metastatic lymph nodes, (2) whether the tumor burden is "microscopic" (i.e., clinically occult and detected pathologically by sentinel lymph node biopsy) or "macroscopic" (i.e., clinically apparent physical or radiographic examination and verified pathologically), (3) features of the primary melanoma in the presence of nodal micrometastasis, and (4) the presence or absence of satellite or in transit metastases.[2,16,40,54,65,73,84–92] Note that primary tumor characteristics, including the presence or absence of ulceration of the primary melanoma, increased mitotic rate, and/or tumor thickness, are significant predictors of an adverse outcome in patients with nodal micrometastases, but does not influence outcome in patients who present with nodal macrometastases (Table 31.7). The 5-year survival rates for patients in each of the N categories subgrouped by presence or absence of primary melanoma ulceration are shown in Figure 31.3.

After accounting for these prognostic features in pathologic Stage III melanoma, there are three definable subgroups with statistically significant differences in survival: Stages IIIA, IIIB, and IIIC (see Figure 31.3 and Table 31.8). Patients with pathologic Stage IIIA are confined to those who have 1–3 lymph nodes with "microscopic" metastases (detected by sentinel or elective lymphadenectomy), and whose primary melanoma is not ulcerated (T1-4aN1aM0 or T1-4aN2aM0). The 5- and 10-year survival rates for such patients are 78% and 68%, respectively. Patients with pathologic Stage IIIB are those with 1–3 lymph nodes with "macroscopic" metastases and a nonulcerated primary melanoma (i.e., T1-4aN1bM0 or T1-4aN2bM0) or those with 1–3 "microscopic" lymph node metastases and an ulcerated primary melanoma (T1-4bN1aM0 or T1-4bN2aM0) or patients with intralymphatic regional metastases but without nodal metastases (T1-4aN2cM0) (see Figure 31.3 and Table 31.8). The estimated 5- and 10-year survival for Stage IIIB patients is 59% and 43%, respectively (see Figure 31.3 and Table 31.8). In the sixth edition version of the melanoma staging database, the survival rates for patients with isolated intralymphatic metastases were similar to that of patients in the other two subgroups of Stage IIIB disease described above. In the 2008 Melanoma Staging Database, the results of the N2c melanoma patients were somewhat better, with 5- and 10-year survival rates of 69% and 52%, respectively; a more favorable outcome than those in the other two subgroups comprising Stage IIIB melanoma (Figure 31.3 and Table 31.8), but still lower than patients with Stage IIIA melanoma.

Patients grouped as Stage IIIC melanoma are defined as those with a 1–3 "macroscopic" lymph node metastases and an ulcerated primary melanoma (T1-4bN1bM0 or T1-4bN2bM0), patients with satellite(s)/in transit metastases arising from an ulcerated primary melanoma (T1-4bN2cM0), or any patient with N3 disease regardless of T status, including patients with any combination of satellites or in transit metastases and nodal metastases. The estimated 5- and 10-year survival rates for pathologic Stage IIIC patients is significantly lower at 40% and 24%, respectively (see Figure 31.3 and Table 31.8).

***Distant Metastases (Stage IV).*** Because the survival differences between the M categories are small, there are no stage subgroups of Stage IV melanoma.

## DEFINITIONS OF TNM

### Primary Tumor (T)

| | |
|---|---|
| TX | Primary tumor cannot be assessed (e.g., curettaged or severely regressed melanoma) |
| T0 | No evidence of primary tumor |
| Tis | Melanoma in situ |
| T1 | Melanomas 1.0 mm or less in thickness |
| T2 | Melanomas 1.01–2.0 mm |
| T3 | Melanomas 2.01–4.0 mm |
| T4 | Melanomas more than 4.0 mm |

*Note*: a and b subcategories of T are assigned based on ulceration and number of mitoses per mm² as shown below:

| T classification | Thickness (mm) | Ulceration Status/Mitoses |
|---|---|---|
| T1 | ≤1.0 | a: w/o ulceration and mitosis <1/mm² |
| | | b: with ulceration or mitoses ≥1/mm² |
| T2 | 1.01–2.0 | a: w/o ulceration |
| | | b: with ulceration |
| T3 | 2.01–4.0 | a: w/o ulceration |
| | | b: with ulceration |
| T4 | >4.0 | a: w/o ulceration |
| | | b: with ulceration |

### Regional Lymph Nodes (N)

| | |
|---|---|
| NX | Patients in whom the regional nodes cannot be assessed (e.g., previously removed for another reason) |
| N0 | No regional metastases detected |
| N1-3 | Regional metastases based upon the number of metastatic nodes and presence or absence of intralymphatic metastases (in transit or satellite metastases) |

*Note*: N1-3 and a–c subcategories assigned as shown below:

| N Classification | No. of Metastatic Nodes | Nodal Metastatic Mass |
|---|---|---|
| N1 | 1 node | a: micrometastasis* |
| | | b: macrometastasis** |
| N2 | 2–3 nodes | a: micrometastasis* |
| | | b: macrometastasis** |
| | | c: in transit met(s)/ satellite(s) *without* metastatic nodes |
| N3 | 4 or more metastatic nodes, or matted nodes, or in transit met(s)/ satellite(s) *with* metastatic node(s) | |

\* Micrometastases are diagnosed after sentinel lymph node biopsy and completion lymphadenectomy (if performed).

\** Macrometastases are defined as clinically detectable nodal metastases confirmed by therapeutic lymphadenectomy or when nodal metastasis exhibits gross extracapsular extension.

### Distant Metastasis (M)

| | |
|---|---|
| M0 | No detectable evidence of distant metastases |
| M1a | Metastases to skin, subcutaneous, or distant lymph nodes |
| M1b | Metastases to lung |
| M1c | Metastases to all other visceral sites or distant metastases to any site combined with an elevated serum LDH |

*Note:* Serum LDH is incorporated into the M category as shown below:

| M Classification | Site | Serum LDH |
|---|---|---|
| M1a | Distant skin, subcutaneous, or nodal mets | Normal |
| M1b | Lung metastases | Normal |
| M1c | All other visceral metastases | Normal |
| | Any distant metastasis | Elevated |

### ANATOMIC STAGE/PROGNOSTIC GROUPS

| Clinical Staging* | | | | Pathologic Staging** | | | |
|---|---|---|---|---|---|---|---|
| Stage 0 | Tis | N0 | M0 | 0 | Tis | N0 | M0 |
| Stage IA | T1a | N0 | M0 | IA | T1a | N0 | M0 |
| Stage IB | T1b | N0 | M0 | IB | T1b | N0 | M0 |
| | T2a | N0 | M0 | | T2a | N0 | M0 |
| Stage IIA | T2b | N0 | M0 | IIA | T2b | N0 | M0 |
| | T3a | N0 | M0 | | T3a | N0 | M0 |
| Stage IIB | T3b | N0 | M0 | IIB | T3b | N0 | M0 |
| | T4a | N0 | M0 | | T4a | N0 | M0 |
| Stage IIC | T4b | N0 | M0 | IIC | T4b | N0 | M0 |
| Stage III | Any T | ≥N1 | M0 | IIIA | T1 – 4a | N1a | M0 |
| | | | | | T1 – 4a | N2a | M0 |
| | | | | IIIB | T1 – 4b | N1a | M0 |
| | | | | | T1 – 4b | N2a | M0 |
| | | | | | T1 – 4a | N1b | M0 |
| | | | | | T1 – 4a | N2b | M0 |
| | | | | | T1 – 4a | N2c | M0 |
| | | | | IIIC | T1 – 4b | N1b | M0 |
| | | | | | T1 – 4b | N2b | M0 |
| | | | | | T1 – 4b | N2c | M0 |
| | | | | | Any T | N3 | M0 |
| Stage IV | Any T | Any N | M1 | IV | Any T | Any N | M1 |

*Clinical staging includes microstaging of the primary melanoma and clinical/radiologic evaluation for metastases. By convention, it should be used after complete excision of the primary melanoma with clinical assessment for regional and distant metastases.

**Pathologic staging includes microstaging of the primary melanoma and pathologic information about the regional lymph nodes after partial or complete lymphadenectomy. Pathologic Stage 0 or Stage IA patients are the exception; they do not require pathologic evaluation of their lymph nodes.

## PROGNOSTIC FACTORS (SITE-SPECIFIC FACTORS)
### (Recommended for Collection)

| | |
|---|---|
| Required for staging | None |
| Clinically significant | Measured thickness<br>Ulceration<br>Serum lactate dehydrogenase (LDH)<br>Mitotic rate<br>Tumor infiltrating lymphocytes (TIL)<br>Level of invasion<br>Vertical growth phase<br>Regression |

## HISTOLOGIC GRADE (G)

Histologic grading is not used in the staging of melanoma.

**31**

## DATA RECORDING CRITERIA

**Stages I and II.** When entering melanoma TNM data into cancer registries for the purposes of stage grouping, the electronic data fields must record the measured tumor thickness (in hundredths of a millimeter), the presence or absence of ulceration (based upon histopathologic examination), and mitotic rate in order to derive stage groupings for localized melanomas. In those circumstances where there has been an incisional (or punch) biopsy, the maximum tumor thickness in *either* the biopsy or definitive excision should be recorded (the measurements cannot be added). A deep shave biopsy or curettage may result in transection of the tumor at the deep margin. The maximal thickness should be recorded without the addition of any residual tumor found in the re-excision. If the total thickness found in the re-excision is greater than the thickness of the original biopsy, then only the maximal thickness in the re-excision should be recorded. Other prognostic features of localized melanomas were not incorporated into the new TNM categories, but are important nevertheless to record in medical records and cancer registries so that the information is available for other types of data analysis, such as for clinical trials. These include the patient's age and gender, the anatomic site of the primary melanoma (i.e., trunk, extremities, or head and neck), regression (if present), and the growth pattern (superficial spreading, nodular, lentigo maligna melanoma, acral lentiginous melanoma, or desmoplastic melanoma).

**Stage III Melanoma.** Electronic data fields for melanoma should incorporate all the information listed above for the primary melanoma. In addition, the total number of metastatic lymph nodes identified by the pathologist (out of a total number of lymph nodes examined), the presence or absence of intralymphatic metastases (satellites or in transits), and the intent of the surgical procedure that led to the detection of the nodal metastases (i.e., a "therapeutic" lymphadenectomy for clinically detectable metastatic lymph nodes or a sentinel lymph node biopsy that detected clinically occult metastases). The former define "macroscopic" nodal disease while the latter would define "microscopic" nodal disease. It is acknowledged that these terms are operational definitions simply used for communicating a level of tumor burden, and are not intended to be used as a more strict definition of microscopic disease that cannot be observed without a microscope. Given the evolving importance of sentinel node microscopic tumor burden in recent reports, pathologists should also consider reporting the diameter of the largest metastasis in the sentinel node and/or the percentage area of the node involved by tumor.

**Stage IV Melanoma.** Electronic fields for patients with Stage IV melanoma should include all the information listed above for the primary melanoma and regional metastases, plus the site(s) of distant metastases as well as the serum LDH level (normal vs. elevated). Additional data to be considered include the number of distant metastases, the patient's age, gender, and performance status.

## BIBLIOGRAPHY

1. Balch CM, Soong SJ, Gershenwald JE, et al. Prognostic factors analysis of 17, 600 melanoma patients: validation of the American Joint Committee on Cancer melanoma staging system. J Clin Oncol. 2001;19:3622–34.
2. Morton DL, Wanek L, Nizze JA, et al. Improved long-term survival after lymphadenectomy of melanoma metastatic to regional nodes. Analysis of prognostic factors in 1134 patients from the John Wayne Cancer Clinic. Ann Surg. 1991;214:491–9; discussion 499–501.
3. Rousseau DL Jr, Ross MI, Johnson MM, et al. Revised American Joint Committee on Cancer staging criteria accurately predict sentinel lymph node positivity in clinically node-negative melanoma patients. Ann Surg Oncol. 2003;10:569–74.
4. Karakousis GC, Gimotty PA, Botbyl JD, et al. Predictors of regional nodal disease in patients with thin melanomas. Ann Surg Oncol. 2006;13:533–41.
5. Vaquerano J, Kraybill WG, Driscoll DL, et al. American Joint Committee on Cancer clinical stage as a selection criterion for sentinel lymph node biopsy in thin melanoma. Ann Surg Oncol. 2006;13:198–204.
6. Paek SC, Griffith KA, Johnson TM, et al. The impact of factors beyond Breslow depth on predicting sentinel lymph node positivity in melanoma. Cancer. 2007;109:100–8.
7. Morton DL, Cochran AJ, Thompson JF, et al. Sentinel node biopsy for early-stage melanoma: accuracy and morbidity in MSLT-I, an international multicenter trial. Ann Surg. 2005;242:302–11; discussion 311–3.
8. Balch CM, Cascinelli N. Sentinel-node biopsy in melanoma. N Engl J Med. 2006;355:1370–1.
9. Carlson GW, Murray DR, Hestley A, et al. Sentinel lymph node mapping for thick (> or = 4-mm) melanoma: should we be doing it? Ann Surg Oncol. 2003;10:408–15.
10. Ferrone CR, Panageas KS, Busam K, et al. Multivariate prognostic model for patients with thick cutaneous melanoma: importance of sentinel lymph node status. Ann Surg Oncol. 2002;9:637–45.

11. Chao C, Wong SL, Ross MI, et al. Patterns of early recurrence after sentinel lymph node biopsy for melanoma. Am J Surg. 2002;184:520–4; discussion 525.

12. Cascinelli N, Bombardieri E, Bufalino R, et al. Sentinel and nonsentinel node status in stage IB and II melanoma patients: two-step prognostic indicators of survival. J Clin Oncol. 2006;24:4464–71.

13. Sondak VK, Taylor JM, Sabel MS, et al. Mitotic rate and younger age are predictors of sentinel lymph node positivity: lessons learned from the generation of a probabilistic model. Ann Surg Oncol. 2004;11:247–58.

14. McMasters KM, Wong SL, Edwards MJ, et al. Factors that predict the presence of sentinel lymph node metastasis in patients with melanoma. Surgery. 2001;130:151–6.

15. Leong SP, Kashani-Sabet M, Desmond RA, et al. Clinical significance of occult metastatic melanoma in sentinel lymph nodes and other high-risk factors based on long-term follow-up. World J Surg. 2005;29:683–91.

16. Gershenwald JE, Thompson W, Mansfield PF, et al. Multi-institutional melanoma lymphatic mapping experience: the prognostic value of sentinel lymph node status in 612 stage I or II melanoma patients. J Clin Oncol. 1999;17:976–83.

17. Cormier JN, Xing Y, Ding M, et al. Population-based assessment of surgical treatment trends for patients with melanoma in the era of sentinel lymph node biopsy. J Clin Oncol. 2005;23:6054–62.

18. Voit C, Kron M, Schafer G, et al. Ultrasound-guided fine needle aspiration cytology prior to sentinel lymph node biopsy in melanoma patients. Ann Surg Oncol. 2006;13:1682–9.

19. Doubrovsky A, Scolyer RA, Murali R, et al. Diagnostic accuracy of fine needle biopsy for metastatic melanoma and its implications for patient management. Ann Surg Oncol. 2008;15:323–332.

20. van Rijk MC, Teertstra HJ, Peterse JL, et al. Ultrasonography and fine-needle aspiration cytology in the preoperative evaluation of melanoma patients eligible for sentinel node biopsy. Ann Surg Oncol. 2006;13:1511–6.

21. Starritt EC, Uren RF, Scolyer RA, et al. Ultrasound examination of sentinel nodes in the initial assessment of patients with primary cutaneous melanoma. Ann Surg Oncol. 2005;12:18–23.

22. Rossi CR, Mocellin S, Scagnet B, et al. The role of preoperative ultrasound scan in detecting lymph node metastasis before sentinel node biopsy in melanoma patients. J Surg Oncol. 2003;83:80–4.

23. Lee JH, Essner R, Torisu-Itakura H, et al. Factors predictive of tumor-positive nonsentinel lymph nodes after tumor-positive sentinel lymph node dissection for melanoma. J Clin Oncol. 2004;22:3677–84.

24. Balch CM, Buzaid AC, Soong SJ, et al. Final version of the American Joint Committee on Cancer staging system for cutaneous melanoma. J Clin Oncol. 2001;19:3635–48.

25. Dessureault S, Soong SJ, Ross MI, et al. Improved staging of node-negative patients with intermediate to thick melanomas (>1 mm) with the use of lymphatic mapping and sentinel lymph node biopsy. Ann Surg Oncol. 2001;8: 766–70.

26. Breslow A. Tumor thickness, level of invasion and node dissection in stage I cutaneous melanoma. Ann Surg. 1975;182:572–5.

27. Breslow A. Thickness, cross-sectional areas and depth of invasion in the prognosis of cutaneous melanoma. Ann Surg. 1970;172:902–8.

28. Spatz A, Cook MG, Elder DE, et al. Interobserver reproducibility of ulceration assessment in primary cutaneous melanomas. Eur J Cancer. 2003;39: 1861–5.

29. Balch CM, Murad TM, Soong SJ, et al. A multifactorial analysis of melanoma: prognostic histopathological features comparing Clark's and Breslow's staging methods. Ann Surg. 1978;188:732–42.

30. Balch CM, Soong SJ, Murad TM, et al. A multifactorial analysis of melanoma. II. Prognostic factors in patients with stage I (localized) melanoma. Surgery. 1979;86:343–51.

31. Balch CM, Wilkerson JA, Murad TM, et al. The prognostic significance of ulceration of cutaneous melanoma. Cancer. 1980;45:3012–7.

32. McGovern VJ, Shaw HM, Milton GW, et al. Ulceration and prognosis in cutaneous malignant melanoma. Histopathology. 1982;6:399–407.

33. Gimotty PA, Elder DE, Fraker DL, et al. Identification of high-risk patients among those diagnosed with thin cutaneous melanomas. J Clin Oncol. 2007;25:1129–34.

34. Kesmodel SB, Karakousis GC, Botbyl JD, et al. Mitotic rate as a predictor of sentinel lymph node positivity in patients with thin melanomas. Ann Surg Oncol. 2005;12:449–58.

35. Busam KJ. The prognostic importance of tumor mitotic rate for patients with primary cutaneous melanoma. Ann Surg Oncol. 2004;11:360–1.

36. Francken AB, Shaw HM, Thompson JF, et al. The prognostic importance of tumor mitotic rate confirmed in 1317 patients with primary cutaneous melanoma and long follow-up. Ann Surg Oncol. 2004;11:426–33.

37. Azzola MF, Shaw HM, Thompson JF, et al. Tumor mitotic rate is a more powerful prognostic indicator than ulceration in patients with primary cutaneous melanoma: an analysis of 3661 patients from a single center. Cancer. 2003;97:1488–98.

37a. Scolyer RA, Shaw HM, Thompson JF, et al. Interobserver reproducibility of histopathologic prognostic variables in primary cutaneous melanomas. Am J Surg Pathol. 2003;27:1571–6.

38. Clark WH Jr, From L, Bernardino EA, et al. The histogenesis and biologic behavior of primary human malignant melanomas of the skin. Cancer Res. 1969;29:705–27.

39. Balch CM, Soong S, Ross MI, et al. Long-term results of a multi-institutional randomized trial comparing prognostic factors and surgical results for intermediate thickness melanomas (1.0 to 4.0 mm). Intergroup Melanoma Surgical Trial. Ann Surg Oncol. 2000;7:87–97.

40. Buzaid AC, Ross MI, Balch CM, et al. Critical analysis of the current American Joint Committee on Cancer staging system for cutaneous melanoma and proposal of a new staging system. J Clin Oncol. 1997;15:1039–51.

41. Breslow A. Problems in the measurement of tumor thickness and level of invasion in cutaneous melanoma. Hum Pathol. 1977;8:1–2.

42. Prade M, Sancho-Garnier H, Cesarini JP, et al. Difficulties encountered in the application of Clark classification and the Breslow thickness measurement in cutaneous malignant melanoma. Int J Cancer. 1980;26: 159–63.

43. Finley JW, Gibbs JF, Rodriguez LM, et al. Pathologic and clinical features influencing outcome of thin cutaneous melanoma: correlation with newly proposed staging system. Am Surg. 2000;66:527–31; discussion 531–2.

44. Salman SM, Rogers GS. Prognostic factors in thin cutaneous malignant melanoma. J Dermatol Surg Oncol. 1990;16:413–8.

45. Shaw HM, McCarthy WH, McCarthy SW, et al. Thin malignant melanomas and recurrence potential. Arch Surg. 1987;122:1147–50.

46. Morton DL, Davtyan DG, Wanek LA, et al. Multivariate analysis of the relationship between survival and the microstage of primary melanoma by Clark level and Breslow thickness. Cancer. 1993;71:3737–43.

47. Marghoob AA, Koenig K, Bittencourt FV, et al. Breslow thickness and clark level in melanoma: support for including level in pathology reports and in American Joint Committee on Cancer Staging. Cancer. 2000;88: 589–95.

48. Mansson-Brahme E, Carstensen J, Erhardt K, et al. Prognostic factors in thin cutaneous malignant melanoma. Cancer. 1994;73:2324–32.

49. Buttner P, Garbe C, Bertz J, et al. Primary cutaneous melanoma. Optimized cutoff points of tumor thickness and importance of Clark's level for prognostic classification. Cancer. 1995;75:2499–506.

50. McGovern VJ, Shaw HM, Milton GW, et al. Is malignant melanoma arising in a Hutchinson's melanotic freckle a separate disease entity? Histopathology. 1980;4:235–42.

51. Kuchelmeister C, Schaumburg-Lever G, Garbe C. Acral cutaneous melanoma in caucasians: clinical features, histopathology and prognosis in 112 patients. Br J Dermatol. 2000;143:275–80.

52. Urist MM, Balch CM, Soong SJ, et al. Head and neck melanoma in 534 clinical Stage I patients. A prognostic factors analysis and results of surgical treatment. Ann Surg. 1984;200:769–75.

53. Slingluff CL Jr, Vollmer R, Seigler HF. Acral melanoma: a review of 185 patients with identification of prognostic variables. J Surg Oncol. 1990;45:91–8.

54. Balch CM. Cutaneous melanoma: prognosis and treatment results worldwide. Semin Surg Oncol. 1992;8:400–14.

55. Posther KE, Selim MA, Mosca PJ, et al. Histopathologic characteristics, recurrence patterns, and survival of 129 patients with desmoplastic melanoma. Ann Surg Oncol. 2006;13:728–39.

56. Cascinelli N, Belli F, Santinami M, et al. Sentinel lymph node biopsy in cutaneous melanoma: the WHO Melanoma Program experience. Ann Surg Oncol. 2000;7:469–74.

57. van Akkooi AC, de Wilt JH, Verhoef C, et al. Clinical relevance of melanoma micrometastases (<0.1 mm) in sentinel nodes: are these nodes to be considered negative? Ann Oncol. 2006;17:1578–85.

58. Scheri RP, Essner R, Turner RR, et al. Isolated tumor cells in the sentinel node affect long-term prognosis of patients with melanoma. Ann Surg Oncol. 2007;14:2861–6.

59. Ohsie SJ, Sarantopoulos GP, Cochran AJ, et al. Immunohistochemical characteristics of melanoma. J Cutan Pathol. 2008;35:433–44.

60. Yu LL, Flotte TJ, Tanabe KK, et al. Detection of microscopic melanoma metastases in sentinel lymph nodes. Cancer. 1999;86:617–27.

61. Spanknebel K, Coit DG, Bieligk SC, et al. Characterization of micrometastatic disease in melanoma sentinel lymph nodes by enhanced pathology: recommendations for standardizing pathologic analysis. Am J Surg Pathol. 2005;29:305–17.

62. Gibbs JF, Huang PP, Zhang PJ, et al. Accuracy of pathologic techniques for the diagnosis of metastatic melanoma in sentinel lymph nodes. Ann Surg Oncol. 1999;6:699–704.

63. Greene FL, Page DL, Fleming ID, et al., editors. AJCC cancer staging manual. 6th ed. New York: Springer-Verlag; 2002.

64. Cascinelli N, Bufalino R, Marolda R, et al. Regional non-nodal metastases of cutaneous melanoma. Eur J Surg Oncol. 1986;12:175–80.

65. Day CL Jr, Harrist TJ, Gorstein F, et al. Malignant melanoma. Prognostic significance of "microscopic satellites" in the reticular dermis and subcutaneous fat. Ann Surg. 1981;194:108–12.

66. Leon P, Daly JM, Synnestvedt M, et al. The prognostic implications of microscopic satellites in patients with clinical stage I melanoma. Arch Surg. 1991;126:1461–8.

**31**

67. Harrist TJ, Rigel DS, Day CL Jr, et al. "Microscopic satellites" are more highly associated with regional lymph node metastases than is primary melanoma thickness. Cancer. 1984;53:2183–7.

68. Pawlik TM, Ross MI, Johnson MM, et al. Predictors and natural history of in-transit melanoma after sentinel lymphadenectomy. Ann Surg Oncol. 2005;12:587–96.

69. Pawlik TM, Ross MI, Thompson JF, et al. The risk of in-transit melanoma metastasis depends on tumor biology and not the surgical approach to regional lymph nodes. J Clin Oncol. 2005;23:4588–90.

70. Rao UN, Ibrahim J, Flaherty LE, et al. Implications of microscopic satellites of the primary and extracapsular lymph node spread in patients with high-risk melanoma: pathologic corollary of Eastern Cooperative Oncology Group Trial E1690. J Clin Oncol. 2002;20:2053–7.

71. Shaikh L, Sagebiel RW, Ferreira CM, et al. The role of microsatellites as a prognostic factor in primary malignant melanoma. Arch Dermatol. 2005;141: 739–42.

72. Nagore E, Oliver V, Botella-Estrada R, et al. Prognostic factors in localized invasive cutaneous melanoma: high value of mitotic rate, vascular invasion and microscopic satellitosis. Melanoma Res. 2005;15:169–77.

73. Balch CM, Soong SJ, Murad TM, et al. A multifactorial analysis of melanoma: III. Prognostic factors in melanoma patients with lymph node metastases (stage II). Ann Surg. 1981;193:377–88.

74. Bowen GM, Chang AE, Lowe L, et al. Solitary melanoma confined to the dermal and/or subcutaneous tissue: evidence for revisiting the staging classification. Arch Dermatol. 2000;136:1397–9.

75. Barth A, Wanek LA, Morton DL. Prognostic factors in 1, 521 melanoma patients with distant metastases. J Am Coll Surg. 1995;181:193–201.

76. Brand CU, Ellwanger U, Stroebel W, et al. Prolonged survival of 2 years or longer for patients with disseminated melanoma. An analysis of related prognostic factors. Cancer. 1997;79:2345–53.

77. Bedikian AY, Johnson MM, Warneke CL, et al. Prognostic factors that determine the long-term survival of patients with unresectable metastatic melanoma. Cancer Invest. 2008;26:624–33.

78. Keilholz U, Martus P, Punt CJ, et al. Prognostic factors for survival and factors associated with long-term remission in patients with advanced melanoma receiving cytokine-based treatments: second analysis of a randomised EORTC Melanoma Group trial comparing interferon-alpha2a (IFNalpha) and interleukin 2 (IL-2) with or without cisplatin. Eur J Cancer. 2002;38:1501–11.

79. Manola J, Atkins M, Ibrahim J, et al. Prognostic factors in metastatic melanoma: a pooled analysis of Eastern Cooperative Oncology Group trials. J Clin Oncol. 2000;18:3782–93.

80. Sirott MN, Bajorin DF, Wong GY, et al. Prognostic factors in patients with metastatic malignant melanoma. A multivariate analysis. Cancer. 1993;72: 3091–8.

81. Cormier JN, Xing Y, Feng L, et al. Metastatic melanoma to lymph nodes in patients with unknown primary sites. Cancer. 2006;106:2012–20.

82. Lee CC, Faries MB, Wanek LA, et al. Improved survival after lymphadenectomy for nodal metastasis from an unknown primary melanoma. J Clin Oncol. 2008;26:535–41.

83. Kopf AW, Salopek TG, Slade J, et al. Techniques of cutaneous examination for the detection of skin cancer. Cancer. 1995;75:684–90.

84. Gershenwald JE, Mansfield PF, Lee JE, et al. Role for lymphatic mapping and sentinel lymph node biopsy in patients with thick (> or = 4 mm) primary melanoma. Ann Surg Oncol. 2000;7:160–5.

85. Bevilacqua RG, Coit DG, Rogatko A, et al. Axillary dissection in melanoma. Prognostic variables in node-positive patients. Ann Surg. 1990;212:125–31.
86. Calabro A, Singletary SE, Balch CM. Patterns of relapse in 1001 consecutive patients with melanoma nodal metastases. Arch Surg. 1989;124:1051–5.
87. Coit DG, Peters M, Brennan MF. A prospective randomized trial of peri-operative cefazolin treatment in axillary and groin dissection. Arch Surg. 1991;126:1366–71; discussion 1371–2.
88. Drepper H, Biess B, Hofherr B, et al. The prognosis of patients with stage III melanoma. Prospective long-term study of 286 patients of the Fachklinik Hornheide. Cancer. 1993;71:1239–46.
89. Slingluff CL Jr, Vollmer R, Seigler HF. Stage II malignant melanoma: presentation of a prognostic model and an assessment of specific active immunotherapy in 1,273 patients. J Surg Oncol. 1988;39:139–47.
90. Gershenwald JE, Colome MI, Lee JE, et al. Patterns of recurrence following a negative sentinel lymph node biopsy in 243 patients with stage I or II melanoma. J Clin Oncol. 1998;16:2253–60.
91. Dale PS, Foshag LJ, Wanek LA, et al. Metastasis of primary melanoma to two separate lymph node basins: prognostic significance. Ann Surg Oncol. 1997;4:13–8.
92. Shaw HM, Balch CM, Soong SJ, et al. Prognostic histopathological factors in malignant melanoma. Pathology. 1985;17:271–4.

**31**

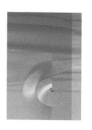

# PART VII
## Breast

# Breast

## *At-A-Glance*

---

**SUMMARY OF CHANGES**

**Tumor (T)**

- Identified specific imaging modalities that can be used to estimate clinical tumor size, including mammography, ultrasound, and magnetic resonance imaging (MRI)

- Made specific recommendations that (1) the microscopic measurement is the most accurate and preferred method to determine pT with a small invasive cancer that can be entirely submitted in one paraffin block, and (2) the gross measurement is the most accurate and preferred method to determine pT with larger invasive cancers that must be submitted in multiple paraffin blocks

- Made the specific recommendation to use the clinical measurement thought to be most accurate to determine the clinical T of breast cancers treated with neoadjuvant therapy. Pathologic (posttreatment) size should be estimated based on the best combination of gross and microscopic histological findings

- Made the specific recommendation to estimate the size of invasive cancers that are unapparent to any clinical modalities or gross pathologic examination by carefully measuring and recording the relative positions of tissue samples submitted for microscopic evaluation and determining which contain tumor

- Acknowledged "ductal intraepithelial neoplasia" (DIN) as uncommon, and still not widely accepted, terminology encompassing both DCIS and ADH, and clarification that only cases referred to as DIN containing DCIS (±ADH) are classified as Tis (DCIS)

- Acknowledged "lobular intraepithelial neoplasia" (LIN) as uncommon, and still not widely accepted, terminology encompassing both LCIS and ALH, and clarification that only cases referred to as LIN containing LCIS (±ALH) are classified as Tis (LCIS)

- Clarification that only Paget's disease NOT associated with an underlying noninvasive (i.e., DCIS and/or LCIS) or invasive breast cancer should be classified as Tis (Paget's) and that Paget's disease associated with an underlying cancer be classified according to the underlying cancer (Tis, T1, etc.)

- Made the recommendation to estimate the size of noninvasive carcinomas (DCIS and LCIS), even though it does not currently change their T classification, because noninvasive cancer size may influence therapeutic decisions, acknowledging that providing a precise size for LCIS may be difficult

- Acknowledged that the prognosis of microinvasive carcinoma is generally thought to be quite favorable, although the clinical impact of multifocal microinvasive disease is not well understood at this time

*continued*

---

## SUMMARY OF CHANGES (CONTINUED)

- Acknowledged that it is not necessary for tumors to be in separate quadrants to be classified as multiple simultaneous ipsilateral carcinomas, providing that they can be unambiguously demonstrated to be macroscopically distinct and measurable using available clinical and pathologic techniques

- Maintained that the term "inflammatory carcinoma" be restricted to cases with typical skin changes involving a third or more of the skin of the breast. While the histologic presence of invasive carcinoma invading dermal lymphatics is supportive of the diagnosis, it is not required, nor is dermal lymphatic invasion without typical clinical findings sufficient for a diagnosis of inflammatory breast cancer

- Recommend that all invasive cancer should be graded using the Nottingham combined histologic grade (Elston-Ellis modification of Scarff–Bloom–Richardson grading system)

### Nodes (N)

- Classification of isolated tumor cell clusters and single cells is more stringent. Small clusters of cells not greater than 0.2 mm, or nonconfluent or nearly confluent clusters of cells not exceeding 200 cells in a single histologic lymph node cross section are classified as isolated tumor cells

- Use of the (sn) modifier has been clarified and restricted. When six or more sentinel nodes are identified on gross examination of pathology specimens the (sn) modifier should be omitted

- Stage I breast tumors have been subdivided into Stage IA and Stage IB; Stage IB includes small tumors (T1) with exclusively micrometastases in lymph nodes (N1mi)

### Metastases (M)

- Created new M0(i+) category, defined by presence of either disseminated tumor cells detectable in bone marrow or circulating tumor cells or found incidentally in other tissues (such as ovaries removed prophylactically) if not exceeding 0.2 mm. However, this category does not change the Stage Grouping. Assuming that they do not have clinically and/or radiographically detectable metastases, patients with M0(i+) are staged according to T and N

### Postneoadjuvant Therapy (yc or ypTNM)

- In the setting of patients who received neoadjuvant therapy, pretreatment clinical T (cT) should be based on clinical or imaging findings

- Postneoadjuvant therapy T should be based on clinical or imaging (ycT) or pathologic findings (ypT)

- A subscript will be added to the clinical N for both node negative and node positive patients to indicate whether the N was derived from clinical examination, fine needle aspiration, core needle biopsy, or sentinel lymph node biopsy

- The posttreatment ypT will be defined as the largest contiguous focus of invasive cancer as defined histopathologically with a subscript to indicate the presence of multiple tumor foci. Note: definition of posttreatment ypT remains controversial and an area in transition

- Posttreatment nodal metastases no greater than 0.2 mm are classified as ypN0(i+) as in patients who have not received neoadjuvant systemic

*continued*

therapy. However, patients with this finding are not considered to have achieved a pathologic complete response (pCR)

* A description of the degree of response to neoadjuvant therapy (complete, partial, no response) will be collected by the registrar with the posttreatment ypTNM. The registrars are requested to describe how they defined response [by physical examination, imaging techniques (mammogram, ultrasound, magnetic resonance imaging (MRI)) or pathologically]

* Patients will be considered to have M1 (and therefore Stage IV) breast cancer if they have had clinically or radiographically detectable metastases, with or without biopsy, prior to neoadjuvant systemic therapy, regardless of their status after neoadjuvant systemic therapy

## PROGNOSTIC FEATURES

New biomarkers are added and recommended for collection in addition to hormone receptors (estrogen receptor, ER; progesterone receptor, PgR). These are HER2 (also designated as erbB2 and c-neu) status and multigene signature "score" or classifications.

**32**

### ANATOMIC STAGE/PROGNOSTIC GROUPS

| Stage 0 | Tis | N0 | M0 |
|---|---|---|---|
| Stage IA | T1* | N0 | M0 |
| Stage IB | T0 | N1mi | M0 |
| | T1* | N1mi | M0 |
| Stage IIA | T0 | N1** | M0 |
| | T1* | N1** | M0 |
| | T2 | N0 | M0 |
| Stage IIB | T2 | N1 | M0 |
| | T3 | N0 | M0 |
| Stage IIIA | T0 | N2 | M0 |
| | T1* | N2 | M0 |
| | T2 | N2 | M0 |
| | T3 | N1 | M0 |
| | T3 | N2 | M0 |
| Stage IIIB | T4 | N0 | M0 |
| | T4 | N1 | M0 |
| | T4 | N2 | M0 |
| Stage IIIC | Any T | N3 | M0 |
| Stage IV | Any T | Any N | M1 |

*Notes:*
*T1 includes T1mi.

**T0 and T1 tumors with nodal micrometastases only are excluded from Stage IIA and are classified Stage IB.

### ICD-O-3 TOPOGRAPHY CODES

| | |
|---|---|
| C50.0 | Nipple |
| C50.1 | Central portion of breast |
| C50.2 | Upper inner quadrant of breast |
| C50.3 | Lower inner quadrant of breast |
| C50.4 | Upper outer quadrant of breast |
| C50.5 | Lower outer quadrant of breast |
| C50.6 | Axillary tail of breast |
| C50.8 | Overlapping lesion of breast |
| C50.9 | Breast, NOS |

### ICD-O-3 HISTOLOGY CODE RANGES

8000–8576, 8940–8950, 8980–8981, 9020

- M0 includes M0(i+).
- The designation pM0 is not valid; any M0 should be clinical.
- If a patient presents with M1 prior to neoadjuvant systemic therapy, the stage is considered stage IV and remains stage IV regardless of response to neoadjuvant therapy.
- Stage designation may be changed if postsurgical imaging studies reveal the presence of distant metastases, provided that the studies are carried out within 4 months of diagnosis in the absence of disease progression and provided that the patient has not received neoadjuvant therapy.
- Postneoadjuvant therapy is designated with "yc" or "yp" prefix. Of note, no stage group is assigned if there is a complete pathologic response (CR) to neoadjuvant therapy, for example, ypT0ypN0cM0.

## INTRODUCTION

This staging system for carcinoma of the breast applies to invasive (also designated infiltrating) as well as in situ carcinomas, with or without microinvasion. Microscopic confirmation of the diagnosis is mandatory, and the histologic type and grade of carcinoma should be recorded. For all sites (T, N, M), clinical staging (c) is determined using information identified prior to surgery or neoadjuvant therapy. Pathologic staging (p) includes information defined at surgery. With neoadjuvant therapy a posttherapy pathologic staging is recorded using the "yp" designator.

The year 2009 marks the 50th anniversary of codification of tumor staging into the TNM system by the American Joint Committee on Cancer (AJCC; originally designated the American Joint Committee for Cancer Staging and End-Results Reporting). Beginning with that initiative, six editions of the AJCC Staging Manual have been published, in which careful definitions of the primary tumor (T), the status of the surrounding lymph nodes (N), and the presence of distant metastases have been refined to reflect updates in technology and clinical evidence.[1] In each case, changes in the TNM system were made cautiously, so as to reflect modern clinical approaches while maintaining connections with the past. The recommendations by the Breast Cancer Task Force for the seventh edition are made in the same spirit.

Rapid advances in both clinical and laboratory science and in translational research have raised questions about the ongoing relevance of TNM staging, especially in breast cancer. For the most part, the TNM system was developed in 1959 in the absence of effective systemic therapy and certainly in a void of the understanding of the biology of breast cancer that exists today. The system was generated to reflect the risk of distant recurrence and death subsequent to local therapy, which at the time was almost universally aggressive surgery (radical mastectomy) and postoperative radiation to the chest wall. Therefore, the primary objective of TNM staging was to provide a standard nomenclature for prognosis of patients with newly diagnosed breast cancer, and its main clinical utility was to prevent apparently futile therapy in those patients who were destined to die rapidly in spite of aggressive local treatments.

Over the succeeding decades, remarkable progress has led to (1) less disfiguring surgery with modified radical mastectomies and breast conserving therapy, (2) dramatic improvements in the delivery and safety of radiation, (3) the recognition that early (adjuvant) systemic therapy reduces recurrences and mortality, and (4) a better understanding of biologic markers of prognosis, and perhaps more importantly, of prediction of response to selective categories of systemic therapy, such as those targeting cancer cells positive for estrogen receptors (ER) and HER2 overexpression.[2] TNM staging has been used as a guide to select whether to apply systemic therapy based on anatomic prognosis. Increasingly, biologic factors, such as ER and HER2, have become important to select which therapy to give.

These advances raise the questions: Is TNM staging still relevant for breast cancer in the twenty-first century and what, exactly, is the objective of TNM staging for patients with this disease? There are three potential answers to the second question: (1) To permit breast cancer investigators to remain linked to the past, in regards to studying categories of patients that accurately reflect prior groupings over the last six decades, (2) to permit current investigators in the field to communicate with one another in the same manner, and/or (3) to improve individual patient care. The AJCC Breast Cancer Task force has struggled with these questions, both for the seventh edition as well as for past editions. Indeed, the Breast Cancer Task Force made a major change from the fifth edition to the sixth edition in recommending that the N staging category be divided into three categories based on the number of axillary lymph nodes involved. In this regard, the current Breast Cancer Task Force came to the conclusion that although the TNM staging system provides insight into whether a patient's prognosis is so favorable the patient might forego systemic therapy, it is becoming anachronistic with regard to making recommendations for specific types of systemic therapy.

Although T, N, and M do still provide some value in determining a patient's future outcome, the average clinician today must take into account multiple factors that relate both to prognosis and prediction. For example, testing for estrogen and progesterone receptor content as well as HER2 status is now considered standard of care.[3] Although these factors do have intrinsic prognostic value in regards to the risk of subsequent recurrence for patients who do not receive systemic therapy, their main utility is to guide whether a patient should or should not receive adjuvant endocrine (anti-estrogen) or anti-HER2 (such as trastuzumab) therapy. The use of these factors as predictive, rather than prognostic, markers is fundamentally important in evaluation and care of patients with newly diagnosed breast cancer, but the Committee found it difficult to devise a scheme in which they might be incorporated into the TNM system.

The situation has become even more complex with the availability of multigene expression assays.[4] One such assay, based on a 70-gene prognostic signature developed by investigators from Amsterdam,[5] has been cleared by the United States Food and Drug Administration for use in women who are less than 61 years old and who have stage I or II, node negative breast cancer, explicitly to "assess a patient's risk for distant metastases." (http://www.accessdata.fda.gov/scripts/cdrh/cfdocs/cfPMN/pmn.cfm?ID=24303). The Tumor Marker Guidelines Committee of the American Society of Clinical Oncology (ASCO) has recommended that a second multigene assay, which is based on expression of 21-genes as determined by RT-PCR (designated the "21-gene recurrence score assay") "can be used" to determine prognosis for patients with ER positive breast cancer and uninvolved lymph nodes who will, at the least, receive adjuvant tamoxifen,[2] and the Breast Committee of the National Comprehensive Cancer Network (NCCN) Guidelines states that "the use of genomic/gene expression arrays which also incorporate additional prognostic/predictive biomarkers (e.g., Oncotype Dx recurrence score) may provide additional prognostic and predictive information beyond anatomic staging and determination of ER/PR and HER2 status."[3] How do such assays become incorporated into the TNM staging system, since they portend future outcomes in several ways? (1) As pure prognostic factors (the profile predicts the odds of recurrence independent of systemic therapy),[6,7] (2) as markers of residual risk assuming the patient will receive endocrine therapy (the profile predicts favorable or unfavorable chances of recurrence presumably due to both prognosis and prediction of benefit or resistance to endocrine therapy),[5,8,9] and (3) perhaps as predictive factors for specific types of, or all, chemotherapies.[10,11]

Should these multiparameter prognostic assays that appear to predict outcomes in newly diagnosed breast cancer patients be included in staging? Since their value may be as much a predictor of response to chemotherapy regardless of TNM stage than as a prognostic factor, should an entirely new category related to prediction of benefit from systemic therapy be incorporated into the TNM staging system? In other words, increasingly in the modern era, many treatment decisions for patients with newly diagnosed breast cancer are not, or will not be, based on TNM stage. Although the size of the invasive cancer is a factor, the type of surgery for an individual patient is usually determined by multicentricity and tumor margins, neither of which is part of TNM. Perhaps the only exception is the almost universal recommendation of mastectomy, regardless of other factors, for patients with inflammatory breast cancer. Large tumor size (T3 vs. T1, 2) and lymph node (N 1, 2, or 3 vs. N0) status do play a role in deciding whether radiation should be used after mastectomy or for directing the fields of radiation for women undergoing breast preservation and in the recommendation for axillary dissection. However, in an era when many invasive cancers are detected at very small sizes when breast screening is used, multicentricity and tumor margins appear to be as important as T or N in determining optimal local treatment approaches. In the past, recommendations for most systemic therapy, especially chemotherapy, have been based on nodal status, and in the absence of involved lymph nodes, tumor size.[12,13] However, biologic features such as ER, progesterone receptor, HER2, and to some extent, grade, all play a role in a complex dance involving both prognosis and prediction for the specific therapies. With ongoing advances in molecular biology and technology, coupled with increasing options for novel systemic therapies, such as agents that interfere with angiogenesis, we anticipate that anatomic staging with tumor size, lymph node status, and the presence of clinical and radiographically evident metastases may play increasingly less important roles than understanding of the biology of the cancer.

While the advances in molecular diagnosis have provided new insights into cancer therapy, the Committee understands that much of this consideration is relevant only to the societies in which resources permit widespread screening, molecular evaluation of tumor tissue, and application of cutting edge biological-directed therapies. Projecting to 2010, the annual global burden of new breast cancer cases will be 1.5 million and an ever-increasing fraction will be from low and middle income countries (LMCs).[14] Despite the common misconception that breast cancer is predominantly a problem of wealthy countries, the majority of breast cancer deaths each year in fact occur in developing rather than developed countries. In this regard, LMCs may simply not be able to afford testing for individual molecular events or multiparameter profiles, nor will they be able to provide expensive therapies directed against HER2 or other emerging targets. Tissue assays as basic as ER and PR may be unavailable in low income settings, even when oral endocrine therapies can be provided. Further complicating these resource limitations, women in LMCs typically present with locally advanced (Stage III) or metastatic disease (Stage IV) at diagnosis. In these settings, downstaging of disease through early detection programs may be the most practical approach to improving cancer outcome at the population level.[14] Thus, anatomic (TNM) staging remains a key aspect of cancer control in LMCs, because it directly reflects the degree to which early detection programs are working. While it is of value to continue education regarding the exciting advances in molecular oncology in LMCs, anatomic staging will remain the fundamental cornerstone on which evaluation and treatment decisions of newly diagnosed breast cancer patients will be made.

Ultimately, and after much deliberation, the Task Force has elected to make minor to modest adjustments to the T, N, and M categories for the seventh edition to reflect new technologies and new clinical outcome data since the sixth edition. The Task Force has also substantially enhanced the "yp" category to distinguish stage after preoperative, or "neoadjuvant" systemic therapy and surgery. This designation has already been used by other disease groups, and its incorporation into the seventh edition seems appropriate in light of the growing application of this strategy.[15]

Nonetheless, the Breast Cancer Task Force does not want to ignore the importance of tumor biology, both in predicting recurrence and benefits from therapy. The Task Force did consider adding a "B" category (for biology), in which the status of ER, PR, HER2, and even multigene expression profiles would be incorporated and ultimately added to the Stage Grouping. However, for the reasons above, the Breast Cancer Task Force decided such a step would add little, since they are already used to care for individual patients. Such a change would, by definition, completely abrogate at least the first objective of TNM staging elucidated above (linkage to the past), and it would almost certainly confuse the second (discussion among peers), since not all clinicians worldwide have access to the necessary assays to determine them, especially the newer multigene assays. Therefore, although the Breast Cancer Task Force has not recommended changes to the TNM staging system to incorporate biology, we have requested that the invasive cancer data, if available, be collected in a highly detailed manner for inclusion into the National Cancer Database (NCDB) and other central registry databases. Although we recognize that the "prognostic" value of these data will be highly confounded by the effects of systemic therapy we hope this inclusion will permit future investigators to further define the role of these important features in future TNM deliberations.

## ANATOMY

**Primary Site.** The mammary gland, situated on the anterior chest wall, is composed of glandular tissue with a dense fibrous stroma. The glandular tissue consists of lobules that group together into 8–15 lobes, occasionally more, arranged approximately in a spoke-like pattern. Multiple major and minor ducts connect the milk-secreting lobular units to the nipple. Small milk ducts course throughout the breast, converging into larger collecting ducts that open into the lactiferous sinus at the base of the nipple. Each duct system has unique anatomy: the smallest systems may comprise only a portion of a quadrant whereas the largest systems may comprise more than a quadrant. The periphery of each system overlaps along their radial boundaries. Most cancers form initially in the terminal duct lobular units of the breast. Carcinoma spreads along the duct system in the radial axis of the lobe; invasive carcinoma is more likely to spread in a centripetal orientation in the breast stroma from the initial locus of invasion, although opportunistic intraductal spread may be enhanced along the radial axes. Glandular tissue is more abundant in the upper outer portion of the breast; as a result, half of all breast cancers occur in this area.

**Chest Wall.** The chest wall includes ribs, intercostal muscles, and serratus anterior muscle, but not the pectoral muscles. Therefore, involvement of the pectoral muscle does not constitute chest wall invasion.

**Regional Lymph Nodes.** The breast lymphatics drain by way of three major routes: axillary, transpectoral, and internal mammary. Intramammary lymph nodes reside within breast tissue and are coded as axillary lymph nodes for staging purposes. Supraclavicular lymph nodes are classified as regional lymph nodes for staging purposes. Metastases to any other lymph node, including cervical or contralateral internal mammary or axillary lymph nodes, are classified as distant (M1) (Figure 32.1.)

The regional lymph nodes are as follows:

1. Axillary (ipsilateral): interpectoral (Rotter's) nodes and lymph nodes along the axillary vein and its tributaries that may be (but are not required to be) divided into the following levels:
   a. Level I (low-axilla): lymph nodes lateral to the lateral border of pectoralis minor muscle.
   b. Level II (mid-axilla): lymph nodes between the medial and lateral borders of the pectoralis minor muscle and the interpectoral (Rotter's) lymph nodes.
   c. Level III (apical axilla): lymph nodes medial to the medial margin of the pectoralis minor muscle and inferior to the clavicle. These are

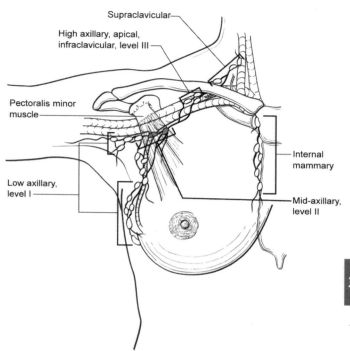

**FIGURE 32.1.** Schematic of the breast and regional lymph nodes.

also known as apical or infraclavicular nodes. Metastases to these nodes portend a worse prognosis. Therefore, the infraclavicular designation will be used hereafter to differentiate these nodes from the remaining (level I, II) axillary nodes.

2. Internal mammary (ipsilateral): lymph nodes in the intercostal spaces along the edge of the sternum in the endothoracic fascia.
3. Supraclavicular: lymph nodes in the supraclavicular fossa, a triangle defined by the omohyoid muscle and tendon (lateral and superior border), the internal jugular vein (medial border), and the clavicle and subclavian vein (lower border). Adjacent lymph nodes outside of this triangle are considered to be lower cervical nodes (M1).
4. Intramammary: lymph nodes within the breast; these are considered axillary lymph nodes for purposes of N classification and staging.

**Metastatic Sites.** Tumor cells may be disseminated by either the lymphatic or the blood vascular system. The four major sites of involvement are bone, lung, brain, and liver, but tumor cells are also capable of metastasizing to many other sites. Bone marrow micrometastases, circulating tumor cells, and tumor deposits no larger than 0.2 mm detected inadvertently, such as in prophylactically removed ovarian tissue, are collectively known as microscopic disseminated tumor cells (DTCs). These deposits do not alone define or constitute metastatic disease, although there are data that demonstrate that, in early stage disease, DTCs correlate with recurrence and mortality risk, and in patients with established M1 disease, circulating tumor cells (CTCs) are prognostic for shorter survival.

## RULES FOR CLASSIFICATION

**Clinical Staging.** Clinical staging includes physical examination, with careful inspection and palpation of the skin, mammary gland, and lymph nodes (axillary, supraclavicular, and cervical), imaging, and pathologic examination of the breast or other tissues as appropriate to establish the diagnosis of breast carcinoma. The extent of tissue examined pathologically for clinical staging is not as great as that required for pathologic staging (see "Pathologic Staging" below). Imaging findings are considered elements of staging if they are collected within 4 months of diagnosis in the absence of disease progression or through completion of surgery, whichever is longer. Such imaging findings would include the size of the primary invasive cancer and of chest wall invasion, and the presence or absence of regional or distant metastases. Imaging and clinical findings obtained after a patient has been treated with neoadjuvant chemotherapy, hormonal therapy, immunotherapy, or radiation therapy are not considered elements of initial clinical staging. If recorded in the medical record, these should be denoted using the modifier prefix "yc."

**Pathologic Staging.** Pathologic staging includes all data used for clinical staging, plus data from surgical exploration and resection as well as pathologic examination (gross and microscopic) of the primary carcinoma, regional lymph nodes, and metastatic sites (if applicable), including not less than excision of the primary carcinoma with no macroscopic tumor in any margin of resection by pathologic examination. A cancer can be classified pT for pathologic stage grouping if there is only microscopic, but not macroscopic, involvement at the margin. If there is transected tumor in the margin of resection by macroscopic examination, the pathologic size of the tumor may be estimated from available information but will not necessarily be the sum of the sizes of multiple resected pieces of tumor.

If the primary tumor is invasive (with a possible exception of microinvasive cancer), resection of at least the low axillary lymph nodes (Level I) – that is, those lymph nodes located lateral to the lateral border of the pectoralis minor muscle – should be performed for pathologic (pN) classification. Such a resection will ordinarily include six or more lymph nodes. Alternatively, one or more sentinel lymph nodes may be resected and examined for pathologic classification [pN(sn)]. Certain histologic invasive cancer types [classic tubular carcinoma <1 cm, classic mucinous carcinoma <1 cm, and microinvasive carcinoma (pT1mi)] have a very low incidence of axillary lymph node metastases and may not require an axillary lymph node dissection, although sentinel lymph node biopsy may be appropriate. Cancerous nodules in the axillary fat adjacent to the breast, without histologic evidence of residual lymph node tissue, are classified as regional lymph node metastases (≥N1). Pathologic stage grouping includes the following two combinations of pathologic and clinical classifications: pT pN pM, or pT pN cM. If surgery occurs after the patient has received neoadjuvant chemotherapy, hormonal therapy, immunotherapy, or radiation therapy, the prefix "yp" should be used with the TNM classification, for example, ypTNM.

## Primary Tumor (T)

***Determining Tumor Size.*** The original size of a primary tumor (T) can be measured based on clinical findings (physical examination and imaging modalities such as mammography, ultrasound, and MRI) and pathologic findings (gross and microscopic measurements). Clinical tumor size (cT) should be based on the clinical findings that are judged to be most accurate for a particular case, although it may still be somewhat inaccurate because the extent of some breast cancers is not always apparent with current imaging techniques, and because tumors are composed of varying proportions of noninvasive and invasive disease, which these techniques are currently unable to distinguish. Pathologic tumor size (pT) based on gross measurement may also be somewhat inaccurate for the same reasons, although microscopic assessment is able to distinguish noninvasive and invasive carcinoma, and microscopically determined pT should be based on measuring *only the invasive component*. For small invasive tumors that can be submitted in one section/paraffin block, the microscopic measurement is the most accurate way to determine pT. If an invasive tumor is too large to be submitted for microscopic evaluation in one tissue section/block, the gross measurement is the preferred method of determining pT. Whichever method is used, pT should be recorded to the nearest millimeter. The size of the primary tumor is measured for T classification before any tissue is removed for special purposes, such as prognostic biomarkers or tumor banking. In patients who have undergone diagnostic core biopsies prior to surgical excision (particularly vacuum-assisted core biopsy sampling), measuring only the residual tumor may result in underclassifying the T component and understaging the tumor, especially with smaller tumors. In such cases, the original invasive cancer size should be estimated and verified based on the best combination of imaging, gross, and microscopic histological findings. Adding the maximum invasive cancer dimension on the core biopsy to the residual invasive tumor in the excision is not recommended as this often overestimates maximum tumor dimension. In general, the maximum dimension in either the core biopsy or the excisional biopsy is used for T classification unless imaging dimensions suggest a larger invasive cancer.

For patients who receive neoadjuvant systemic or radiation therapy, it is not possible to determine a pretreatment pathologic size. Therefore, pretreatment T is defined as clinical (cT). Pretreatment staging is clinical, and the clinical measurement defined from examination and imaging is recorded (cT). Posttreatment (ypT) size should be estimated based on the best combination of imaging, gross, and microscopic histological findings. The size of some invasive cancers, regardless of previous biopsy or chemotherapy, may be unapparent to any imaging modalities or gross pathologic examination. In these cases, invasive cancer size can be estimated by carefully measuring and recording the relative positions of tissue samples submitted for microscopic evaluation and determining which contain invasive cancer.

**32**

*Tis Classification.* Pure noninvasive carcinoma, or carcinoma in situ, is classified as Tis, with an additional parenthetical subclassification indicating the subtype. Three subtypes are currently recognized, including ductal carcinoma in situ (DCIS), lobular carcinoma in situ (LCIS), and Paget's disease of the nipple with no underlying invasive cancer. These are categorized as Tis (DCIS), Tis (LCIS), and Tis (Paget's), respectively. "Intraductal carcinoma" is an outmoded term for DCIS, which is still used occasionally, and tumors referred to in this manner (which is discouraged) should be categorized as Tis (DCIS). "Ductal intraepithelial neoplasia" (DIN) is a recently proposed but uncommonly used terminology encompassing both DCIS and atypical ductal hyperplasia (ADH), and only cases referred to as DIN containing DCIS (±ADH) should be classified as Tis (DCIS).[16,17] Similarly, "lobular intraepithelial neoplasia" (LIN) is an uncommon terminology encompassing both atypical lobular hyperplasia (ALH) and LCIS, and only cases referred to as LIN containing LCIS (±ALH) should be classified as Tis (LCIS).[18] DIN and LIN are not widely accepted terminology. "Lobular neoplasia in situ" is an outmoded term also encompassing both ALH and LCIS, and only tumors referred to in this manner (which is discouraged) containing LCIS (±ALH) should be classified as Tis (LCIS). If DCIS and LCIS are both present, the tumor is currently classified as Tis (DCIS). A recently published Cancer Protocol and Checklist from the College of American Pathology provides much greater detail regarding definition and evaluation of in situ cancer of the breast[19] (http://www.cap.org).

Paget's disease is characterized clinically by an exudate or crust of the nipple and areola caused by infiltration of the epidermis by noninvasive breast cancer epithelial cells. This condition usually occurs in one of the following three settings[20]: (1) Associated with an invasive carcinoma in the underlying breast parenchyma. The T classification should be based on the size of the invasive disease. (2) Associated with an underlying noninvasive carcinoma, usually DCIS but rarely LCIS. T classification should be based on the underlying tumor as Tis (DCIS) or Tis (LCIS), accordingly. However, the presence of Paget's disease associated with invasive or noninvasive carcinomas should still be recorded. (3) Not associated with identifiable underlying invasive or noninvasive disease. These are the only lesions that should be classified as Tis (Paget's).

The size of noninvasive carcinomas does not change their T classification. However, because tumor size may influence therapeutic decisions, an estimate of size should be still provided based on the best combination of imaging, gross, and microscopic histological findings.[19] Sizing of LCIS may be difficult, but an attempt to do so, based on either clinical/radiographic and/or pathologic features, is recommended.

*Microinvasive Carcinoma.* Microinvasive carcinoma is defined as an invasive carcinoma with no focus measuring >1 mm. In cases with only one focus, its microscopic measurement should be provided. In cases with multiple foci, the pathologist should attempt to quantify the number of foci and the range of their sizes, including the largest, but should not report the size of the tumor as the sum of the sizes. If there are multiple foci, reporting of the number may be difficult. In these cases, it is recommended that an estimate of the number be provided, or alternatively a note that the number of foci of microinvasion is too numerous to quantify, but that no identified focus is larger than 1.0 mm. Microinvasive carcinoma is nearly always encountered in a setting of DCIS (or, less often, LCIS) where small foci of tumor cells have invaded through the basement membrane into the surrounding stroma, although rare cases are encountered in the absence of noninvasive disease. The prognosis of microinvasive carcinoma is generally thought to be quite favorable, although the clinical impact of multifocal microinvasive disease is not well understood at this time.

***Multiple Simultaneous Ipsilateral Primary Carcinomas.*** Multiple simultaneous ipsilateral primary carcinomas are defined as infiltrating carcinomas in the same breast, which are grossly or macroscopically distinct and measurable using available clinical and pathologic techniques. T stage assignment in this setting should be based only on the largest tumor, and the sum of the sizes should not be used. However, the presence and sizes of the smaller tumor(s) should be recorded using the "(m)" modifier as defined by the TNM rules in Chap. 1.

Invasive cancers that are in close proximity, but are apparently separate grossly, may represent truly separate tumors or one tumor with a complex shape. Distinguishing these two situations may require judgment and close correlation between pathologic and clinical findings (especially imaging), and preference should be given to the modality thought to be the most accurate in a specific case. When macroscopically apparently distinct tumors are very close (e.g., <5 mm), especially if they are similar histologically, they are most likely one tumor with a complex shape, and their T category should be based on the largest combined dimension. Careful and comprehensive microscopic evaluation often reveals subtle areas of continuity between tumor foci in this setting. However, contiguous uniform tumor density in the intervening tissue is needed to justify adding two grossly distinct masses. These criteria apply to multiple macroscopically measurable tumors and do not apply to one macroscopic carcinoma associated with multiple separate microscopic (satellite) foci. Tumors along the same approximate radial axis are frequently related and have arisen in the same duct system.

***Simultaneous Bilateral Primary Carcinomas.*** Each carcinoma is staged as a separate primary carcinoma in a separate organ based on its own characteristics, including T category as specified in the TNM rules (see Chap. 1).

***Inflammatory Carcinoma.*** Inflammatory carcinoma is a clinical-pathologic entity characterized by diffuse erythema and edema (peau d'orange) involving a third or more of the skin of the breast.[21] The tumor of inflammatory carcinoma is classified T4d. It is important to remember that inflammatory carcinoma is primarily a clinical diagnosis. On imaging, there may be a detectable mass and characteristic thickening of the skin over the breast. An underlying mass may or may not be palpable, although imaging modalities often reveal one. The skin changes are due to lymphedema caused by tumor emboli within dermal lymphatics, which may or may not be obvious in a small skin biopsy. However, a tissue diagnosis is still necessary to demonstrate an invasive carcinoma in the underlying breast parenchyma or at least in the dermal lymphatics, as well as to determine biologic markers, such as estrogen receptor, progesterone receptor, and HER2 status. Tumor emboli in dermal lymphatics without the clinical skin changes described above do not qualify as inflammatory carcinoma. Locally advanced breast cancers directly invading the dermis or ulcerating the skin without the clinical skin changes and tumor emboli in dermal lymphatics also do not qualify as inflammatory carcinoma. Thus, the term *inflammatory carcinoma* should not be applied to a patient with neglected locally advanced cancer of the breast presenting late in the course of her disease. The rare case that exhibits all the features of inflammatory breast carcinoma, but in which skin changes involve less than one third of the skin, should be classified as T4b or T4c.

***Skin of Breast.*** Dimpling of the skin, nipple retraction, or any other skin change except those described under T4b and T4d may occur in T1, T2, or T3 without changing the classification.

### Regional Lymph Nodes (N)

***Macrometastases.*** Cases in which regional lymph nodes cannot be assessed (previously removed or not removed for pathologic examination) are designated NX or pNX. Cases in which no regional lymph node metastases are detected are designated cN0 or pN0.

For patients who are clinically node-positive, cN1 designates metastases to one or more movable ipsilateral level I, II axillary lymph nodes, cN2a designates metastases to level I, II axillary lymph nodes that are fixed to each other (matted) or to other structures, and cN3a indicates metastases to ipsilateral infraclavicular (level III axillary) lymph nodes. Metastases to the ipsilateral internal mammary nodes are designated as cN2b when they are detected by imaging studies (including CT scan and ultrasound, but excluding lymphoscintigraphy) or by clinical examination and when they do not occur in conjunction with metastases to the level I, II axillary lymph nodes. Metastases to the ipsilateral internal mammary nodes are designated as cN3b when they are detected by imaging studies or by clinical examination and when they occur in conjunction with metastases to the level I, II axillary lymph nodes. Metastases to the ipsilateral supraclavicular lymph nodes are designated as cN3c regardless of the presence or absence of axillary or internal mammary nodal involvement. Since lymph nodes that are detected by clinical or imaging examination are frequently larger than 1.0 cm, the presence of tumor deposits should be confirmed by fine needle aspirate or core biopsy with cytologic/histologic examination if possible. Lymph nodes classified as malignant by clinical or imaging characteristics alone, or only by fine needle aspirate cytology examination or core biopsy, and not by formal surgical dissection and pathologic review, are presumed to contain macrometastases for purposes of clinical staging classification. When confirmed by fine needle aspirate or core biopsy, the (f) modifier should be used to indicate cytologic/histologic confirmation, for example, cN2a(f). Pathologic classification rules apply when lymph nodes are removed by surgical excisional biopsy and examined histopathologically.

For patients who are pathologically node-positive with macrometastases, at least one node must contain a tumor deposit greater than 2 mm and all remaining quantified nodes must contain tumor deposits greater than 0.2 mm (at least micrometastases); nodes containing only tumor deposits ≤0.2 mm (ITCs) are excluded from the positive node count for purposes of N classification but should be recorded as additional ITC involved nodes and should be included in the total nodes evaluated. Cases with 1–3 positive level I/II axillary lymph nodes are classified pN1a; cases with 4–9 positive axillary lymph nodes are classified pN2a, and cases with 10 or more positive axillary lymph nodes are classified pN3a. Cases with histologically confirmed metastases to the internal mammary nodes, detected by sentinel lymph node dissection but not by clinical examination or imaging studies (excluding lymphoscintigraphy), are classified as pN1b if occurring in the *absence* of metastases to the axillary lymph nodes and as pN1c if occurring in the *presence* of metastases to 1–3 axillary lymph nodes. If four or more axillary lymph nodes are involved, and internal mammary sentinel nodes are involved, the classification pN3b is used. Pathologic classification is used when axillary nodes have been histologically examined and clinical involvement of the ipsilateral internal mammary nodes is detected by imaging studies (excluding lymphoscintigraphy); in the absence or presence of axillary nodal metastases, pN2b and pN3b classification is used, respectively.

Histologic evidence of metastases in ipsilateral supraclavicular lymph node(s) is classified as pN3c. A classification of pN3, regardless of primary tumor size or grade, is classified as Stage IIIC. A case in which the classification is based only on sentinel lymph node biopsy is given the additional designation (sn) for "sentinel node" – for example, pN1(sn). For a case in which an initial classification is based on a sentinel lymph node biopsy but a standard axillary lymph node dissection is subsequently performed, the classification is based on the total results of both the axillary lymph node dissection and the sentinel node biopsy, and the (sn) modifier is removed. The (sn) modifier indicates that nodal classification is based on less than an axillary dissection. When the combination of sentinel and nonsentinel nodes removed is less than a standard low axillary dissection (less than six nodes) the (sn) modifier is used. The number of quantified nodes for staging is generally the number of grossly identified, histologically confirmed lymph nodes. Care should be taken to avoid overcounting sectioned nodes or sectioned adipose tissue with no grossly apparent nodes.

The first priority in pathologic evaluation of lymph nodes is to identify all macrometastases (metastases larger than 2.0 mm). The entire lymph node should be submitted for evaluation and larger nodes should be bisected or thinly sliced no thicker than 2.0 mm. A single histologic section of each slice has a high probability of detecting all macrometastases present although the largest dimension of the metastases may not be represented. More comprehensive evaluation of lymph node paraffin blocks is not required for staging; however, techniques such as multilevel sectioning and immunohistochemistry will identify additional tumor deposits, typically less than or equal to 2.0 mm [micrometastases and isolated tumor cell clusters (ITCs)]. It is not recommended that nodal tissue that may contain a macrometastasis be diverted for experimental or alternative testing,

**32**

such as molecular analysis, if this diversion would potentially result in the pathologist missing macrometastases detectable by routine microscopic examination.

*Isolated Tumor Cell Clusters and Micrometastases.* ITCs are defined as small clusters of cells not greater than 0.2 mm in largest dimension, or single cells, usually with little if any histologic stromal reaction. ITCs may be detected by routine histology or by immunohistochemical (IHC) methods. When no single metastasis larger than 0.2 mm is identified, regardless of the number of nodes containing ITCs, the regional lymph nodes should be designated as pN0(i+) or pN0(i+)(sn), as appropriate, and the number of ITC-involved nodes should be noted.

Approximately 1,000 tumor cells are contained in a three-dimensional 0.2-mm cluster. Thus, if more than 200 individual tumor cells are identified as single dispersed tumor cells or as a nearly confluent elliptical or spherical focus in a single histologic section of a lymph node there is a high probability that more than 1,000 cells are present in the lymph node. In these situations, the node should be classified as containing a micrometastasis (pN1mi). Cells in different lymph node cross or longitudinal sections or levels of the block are not added together; the 200 cells must be in a single node profile even if the node has been thinly sectioned into multiple slices. It is recognized that there is substantial overlap between the upper limit of the ITC and the lower limit of the micrometastasis categories due to inherent limitations in pathologic nodal evaluation and detection of minimal tumor burden in lymph nodes. Thus, the threshold of 200 cells in a single cross-section is a guideline to help pathologists distinguish between these two categories. The pathologist should use judgment regarding whether it is likely that the cluster of cells represents a true micrometastasis or is simply a small group of isolated tumor cells.

Micrometastases are defined as tumor deposits greater than 0.2 mm but not greater than 2.0 mm in largest dimension. Cases in which at least one micrometastasis is detected but no metastases greater than 2 mm (macrometastases) are detected, regardless of the number of involved nodes, are classified pN1mi or pN1mi(sn), as appropriate, and the number of involved nodes should be noted.

The size of a tumor deposit is determined by measuring the largest dimension of any group of cells that are touching one another (confluent or contiguous tumor cells) regardless of whether the deposit is confined to the lymph node, extends outside the node (extranodal or extracapsular extension), or is totally present outside the lymph node and invading adipose. When there are multiple tumor deposits in a lymph node, whether ITCs or micrometastases, the size of only the largest contiguous tumor deposit is used to classify the node; do not use the sum of all individual tumor deposits. When a tumor deposit has induced a fibrous (desmoplastic) stromal reaction, the combined contiguous dimension of tumor cells and fibrosis determines size of the metastasis. When a single case contains multiple positive lymph nodes and the largest tumor deposit in each node is categorically distinct, the number of nodes in each category (macrometastases, micrometastases, ITCs) may be recorded separately to facilitate N classification as described previously.

If histologically negative lymph nodes are examined for evidence of unique tumor or epithelial cell markers using molecular methods [reverse transcriptase–polymerase chain reaction (RT-PCR)] and these markers are detected, the regional lymph nodes are classified as pN0(mol+) or pN0(mol+)(sn), as appropriate. Sacrificing lymph node tissue for molecular analysis that would otherwise be available for histologic evaluation and staging is not recommended particularly when the size of the sacrificed tissue is large enough to contain a macrometastasis. If these data are generated, they should be collected by the registrar.

**Distant Metastases (M).** Cases in which there are no distant metastases as determined by clinical and/or radiographic methods are designated cM0, and cases in which one or more distant metastases are identified by clinical and/or radiographic methods are designated cM1. Positive supraclavicular lymph nodes are classified as N3 (see previous discussion). A case is classified as clinically free of metastases (cM0) unless there is documented evidence of metastases by clinical means (cM1) or by biopsy of a metastatic site (pM1). M stage of breast cancer refers to the classification of clinically significant distant metastases, which typically distinguishes whether or not there is a potential for long-term cure. The ascertainment of M stage requires evaluations consisting of a review of systems, physical examination and often also includes radiographic imaging, blood work, and tissue biopsy. The types of examinations needed in each case may vary and guidelines for these are available.[22] M classification is based on best clinical and radiographic interpretation, but pathologic confirmation is recommended, although it may not be obtained for reasons of feasibility or safety. Additionally, M stage assessment may not yield a definitive answer on the initial set of evaluations, and follow-up studies may be needed such that the final determination is a recursive and iterative process, assuming that the area of question was present at the time of diagnosis of the primary breast cancer. In these cases, the designated stage should remain M0 unless a definitive designation is made that the patient truly had detectable metastases at the time of diagnosis, based on the guidelines that follow. Subsequent development of new metastases in areas not previously thought to be suspicious does not change the patient's original stage and the patient would now be considered to have converted to recurrent Stage IV, which is considered recurrent disease without altering the original stage.

*Physical Examination.* Detection of metastatic disease by clinical exam should include a full physical examination with focused detail based on symptoms and radiographic findings. When appropriate, serial physical examinations based on evolving symptoms, physical findings, radiographic findings, and/or laboratory findings should be done on an iterative basis. Physical findings alone rarely will provide the basis for assigning M1 stage, and radiographic studies are almost always required. Whenever feasible, biopsy confirmation should be performed.

*Radiographic Studies.* It is not necessary for the patient to have radiological evaluation of distant sites to be classified as clinically free of metastases. The indication for the indicated radiographic evaluation for the presence of an M lesion in the staging of breast cancer is uncertain and varies by T and

N stage category. Certainly, all guidelines stipulate that suspicious findings in the history or physical examination, and/or elevated serologic tests for liver or bone function, are indications to proceed with radiographic systemic imaging, such as bone or body scintigraphy or anatomic, cross-sectional imaging. Most experts agree that systemic radiographic staging evaluation for metastases is not warranted in asymptomatic patients with normal blood tests who have T1-2, N0 breast cancer, and likewise most experts agree that staging is appropriate for patients with Stage III disease (clinical or pathologic). Recommendations are mixed for patients with T2N1.

Regardless, staging studies should focus on common sites of metastatic disease and/or sites indicated by symptoms or blood tests. Certain findings such as multiple lesions with classical characteristics of metastases, and clear changes from earlier studies may provide a very high index of suspicion and result in M1 classification. With radiographic screening or evaluation for another cause, false positive staging studies in patients with newly diagnosed breast cancer are relatively common. Pathologic confirmation of metastatic disease should be performed whenever feasible.

***Tissue Biopsy.*** The type of biopsy of a suspicious lesion should be guided by the location of the suspected metastases along with patient preference, safety, and the expertise and equipment available to the care team. Fine needle aspiration (FNA) is adequate, especially for visceral lesions and with the availability of experienced cytopathologic interpretation. Negative FNA or cellular atypia might carry a significant risk of false negativity, especially in bony or scirrhous lesions, so consideration of repeat FNA or other biopsy techniques such as core needle or open surgical biopsy may be warranted. Histopathologic examination should include standard H&E staining and in some cases may require additional immunohistochemical staining or other specialized testing for confirmation of breast cancer or other cancer type. If adequate biomarker data (estrogen receptor, progesterone receptor, HER2) are not available from the primary tumor, these should be obtained on any other biopsy that shows cancer on H&E staining. Special caution should be taken with evaluation of tumor markers in tissue collected from bone biopsies. Decalcification procedures may create false negative results for both immunohistochemistry (IHC) and fluorescent in situ hybridization (FISH). Incidentally detected cancer cells, clusters of cancer cells or foci ≤0.2 mm, or circulating tumor cells that are otherwise clinically and radiographically silent should not alone constitute M1 disease and are discussed below.

***Laboratory Abnormalities.*** Patients with abnormal liver function tests should undergo liver imaging, whereas those with elevated alkaline phosphatase or calcium levels, or suggestive symptoms, should undergo bone imaging and/or scintigraphy. Unexplained anemia and other cytopenias require a full hematologic evaluation (e.g., examination of the peripheral smear, iron studies, B12/folate levels) and should be investigated with bone imaging and a bone marrow biopsy depending on the results of the evaluation. Other unexplained laboratory abnormalities such as elevations in renal function should also prompt appropriate imaging tests. Elevated tumor markers are known to be associated with variable degrees of false positivity and their use has not been shown to improve outcome. The routine ordering of these tests, such as CA 15-3, CA 27.29, CEA, and other protein-based markers for staging is not indicated.[2]

***Circulating Tumor Cells, Bone Marrow Micrometastases, and Disseminated Tumor Cells.*** The presence of circulating tumor cells (CTCs) in the blood or micrometastases (≤0.2 mm) in the bone marrow or other nonregional nodal tissues should not be used to define M stage in the absence of other apparent clinical and/or radiographic findings that correspond to pathologic findings. However, an increasing number of studies are showing microscopic bone marrow and circulating tumor cells in M0 disease to be prognostic for recurrence or survival. Thus, denotation of histologically visible micrometastases in bone marrow, blood, or other organs distant from the breast and regional lymph nodes should be denoted by the term M0(i+). For M1 stage breast cancer (clinically and/or radiographically detectable metastases), the enumeration of CTCs at the time of diagnosis of metastatic disease has been shown to strongly correlate with survival, but neither the presence nor the number of CTCs will change the overall classification.

## OUTCOMES

Figure 32.2 shows percent survival at 5 years by size of primary tumor and number of nodes involved. Figure 32.3 shows observed survival rates for 211,645 cases with carcinoma of the breast diagnosed in years 2001–2002.

**32**

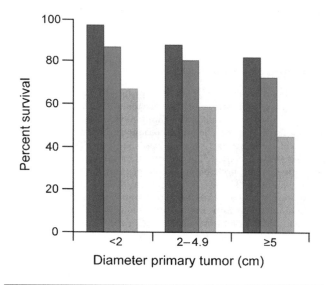

**FIGURE 32.2.** Percent survival at 5 years by size of primary tumor and number of nodes involved.

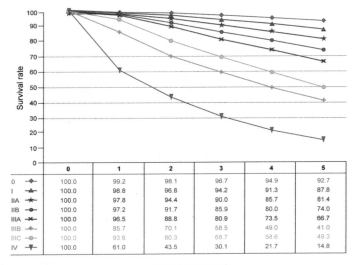

| | 0 | 1 | 2 | 3 | 4 | 5 |
|---|---|---|---|---|---|---|
| 0 | 100.0 | 99.2 | 98.1 | 96.7 | 94.9 | 92.7 |
| I | 100.0 | 98.8 | 96.8 | 94.2 | 91.3 | 87.8 |
| IIA | 100.0 | 97.8 | 94.4 | 90.0 | 85.7 | 81.4 |
| IIB | 100.0 | 97.2 | 91.7 | 85.9 | 80.0 | 74.0 |
| IIIA | 100.0 | 96.5 | 88.8 | 80.9 | 73.5 | 66.7 |
| IIIB | 100.0 | 85.7 | 70.1 | 58.5 | 49.0 | 41.0 |
| IIIC | 100.0 | 93.6 | 80.3 | 68.7 | 58.6 | 49.3 |
| IV | 100.0 | 61.0 | 43.5 | 30.1 | 21.7 | 14.8 |

Years from diagnosis

**FIGURE 32.3.** Observed survival rates for 211,645 cases with carcinoma of the breast. Data from the National Cancer Data Base (Commission on Cancer of the American College of Surgeons and the American Cancer Society) diagnosed in years 2001–2002. Stage 0 includes 30,263; Stage I, 85,278; Stage IIA, 43,047; Stage IIB, 17,665; Stage IIIA, 13,983; Stage IIIB, 4,533; Stage IIIC, 6,741; and Stage IV, 10,135.

## DEFINITIONS OF TNM

The increasing use of neoadjuvant therapy in breast cancer and the documented prognostic impact of postneoadjuvant extent of disease and response to therapy warrant clear definitions of the use of the "yp" prefix and response to therapy. The use of neoadjuvant therapy does not change the clinical (pretreatment) stage. As per TNM rules, the clinical stage is identified with the prefix "c". In addition, the use of fine needle aspiration and sentinel lymph node biopsy before neoadjuvant therapy is denoted with the subscripts "f" and "sn," respectively. Nodal metastases detected by FNA or core biopsy are classified as macrometastases (N1) regardless of the size of the tumor focus in the final pathologic specimen. For example, if, prior to neoadjuvant systemic therapy, a patient has no palpable nodes but has an ultrasound-guided FNA biopsy of an axillary lymph node that is positive, the patient will be categorized as cN1 (f) for her clinical (pretreatment) staging and would be considered as stage IIA. Likewise, if the patient has a positive axillary sentinel node identified prior to neoadjuvant systemic therapy, the patient will be categorized as cN1 (sn) (Stage IIA).

As per TNM rules, with the absence of pathologic T evaluation (removal of the primary tumor), microscopic evaluation of nodes before neoadjuvant therapy is still classified as clinical "c."

### Primary Tumor (T)

The T classification of the primary tumor is the same regard~~[ ]~~ ther it is based on clinical or pathologic criteria, or both. S~~[ ]~~ measured to the nearest millimeter. If the tumor size is slightly ~~[ ]~~ or greater than a cutoff for a given T classification, it is recommended ~~[ ]~~ the size be rounded to the millimeter reading that is closest to the cutoff. For example, a reported size of 1.1 mm is reported as 1 mm, or a size of 2.01 cm is reported as 2.0 cm. Designation should be made with the subscript "c" or "p" modifier to indicate whether the T classification was determined by clinical (physical examination or radiologic) or pathologic measurements, respectively. In general, pathologic determination should take precedence over clinical determination of T size.

| | |
|---|---|
| TX | Primary tumor cannot be assessed |
| T0 | No evidence of primary tumor |
| Tis | Carcinoma in situ |
| Tis (DCIS) | Ductal carcinoma in situ |
| Tis (LCIS) | Lobular carcinoma in situ |
| Tis (Paget's) | Paget's disease of the nipple NOT associated with invasive carcinoma and/or carcinoma in situ (DCIS and/or LCIS) in the underlying breast parenchyma. Carcinomas in the breast parenchyma associated with Paget's disease are categorized based on the size and characteristics of the parenchymal disease, although the presence of Paget's disease should still be noted |
| T1 | Tumor ≤20 mm in greatest dimension |
| T1mi | Tumor ≤1 mm in greatest dimension |
| T1a | Tumor >1 mm but ≤5 mm in greatest dimension |
| T1b | Tumor >5 mm but ≤10 mm in greatest dimension |
| T1c | Tumor >10 mm but ≤20 mm in greatest dimension |
| T2 | Tumor >20 mm but ≤50 mm in greatest dimension |
| T3 | Tumor >50 mm in greatest dimension |
| T4 | Tumor of any size with direct extension to the chest wall and/or to the skin (ulceration or skin nodules). |

*Note*: Invasion of the dermis alone does not qualify as T4

| | |
|---|---|
| T4a | Extension to the chest wall, not including only pectoralis muscle adherence/invasion |
| T4b | Ulceration and/or ipsilateral satellite nodules and/or edema (including peau d'orange) of the skin, which do not meet the criteria for inflammatory carcinoma |
| T4c | Both T4a and T4b |
| T4d | Inflammatory carcinoma (see "Rules for Classification") |

***Posttreatment ypT.*** Clinical (pretreatment) T will be defined by clinical and radiographic findings, while y pathologic (posttreatment) T will be determined by pathologic size and extension. The ypT will be measured as the largest single focus of invasive tumor, with the modifier "m" indicating multiple foci. The measurement of the largest tumor focus should not include areas of fibrosis within the tumor bed. The inclusion of additional information in the pathology report such as the distance over which tumor

extend, the number of tumor foci present, or the number of slides/
blocks in which tumor appears may assist the clinician in estimating the
extent of disease. A comparison of the cellularity in the initial biopsy to that
in the posttreatment specimen may also aid in the assessment of response.

*Note*: If a cancer was designated as inflammatory before neoadjuvant
chemotherapy, the patient will be designated to have inflammatory breast
cancer throughout, even if the patient has complete resolution of inflammatory findings.

### Regional Lymph Nodes (N)

*Clinical*

| | |
|---|---|
| NX | Regional lymph nodes cannot be assessed (e.g., previously removed) |
| N0 | No regional lymph node metastases |
| N1 | Metastases to movable ipsilateral level I, II axillary lymph node(s) |
| N2 | Metastases in ipsilateral level I, II axillary lymph nodes that are clinically fixed or matted; or in clinically detected* ipsilateral internal mammary nodes in the *absence* of clinically evident axillary lymph node metastases |
| N2a | Metastases in ipsilateral level I, II axillary lymph nodes fixed to one another (matted) or to other structures |
| N2b | Metastases only in clinically detected* ipsilateral internal mammary nodes and in the *absence* of clinically evident axillary lymph node metastases |
| N3 | Metastases in ipsilateral infraclavicular (level III axillary) lymph node(s) with or without level I, II axillary lymph node involvement; or in clinically detected* ipsilateral internal mammary lymph node(s) with clinically evident level I, II axillary lymph node metastases; or metastases in ipsilateral supraclavicular lymph node(s) with or without axillary or internal mammary lymph node involvement |
| N3a | Metastases in ipsilateral infraclavicular lymph node(s) |
| N3b | Metastases in ipsilateral internal mammary lymph node(s) and axillary lymph node(s) |
| N3c | Metastases in ipsilateral supraclavicular lymph node(s) |

*Note: *Clinically detected* is defined as detected by imaging studies (excluding
lymphoscintigraphy) or by clinical examination and having characteristics
highly suspicious for malignancy or a presumed pathologic macrometastasis based on fine needle aspiration biopsy with cytologic examination.
Confirmation of clinically detected metastatic disease by fine needle aspiration without excision biopsy is designated with an (f) suffix, for example, cN3a(f). Excisional biopsy of a lymph node or biopsy of a sentinel
node, in the absence of assignment of a pT, is classified as a clinical N, for
example, cN1. Information regarding the confirmation of the nodal status
will be designated in site-specific factors as clinical, fine needle aspiration,
core biopsy, or sentinel lymph node biopsy. Pathologic classification (pN)
is used for excision or sentinel lymph node biopsy only in conjunction with
a pathologic T assignment.

pNX      Regional lymph nodes cannot be assessed (e.g., previou
          or not removed for pathologic study)

pN0       No regional lymph node metastasis identified histolog

*Note*: Isolated tumor cell clusters (ITC) are defined as small clusters of cells not greater than 0.2 mm, or single tumor cells, or a cluster of fewer than 200 cells in a single histologic cross-section. ITCs may be detected by routine histology or by immunohistochemical (IHC) methods. Nodes containing only ITCs are excluded from the total positive node count for purposes of N classification but should be included in the total number of nodes evaluated.

pN0(i−)     No regional lymph node metastases histologically, negative IHC

pN0(i+)     Malignant cells in regional lymph node(s) no greater than 0.2 mm (detected by H&E or IHC including ITC)

pN0(mol−)   No regional lymph node metastases histologically, negative molecular findings (RT-PCR)

pN0(mol+)   Positive molecular findings (RT-PCR),** but no regional lymph node metastases detected by histology or IHC

pN1        Micrometastases; or metastases in 1–3 axillary lymph nodes; and/or in internal mammary nodes with metastases detected by sentinel lymph node biopsy but not clinically detected***

pN1mi     Micrometastases (greater than 0.2 mm and/or more than 200 cells, but none greater than 2.0 mm)

pN1a      Metastases in 1–3 axillary lymph nodes, at least one metastasis greater than 2.0 mm

pN1b      Metastases in internal mammary nodes with micrometastases or macrometastases detected by sentinel lymph node biopsy but not clinically detected***

pN1c      Metastases in 1–3 axillary lymph nodes and in internal mammary lymph nodes with micrometastases or macrometastases detected by sentinel lymph node biopsy but not clinically detected

pN2        Metastases in 4–9 axillary lymph nodes; or in clinically detected**** internal mammary lymph nodes in the *absence* of axillary lymph node metastases

pN2a      Metastases in 4–9 axillary lymph nodes (at least one tumor deposit greater than 2.0 mm)

pN2b      Metastases in clinically detected**** internal mammary lymph nodes in the *absence* of axillary lymph node metastases

pN3        Metastases in ten or more axillary lymph nodes; or in infraclavicular (level III axillary) lymph nodes; or in clinically detected**** ipsilateral internal mammary lymph nodes in the *presence* of one or more positive level I, II axillary lymph nodes; or in more than three axillary lymph nodes and in internal mammary lymph nodes with micrometastases or macrometastases detected by sentinel lymph node biopsy but not clinically detected***; or in ipsilateral supraclavicular lymph nodes

**32**

| $\jmath$ | Metastases in ten or more axillary lymph nodes (at least one tumor deposit greater than 2.0 mm); or metastases to the infraclavicular (level III axillary lymph) nodes |
| pN3b | Metastases in clinically detected**** ipsilateral internal mammary lymph nodes in the *presence* of one or more positive axillary lymph nodes; or in more than three axillary lymph nodes and in internal mammary lymph nodes with micrometastases or macrometastases detected by sentinel lymph node biopsy but not clinically detected*** |
| pN3c | Metastases in ipsilateral supraclavicular lymph nodes |

*Notes*:

*Classification is based on axillary lymph node dissection with or without sentinel lymph node biopsy. Classification based solely on sentinel lymph node biopsy without subsequent axillary lymph node dissection is designated (sn) for "sentinel node," for example, pN0(sn).

** RT-PCR: reverse transcriptase/polymerase chain reaction.

*** "Not clinically detected" is defined as not detected by imaging studies (excluding lymphoscintigraphy) or not detected by clinical examination.

**** "Clinically detected" is defined as detected by imaging studies (excluding lymphoscintigraphy) or by clinical examination and having characteristics highly suspicious for malignancy or a presumed pathologic macrometastasis based on fine needle aspiration biopsy with cytologic examination.

### Posttreatment ypN

- Post-treatment yp "N" should be evaluated as for clinical (pretreatment) "N" methods above. The modifier "sn" is used only if a sentinel node evaluation was performed after treatment. If no subscript is attached, it is assumed that the axillary nodal evaluation was by axillary node dissection (AND).
- The X classification will be used (ypNX) if no yp posttreatment SN or AND was performed
- N categories are the same as those used for pN.

| Distant Metastases (M) | |
| --- | --- |
| M0 | No clinical or radiographic evidence of distant metastases |
| cM0(i+) | No clinical or radiographic evidence of distant metastases, but deposits of molecularly or microscopically detected tumor cells in circulating blood, bone marrow, or other nonregional nodal tissue that are no larger than 0.2 mm in a patient without symptoms or signs of metastases |
| M1 | Distant detectable metastases as determined by classic clinical and radiographic means and/or histologically proven larger than 0.2 mm |

**Posttreatment yp M classification.** The M category for patients treated with neoadjuvant therapy is the category assigned in the clinical stage, prior to initiation of neoadjuvant therapy. Identification of distant metastases after the start of therapy in cases where pretherapy evaluation showed no metastases is considered progression of disease. If a patient was designated to have detectable distant metastases (M1) before chemotherapy, the patient will be designated as M1 throughout.

## ANATOMIC STAGE/PROGNOSTIC GROUPS

| Stage 0 | Tis | N0 | M0 |
|---|---|---|---|
| Stage IA | T1* | N0 | M0 |
| Stage IB | T0 | N1mi | M0 |
| | T1* | N1mi | M0 |
| Stage IIA | T0 | N1** | M0 |
| | T1* | N1** | M0 |
| | T2 | N0 | M0 |
| Stage IIB | T2 | N1 | M0 |
| | T3 | N0 | M0 |
| Stage IIIA | T0 | N2 | M0 |
| | T1* | N2 | M0 |
| | T2 | N2 | M0 |
| | T3 | N1 | M0 |
| | T3 | N2 | M0 |
| Stage IIIB | T4 | N0 | M0 |
| | T4 | N1 | M0 |
| | T4 | N2 | M0 |
| Stage IIIC | Any T | N3 | M0 |
| Stage IV | Any T | Any N | M1 |

*Notes*:
*T1 includes T1mi.

**T0 and T1 tumors with nodal micrometastases only are excluded from Stage IIA and are classified Stage IB.

- M0 includes M0(i+).
- The designation pM0 is not valid; any M0 should be clinical.
- If a patient presents with M1 prior to neoadjuvant systemic therapy, the stage is considered Stage IV and remains Stage IV regardless of response to neoadjuvant therapy.
- Stage designation may be changed if postsurgical imaging studies reveal the presence of distant metastases, provided that the studies are carried out within 4 months of diagnosis in the absence of disease progression and provided that the patient has not received neoadjuvant therapy.
- Postneoadjuvant therapy is designated with "yc" or "yp" prefix. Of note, no stage group is assigned if there is a complete pathologic response (CR) to neoadjuvant therapy, for example, ypT0ypN0cM0.

## PROGNOSTIC FACTORS (SITE-SPECIFIC FACTORS)
### (Recommended for Collection)

| | |
|---|---|
| Required for staging | None |
| Clinically significant | Paget's disease |
| | Tumor grade (Scarff–Bloom–Richardson system) |

Estrogen receptor and test method (IHC, RT-PCR, other)

Progesterone receptor and test method (IHC, RT-PCR, other)

HER2 status and test method (IHC, FISH, CISH, RT-PCR, other)

Method of lymph node assessment (e.g., clinical, fine needle aspiration; core biopsy; sentinel lymph node biopsy)

IHC of regional lymph nodes

Molecular studies regional lymph nodes

Distant metastases method of detection (clinical, radiographic, biopsy)

Circulating tumor cells (CTC) and method of detection (RT-PCR, immunomagnetic separation, other)

Disseminated tumor cells (DTC; bone marrow micrometastases) and method of detection (RT-PCR, immunohistochemical, other)

Multigene signature score

| | |
|---|---|
| Response to neoadjuvant therapy | Will be collected in the registry but does not affect the postneoadjuvant stage |
| Complete response (CR) | Pathologic complete response can only be determined by histopathologic evaluation and is defined by the absence of invasive carcinoma in the breast and lymph nodes.<br><br>Residual in situ cancer, in the absence of invasive disease, constitutes a pCR.<br><br>Patients with isolated tumor foci in lymph nodes are not classified as having a CR. The presence of axillary nodal tumor deposits of any size, including cell clusters less than or equal to 0.2 mm, excludes a complete response. These patients will be categorized as ypN0(i+). |
| Partial response (PR) | A decrease in either or both the T or N category compared to the pretreatment T or N, and no increase in either T or N. After chemotherapy, one should use the method that most clearly defined tumor dimensions at baseline for this comparison, although prechemotherapy pT cannot be measured.<br><br>Clinical (pretreatment) T will be defined by clinical and radiographic findings. y pathologic (posttreatment) T will be determined by pathologic size and extension.<br><br>Nodal response should be determined by physical examination or radiologic evaluation, if the nodes are palpable or visible before chemotherapy. |

If prechemotherapy pathologic lymph node involvement is demonstrated by fine needle aspiration, core biopsy, or sentinel node biopsy, it should be recorded as such. Absence of posttreatment pathologic nodal involvement should be used to document pathologic complete response, and should be recorded, but does not necessarily represent a true "response" since one does not know whether lymph nodes removed surgically postchemotherapy were involved prior to chemotherapy.

No response (NR)

No apparent change in either the T or N categories compared to the clinical (pretreatment) assignment or an increase in the T or N category at the time of y pathologic evaluation.

Clinical (pretreatment) T will be defined by clinical and radiographic findings.

yp (posttreatment) T will be determined by pathologic size.

The response category will be appended to the y stage description. For example:

- ypTisypN0cM0CR; ypT1ypN0cM0PR; ypT2ypN-1cM0NR

## HISTOLOGIC GRADE (G)

All invasive breast carcinomas should be graded. The Nottingham combined histologic grade (Elston-Ellis modification of Scarff–Bloom–Richardson grading system) is recommended.[2,23] The grade for a tumor is determined by assessing morphologic features (tubule formation, nuclear pleomorphism, and mitotic count), assigning a value of 1 (favorable) to 3 (unfavorable) for each feature, and adding together the scores for all three categories. A combined score of 3–5 points is designated as grade 1; a combined score of 6–7 points is grade 2; a combined score of 8–9 points is grade 3.

## HISTOLOGIC GRADE (NOTTINGHAM COMBINED HISTOLOGIC GRADE IS RECOMMENDED)

GX  Grade cannot be assessed
G1  Low combined histologic grade (favorable)
G2  Intermediate combined histologic grade (moderately favorable)
G3  High combined histologic grade (unfavorable)

## HISTOPATHOLOGIC TYPE

The histopathologic types are the following:

### In situ Carcinomas

NOS (not otherwise specified)
Intraductal
Paget's disease and intraductal

### Invasive Carcinomas

NOS
Ductal
Inflammatory
Medullary, NOS
Medullary with lymphoid stroma
Mucinous
Papillary (predominantly micropapillary pattern)
Tubular
Lobular
Paget's disease and infiltrating
Undifferentiated
Squamous cell
Adenoid cystic
Secretory
Cribriform

## SPECIFIC CONSIDERATIONS FOR EVIDENCE-BASED CHANGES TO THE *AJCC CANCER STAGING MANUAL*, SEVENTH EDITION

### Revisit of Considerations Between Fifth and Sixth Editions

**Q:** *Should histologic grade (Nottingham combined histologic grade recommended) be incorporated into the TNM classification system?*
**A:** No; see "Considerations" below; T category.

**Q:** *Should the classification of pathologic lymph node status in node-negative patients be amplified to include information about isolated tumor cells detected by immunohistochemical techniques?*
**A:** Yes, in part and now further clarified; see "Considerations" below; N category

**Q:** *Should micrometastases (pN1mi) detected by immunohistochemical staining and not verified by H&E staining be classified as pN1?*
**A:** Yes; see "Considerations" below; N category. The definition is now based on size, NOT how they were detected.

**Q:** *Should size criteria be used to distinguish between isolated tumor cells and micrometastases?*
**A:** Yes; see "Considerations" below; N category. The definition is now based on size, NOT how they were detected.

**Q:** *How should RT-PCR be used in the detection of small tumor deposits?*
**A:** If collected, it should be collected by the registrar, but not used for staging; see "Considerations" below; N category

**Q:** *Should the classification of pathologic lymph node status in node-positive (all nodes with deposits greater than 0.2 mm) patients be changed to reflect more clearly the prognostic significance of number of affected nodes?*
**A:** It was changed in sixth edition; no change in seventh edition.

**Q:** *Should a finding of positive internal mammary lymph nodes retain a current classification of N3?*

**A:** It was reclassified pN2b in the sixth edition. In the seventh edition, if positive internal mammary lymph nodes are identified in the absence of axillary lymph node positivity, then it is classified N2b. If positive lymph nodes are identified in the presence of axillary lymph node positivity, then it is classified N3b.

**Q:** *Should a finding of positive supraclavicular lymph nodes be classified as N3 rather than M1?*

**A:** It was reclassified pN3 from M1 in the sixth edition. No change in the seventh edition.

**Q:** *Are there other prognostic factors that are powerful enough to consider for inclusion in the TNM grading system?*

**A:** No. See "Considerations" below; B category regarding multiparameter assays.

**New Considerations Between Sixth and Seventh Editions.** The Breast Cancer Task Force deliberated many important issues regarding the TNM staging system for the seventh edition. These can be divided into subtle, but important changes in rules regulating how to collect or interpret already existing factors, such as T, N, and M, and whether new markers and/or technologies should be incorporated into any of these categories. The following discussions highlight these considerations and justify the changes that have been recommended.

Of note, the Breast Cancer Task Force did not feel that any new factors have reached a level of evidence to justify inclusion into the staging system. Indeed, a literature search using the terms "breast cancer" and "prognostic factors" yielded over 1,800 publications in the English literature during the 5-year period 2003–2007. These factors included ethnic origin, pre- and post-diagnostic life styles and body habitus, means of diagnosis and apparent radiographic character of the tumor, germ line polymorphisms in candidate genes related to tumor behavior and/or distribution and activity of therapeutic agents, somatic biologic changes in the primary cancer, and evidence of distant, microscopic metastases using sensitive radiographic, molecular, and cellular detection systems. In most, if not all of these studies, the authors conclude that the investigational factor was statistically significantly associated with outcome. However, the studies were often conducted using datasets and tissue specimens that were conveniently available rather than as prospective, well-designed investigations. Importantly, the effects of systemic therapy, either in the adjuvant or metastatic settings, were often ignored or not even considered. Therefore, one is unable to determine if differential outcomes between those patients who were positive vs. those who were negative occurred because of, or in spite of, the marker. Such considerations must be taken into account in the design, conduct, analysis, and reporting of tumor marker studies.[24–30]

## Primary Tumor (T)

*Should histologic grade (Nottingham combined histologic grade recommended) be incorporated into the TNM classification system?*

As noted, the issue of inclusion of histologic grade was very seriously considered by the Breast Cancer Task Force in preparation of the sixth edition. Ultimately, after careful deliberation of all of the identified published literature on the subject, the Task Force elected not to include grade as a stage modifying factor in the TNM system.[23] The Task Force acknowledged the consistent differences in outcomes between women whose tumors were grade 1 vs. those that were grade 3, using the modified Scarff–Bloom–Richardson scoring system. However, the majority of breast cancers are classified as grade 2, and the prognostic significance of this category inconsistently tracked with either of the other two grades, depending on the study. Moreover, persistent concerns about grading inconsistency between observers contributed to the decision not to include grade.

Several new studies have been published since the sixth edition, but none has clarified the issue any further than what were available to the Task Force at that time. Additionally, several authors have addressed specific molecular components of grade, such as proliferative markers and multigene expression arrays that appear to reflect grade.[31–33] However, these assays are either not widely available, or, like standard histopathologic analyses, reproducibility has been an issue. However, the Task Force does recommend collection of tumor grade, using the standardized Nottingham combined histologic score with calibrated mitotic counts, for inclusion in registry databases.

*Should T4 be distilled to inflammatory carcinoma only?*

Recent studies have suggested that the T4 designation should be restricted to inflammatory carcinoma (T4d) only, with the consideration that T4 a, b, and c categories have outcomes similar to those in the T3 category, and substantially better than those with true inflammatory breast cancer, if carefully defined.[34–36] In this case, the other subcategories (T4a, T4b, T4c) would then be categorized based on the size of the tumor in each case, regardless of skin or chest wall involvement.

The Breast Cancer Task Force concluded that the data from the main study suggesting this change were interesting, but size of the study was modest and the analyses were not comprehensive. Therefore, the Task Force requested an analysis of 5-year survival rates in T4 lesions in the National Cancer Database from 1998 to 2000. In this analysis of 9,865 cases, significantly different outcomes were observed for each of the T4 categories (T4a = 47%, T4b = 40%, T4c = 28%, T4d = 34%; $p < 0.0001$ all pair-wise comparisons). However, without a comprehensive comparison to tumors of similar size/stage but <T4, the Task Force could not conclude that restricting T4 to T4d was appropriate. The group concluded that the data were insufficient at this time to recommend a change, but that they do warrant further study and future consideration.

*Should the term "inflammatory carcinoma" be restricted to cases with typical clinical skin changes AND the presence of histologically confirmed invasive carcinoma involving dermal lymphatics?*

The Task Force carefully considered this issue and elected not to recommend changes in the seventh edition. The definition of inflammatory breast cancer will remain clinical and does not require the finding of dermal lymphatic involvement, although it does, of course, require histologic confirmation of cancer either in breast parenchyma or skin. Dermal lymphatic involvement supports the diagnosis of inflammatory breast cancer but is not necessary, nor is it sufficient, in the absence of classical clinical findings, for the diagnosis of inflammatory breast cancer. The Task Force acknowledges that this recommendation is not based so much on new data but rather a perceived need to clarify the definition in the sixth edition, which was considered ambiguous.

### Should the size of multiple separate ipsilateral tumors be taken into account when determining T category and Stage?

In prior editions of the *Staging Manual*, T stage assignment for patients with multiple, concurrent ipsilateral breast cancers has been based only on the largest tumor, and the sum of the sizes has not been used. Although some studies suggest that multiple tumors may have a somewhat worse prognosis than single tumors in the same T category, the data are insufficient to change the current rules for staging.[37] However, the presence and sizes of the smaller tumor(s) should be recorded. The Breast Cancer Task Force does express concern about this issue and suggests it warrants further study.

**Regional Lymph Nodes (N)**

### Should the size thresholds for isolated tumor cell clusters and micrometastases be changed from the current limits of 0.2 and 2.0 mm?

The prognostic significance of axillary metastases above a 2.0-mm threshold was confirmed by two studies reported over 3 decades ago.[38,39] Following the first study, a subcategory for micrometastases was added to the *Cancer Staging Manual*. The introduction of sentinel lymph node biopsy and widespread use of immunohistochemistry facilitated detection of minimal disease in axillary lymph nodes and the sixth edition of the *Staging Manual* established a lower limit for micrometastases of >0.2 mm creating a new category of minimal nodal disease. This limit was ten times smaller than the upper limit for micrometastases and had been tested in one retrospective study of occult metastases.[40] It was not a limit based on firm medical evidence and should be periodically reevaluated.

Testing these thresholds is not an easy task. Doing so requires excluding the presence of metastases above the suggested threshold prior to comparing differences in outcome for subgroups with smaller metastases, and then either accepting the confounding effects of systemic therapy or identifying datasets of untreated patients. To date, no study has evaluated differences in disease free or overall survival for metastases above and below a 1.0-mm threshold after excluding all metastases above 2.0 mm. When these data become available, the upper limit of 2.0 mm for micrometastases could be reconsidered.

Evaluating the upper limit for isolated tumor cell clusters is more problematic because it requires excluding all patients with metastases larger than 0.2 mm prior to comparing subgroups with metastases below this threshold. Creating a "true node negative" comparison group is probably not practical with standard histologic techniques. In other words, any "node negative" group will contain some patients with occult metastatic disease. Two limiting principles emerge when evaluating these thresholds; the first is lymph node sectioning strategies and the second is section screening. The possibility of missing a metastasis is proportional to the thickness of unexamined tissue, the number of sections examined, and the capability of the slide screening system to detect disease.[41-44] For example, if evaluation of serial sections from a lymph node is negative, but if a pathologist leaves 1.0 mm of unexamined tissue in the paraffin lymph node block, one can only conclude that there is no metastasis larger than 1.0 mm; there is no guarantee the node does not contain occult disease. Single cells are routinely detected on histologic sections, but metastases as large as 0.1 mm may be missed by a pathologist screening slides.[43,44]

It has been theorized that isolated tumor cell clusters should be distinguishable from micrometastases on the basis of metastatic characteristics, such as proliferation or stromal reaction, and indeed this observation was included in the sixth edition.[23,45] However, in consideration of the seventh edition, the Breast Cancer Task Force perceived that this distinction can be highly subjective and expressed concern that replication among pathologists and among institutions may be difficult. For the seventh edition, the Breast Cancer Task Force continues to define isolated tumor cell clusters as not greater than 0.2 mm in diameter and micrometastases as greater than 0.2 mm and not greater than 2.0 mm in diameter. However, the Task Force has recommended additional stringency to the isolated tumor cell cluster (ITC) category. A 0.2-mm metastasis contains approximately 1,000 tumor cells and a 2.0-mm metastasis contains approximately one million tumor cells. The use of 0.2 mm as a lower limit was selected because it significantly reduces the likelihood that ITCs will be recorded as micrometastases without making it necessary to estimate actual cell number counts in ITCs. However, pathologists have had difficulty applying the size criterion when a large number of nonconfluent tumor cells are present in a lymph node such as may occur in some invasive lobular carcinomas.[46] For this reason, additional guidance has been incorporated in this edition. When more than 200 nonconfluent or nearly confluent tumor cells are present in a single histologic cross section of a lymph node, there is a high probability that more than 1,000 cells are present in the node, that the cumulative volume of these cells exceeds the volume of an ITC, and the node should be classified as containing a micrometastasis. The classification of patients with metastatic tumor deposits no greater than 0.2 mm as pN0 is consistent with the low recurrence rates typically seen in this patient group. The use of 2.0 mm as an upper size limit for micrometastases, originally proposed by Huvos and colleagues in 1971, is consistent with standards already used in the AJCC staging system.[38] These thresholds are meant to be guidelines, and not absolute cutoffs, to help pathologists determine if the tumor burden in a given lymph node is likely to be clinically important or not. The pathologist should use judgment, and not an absolute cutoff of 0.2 mm or exactly 200 cells, in determining the likelihood of whether the cluster of cells is an ITC or a true micrometastasis.

There is significant theoretic overlap in nodal tumor burden at the upper limit of the ITC category and the lower limit of the micrometastasis category that is due to practical and economic constraints in the pathologic evaluation of lymph nodes. After considering these limitations in lymph node examination and the absence of outcome data on clinical significance of isolated tumor cell clusters and micrometastases *after* systematic exclusion of macrometastases, the Breast Cancer Task Force perceived no compelling reason to change the current thresholds.

### Should nodal micrometastases be considered different from nodal macrometastases for purposes of overall stage grouping?

The *AJCC Cancer Staging Manual* has traditionally grouped breast cancer cases with exclusively nodal micrometastases (pN1mi) as having the same prognostic significance as macrometastases with respect to assigning an overall stage grouping based on T, N, and M categorical classifications. A recent analysis of data in the United States Surveillance, Epidemiology, and End Results (SEER) national cancer database has demonstrated that when nodal tumor deposits no larger than 2.0 mm are the only finding in lymph nodes and the primary tumor is less than or equal to 2 cm (pT1) the incremental decrease in survival at 5 and 10 years was only 1% compared to patients with no nodal metastases detected.[47] Patients with tumors no larger than 2.0 cm (T1) represented 70% of the total population in the analysis, and in this subset calculated 10-year survival decreased from 78% to 77% to 73% for pN0, pN1mi, and pN1a, respectively. This does not justify classifying pN1mi cases with Stage II tumors. This analysis included data from 1992 to 2003 spanning the introduction and widespread adoption of sentinel lymph node biopsy. In this edition of the manual, T1 tumors with nodal micrometastases (pN1mi) will be classified as Stage IB to indicate the better prognosis for the subset of breast cancer patients and to facilitate further investigation.

### How should RT-PCR be classified in the detection of nodal tumor deposits?

An even finer level of resolution in the detection of isolated tumor cells and micrometastases is available with the use of reverse transcriptase-polymerase chain reaction (RT-PCR). This technique was able to identify epithelial markers in a significant percentage of sentinel nodes that were negative for disease by both histologic and immunohistochemical staining.[48] This is not surprising given that RT-PCR is theoretically capable of identifying single cells. However, it seems unlikely that minimal tumor burden would be as significant as clinically detected disease or macrometastases. Furthermore, because lymph node tissue is digested and consumed in preparation for RT-PCR, it is technically challenging to determine the exact size of the original metastatic focus. RT-PCR assays have been offered as an adjunct to standard histological analysis of sentinel lymph node biopsy to assist in intraoperative decision making regarding the performance of completion axillary node dissection.[49] The prognostic or staging significance of such RT-PCR assay results remains unclear. There is evidence that such highly-sensitive tests produce false positive results despite efforts to calibrate RT-PCR results with traditional histologic measurements.[41] Correlation between RT-PCR testing and histology has been performed but there is continued and justified concern that RT-PCR assays do not provide the same data as routine histologic measurement and categorization of nodal metastases. A lymph node that is exclusively positive by molecular assay alone (mol+) may contain isolated tumor cell clusters, micrometastases, macrometastases, or be a false positive result due to sampling, contamination, or features intrinsic to the assay. Presently, there are insufficient data to suggest that RT-PCR assay of lymph nodes should replace or substitute for traditional histologic evaluation of lymph nodes. Staging is further complicated when some nodes or portions of some nodes are evaluated by RT-PCR and other nodes are evaluated by histology.

Pending further developments in this area, this edition of the *AJCC Cancer Staging Manual* will continue to classify any lesion identified by RT-PCR alone as pN0 for the purposes of staging. In addition, any case that is histologically negative for regional lymph node metastases and in which examination for epithelial markers was made with RT-PCR and the examination was considered positive will have the appended designation (mol+). It is recommended that the first priority in evaluating lymph nodes is histologic identification of macrometastases (metastases larger than 2.0 mm). Thus, it is not recommended to divert portions of nodal tissue for molecular analysis that might contain a macrometastasis. When lymph nodes contain tumor deposits detected by histologic evaluation and molecular techniques, N classification based on histologic findings and measurements is utilized.

## Distant Metastases (M)

*How should circulating tumor cells or microscopic tumor cells be handled in the absence of overt clinical finding?*
Circulating tumor cells (CTCs) and microscopic tumor cells detected in the bone marrow are collectively designated as DTCs. Several studies have shown a relationship between bone marrow DTCs and recurrence risk and mortality in M0 stage breast cancer.[50,51] However, the Breast Cancer Task Force concluded that although the presence of positive bone marrow micrometastases has been statistically significantly associated with worse outcomes, the difference in recurrence and mortality rates between patients who have them and those who do not was not sufficiently large to recommend a change in the M staging system. In particular, patients who already have a favorable prognosis (T1, N0) do not appear to have a substantially worse outcome if they have positive bone marrow micrometastases.[50]

Although several recent studies have suggested that CTC are commonly detected in patients with early stage breast cancer and may be prognostic, the Task Force concluded that most of these studies were small with short follow-up and were confounded by the effects of systemic therapy.[2,28,52–60]

In summary, the designation of M1 has generally been used to determine a relative, or even, absolute state of incurability. Thus, many clinicians revert to a philosophy of palliative, rather than curative intent, for patients who are designated M1. There are no data to suggest that detection of DTCs in any tissue (bone marrow, ovary, blood) in the absence of clinical and/or radiographic findings confers incurability. Therefore, the Task Force recommends that in the absence of overt metastases detected by clinical examination or imaging abnormalities, DTCs should not affect M staging.

The Task Force has recommended that, for data collection purposes, the DTC designation should be expanded to include any cluster of malignant cells not greater than 0.2 mm found in any tissue outside of the breast and surrounding regional lymph nodes in the absence of clinical or radiographic signs of metastases. DTC assessment is not required or recommended as part of staging at the current time outside of the investigational setting in patients with clinical M0 disease. However, if DTCs are detected, the staging category should be denoted as M0(i+) and the data should be collected by the registrars.

### Should DTC (bone marrow micrometastases or CTC) be incorporated to subdivide the M1 category?

The Task Force considered whether the TNM system might be used to further subdivide patients with M1 disease. In patients with overt metastases (M1), the presence and number of CTCs at the time of diagnosis have been shown to be prognostic for both disease progression and mortality.[51,58,61–67] Changes in CTCs after treatment are also predictive of response to therapy and prognostic for recurrence and mortality, although the American Society of Clinical Oncology Tumor Marker Guidelines Panel has not recommended routine use of CTC in management of patients with metastatic breast cancer, since the utility of this assay in patient management decisions has not been demonstrated.[2] After careful deliberation, the Task Force decided that the TNM system has not, in the past, dealt with prognosis in those patients with established, clinically or radiographically detectable metastases, and the Task Force elected not to recommend that CTC presence or number be used to further subclassify M1 staging.

### y Pathologic (Postneoadjuvant) Systemic Therapy

### Why add a postneoadjuvant systemic therapy staging system?

Neoadjuvant therapy, also designated preoperative, presurgical, or primary adjuvant systemic therapy, has been increasingly studied and applied for patients with operable, as well as traditionally inoperable breast cancer.[68] While most commonly considered for chemotherapy, neo- or preoperative adjuvant endocrine therapy has also been studied extensively.[68] The increasing importance of this strategy mandates that the staging system provide the information necessary to assess prognosis in this diverse group of patients. Clearly, outcomes after neoadjuvant systemic therapy differ among patients, so that a staging system should reflect potential prognosis. Thus, the Breast Cancer Task Force has included a staging system to be applied for patients treated in this manner, which will be designated with the prefix y, y pathologic or yp, in accordance with AJCC policy in other disease sites.

### What is the proper definition of complete response after neoadjuvant systemic therapy?

The prognostic importance of a histologic complete response (CR) to neoadjuvant chemotherapy was first documented in patients with locally advanced breast cancer.[69] This observation was subsequently confirmed in randomized trials involving patients with operable disease.[70] In several studies, a variety of different definitions of CR have been employed, making a comparison of the outcomes of different treatment regimens difficult. For this reason, the Task Force proposed a standard set of response definitions to be included with the posttreatment stage.

Although an international expert panel proposed that a CR be defined as the absence of invasive and *noninvasive* tumor in the breast,[71] the Task Force recommends that the AJCC definition of CR should be the absence of invasive carcinoma in the breast and the axillary nodes, since the presence of noninvasive cancer, while important in the selection of local therapy, is not a determinant of survival. A retrospective review from the MD Anderson Cancer Center compared the outcome of 78 patients with a pathologic CR and no residual tumor of any kind to that of 199 patients with residual DCIS only and 2,025 patients with residual invasive cancer. The 5 and 10 year disease-free and overall survival rates for patients with a pathologic CR with and without DCIS did not differ significantly, but were significantly better than the survival rates of patients with invasive cancer.[72] Similar findings were reported by Jones et al. in a study of 435 patients.[73]

### What is the optimal method of determining T after neoadjuvant systemic therapy?

An unresolved problem in defining the yp posttreatment stage is how to determine the best method for measuring tumor size after neoadjuvant/preoperative chemotherapy. In the absence of a CR, the assessment of the extent of response in the tumor and the measurement of tumor size remain problematic. Partial response in the NSABP protocol B18[74] and in the grading system proposed by Chevillard et al.[75] is identified by nests of tumor in a desmoplastic or fibrotic stroma. In contrast, the Miller–Payne grading system[76] and a system used at the M.D. Anderson Cancer Center[77] rely upon loss of cellularity to describe the degree of response. No single method of assessing response has been shown to be a superior predictor of outcome, and concerns about reproducibility exist for all these measures. The combination of tumor size and an assessment of changes in cellularity are useful in documenting pathologic evidence of response. However, pretreatment biopsies are not always available to the pathologist assessing the posttreatment specimen. For this reason, the Breast Cancer Task Force has defined the pathologic T size by the largest contiguous tumor focus, with a suffix to alert the clinician when multiple scattered tumor foci are observed. When nests of tumor cells in fibrotic stroma are observed posttreatment, the T should be determined based on the largest contiguous area of invasive carcinoma, excluding surrounding areas of fibrosis. This method of T determination has been shown to correlate with survival in the study of Carey et al.[78] Additional information that is important for planning local therapy such as the distance over which the tumor extends (when scattered foci are present) or the number of slides/blocks in which tumor is seen should be included in the pathology report, but is not part of TNM.

### How should isolated tumor cells be considered after neoadjuvant therapy?

In patients who have not received neoadjuvant therapy, nodes with ITCs are classified pN0, reflecting uncertainty about their prognostic significance. After neoadjuvant therapy, ITCs could represent the presence of minimal nodal disease pre-treatment which did not respond to therapy or the remnants of macroscopic nodal disease which has had a partial response. Until further data are available to address the prognostic significance of ITCs post-treatment, the presence of ITC precludes classifying the patient as having a complete response to therapy. However, these patients will be classified as ypN0(i+) to maintain standard definitions throughout the TNM system.

### Should the same considerations be used for preoperative endocrine (anti-estrogen) or other targeted therapy?

The overwhelming majority of the available information regarding the prognostic significance of CR comes from patients treated with chemotherapy. Limited information is available about the prognostic significance of the degree of response when targeted therapies directed against ER or HER2 are used. Pathologic CR is rarely seen in patients receiving 3–4 months of neoadjuvant endocrine therapy, and its absence should not be considered evidence of endocrine resistance or poor prognosis.[79,80] Complete response in patients overexpressing HER2 and treated with trastuzumab plus chemotherapy was associated with a significant survival improvement compared with that in women who did not have pathologic CR.[81] Additional information regarding the relationship between response and survival is needed for the newer targeted therapies, and therefore the Breast Cancer Task Force recommends collection of postneoadjuvant therapy TNM data by the registrars.

### What are the difficulties in evaluating partial response?

The Breast Cancer Task Force recognizes that the definition of partial response (PR), requiring a decrease in the T or N category, may fail to capture some patients with a reduction in tumor volume. However, modalities such as physical examination, mammography, ultrasound, and MRI, which may be used to determine the clinical (pretreatment) tumor size, have been demonstrated to significantly overestimate and underestimate the extent of tumor when compared with pathologic examination,[82] making definitions of response based on small changes in the clinically determined pretreatment tumor size compared to the y pathologic posttreatment tumor size potentially inaccurate. In this regard, the most accurate predictor of outcome after neoadjuvant chemotherapy is pathologic complete response.[68,79] However, a rough estimate of response should be determined comparing posttreatment clinical, radiographic, and pathologic assessments with those made prior to initiation of systemic therapy, and this should be recorded.

### Should TNM stage prior to neoadjuvant systemic (clinical stage) be considered in y pathologic posttreatment staging?

An increasing body of data suggests that prognosis after neoadjuvant therapy is determined by the posttreatment pathologic stage, degree of response, and the pretreatment stage. Carey et al. demonstrated that the AJCC TNM posttreatment (yp) stage was a significant predictor of both 5-year disease-free and overall survival.[78] However, even in patients with a pathologic CR, the clinical TNM at presentation provides valuable prognostic information. In a group of 226 patients treated at the MD Anderson Cancer Center and having a pathologic CR to neoadjuvant therapy, statistically significant differences in the 10-year metastases-free survival were noted on the basis of stage at presentation.[83] Similar findings were noted for locoregional recurrence (LRR), with patients with clinical Stage I or II disease and a pathologic CR to neoadjuvant therapy having a 0% 10-year incidence of LRR without radiation therapy compared with 33% for those with clinical Stage III disease and a pathologic CR treated without radiotherapy.[10] The relative importance of pretreatment stage, posttreatment stage, and degree of response in predicting survival remains to be defined, and therefore the Task Force does not recommend inclusion of pretreatment TNM data in calculating a posttreatment stage ("yp"), unless the patient was M1 prior to initiation of therapy. In this case, her M status is considered M1 regardless of response to therapy. However, the Task Force does recommend inclusion of response in the data routinely collected in patients receiving neoadjuvant therapy and the definition of the method of determining pretreatment nodal status will allow these relationships to be more carefully assessed.

## REFERENCES

1. AJCC. AJCC Cancer Staging Atlas. New York: Springer; 2006.
2. Harris L, Fritsche H, Mennel R, et al. American Society of Clinical Oncology 2007 update of recommendations for the use of tumor markers in breast cancer. J Clin Oncol. 2007;25:5287–312.
3. Carlson RW, Allred DC, Anderson BO, et al. Breast cancer. J Natl Compr Canc Netw. 2009;7:122–92.
4. Van't Veer LJ, Paik S, Hayes DF. Gene expression profiling of breast cancer: a new tumor marker. J Clin Oncol. 2005;23:1631–5.
5. Buyse M, Loi S, van't Veer L, et al. Validation and clinical utility of a 70-gene prognostic signature for women with node-negative breast cancer. J Natl Cancer Inst. 2006;98:1183–92.
6. van de Vijver MJ, He YD, van't Veer LJ, et al. A gene-expression signature as a predictor of survival in breast cancer. N Engl J Med. 2002;347:1999–2009.
7. Wang Y, Klijn JG, Zhang Y, et al. Gene-expression profiles to predict distant metastasis of lymph-node-negative primary breast cancer. Lancet. 2005;365:671–9.
8. Paik S, Shak S, Tang G, et al. A multigene assay to predict recurrence of tamoxifen-treated, node-negative breast cancer. N Engl J Med. 2004;351: 2817–26.
9. Dowsett M, Cuzick J, Wale C, et al. Risk of distant recurence using Oncotype DX in postmenopausal primary breast cancer patients treated with anastrozole or tamoxifen: a TransATAC study. Proceedings of the San Antonio Breast Cancer Symposium, 2008.
10. Paik S, Tang G, Shak S, et al. Gene expression and benefit of chemotherapy in women with node-negative, estrogen receptor-positive breast cancer. J Clin Oncol. 2006;24:3726–34.
11. Albain K, Barlow W, Shak S, et al. Prognostic and predictive value of the 21-gene recurrence score assay in postmenopausal, node-positive, ER-poisitive breast cancer (S8814, INT0100). Breast Cancer Res Treat. 2007;106 (suppl 1):late breaking abstract, no. 10.
12. NCCN. NCCN Clinical practice guidelines in oncology. In: Winn R, editor. Jenkintown, PA: National Comprehensive Cancer Network; 2008.
13. Goldhirsch A, Wood WC, Gelber RD, et al. Progress and promise: highlights of the international expert consensus on the primary therapy of early breast cancer 2007. Ann Oncol. 2007;18:1133–44.
14. Anderson BO, Yip CH, Smith RA, Shyyan R, Sener SF, Eniu A, et al. Guideline implementation for breast healthcare in low-income and middle-income

countries : overview of the Breast Health Global Initiative Global Summit 2007. Cancer. 2008;113(8 Suppl):2221–43.

15. Schwartz GF, Hortobagyi GN. Proceedings of the consensus conference on neoadjuvant chemotherapy in carcinoma of the breast, April 26–28, 2003, Philadelphia, Pennsylvania. Cancer. 2004;100:2512–32.

16. Tavassoli FA. Ductal carcinoma in situ: introduction of the concept of ductal intraepithelial neoplasia. Mod Pathol. 1998;11:140–54.

17. Tavassoli FA. Breast pathology: rationale for adopting the ductal intraepithelial neoplasia (DIN) classification. Nat Clin Pract Oncol. 2005;2:116–7.

18. Bratthauer GL, Tavassoli FA. Lobular intraepithelial neoplasia: previously unexplored aspects assessed in 775 cases and their clinical implications. Virchows Arch. 2002;440:134–8.

19. Lester SC, Bose S, Chen YY, et al. Protocol for the examination of specimens from patients with ductal carcinoma in situ of the breast. Arch Pathol Lab Med. 2009;133:15–25.

20. Chen CY, Sun LM, Anderson BO. Paget disease of the breast: changing patterns of incidence, clinical presentation, and treatment in the U.S. Cancer. 2006;107:1448–58.

21. Walshe JM, Swain SM. Clinical aspects of inflammatory breast cancer. Breast Dis. 2005–2006;22:35–44.

22. Network NCC. NCCN Practice Guidelines in Oncology. Fort Washington, PA: NCCN; 2008.

23. Singletary SE, Allred C, Ashley P, et al. Revision of the American Joint Committee on Cancer staging system for breast cancer. J Clin Oncol. 2002;20: 3628–36.

24. Simon R, Altman DG. Statistical aspects of prognostic factor studies in oncology. Br J Cancer. 1994;69:979–85.

25. Hayes DF, Bast RC, Desch CE, et al. Tumor marker utility grading system: a framework to evaluate clinical utility of tumor markers. J Natl Cancer Inst. 1996;88:1456–66.

26. Ransohoff DF. Rules of evidence for cancer molecular-marker discovery and validation. Nat Rev Cancer. 2004;4:309–14.

27. Sauerbrei W. Prognostic factors. Confusion caused by bad quality design, analysis and reporting of many studies. Adv Otorhinolaryngol. 2005;62:184–200.

28. Altman DG, Riley RD. Primer: an evidence-based approach to prognostic markers. Nat Clin Pract Oncol. 2005;2:466–72.

29. McShane LM, Altman DG, Sauerbrei W, et al. Reporting recommendations for tumor marker prognostic studies (REMARK). J Natl Cancer Inst. 2005;97:1180–4.

30. Henry NL, Hayes DF. Uses and abuses of tumor markers in the diagnosis, monitoring, and treatment of primary and metastatic breast cancer. Oncologist. 2006;11:541–52.

31. Colozza M, Azambuja E, Cardoso F, et al. Proliferative markers as prognostic and predictive tools in early breast cancer: where are we now? Ann Oncol. 2005;16:1723–39.

32. Sotiriou C, Neo SY, McShane LM, et al. Breast cancer classification and prognosis based on gene expression profiles from a population-based study. Proc Natl Acad Sci USA. 2003;100:10393–8.

33. Sotiriou C, Wirapati P, Loi S, et al. Gene expression profiling in breast cancer: understanding the molecular basis of histologic grade to improve prognosis. J Natl Cancer Inst. 2006;98:262–72.

34. Guth U, Jane Huang D, Holzgreve W, et al. T4 breast cancer under closer inspection: a case for revision of the TNM classification. Breast. 2007;16: 625–36.

**32**

35. Guth U, Singer G, Schotzau A, et al. Scope and significance of non-uniform classification practices in breast cancer with non-inflammatory skin involvement: a clinicopathologic study and an international survey. Ann Oncol. 2005;16:1618–23.

36. Guth U, Wight E, Schotzau A, et al. A new approach in breast cancer with non-inflammatory skin involvement. Acta Oncol. 2006;45:576–83.

37. Jain S, Rezo A, Shadbolt B, et al. Synchronous multiple ipsilateral breast cancers: implications for patient management. Pathology. 2009;41:57–67.

38. Huvos AG, Hutter RV, Berg JW. Significance of axillary macrometastases and micrometastases in mammary cancer. Ann Surg. 1971;173:44–6.

39. Fisher ER, Palekar A, Rockette H, et al. Pathologic findings from the National Surgical Adjuvant Breast Project (Protocol No. 4). V. Significance of axillary nodal micro- and macrometastases. Cancer. 1978;42:2032–8.

40. Nasser IA, Lee AK, Bosari S, et al. Occult axillary lymph node metastases in "node-negative" breast carcinoma. Hum Pathol. 1993;24:950–7.

41. Viale G, Dell'Orto P, Biasi MO, et al. Comparative evaluation of an extensive histopathologic examination and a real-time reverse-transcription-polymerase chain reaction assay for mammaglobin and cytokeratin 19 on axillary sentinel lymph nodes of breast carcinoma patients. Ann Surg. 2008;247:136–42.

42. Weaver DL. Pathological evaluation of sentinel lymph nodes in breast cancer: a practical academic perspective from America. Histopathology. 2005;46:702–6.

43. Weaver DL. Assessing the significance of occult micrometastases in axillary lymph nodes from breast cancer patients. Breast J. 2006;12:291–3.

44. Weaver DL, Krag DN, Manna EA, et al. Detection of occult sentinel lymph node micrometastases by immunohistochemistry in breast cancer. An NSABP protocol B-32 quality assurance study. Cancer. 2006;107:661–7.

45. Hermanek P, Sobin LH, Wittekind C. How to improve the present TNM staging system. Cancer. 1999;86:2189–91.

46. Turner RR, Weaver DL, Cserni G, et al. Nodal stage classification for breast carcinoma: improving interobserver reproducibility through standardized histologic criteria and image-based training. J Clin Oncol. 2008;26:258–63.

47. Chen SL, Hoehne FM, Giuliano AE. The prognostic significance of micrometastases in breast cancer: a SEER population-based analysis. Ann Surg Oncol. 2007;14:3378–84.

48. Min CJ, Tafra L, Verbanac KM. Identification of superior markers for polymerase chain reaction detection of breast cancer metastases in sentinel lymph nodes. Cancer Res. 1998;58(20):4581–4.

49. Blumencranz P, Whitworth PW, Deck K, et al. Scientific impact recognition award. Sentinel node staging for breast cancer: intraoperative molecular pathology overcomes conventional histologic sampling errors. Am J Surg. 2007;194:426–32.

50. Braun S, Vogl FD, Naume B, et al. A pooled analysis of bone marrow micrometastasis in breast cancer. N Engl J Med. 2005;353:793–802.

51. Hayes DF, Smerage J. Is there a role for circulating tumor cells in the management of breast cancer? Clin Cancer Res. 2008;14:3646–50.

52. Rack K, Schindlbeck C, Hofmann S, et al. Circulating tumor cells (CTCs) in peripheral blood of primary breast cancer patients. Proc Am Soc Clin Oncol. 2007;25S:abs 10595.

53. Nakagawa T, Martinez SR, Goto Y, et al. Detection of circulating tumor cells in early-stage breast cancer metastasis to axillary lymph nodes. Clin Cancer Res. 2007;13:4105–10.

54. Iakovlev VV, Goswami RS, Vecchiarelli J, et al. Quantitative detection of circulating epithelial cells by Q-RT-PCR. Breast Cancer Res Treat. 2008;107:145–54.

55. Apostolaki S, Perraki M, Pallis A, et al. Circulating HER2 mRNA-positive cells in the peripheral blood of patients with stage I and II breast cancer after the administration of adjuvant chemotherapy: evaluation of their clinical relevance. Ann Oncol. 2007;18:851–8.

56. Ntoulia M, Stathopoulou A, Ignatiadis M, et al. Detection of Mamma-globin A-mRNA-positive circulating tumor cells in peripheral blood of patients with operable breast cancer with nested RT-PCR. Clin Biochem. 2006;39:879–87.

57. Ignatiadis M, Kallergi G, Ntoulia M, et al. Prognostic value of the molecular detection of circulating tumor cells using a multimarker reverse transcription-PCR assay for cytokeratin 19, mammaglobin A, and HER2 in early breast cancer. Clin Cancer Res. 2008;14:2593–600.

58. Ignatiadis M, Georgoulias V, Mavroudis D. Circulating tumor cells in breast cancer. Curr Opin Obstet Gynecol. 2008;20:55–60.

59. Kallergi G, Mavroudis D, Georgoulias V, et al. Phosphorylation of FAK, PI-3K, and impaired actin organization in CK-positive micrometastatic breast cancer cells. Mol Med. 2007;13:79–88.

60. Ignatiadis M, Xenidis N, Perraki M, et al. Different prognostic value of cytokeratin-19 mRNA positive circulating tumor cells according to estrogen receptor and HER2 status in early-stage breast cancer. J Clin Oncol. 2007;25:5194–202.

61. Cristofanilli M, Budd GT, Ellis MJ, et al. Circulating tumor cells, disease progression, and survival in metastatic breast cancer. N Engl J Med. 2004;351:781–91.

62. Kahn HJ, Presta A, Yang LY, et al. Enumeration of circulating tumor cells in the blood of breast cancer patients after filtration enrichment: correlation with disease stage. Breast Cancer Res Treat. 2004;86:237–47.

63. Schwarzenbach H, Muller V, Stahmann N, et al. Detection and characterization of circulating microsatellite-DNA in blood of patients with breast cancer. Ann N Y Acad Sci. 2004;1022:25–32.

64. Cristofanilli M, Hayes DF, Budd GT, et al. Circulating tumor cells: a novel prognostic factor for newly diagnosed metastatic breast cancer. J Clin Oncol. 2005;23:1420–30.

65. Budd GT, Cristofanilli M, Ellis MJ, et al. Circulating tumor cells versus imaging–predicting overall survival in metastatic breast cancer. Clin Cancer Res. 2006;12:6403–9.

66. Hayes DF, Cristofanilli M, Budd GT, et al. Circulating tumor cells at each follow-up time point during therapy of metastatic breast cancer patients predict progression-free and overall survival. Clin Cancer Res. 2006;12:4218–24.

67. Alix-Panabieres C, Muller V, Pantel K. Current status in human breast cancer micrometastasis. Curr Opin Oncol. 2007;19:558–63.

68. Gralow JR, Zujewski JA, Winer E. Preoperative therapy in invasive breast cancer: reviewing the state of the science and exploring new research directions. J Clin Oncol. 2008;26:696–7.

69. Feldman LD, Hortobagyi GN, Buzdar AU, et al. Pathological assessment of response to induction chemotherapy in breast cancer. Cancer Res. 1986;46:2578–81.

70. Fisher B, Bryant J, Wolmark N, et al. Effect of preoperative chemotherapy on the outcome of women with operable breast cancer. J Clin Oncol. 1998;16:2672–85.

71. Kaufmann M, Hortobagyi GN, Goldhirsch A, et al. Recommendations from an international expert panel on the use of neoadjuvant (primary) systemic treatment of operable breast cancer: an update. J Clin Oncol. 2006;24:1940–9.

72. Mazouni C, Peintinger F, Wan-Kau S, et al. Residual ductal carcinoma in situ in patients with complete eradication of invasive breast cancer after neoadjuvant chemotherapy does not adversely affect patient outcome. J Clin Oncol. 2007;25:2650–5.

73. Jones RL, Lakhani SR, Ring AE, et al. Pathological complete response and residual DCIS following neoadjuvant chemotherapy for breast carcinoma. Br J Cancer. 2006;94:358–62.

74. Fisher ER, Wang J, Bryant J, et al. Pathobiology of preoperative chemotherapy: findings from the National Surgical Adjuvant Breast and Bowel (NSABP) protocol B-18. Cancer. 2002;95:681–95.

75. Chevillard S, Vielh P, Pouillart P. Tumor response of breast cancer patients treated by neaoadjuvant chemotherapy may be predicted by measuring the early level of MDR1 gene expression. Proc Am Soc Clin Oncol. 1993;12:59.

76. Ogston KN, Miller ID, Payne S, et al. A new histological grading system to assess response of breast cancers to primary chemotherapy: prognostic significance and survival. Breast. 2003;12:320–7.

77. Symmans WF, Peintinger F, Hatzis C, et al. Measurement of residual breast cancer burden to predict survival after neoadjuvant chemotherapy. J Clin Oncol. 2007;25:4414–22.

78. Carey LA, Metzger R, Dees EC, et al. American Joint Committee on cancer tumor-node-metastasis stage after neoadjuvant chemotherapy and breast cancer outcome. J Natl Cancer Inst. 2005;97:1137–42.

79. Wolff AC, Berry D, Carey LA, et al. Research issues affecting preoperative systemic therapy for operable breast cancer. J Clin Oncol. 2008;26:806–13.

80. Eiermann W, Paepke S, Appfelstaedt J, et al. Preoperative treatment of postmenopausal breast cancer patients with letrozole: a randomized double-blind multicenter study. Ann Oncol. 2001;12:1527–32.

81. Buzdar AU, Valero V, Ibrahim NK, et al. Neoadjuvant therapy with paclitaxel followed by 5-fluorouracil, epirubicin, and cyclophosphamide chemotherapy and concurrent trastuzumab in human epidermal growth factor receptor 2-positive operable breast cancer: an update of the initial randomized study population and data of additional patients treated with the same regimen. Clin Cancer Res. 2007;13:228–33.

82. Berg WA, Gutierrez L, NessAiver MS, et al. Diagnostic accuracy of mammography, clinical examination, US, and MR imaging in preoperative assessment of breast cancer. Radiology. 2004;233:830–49.

83. Gonzalez-Angulo AM, McGuire SE, Buchholz TA, et al. Factors predictive of distant metastases in patients with breast cancer who have a pathologic complete response after neoadjuvant chemotherapy. J Clin Oncol. 2005;23:7098–104.

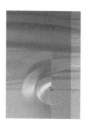

# PART VIII
# Gynecologic Sites

Cervix uteri, corpus uteri, ovary, vagina, vulva, fallopian tube, and gestational trophoblastic tumors are the sites included in this section. Cervix uteri and corpus uteri were among the first sites to be classified by the TNM system. The League of Nations stages for carcinoma of the cervix were first introduced more than 70 years ago, and since 1937 the Fédération Internationale de Gynécologie et d'Obstétrique (FIGO) has continued to modify these staging systems and collect outcomes data from throughout the world. The TNM categories have therefore been defined to correspond to the FIGO stages. Some amendments have been made in collaboration with FIGO, and the classifications now published have the approval of FIGO, the American Joint Committee on Cancer (AJCC), and all other national TNM committees of the International Union Against Cancer (UICC).

# Vulva

*(Mucosal malignant melanoma is not included)*

## *At-A-Glance*

| SUMMARY OF CHANGES |
|---|
| • The definition of TNM and the Stage Grouping for this chapter have changed from the Sixth Edition and reflect new staging adopted by the International Federation of Gynecology and Obstetrics (FIGO) (2008) |

| ANATOMIC STAGE/PROGNOSTIC GROUPS | | | |
|---|---|---|---|
| Stage 0* | Tis | N0 | M0 |
| Stage I | T1 | N0 | M0 |
| Stage IA | T1a | N0 | M0 |
| Stage IB | T1b | N0 | M0 |
| Stage II | T2 | N0 | M0 |
| Stage IIIA | T1, T2 | N1a, N1b | M0 |
| Stage IIIB | T1, T2 | N2a, N2b | M0 |
| Stage IIIC | T1, T2 | N2c | M0 |
| Stage IVA | T1, T2 | N3 | M0 |
| | T3 | Any N | M0 |
| Stage IVB | Any T | Any N | M1 |

*Note: FIGO no longer includes Stage 0 (Tis).

**ICD-O-3 TOPOGRAPHY CODES**

| | |
|---|---|
| C51.0 | Labium majus |
| C51.1 | Labium minus |
| C51.2 | Clitoris |
| C51.8 | Overlapping lesion of vulva |
| C51.9 | Vulva, NOS |

**ICD-O-3 HISTOLOGY CODE RANGES**

8000–8246, 8248–8276, 8940–8950, 8980–8981

## ANATOMY

**Primary Site.** The vulva is the anatomic area immediately external to the vagina. It includes the labia and the perineum. The tumor may extend to involve the vagina, urethra, or anus. It may be fixed to the pubic bone. Changes to the staging classification reflect a belief that tumor size independent of other factors (spread to adjacent structures, nodal metastases) is less important in predicting survival.

**Regional Lymph Nodes.** The femoral and inguinal nodes are the sites of regional spread. For pN, histologic examination of regional lymphadenectomy specimens will ordinarily include six or more lymph nodes. For TNM staging, cases with fewer than six resected nodes should be classified using the TNM pathologic classification according to the status of those nodes (e.g., pN0; pN1) as per the general rules of TNM. The number of resected and positive nodes should be recorded (note that FIGO classifies cases with less than six nodes resected as pNX). The concept of sentinel lymph node mapping where only one or two key nodes are removed is currently being investigated. In most cases, a surgical assessment of regional lymph nodes (inguinal-femoral lymphadenectomy) is performed. Rarely, assessment of lymph nodes will be made by radiologic guided fine-needle aspiration or use of imaging techniques [computerized tomography (CT), magnetic resonance imaging (MRI), or positron emission tomography (PET)]. The current revisions to staging adopted reflect a recognition that the number and size of lymph node metastases more accurately reflect prognosis.

**Metastatic Sites.**  The metastatic sites include any site beyond the area of the regional lymph nodes. Tumor involvement of pelvic lymph nodes, including internal iliac, external iliac, and common iliac lymph nodes, is considered distant metastasis.

## RULES FOR CLASSIFICATION

**Clinical Staging.**  Cases should be classified as carcinoma of the vulva when the primary site of the growth is in the vulva. Tumors present on the vulva as secondary growths from either a genital or an extragenital site should be excluded. This classification does not apply to mucosal malignant melanoma. There should be histologic confirmation of the tumor.

**Pathologic Staging.**  FIGO uses surgical/pathologic staging for vulvar cancer. Stage should be assigned at the time of definitive surgical treatment or prior to radiation or chemotherapy if either of these is the initial mode of therapy. The stage cannot be changed on the basis of disease progression or recurrence or on the basis of response to initial radiation or chemo-therapy that precedes primary tumor resection.

## PROGNOSTIC FEATURES

Vulvar cancer is a surgically staged malignancy. Surgical-pathologic staging provides specific information about primary tumor size and lymph node status, which are the most important prognostic factors in vulvar cancer. Other commonly evaluated items, such as histologic type, differentiation, DNA ploidy, and S-phase fraction analysis, as well as age, are not uniformly identified as important prognostic factors in vulvar cancer.

## DEFINITIONS OF TNM

The definitions of the T categories correspond to the stages accepted by the Fédération Internationale de Gynécologie et d'Obstétrique (FIGO). Both systems are included for comparison.

### Primary Tumor (T)

| TNM Categories | FIGO Stages | |
|---|---|---|
| TX | | Primary tumor cannot be assessed |
| T0 | | No evidence of primary tumor |
| Tis* | | Carcinoma in situ (preinvasive carcinoma) |
| T1a | IA | Lesions 2 cm or less in size, confined to the vulva or perineum and with stromal invasion 1.0 mm or less** |
| T1b | IB | Lesions more than 2 cm in size *or* any size with stromal invasion more than 1.0 mm, confined to the vulva or perineum |
| T2*** | II | Tumor of any size with extension to adjacent perineal structures (lower/distal 1/3 urethra, lower/distal 1/3 vagina, anal involvement) |
| T3**** | IVA | Tumor of any size with extension to any of the following: upper/proximal 2/3 of urethra, upper/proximal 2/3 vagina, bladder mucosa, rectal mucosa, or fixed to pelvic bone |

*Note: FIGO no longer includes Stage 0 (Tis).

**Note: The depth of invasion is defined as the measurement of the tumor from the epithelial–stromal junction of the adjacent most superficial dermal papilla to the deepest point of invasion.

***FIGO uses the classification T2/T3. This is defined as T2 in TNM.

**** FIGO uses the classification T4. This is defined as T3 in TNM.

### Regional Lymph Nodes (N)

| TNM Categories | FIGO Stages | |
|---|---|---|
| NX | | Regional lymph nodes cannot be assessed |
| N0 | | No regional lymph node metastasis |
| N1 | | One or two regional lymph nodes with the following features |
| N1a | IIIA | One lymph node metastasis each 5 mm or less |
| N1b | IIIA | One lymph node metastasis 5 mm or greater |
| N2 | IIIB | Regional lymph node metastasis with the following features |
| N2a | IIIB | Three or more lymph node metastases each less than 5 mm |
| N2b | IIIB | Two or more lymph node metastases 5 mm or greater |
| N2c | IIIC | Lymph node metastasis with extracapsular spread |
| N3 | IVA | Fixed or ulcerated regional lymph node metastasis |

An effort should be made to describe the site and laterality of lymph node metastases.

| Distant Metastasis (M) | | |
|---|---|---|
| TNM Categories | FIGO Stages | |
| M0 | | No distant metastasis |
| M1 | IVB | Distant metastasis (including pelvic lymph node metastasis) |

## ANATOMIC STAGE/PROGNOSTIC GROUPS

| Stage 0* | Tis | N0 | M0 |
|---|---|---|---|
| Stage I | T1 | N0 | M0 |
| Stage IA | T1a | N0 | M0 |
| Stage IB | T1b | N0 | M0 |
| Stage II | T2 | N0 | M0 |
| Stage IIIA | T1, T2 | N1a, N1b | M0 |
| Stage IIIB | T1, T2 | N2a, N2b | M0 |
| Stage IIIC | T1, T2 | N2c | M0 |
| Stage IVA | T1, T2 | N3 | M0 |
| | T3 | Any N | M0 |
| Stage IVB | Any T | Any N | M1 |

*Note: FIGO no longer includes Stage 0 (Tis).

## PROGNOSTIC FACTORS (SITE-SPECIFIC FACTORS)
## (Recommended for Collection)

| Required for staging | None |
|---|---|
| Clinically significant | FIGO Stage |
| | Pelvic nodal status and method of assessment |
| | Femoral-inguinal nodal status and method of assessment |

## HISTOLOGIC GRADE (G)

Grade is reported in registry systems by the grade value. A two-grade, three-grade, or four-grade system may be used. If a grading system is not specified, generally the following system is used:

GX    Grade cannot be assessed
G1    Well differentiated
G2    Moderately differentiated
G3    Poorly differentiated
G4    Undifferentiated

## HISTOPATHOLOGIC TYPE

Squamous cell carcinoma is the most frequent form of cancer of the vulva. This staging classification does not apply to malignant melanoma.

The common histopathologic types are as follows:

Squamous cell carcinoma
Verrucous carcinoma
Paget's disease of vulva
Adenocarcinoma, NOS
Basal cell carcinoma, NOS
Bartholin's gland carcinoma

The presence or absence of lymphovascular space invasion should be noted in the pathology report.

## BIBLIOGRAPHY

Beller U, Sideri M, Maisonneuve P, et al. Carcinoma of the vulva. FIGO annual report. J Epidemiol Biostat. 2001;6:153–74.

Chan JK, Sugiyama V, Pham H, Gu M, et al. Margin distance and other clinico-pathologic prognostic factors in vulvar carcinoma: a multivariate analysis. Gynecol Oncol. 2007;104:636–41.

Grendys EC Jr, Fiorica JV. Innovations in the management of vulvar carcinoma. Curr Opin Obstet Gynecol. 2000;12:15–20.

Homesley HD, Bundy BN, Sedlis A, Yordan E, Berek JS, Jahshan A, Mortel R. Assessment of current International Federation of Gynecology and Obstetrics staging of vulvar carcinoma relative to prognostic factors for survival (a Gynecologic Oncology Group study). Am J Obstet Gynecol. 1991;164:997–1004.

Magrina JF, Gonzalez-Bosquet J, Weaver AL, et al. Squamous cell carcinoma of the vulva stage IA: long-term results. Gynecol Oncol. 2000;76:24–7.

Moore DH, Thomas GM, Montana GS, et al. Preoperative chemoradiation for advanced vulvar cancer: a phase II study of the Gynecologic Oncology Group. Int J Radiat Oncol Biol Phys. 1998;42:79–85.

Nash JD, Curry S. Vulvar cancer. Surg Oncol Clin North Am. 1998;7:335–46.

Origoni M, Sideri M, Garsia S, Carinelli SG, Ferrari AG. Prognostic value of pathological patterns of lymph node positivity in squamous cell carcinoma of the vulva Stage III and IVA FIGO. Gynecol Oncol. 1992;45:313–6.

Paladini D, Cross P, Lopes A, Monaghan JM. Prognostic significance of lymph node variables in squamous cell carcinoma of the vulva. Cancer. 1994;74:2491–6.

van der Velden J, van Lindert AC, Lammes FB, ten Kate FJ, Sie-Go DM, Oosting H, Heintz AP. Extracapsular growth of lymph node metastases in squamous cell carcinoma of the vulva. The impact on recurrence and survival. Cancer. 1995;75:2885–90.

**33**

## At-A-Glance

### SUMMARY OF CHANGES

- The definition of TNM and the Stage Grouping for this chapter have not changed from the Sixth Edition

### ANATOMIC STAGE/PROGNOSTIC GROUPS

| Stage 0* | Tis | N0 | M0 |
|---|---|---|---|
| Stage I | T1 | N0 | M0 |
| Stage II | T2 | N0 | M0 |
| Stage III | T1–T3 | N1 | M0 |
| | T3 | N0 | M0 |
| Stage IVA | T4 | Any N | M0 |
| Stage IVB | Any T | Any N | M1 |

*Note: FIGO no longer includes Stage 0 (Tis).

ICD-O-3
TOPOGRAPHY
CODES
C52.9    Vagina, NOS

ICD-O-3 HISTOLOGY
CODE RANGES
8000–8576, 8800–8801,
8940–8950, 8980–8981

## ANATOMY

**Primary Site.** The vagina extends from the vulva upward to the uterine cervix. It is lined by squamous epithelium with only rare glandular structures. The vagina is drained by lymphatics toward the pelvic nodes in its upper two-thirds and toward the inguinal nodes in its lower third.

**Regional Lymph Nodes.** The upper two-thirds of the vagina is drained by lymphatics to the pelvic nodes, including the following:

Obturator
Internal iliac (hypogastric)
External iliac
Pelvic, NOS

The lower third of the vagina is drained to the groin nodes, including the following:

Inguinal
Femoral

**Metastatic Sites.** The most common sites of distant spread include the aortic lymph nodes, lungs, and skeleton.

## RULES FOR CLASSIFICATION

There should be histologic verification of the disease. The classification applies to primary carcinoma only. Cases should be classified as carcinoma of the vagina when the primary site of the growth is in the vagina. Tumors present in the vagina as secondary growths from either genital or extragenital sites should not be included. A growth that involves the cervix, including the external os, should always be assigned to carcinoma of the cervix. A growth limited to the urethra should be classified as carcinoma of the urethra. Tumor involving the vulva and extending to the vagina should be classified as carcinoma of the vulva.

**Clinical Staging.** FIGO uses clinical staging for cancer of the vagina. All data available prior to first definitive treatment should be used. The results of biopsy or fine-needle aspiration of inguinal/femoral or other nodes may be included in the clinical staging. The rules of staging are similar to those for carcinoma of the cervix.

**Pathologic Staging.** In addition to data used for clinical staging, information available from examination of the resected specimen, including pelvic and retroperitoneal lymph nodes, is to be used. The pT, pN, and pM categories correspond to the T, N, and M categories.

## PROGNOSTIC FEATURES

The most significant prognostic factor is anatomic staging, which reflects the extent of invasion into the surrounding tissue or of metastatic spread.

## DEFINITIONS OF TNM

The definitions of the T categories correspond to the stages accepted by the Fédération Internationale de Gynécologie et d'Obstétrique (FIGO). Both systems are included for comparison.

| *Primary Tumor (T)* | | |
|---|---|---|
| TNM Categories | FIGO Stages | |
| TX | | Primary tumor cannot be assessed |
| T0 | | No evidence of primary tumor |
| Tis* | | Carcinoma in situ (preinvasive carcinoma) |
| T1 | I | Tumor confined to vagina |
| T2 | II | Tumor invades paravaginal tissues but not to pelvic wall |
| T3 | III | Tumor extends to pelvic wall** |
| T4 | IVA | Tumor invades mucosa of the bladder or rectum and/or extends beyond the true pelvis (bullous edema is not sufficient evidence to classify a tumor as T4) |

*Note: FIGO no longer includes Stage 0 (Tis).

**Note: Pelvic wall is defined as muscle, fascia, neurovascular structures, or skeletal portions of the bony pelvis. On rectal examination, there is no cancer-free space between the tumor and pelvic walls.

### Regional Lymph Nodes (N)

| TNM Categories | FIGO Stages | |
|---|---|---|
| NX | | Regional lymph nodes cannot be assessed |
| N0 | | No regional lymph node metastasis |
| N1 | III | Pelvic or inguinal lymph node metastasis |

### Distant Metastasis (M)

| TNM Categories | FIGO Stages | |
|---|---|---|
| M0 | | No distant metastasis |
| M1 | IVB | Distant metastasis |

### ANATOMIC STAGE/PROGNOSTIC GROUPS

| Stage 0* | Ti | N0 | M0 |
|---|---|---|---|
| Stage I | T1 | N0 | M0 |
| Stage II | T2 | N0 | M0 |
| Stage III | T1–T3 | N1 | M0 |
| | T3 | N0 | M0 |
| Stage IVA | T4 | Any N | M0 |
| Stage IVB | Any T | Any N | M1 |

*Note: FIGO no longer includes Stage 0 (Tis).

## PROGNOSTIC FACTORS (SITE-SPECIFIC FACTORS)
### (Recommended for Collection)

| | |
|---|---|
| Required for staging | None |
| Clinically significant | FIGO Stage |
| | Pelvic nodal status and method of assessment |
| | Para-aortic nodal status and method of assessment |
| | Distant (mediastinal, scalene) nodal status and method of assessment |

## HISTOLOGIC GRADE (G)

Grade is reported in registry systems by the grade value. A two-grade, three-grade, or four-grade system may be used. If a grading system is not specified, generally the following system is used:

| GX | Grade cannot be assessed |
|---|---|
| G1 | Well differentiated |
| G2 | Moderately differentiated |
| G3 | Poorly differentiated |
| G4 | Undifferentiated |

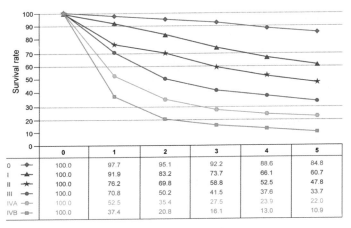

| | | 0 | 1 | 2 | 3 | 4 | 5 |
|---|---|---|---|---|---|---|---|
| 0 | ◆ | 100.0 | 97.7 | 95.1 | 92.2 | 88.6 | 84.8 |
| I | ▲ | 100.0 | 91.9 | 83.2 | 73.7 | 66.1 | 60.7 |
| II | ★ | 100.0 | 76.2 | 69.8 | 58.8 | 52.5 | 47.8 |
| III | ● | 100.0 | 70.8 | 50.2 | 41.5 | 37.6 | 33.7 |
| IVA | ● | 100.0 | 52.5 | 35.4 | 27.5 | 23.9 | 22.0 |
| IVB | ■ | 100.0 | 37.4 | 20.8 | 16.1 | 13.0 | 10.9 |

Years from diagnosis

**FIGURE 34.1.** Observed survival rates for 4,114 cases with carcinoma of the vagina. Data from the National Cancer Data Base (Commission on Cancer of the American College of Surgeons and the American Cancer Society) diagnosed in years 1998–2002. Stage 0 includes 1,458 patients; Stage I, 883; Stage II, 901; Stage III, 459; Stage IVA, 203; and Stage IVB, 210.

## HISTOPATHOLOGIC TYPE

Squamous cell carcinoma is the most common type of cancer occurring in the vagina. Approximately 10% of vaginal cancers are adenocarcinoma; melanoma and sarcoma occur rarely.

## OUTCOMES RESULTS

Overall survival data from large series are not available because of the rarity of this malignancy. However, FIGO 5-year survival data by clinical stage in patients managed with a variety of modalities are shown in Figure 34.1.

## BIBLIOGRAPHY

Beller U, Sideri M, Maisonneuve P, et al. Carcinoma of the vagina. FIGO annual report. J Epidemiol Biostat. 2001;6:141–52.

Foroudi F, Bull CA, Gebski V. Primary invasive cancer of the vagina: outcome and complications of therapy. Australas Radiol. 1999;43:472–5.

Goodman A. Primary vaginal cancer. Surg Oncol Clin North Am. 1998;7:347–61.

Pingley S, Shrivastava SK, Sarin R, et al. Primary carcinoma of the vagina: Tata Memorial Hospital experience. Int J Radiat Oncol Biol Phys. 2000;46:101–8.

Stock RG, Chen AS, Seski J. A 30-year experience in the management of primary carcinoma of the vagina: analysis of prognostic factors and treatment modalities. Gynecol Oncol. 1995;56:45–52.

Sulak P, Barnhill D, Heller P, et al. Nonsquamous cancer of the vagina. Gynecol Oncol. 1988;29:346–53.

# Cervix Uteri

## *At-A-Glance*

---

**SUMMARY OF CHANGES**

• The definition of TNM and the Stage Grouping for this chapter have changed from the Sixth Edition and reflect new staging adopted by the International Federation of Gynecology and Obstetrics (FIGO) (2008)

---

**ANATOMIC STAGE/PROGNOSTIC GROUPS (FIGO 2008)**

| Stage 0* | Tis | N0 | M0 |
|---|---|---|---|
| Stage I | T1 | N0 | M0 |
| Stage IA | T1a | N0 | M0 |
| Stage IA1 | T1a1 | N0 | M0 |
| Stage IA2 | T1a2 | N0 | M0 |
| Stage IB | T1b | N0 | M0 |
| Stage IB1 | T1b1 | N0 | M0 |
| Stage IB2 | T1b2 | N0 | M0 |
| Stage II | T2 | N0 | M0 |
| Stage IIA | T2a | N0 | M0 |
| Stage IIA1 | T2a1 | N0 | M0 |
| Stage IIA2 | T2a2 | N0 | M0 |
| Stage IIB | T2b | N0 | M0 |
| Stage III | T3 | N0 | M0 |
| Stage IIIA | T3a | N0 | M0 |
| Stage IIIB | T3b | Any N | M0 |
| | T1-3 | N1 | M0 |
| Stage IVA | T4 | Any N | M0 |
| Stage IVB | Any T | Any N | M1 |

*Note: FIGO no longer includes Stage 0 (Tis).

ICD-O-3 TOPOGRAPHY CODES

| C53.0 | Endocervix |
|---|---|
| C53.1 | Exocervix |
| C53.8 | Overlapping lesion of cervix uteri |
| C53.9 | Cervix uteri |

ICD-O-3 HISTOLOGY CODE RANGES
8000–8576, 8940–8950, 8980–8981

---

## ANATOMY

**Primary Site.** The cervix is the lower third of the uterus. It is roughly cylindrical in shape and projects into the upper vagina. The endocervical canal is lined by glandular or columnar epithelium. Through the cervix runs the endocervical canal, which is the passageway connecting the vagina with the uterine cavity. The vaginal portion of the cervix, known as the exocervix, is covered by squamous epithelium. The squamocolumnar junction is usually located at the external cervical os, where the endocervical canal begins. Cancer of the cervix may originate from the squamous epithelium of the exocervix or the glandular epithelium of the canal.

**Regional Lymph Nodes.** The cervix is drained by parametrial, cardinal, and uterosacral ligament routes into the following regional lymph nodes:

> Parametrial
> Obturator
> Internal iliac (hypogastric)
> External iliac
> Common iliac
> Sacral
> Presacral

For pN, histologic examination of regional lymphadenectomy specimens will ordinarily include six or more lymph nodes. For TNM staging, cases with fewer than six resected nodes should be classified using the TNM pathologic classification according to the status of those nodes (e.g., pN0; pN1) as per the general rules of TNM. The number of resected and positive nodes should be recorded (note that FIGO classifies cases with less than six nodes resected as pNX).

**Metastatic Sites.** The most common sites of distant spread include the paraaortic and mediastinal nodes, lungs, peritoneal cavity, and skeleton. Mediastinal or supraclavicular node involvement is considered distant metastasis and is coded M1.

## RULES FOR CLASSIFICATION

The classification applies only to carcinoma. There should be histologic confirmation of the disease.

**Clinical Staging.** Because many patients with cervical cancer are treated by radiation and never undergo surgical-pathologic staging, clinical staging of all patients provides uniformity and is therefore preferred. FIGO staging of cervical cancer is clinical.

The clinical stage should be determined prior to the start of definitive therapy. The clinical stage must not be changed because of subsequent findings once treatment has started. When there is doubt about to which stage a particular cancer should be allocated, the lesser stage should be utilized. Careful clinical examination should be performed in all cases, preferably by an experienced examiner and with the patient under anesthesia. A description of the cervical tumor size is important, especially for stage I–II cancers where tumor size has shown prognostic utility. The 2008 FIGO staging classification has adopted T subclassifications based on tumor size ≤4 cm (T2a1) and >4 cm (T2a2) for cervical carcinoma spreading beyond the cervix but not to the pelvic side wall or lower one-third of the vagina (T2 lesions). The following examinations are recommended for staging purposes: palpation, inspection, colposcopy, endocervical curettage, hysteroscopy, cystoscopy, proctoscopy, intravenous urography, and X-ray examination of the lungs and skeleton. Suspected involvement of the bladder mucosa or rectal mucosa must be confirmed by biopsy and histology. Lymph node status may be assessed by surgical means (radiologic guided fine-needle aspiration, laparoscopic or extraperitoneal biopsy, or lymphadenectomy) or by imagining technologies [computerized tomography (CT), magnetic resonance imaging (MRI), positron emission tomography (PET), or lymphangiography]. The results of these additional examinations or procedures may *not* be used to determine clinical staging because these techniques are not universally available. They may, however, be used to develop a treatment plan and may provide prognostic information. When nodal metastases are identified it is important to identify the extent of nodal involvement (pelvic lymph nodes and/or para-aortic lymph nodes) and the methodology by which the diagnosis was established (pathologic or radiologic).

**Pathologic Staging.** In cases treated by surgical procedures, the pathologist's findings in the removed tissues can be the basis for extremely accurate statements on the extent of disease. These findings should not be allowed to change the clinical staging but should be recorded in the manner described for the pathologic staging of disease. The pTNM nomenclature is appropriate for this purpose and corresponds to the T, N, and M categories. Infrequently, hysterectomy is carried out in the presence of unsuspected invasive cervical carcinoma. Such cases cannot be clinically staged or included in therapeutic statistics; they should be reported separately.

## PROGNOSTIC FEATURES

Current data suggest that more than 90% of squamous cervical cancer contains human papilloma virus (HPV) DNA, most frequently types 16 and 18. In addition to extent or stage of disease, prognostic factors include histology and tumor differentiation. Small cell, neuroendocrine, and clear cell lesions have a worse prognosis, as do poorly differentiated cancers. Women with cervical cancer who are infected with human immunodeficiency virus (HIV) are defined as having autoimmune deficiency syndrome (AIDS), and they have a very poor prognosis, often with rapidly progressive cancer.

## DEFINITIONS OF TNM

The definitions of the T categories correspond to the stages accepted by the Fédération Internationale de Gynécologie et d'Obstétrique (FIGO). Both systems are included for comparison.

35

## Primary Tumor (T)

| TNM Categories | FIGO Stages | |
|---|---|---|
| TX | | Primary tumor cannot be assessed |
| T0 | | No evidence of primary tumor |
| Tis* | | Carcinoma in situ (preinvasive carcinoma) |
| T1 | I | Cervical carcinoma confined to uterus (extension to corpus should be disregarded) |
| T1a** | IA | Invasive carcinoma diagnosed only by microscopy. Stromal invasion with a maximum depth of 5.0 mm measured from the base of the epithelium and a horizontal spread of 7.0 mm or less. Vascular space involvement, venous or lymphatic, does not affect classification |
| T1a1 | IA1 | Measured stromal invasion 3.0 mm or less in depth and 7.0 mm or less in horizontal spread |
| T1a2 | IA2 | Measured stromal invasion more than 3.0 mm and not more than 5.0 mm with a horizontal spread 7.0 mm or less |
| T1b | IB | Clinically visible lesion confined to the cervix or microscopic lesion greater than T1a/IA2 |
| T1b1 | IB1 | Clinically visible lesion 4.0 cm or less in greatest dimension |
| T1b2 | IB2 | Clinically visible lesion more than 4.0 cm in greatest dimension |
| T2 | II | Cervical carcinoma invades beyond uterus but not to pelvic wall or to lower third of vagina |
| T2a | IIA | Tumor without parametrial invasion |
| T2a1 | IIA1 | Clinically visible lesion 4.0 cm or less in greatest dimension |
| T2a2 | IIA2 | Clinically visible lesion more than 4.0 cm in greatest dimension |
| T2b | IIB | Tumor with parametrial invasion |
| T3 | III | Tumor extends to pelvic wall and/or involves lower third of vagina, and/or causes hydronephrosis or nonfunctioning kidney |
| T3a | IIIA | Tumor involves lower third of vagina, no extension to pelvic wall |
| T3b | IIIB | Tumor extends to pelvic wall and/or causes hydronephrosis or nonfunctioning kidney |
| T4 | IVA | Tumor invades mucosa of bladder or rectum, and/or extends beyond true pelvis (bullous edema is not sufficient to classify a tumor as T4) |

*Note: FIGO no longer includes Stage 0 (Tis).

**Note: All macroscopically visible lesions – even with superficial invasion – are T1b/IB.

### Regional Lymph Nodes (N)

| TNM Categories | FIGO Stages | |
|---|---|---|
| NX | | Regional lymph nodes cannot be assessed |
| N0 | | No regional lymph node metastasis |
| N1 | IIIB | Regional lymph node metastasis |

### Distant Metastasis (M)

| TNM Categories | FIGO Stages | |
|---|---|---|
| M0 | | No distant metastasis |
| M1 | IVB | Distant metastasis (including peritoneal spread, involvement of supraclavicular, mediastinal, or paraaortic lymph nodes, lung, liver, or bone) |

### ANATOMIC STAGE/PROGNOSTIC GROUPS (FIGO 2008)

| | | | |
|---|---|---|---|
| Stage 0* | Tis | N0 | M0 |
| Stage I | T1 | N0 | M0 |
| Stage IA | T1a | N0 | M0 |
| Stage IA1 | T1a1 | N0 | M0 |
| Stage IA2 | T1a2 | N0 | M0 |
| Stage IB | T1b | N0 | M0 |
| Stage IB1 | T1b1 | N0 | M0 |
| Stage IB2 | T1b2 | N0 | M0 |
| Stage II | T2 | N0 | M0 |
| Stage IIA | T2a | N0 | M0 |
| Stage IIA1 | T2a1 | N0 | M0 |
| Stage IIA2 | T2a2 | N0 | M0 |
| Stage IIB | T2b | N0 | M0 |
| Stage III | T3 | N0 | M0 |
| Stage IIIA | T3a | N0 | M0 |
| Stage IIIB | T3b | Any N | M0 |
| | T1-3 | N1 | M0 |
| Stage IVA | T4 | Any N | M0 |
| Stage IVB | Any T | Any N | M1 |

*Note: FIGO no longer includes Stage 0 (Tis).

35

## PROGNOSTIC FACTORS (SITE-SPECIFIC FACTORS)
### (Recommended for Collection)

Required for staging     None

Clinically significant     FIGO Stage
Pelvic nodal status and method of assessment
Distant (paraaortic) nodal status and method of assessment
Distant (mediastinal, scalene) nodal status and method of assessment

## HISTOLOGIC GRADE (G)

GX     Grade cannot be assessed
G1     Well differentiated
G2     Moderately differentiated
G3     Poorly differentiated
G4     Undifferentiated

## HISTOPATHOLOGIC TYPE

Cases should be classified as carcinoma of the cervix if the primary growth is in the cervix. All carcinomas should be included. Grading is encouraged but is not a basis for modifying the stage groupings. When surgery is the primary treatment, the histologic findings permit the case to have pathologic staging, and the pTNM nomenclature is to be used. The histopathologic types are as follows:

Cervical intraepithelial neoplasia, grade III
Squamous cell carcinoma *in situ*
Squamous cell carcinoma
      Invasive
      Keratinizing
      Nonkeratinizing
      Verrucous
Adenocarcinoma *in situ*
Adenocarcinoma, invasive
Endometrioid adenocarcinoma
Clear cell adenocarcinoma
Adenosquamous carcinoma
Adenoid cystic carcinoma
Adenoid basal cell carcinoma
Small cell carcinoma
Neuroendocrine
Undifferentiated carcinoma

## OUTCOMES RESULTS

The overall survival by stage of more than 15,070 patients treated from 2000 to 2002 is shown in Figure 35.1.

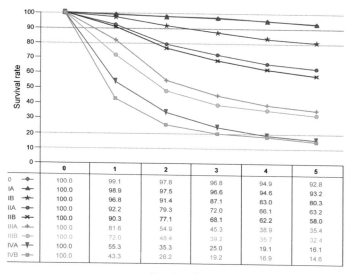

| | | 0 | 1 | 2 | 3 | 4 | 5 |
|---|---|---|---|---|---|---|---|
| 0 | ◆ | 100.0 | 99.1 | 97.8 | 96.8 | 94.9 | 92.8 |
| IA | ▲ | 100.0 | 98.9 | 97.5 | 96.6 | 94.6 | 93.2 |
| IB | ★ | 100.0 | 96.8 | 91.4 | 87.1 | 83.0 | 80.3 |
| IIA | ● | 100.0 | 92.2 | 79.3 | 72.0 | 66.1 | 63.2 |
| IIB | ✕ | 100.0 | 90.3 | 77.1 | 68.1 | 62.2 | 58.0 |
| IIIA | ▲ | 100.0 | 81.6 | 54.9 | 45.3 | 38.9 | 35.4 |
| IIIB | ● | 100.0 | 72.0 | 48.4 | 39.2 | 35.7 | 32.4 |
| IVA | ▼ | 100.0 | 55.3 | 35.3 | 25.0 | 19.1 | 16.1 |
| IVB | ■ | 100.0 | 43.3 | 26.2 | 19.2 | 16.9 | 14.6 |

Years from diagnosis

**FIGURE 35.1.** Observed survival rates for 15,070 cases with carcinoma of the cervix uterus. Data from the National Cancer Data Base (Commission on Cancer of the American College of Surgeons and the American Cancer Society) diagnosed in years 2000–2002. Stage 0 includes 7,119 patients; Stage IA, 1,530; Stage IB, 2,249; Stage IIA, 453; Stage IIB, 1,518; Stage IIIA, 191; Stage IIIB, 1,009; Stage IVA, 213; and Stage IVB, 788.

## BIBLIOGRAPHY

Benedet JL, Odicino F, Maisonneuve P, et al. Carcinoma of the cervix. FIGO annual report. J Epidemiol Biostat. 2001;6:5–44.

Bodurka-Bevers D, Morris M, Eifel PJ, et al. Posttherapy surveillance of women with cervical cancer: an outcomes analysis. Gynecol Oncol. 2000;78:187–93.

Coucke PA, Maingon P, Ciernik IF, et al. A survey on staging and treatment in uterine cervical carcinoma in the Radiotherapy Cooperative Group of the European Organization for Research and Treatment of Cancer. Radiat Oncol. 2000;54:221–8.

FIGO Committee on Gynecologic Cancer. Revised FIGO staging for carcinoma of the vulva, cervix, and endometrium. Int J Gynecol Obstet. 2009;105:105–6.

Koh WJ, Panwala K, Greer B. Adjuvant therapy for high-risk, early stage cervical cancer. Semin Radiat Oncol. 2000;10:51–60.

Perez CA, Grigsby PW, Chao KS, et al. Tumor size, irradiation dose, and long-term outcome of carcinoma of uterine cervix. Int J Radiat Oncol Biol Phys. 1998;41:307–317.

Zaino RJ. Glandular lesions of the uterine cervix. Mod Pathol. 2000;13:261–74.

35

# Corpus Uteri

## *At-A-Glance*

**SUMMARY OF CHANGES**

- The definition of TNM and the Stage Grouping for this chapter have changed from the Sixth Edition and reflect new staging adopted by the International Federation of Gynecology and Obstetrics (FIGO) (2008)

- A separate staging schema adopted by FIGO for uterine sarcoma has been added

**ANATOMIC STAGE/PROGNOSTIC GROUPS**

*Carcinomas\**

| Stage 0** | Tis | N0 | M0 |
|---|---|---|---|
| Stage I | T1 | N0 | M0 |
| Stage IA | T1a | N0 | M0 |
| Stage IB | T1b | N0 | M0 |
| Stage II | T2 | N0 | M0 |
| Stage III | T3 | N0 | M0 |
| Stage IIIA | T3a | N0 | M0 |
| Stage IIIB | T3b | N0 | M0 |
| Stage IIIC1 | T1-T3 | N1 | M0 |
| Stage IIIC2 | T1-T3 | N2 | M0 |
| Stage IVA | T4 | Any N | M0 |
| Stage IVB | Any T | Any N | M1 |

*Carcinosarcomas should be staged as carcinoma.

**Note: FIGO no longer includes Stage 0 (Tis).

*Sarcomas*

| Stage I | T1 | N0 | M0 |
|---|---|---|---|
| Stage IA* | T1a | N0 | M0 |
| Stage IB* | T1b | N0 | M0 |
| Stage IC** | T1c | N0 | M0 |
| Stage II | T2 | N0 | M0 |
| Stage IIIA | T3a | N0 | M0 |
| Stage IIIB | T3b | N0 | M0 |

**ICD-O-3 TOPOGRAPHY CODES**

| C54.0 | Isthmus uteri |
|---|---|
| C54.1 | Endometrium |
| C54.2 | Myometrium |
| C54.3 | Fundus uteri |
| C54.8 | Overlapping lesion of corpus uteri |
| C54.9 | Corpus uteri |
| C55.9 | Uterus, NOS |

**ICD-O-3 HISTOLOGY CODE RANGES**

8000–8576, 8890–8898, 8930–8933, 8940–8950, 8980–8981

36

*Stage IA and IB differ from those applied for leiomyo-sarcoma and endometrial stromal sarcoma

** *Note*: Stage IC does not apply for leiomyosarcoma and endometrial stromal sarcoma.

## INTRODUCTION

The classification for uterine cancers has been subdivided for the seventh edition of TNM in accordance with changes adopted by the International Federation of Gynecology and Obstetrics (FIGO) to have separate systems for endometrial adenocarcinomas and uterine sarcomas. The new schemas for sarcomas are fully described in publications by FIGO.

## ANATOMY

**Primary Site.** The upper two-thirds of the uterus above the level of the internal cervical os is referred to as the uterine corpus. The oviducts (fallopian tubes) and the round ligaments enter the uterus at the upper and outer corners (cornu) of the pear-shaped organ. The portion of the uterus that is above a line connecting the tubo-uterine orifices is referred to as the uterine fundus. The lower third of the uterus is called the cervix and lower uterine segment. Tumor involvement of the cervical stroma is prognostically important and affects staging (T2). The new staging system no longer distinguishes endocervical mucosal/glandular involvement (formerly stage IIA). The location of the tumor must be carefully evaluated and recorded by the pathologist. The depth of tumor invasion into the myometrium is also of prognostic significance and should be included in the pathology report. Involvement of the ovaries by direct extension or metastases, or penetration of tumor to the uterine serosa is important to identify and classify the tumor as T3a.

Malignant cells in peritoneal cytology samples have been documented in approximately 10% of cases of presumed uterine confined endometrial cancer cases. The prognostic importance of positive cytology has been debated. Depth of myometrial invasion, tumor grade, and presence of extrauterine disease are felt to be more prognositically significant, and as such the 2008 FIGO staging system will no longer use peritoneal cytology for the purposes of staging (formerly T3a, FIGO stage IIIA). T3b lesions reflect regional extension of disease and include extension of the tumor through the myometrial wall of the uterus into the parametrium and/or extension/metastatic involvement of the vagina.

**Regional Lymph Nodes.** The regional lymph nodes are paired and each of the paired sites should be examined. The regional nodes are as follows:

Obturator
Internal iliac (hypogastric)
External iliac
Common iliac
Para-aortic
Presacral
Parametrial

For adequate evaluation of the regional lymph nodes, a representative evaluation of bilateral para-aortic and pelvic lymph nodes (including external iliac, internal iliac, and obturator nodes) should be documented in the operative and surgical pathology reports. Parametrial nodes are not commonly detected unless a radical hysterectomy is performed for cases with gross cervical stromal invasion.

For pN, histologic examination of regional lymphadenectomy specimens will ordinarily include six or more lymph nodes. For TNM staging, cases with fewer than six resected nodes should be classified using the TNM pathologic classification according to the status of those nodes (e.g., pN0; pN1) as per the general rules of TNM. The number of resected and positive nodes should be recorded (note that FIGO classifies cases with less than six nodes resected as pNX).

**Metastatic Sites.** The vagina and lung are the common metastatic sites. Intra-abdominal metastases to peritoneal surfaces or the omentum are seen particularly with serous and clear cell tumors.

## RULES FOR CLASSIFICATION

The classification applies only to carcinoma and malignant mixed mesodermal tumors. There should be histologic verification and grading of the tumor.

**Clinical Staging.** If the surgeon feels that systematic regional lymph node sampling imposes an unfavorable risk-to-benefit ratio, clinical assessment of the pertinent node groups (obturator, para-aortic groups, internal iliac, common iliac, and external iliac) should be performed and specifically annotated in the operative report and recorded as cN.

**36**

**Pathologic Staging.** FIGO uses surgical/pathologic staging for corpus uteri cancer. Stage should be assigned at the time of definitive surgical treatment or prior to radiation or chemotherapy if those are the initial modes of therapy. The stage should not be changed on the basis of disease progression or recurrence or on the basis of response to initial radiation or chemotherapy that precedes primary tumor resections. Ideally, the depth of myometrial invasion (in millimeters) should be recorded, along with the thickness of the myometrium at that level (recorded as a percentage of myometrial invasion).

The presence of carcinoma in the regional lymph nodes is a clinically critical prognostic variable. Multiple studies have confirmed the inaccuracy of clinical assessment of regional nodal metastasis in many anatomic sites. For this reason, surgical/pathologic assessment of the regional lymph nodes is strongly advocated for all patients with corpus uteri cancer. This is also the recommendation of FIGO. The therapeutic effect of nodal dissection has not been demonstrated in two randomized controlled clinical trials (ASTEC, CONSORT); however, routine nodal dissection increased the frequency of which patients with node involved disease were identified.

Fractional curettage is not adequate to establish cervical involvement or to distinguish between Stages I and II. That distinction can best be made by histologic verification of clinically suspicious cervical involvement or histopathologic examination of the removed uterus.

The pT, pN, and pM categories correspond to the T, N, and M categories and are used to designate cases where adequate pathologic specimens are available for accurate stage groupings. When there are insufficient surgical-pathologic findings, the clinical cT, cN, cM categories should be used on the basis of clinical evaluation.

## PROGNOSTIC FEATURES

The presence or absence of metastatic disease in the regional lymph nodes is the most important prognostic factor in carcinomas clinically confined to the uterus. The AJCC strongly advocates the use of surgical/pathologic assessment of nodal status whenever possible. Palpation of regional nodes is well recognized to be much less accurate than pathologic evaluation of the nodes.

Historically, the factors of grade of the tumor and depth of myometrial invasion have been recognized as important prognostic factors. In surgically staged patients, using multivariate analysis, these factors are surrogates for the probability of nodal metastasis. Preoperative endometrial biopsy does not accurately correlate with tumor grade and depth of myometrial invasion.

The presence or absence of lymphovascular space involvement of the myometrium is important in most, but not all, series. When present, lymphovascular space involvement increases the probability of metastatic involvement of the regional lymph nodes. The presence or absence of lymphovascular space involvement should be recorded in the pathology report.

The importance of tumor cells in peritoneal "washings" and the presence of metastatic foci in adnexal structures may have an adverse impact on prognosis, but they remain controversial and require further study. The newly adopted staging system (FIGO 2008) no longer utilizes positive cytology to alter stage. When collected, cytology results should be recorded.

Serous papillary and clear cell adenocarcinomas have a higher incidence of extrauterine disease at detection than endometrioid adenocarcinomas. The risk of extrauterine disease does not correlate with the depth of myometrial invasion, because nodal or intraperitoneal mestastases can be found even when there is no myometrial invasion. For this reason, they are classified as Grade 3 tumors.

In malignancies with squamous elements, the aggressiveness of the tumor seems to be related to the degree of differentiation of the glandular component rather than the squamous element. Clinicopathologic and immunohistochemical studies support classifying malignant mixed mesodermal tumors as high-grade (G3) malignancies of epithelial origin rather than as sarcomas with mixed epithelial and mesenchymal differentiation, as in earlier classification systems.

The data regarding the impact of DNA ploidy, estrogen and progesterone receptor status, and tumor suppressor gene and oncogene expression are not sufficiently mature to incorporate into the stage grouping at this time.

## DEFINITIONS OF TNM

The definitions of the T categories correspond to the stages accepted by FIGO.

### Uterine Carcinomas

Carcinosarcomas should be staged as carcinoma.

FIGO stages are further subdivided by histologic grade of tumor – for example, Stage IC G2. Both systems are included for comparison.

*Primary Tumor (T) (Surgical-Pathologic Findings)*

| TNM Categories | FIGO Stages | |
|---|---|---|
| TX | | Primary tumor cannot be assessed |
| T0 | | No evidence of primary tumor |
| Tis* | | Carcinoma in situ (preinvasive carcinoma) |
| T1 | I | Tumor confined to corpus uteri |
| T1a | IA | Tumor limited to endometrium or invades less than one-half of the myometrium |
| T1b | IB | Tumor invades one-half or more of the myometrium |
| T2 | II | Tumor invades stromal connective tissue of the cervix but does not extend beyond uterus** |
| T3a | IIIA | Tumor involves serosa and/or adnexa (direct extension or metastasis) |
| T3b | IIIB | Vaginal involvement (direct extension or metastasis) or parametrial involvement |
| T4 | IVA | Tumor invades bladder mucosa and/or bowel mucosa (bullous edema is not sufficient to classify a tumor as T4) |

*Note: FIGO no longer includes Stage 0 (Tis).
**Endocervical glandular involvement only should be considered as Stage I and not as Stage II.

## Regional Lymph Nodes (N)

| TNM Categories | FIGO Stages | |
|---|---|---|
| NX | | Regional lymph nodes cannot be assessed |
| N0 | | No regional lymph node metastasis |
| N1 | IIIC1 | Regional lymph node metastasis to pelvic lymph nodes |
| N2 | IIIC2 | Regional lymph node metastasis to para-aortic lymph nodes, with or without positive pelvic lymph nodes |

## Distant Metastasis (M)

| TNM Categories | FIGO Stages | |
|---|---|---|
| M0 | | No distant metastasis |
| M1 | IVB | Distant metastasis (includes metastasis to inguinal lymph nodes intraperitoneal disease, or lung, liver, or bone. It excludes metastasis to para-aortic lymph nodes, vagina, pelvic serosa, or adnexa) |

## ANATOMIC STAGE/PROGNOSTIC GROUPS

Carcinomas*

| | | | |
|---|---|---|---|
| Stage 0** | Tis | N0 | M0 |
| Stage I | T1 | N0 | M0 |
| Stage IA | T1a | N0 | M0 |
| Stage IB | T1b | N0 | M0 |
| Stage II | T2 | N0 | M0 |
| Stage III | T3 | N0 | M0 |
| Stage IIIA | T3a | N0 | M0 |
| Stage IIIB | T3b | N0 | M0 |
| Stage IIIC1 | T1-T3 | N1 | M0 |
| Stage IIIC2 | T1-T3 | N2 | M0 |
| Stage IVA | T4 | Any N | M0 |
| Stage IVB | Any T | Any N | M1 |

*Carcinosarcomas should be staged as carcinoma.

**Note: FIGO no longer includes Stage 0 (Tis).

## PROGNOSTIC FACTORS (SITE-SPECIFIC FACTORS)
### (Recommended for Collection for Carcinomas and Sarcomas)

| | |
|---|---|
| Required for staging | None |
| Clinically significant | FIGO Stage |
| | Peritoneal cytology results |
| | Pelvic nodal dissection with number of nodes positive/ examined |
| | Para-aortic nodal dissection with number of nodes positive/examined |
| | Percentage of nonendometrioid cell type in mixed histology tumors |
| | Omentectomy performed |

## HISTOLOGIC GRADE (G)

| | |
|---|---|
| GX | Grade cannot be assessed |
| G1 | Well differentiated |
| G2 | Moderately differentiated |
| G3–4 | Poorly differentiated or undifferentiated |

**Histopathology: Degree of Differentiation.** Cases of carcinoma of the corpus uteri should be grouped according to the degree of differentiation of the adenocarcinoma as follows:

| | |
|---|---|
| G1 | 5% or less of a nonsquamous or nonmorular solid growth pattern |
| G2 | 6–50% of a nonsquamous or nonmorular solid growth pattern |
| G3 | More than 50% of a nonsquamous or nonmorular solid growth pattern |

### Notes on Pathologic Grading

1. Notable nuclear atypia, inappropriate for the architectural grade, raises the grade to 3.
2. Serous, clear cell, and mixed mesodermal tumors are *high risk* and considered Grade 3.
3. Adenocarcinomas with benign squamous elements (squamous metaplasia) are graded according to the nuclear grade of the glandular component.

**Uterine Sarcomas.** (Includes Leiomyosarcoma, Endometrial Stromal Sarcoma, Adenosarcoma)

### Leiomyosarcoma and Endometrial Stromal Sarcoma

| Primary Tumor (T) | | |
|---|---|---|
| TNM Categories | FIGO Stages | Definition |
| TX | | Primary tumor cannot be assessed |
| T0 | | No evidence of primary tumor |
| T1 | I | Tumor limited to the uterus |

36

## Primary Tumor (T) (continued)

| | | |
|---|---|---|
| T1a | IA | Tumor 5 cm or less in greatest dimension |
| T1b | IB | Tumor more than 5 cm |
| T2 | II | Tumor extends beyond the uterus, within the pelvis |
| T2a | IIA | Tumor involves adnexa |
| T2b | IIB | Tumor involves other pelvic tissues |
| T3 | III* | Tumor infiltrates abdominal tissues |
| T3a | IIIA | One site |
| T3b | IIIB | More than one site |
| T4 | IVA | Tumor invades bladder or rectum |

*Note*: Simultaneous tumors of the uterine corpus and ovary/pelvis in association with ovarian/pelvic endometriosis should be classified as independent primary tumors.

* In this stage lesions must infiltrate abdominal tissues and not just protrude into the abdominal cavity.

## Regional Lymph Nodes (N)

| | | |
|---|---|---|
| NX | | Regional lymph nodes cannot be assessed |
| N0 | | No regional lymph node metastasis |
| N1 | IIIC | Regional lymph node metastasis |

## Distant Metastasis (M)

| | | |
|---|---|---|
| M0 | | No distant metastasis |
| M1 | IVB | Distant metastasis (excluding adnexa, pelvic, and abdominal tissues) |

### Adenosarcoma

## Primary Tumor (T)

| TNM Categories | FIGO Stages | Definition |
|---|---|---|
| TX | | Primary tumor cannot be assessed |
| T0 | | No evidence of primary tumor |
| T1 | I | Tumor limited to the uterus |
| T1a | IA | Tumor limited to the endometrium/endocervix |
| T1b | IB | Tumor invades to less than half of the myometrium |
| T1c | IC | Tumor invades more than half of the myometrium |
| T2 | II | Tumor extends beyond the uterus, within the pelvis |
| T2a | IIA | Tumor involves adnexa |
| T2b | IIB | Tumor involves other pelvic tissues |
| T3 | III* | Tumor involves abdominal tissues |
| T3a | IIIA | One site |
| T3b | IIIB | More than one site |
| T4 | IVA | Tumor invades bladder or rectum |

*Note*: Simultaneous tumors of the uterine corpus and ovary/pelvis in association with ovarian/pelvic endometriosis should be classified as independent primary tumors.

* In this stage lesions must infiltrate abdominal tissues and not just protrude into the abdominal cavity.

### Regional Lymph Nodes (N)

| | | |
|---|---|---|
| NX | | Regional lymph nodes cannot be assessed |
| N0 | | No regional lymph node metastasis |
| N1 | IIIC | Regional lymph node metastasis |

### Distant Metastasis (M)

| | | |
|---|---|---|
| M0 | | No distant metastasis |
| M1 | IVB | Distant metastasis (excluding adnexa, pelvic and abdominal tissues) |

## Uterine Sarcomas

### ANATOMIC STAGE/PROGNOSTIC GROUPS

| Stage I | T1 | N0 | M0 |
|---|---|---|---|
| Stage IA* | T1a | N0 | M0 |
| Stage IB* | T1b | N0 | M0 |
| Stage IC** | T1c | N0 | M0 |
| Stage II | T2 | N0 | M0 |
| Stage IIIA | T3a | N0 | M0 |
| Stage IIIB | T3b | N0 | M0 |
| Stage IIIC | T1, T2, T3 | N1 | M0 |
| Stage IVA | T4 | Any N | M0 |
| Stage IVB | Any T | Any N | M1 |

*Stage IA and IB differ from those applied for leiomyosarcoma and endometrial stromal sarcoma

**Note: Stage IC does not apply for leiomyosarcoma and endometrial stromal sarcoma.

## HISTOPATHOLOGIC TYPE

Endometrioid carcinomas
Villoglandular adenocarcinoma
Adenocarcinoma with benign squamous elements, squamous metaplasia, or squamous differentiation (adenoacanthoma)
Adenosquamous carcinoma (mixed adenocarcinoma and squamous cell carcinoma)
Mucinous adenocarcinoma
Serous adenocarcinoma (papillary serous)
Clear cell adenocarcinoma
Squamous cell carcinoma
Undifferentiated carcinoma
Malignant mixed mesodermal tumors
Sarcomas: leiomyosarcomas, endometrial stromal sarcomas, adenosarcomas, carcinosarcomas

**36**

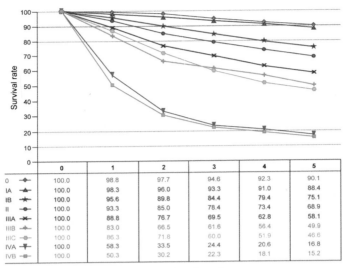

| | 0 | 1 | 2 | 3 | 4 | 5 |
|---|---|---|---|---|---|---|
| 0 | 100.0 | 98.8 | 97.7 | 94.6 | 92.3 | 90.1 |
| IA | 100.0 | 98.3 | 96.0 | 93.3 | 91.0 | 88.4 |
| IB | 100.0 | 95.6 | 89.8 | 84.4 | 79.4 | 75.1 |
| II | 100.0 | 93.3 | 85.0 | 78.4 | 73.4 | 68.9 |
| IIIA | 100.0 | 88.8 | 76.7 | 69.5 | 62.8 | 58.1 |
| IIIB | 100.0 | 83.0 | 66.5 | 61.6 | 56.4 | 49.9 |
| IIIC | 100.0 | 86.3 | 71.8 | 60.0 | 51.9 | 46.6 |
| IVA | 100.0 | 58.3 | 33.5 | 24.4 | 20.6 | 16.8 |
| IVB | 100.0 | 50.3 | 30.2 | 22.3 | 18.1 | 15.2 |

Years from diagnosis

**FIGURE 36.1.** Observed survival rates for 21,904 cases with carcinoma of the corpus uteri. Data from the National Cancer Data Base (Commission on Cancer of the American College of Surgeons and the American Cancer Society) diagnosed in years 2000–2002. Stage 0 includes 415 patients; Stage IA, 12,868; Stage IB, 2,559; Stage II, 2,098; Stage IIIA, 929; Stage IIIB, 91; Stage IIIC, 1,353; Stage IVA, 229; and Stage IVB, 1,362.

## OUTCOMES RESULTS

The significance of clinical compared with surgical/pathologic staging is shown in Figure 36.1. The prognosis for patients with clinical Stage I disease is similar to that for women with surgical Stage III, and those with clinical Stage III cancers have the same prognosis as patients with surgical Stage IV lesions. These findings also emphasize the importance of clearly separating patients who are staged clinically from those who have more accurate surgical/pathologic staging recommended by AJCC and FIGO.

## BIBLIOGRAPHY

Cirisano FD, Robboy SF, Dodge RK, et al. The outcome of stage I–II clinically and surgically staged papillary serous and clear cell endometrial cancers when compared with endometrioid carcinoma. Gynecol Oncol. 2000;77:55–65.

Colombi RP. Sarcomatoid carcinomas of the female genital tract (malignant mixed mullerian tumors). Semin Diagn Pathol. 1993;10:169–75.

Creasman W, Morrow P, Bundy B, Homesley H, Graham J, Heller P. Surgical pathologic spread patterns of endometrial cancer: a Gynecologic Oncology Group study. Cancer. 1987;60:2035–41.

Creasman W, Odicino F, Maisonneuve P, et al. Carcinoma of the corpus uteri: FIGO Annual Report. J Epidemiol Biostat. 2001;6:45–86.

Creutzberg CL, van Patten LE, Koper PC, et al. Surgery and postop radiotherapy vs surgery alone for patients with stage I endometrial carcinoma: multicenter randomized trial. PORTEC Study Group. Lancet. 2000;355:1404–11.

FIGO Committee on Gynecologic Cancer. Revised FIGO staging for carcinoma of the vulva, cervix, and endometrium. Int J Gynecol Obstet. 2009;105:103–4.

FIGO Committee on Gyn Onc Report. FIGO staging for uterine sarcomas. Int J Gynaecol Obstet. 2009;104:179.

Gershenson DM, editor. Guidelines for referral to a gynecologic oncologist: rationale and benefits. Gynecol Oncol. 2000;78:S1–13.

Mariani A, Webb M, Keeney G, Aletti G, Podratz K. Assessment of prognostic factors in stage IIIA endometrial cacer. Gynecol Oncol. 2002;86:38–44.

Marth C, Windbichler G, Petru E, et al. Parity as an independent prognostic factor in malignant mixed mesodermal tumors of the endometrium. Gynecol Oncol. 1997;64:121–5.

Panici PB, Basile S, Maneschi F, et al. Systemic pelvic lymphadenectomy vs no lymphadenectomy in early-stage endometrial carcinoma: randomized clinical trial. J Natl Cancer Inst. 2008;100(23):1707.

Prat J. FIGO staging for uterine sarcomas. Int J Gynaecol Obstet. 2009;104:177–178.

Wheeler DT, Bell KA, Kurman RJ, et al. Minimal uterine serous carcinoma: diagnosis and clinicopathologic correlation. Am J Surg Pathol. 2000;24:797–806.

The Writing Committee on behalf of the ASTEC Study Group. Efficacy of systematic pelvic lymphadenectomy in endometrial cancer (MRC ASTEC trial): a randomised study. Lancet. 2009;373(9658):125.

Zaino RJ, Kurman RJ, Diana KL, et al. The utility of the revised International Federation of Gynecology and Obstetrics histologic grading of endometrial adenocarcinoma using a defined nuclear grading system. Cancer. 1995;75:81–6.

Zerba MJ, Bristow R, Grumbine FC, et al. Inability of preoperative computed tomography scans to accurately predict the extent of myometrial invasion and extracorporal spread in endometrial cancer. Gynecol Oncol. 2000;78:67–70.

36

# Ovary and Primary Peritoneal Carcinoma

## At-A-Glance

---

**SUMMARY OF CHANGES**

- The definition of TNM and the Stage Grouping for this chapter have not changed from the Sixth Edition
- Primary peritoneal carcinoma has been included in this chapter

---

| ANATOMIC STAGE/PROGNOSTIC GROUPS | | | |
|---|---|---|---|
| Stage I | T1 | N0 | M0 |
| Stage IA | T1a | N0 | M0 |
| Stage IB | T1b | N0 | M0 |
| Stage IC | T1c | N0 | M0 |
| Stage II | T2 | N0 | M0 |
| Stage IIA | T2a | N0 | M0 |
| Stage IIB | T2b | N0 | M0 |
| Stage IIC | T2c | N0 | M0 |
| Stage III | T3 | N0 | M0 |
| Stage IIIA | T3a | N0 | M0 |
| Stage IIIB | T3b | N0 | M0 |
| Stage IIIC | T3c | N0 | M0 |
| | Any T | N1 | M0 |
| Stage IV | Any T | Any N | M1 |

**ICD-O-3 TOPOGRAPHY CODES**

| | |
|---|---|
| C56.9 | Ovary |
| C48.1 | Specified parts of peritoneum (female only) |
| C48.2 | Peritoneum (female only) |
| C48.8 | Overlapping lesion of retroperitoneum and peritoneum (female only) |

**ICD-O-3 HISTOLOGY CODE RANGES**

8000–8576, 8930–9110

## ANATOMY

**Primary Site.** The ovaries are a pair of solid, flattened ovoids 2–4 cm in diameter that are connected by a peritoneal fold to the broad ligament and by the infundibulopelvic ligament to the lateral wall of the pelvis. They are attached medially to the uterus by the utero-ovarian ligament.

In some cases, an adenocarcinoma is primary in the peritoneum. The ovaries are not involved or are only involved with minimal surface implants. The clinical presentation, surgical therapy, chemotherapy, and prognosis of these peritoneal tumors mirror those of papillary serous carcinoma of the ovary. Patients who undergo prophylactic oophorectomy for a familial history of ovarian cancer appear to retain a 1–2% chance of developing peritoneal adenocarcinoma, which is histopathologically and clinically similar to primary ovarian cancer.

**Regional Lymph Nodes.** The lymphatic drainage occurs by the infundibulopelvic and round ligament trunks and an external iliac accessory route into the following regional nodes:

External iliac
Internal iliac (hypogastric)
Obturator
Common iliac
Para-aortic
Inguinal
Pelvic, NOS
Retroperitoneal, NOS

For pN0, histologic examination should include both pelvic and para-aortic lymph nodes.

**Metastatic Sites.** The peritoneum, including the omentum and the pelvic and abdominal visceral and parietal peritoneum, comprises common sites for seeding. Diaphragmatic and liver surface involvement are also common. However, to be consistent with FIGO staging, these implants within the abdominal cavity (T3) are not considered distant metastases. Extraperitoneal sites, including parenchymal liver, lung, skeletal metastases, and supraclavicular and axillary nodes, are M1.

## RULES FOR CLASSIFICATION

Ovarian cancer is surgically/pathologically staged. There should be histologic confirmation of the ovarian disease. Laparotomy or operative laparoscopy with resection of the ovarian mass, as well as hysterectomy, form the basis for staging. Biopsies of all frequently involved sites, such as omentum, mesentery, diaphragm, peritoneal surfaces, pelvic nodes, and para-aortic nodes, are required for ideal staging of early disease. For example, in order to stage a patient confidently as Stage IA (T1 N0 M0), negative biopsies of all of the above sites should be obtained to exclude microscopic metastases. On the other hand, a single biopsy from an omental mass 2 cm or greater showing metastatic adenocarcinoma is adequate to classify a patient as Stage IIIC, thus making other biopsies unnecessary from a staging standpoint. The final histologic and cytologic findings after surgery are to be considered in the staging. Operative findings prior to tumor debulking determine stage, which may be modified by histopathologic as well as clinical or radiologic evaluation (palpable supraclavicular node or pulmonary metastases on chest X-ray, for example).

**Clinical Staging.** Although clinical studies similar to those for other sites may be used, surgical-pathologic evaluation of the abdomen and pelvis is necessary to establish a definitive diagnosis of ovarian cancer and rule out other primary malignancies (such as bowel, uterine, and pancreatic cancers or occasionally lymphoma) that may present with similar pre-operative findings. A laparotomy is the most widely accepted procedure used for surgical-pathologic staging, but occasionally laparoscopy can be used. Occasionally, patients with advanced disease and/or women who are medically unsuitable candidates for surgery may be presumed to have ovarian cancer on the basis of cytology of ascites or pleural effusion showing typical adenocarcinoma, combined with imaging studies demonstrating enlarged ovaries. Such patients are usually considered as unstaged (TX), although positive cytology of a pleural effusion or supraclavicular lymph node occasionally allows designation of M1 or FIGO Stage IV disease. The presence of ascites does not affect staging unless malignant cells are present.

Imaging studies are often done in conjunction with definitive abdominal-pelvic surgery, and chest X-ray, bone scans, computerized scanning (CT), or positron emission tomography (PET) may identify lung, bone, or brain metastases that should be considered in the final stage. Pleural effusions should be evaluated with cytology.

As with all gynecologic cancers, the final stage should be established at the time of initial treatment. It should not be modified or changed on the basis of subsequent findings.

Second-look laparotomies and laparoscopy after initial chemotherapy are occasionally utilized because of the limitation of routine examinations in detecting early recurrence. Findings related to these procedures do not change the patient's original stage.

**Pathologic Staging.** Surgery and biopsy of all suspected sites of involvement provide the basis for staging. Histologic and cytologic data are required. This is the preferred method of staging for ovarian cancer. The operative note and/or the pathology report should describe the location and size of metastatic lesions and the primary tumors for optimal staging. In addition, the determination of tumor size outside of the pelvis must be noted and documented in the operative report. This is reported in centimeters and represents the largest implant, whether resected or not at the time of surgical exploration.

## PROGNOSTIC FEATURES

Histology and grade are important prognostic factors. Women with borderline tumors (low malignant potential) have an excellent prognosis, even when extraovarian disease is found. In patients with invasive ovarian cancer, well-differentiated lesions have a better prognosis than poorly differentiated tumors, stage for stage. Histologic type is also extremely important, because some stromal tumors (theca cell, granulosa) have an excellent prognosis, whereas epithelial tumors in general have a less favorable outcome. For this reason, epithelial cell types are generally reported together, and sex-cord stromal tumors and germ cell tumors are reported separately. Tumor cell type also helps to guide the type of chemotherapy that is recommended.

In advanced disease, the most important prognostic factor is the residual disease after the initial surgical management. Even with advanced stage, patients with no gross residual after the surgical debulking have a considerably better prognosis than those with minimal or extensive residual. Not only is the size of the residual important, but the number of sites of residual tumor also appears to be important (tumor volume).

The tumor marker CA-125 is useful for following the response to therapy in patients with epithelial ovarian cancer who have elevated levels of this marker. The rate of regression during chemotherapy treatment may have prognostic significance. Women with germ cell tumors may also have elevated serum tumor markers – alpha fetoprotein (AFP) or human chorionic gonadotropin (β-hCG). Other factors, such as growth factors and oncogene amplification, are currently under investigation.

## DEFINITIONS OF TNM

The definitions of the T categories correspond to the stages accepted by the Fédération Internationale de Gynécologie et d'Obstétrique (FIGO). Both systems are included for comparison.

| Primary Tumor (T) | | |
|---|---|---|
| TNM Categories | FIGO Stages | |
| TX | | Primary tumor cannot be assessed |
| T0 | | No evidence of primary tumor |
| T1 | I | Tumor limited to ovaries (one or both) |
| T1a | IA | Tumor limited to one ovary; capsule intact, no tumor on ovarian surface. No malignant cells in ascites or peritoneal washings |
| T1b | IB | Tumor limited to both ovaries; capsules intact, no tumor on ovarian surface. No malignant cells in ascites or peritoneal washings |
| T1c | IC | Tumor limited to one or both ovaries with any of the following: capsule ruptured, tumor on ovarian surface, malignant cells in ascites or peritoneal washings |
| T2 | II | Tumor involves one or both ovaries with pelvic extension |
| T2a | IIA | Extension and/or implants on uterus and/or tube(s). No malignant cells in ascites or peritoneal washings |
| T2b | IIB | Extension to and/or implants on other pelvic tissues. No malignant cells in ascites or peritoneal washings |
| T2c | IIC | Pelvic extension and/or implants (T2a or T2b) with malignant cells in ascites or peritoneal washings |
| T3 | III | Tumor involves one or both ovaries with microscopically confirmed peritoneal metastasis outside the pelvis |

| T3a | IIIA | Microscopic peritoneal metastasis beyond pelvis (no macroscopic tumor) |
| T3b | IIIB | Macroscopic peritoneal metastasis beyond pelvis 2 cm or less in greatest dimension |
| T3c | IIIC | Peritoneal metastasis beyond pelvis more than 2 cm in greatest dimension and/or regional lymph node metastasis |

*Note*: Liver capsule metastasis T3/Stage III; liver parenchymal metastasis M1/Stage IV. Pleural effusion must have positive cytology for M1/Stage IV.

### Regional Lymph Nodes (N)

| TNM Categories | FIGO Stages | |
|---|---|---|
| NX | | Regional lymph nodes cannot be assessed |
| N0 | | No regional lymph node metastasis |
| N1 | IIIC | Regional lymph node metastasis |

### Distant Metastasis (M)

| TNM Categories | FIGO Stages | |
|---|---|---|
| M0 | | No distant metastasis |
| M1 | IV | Distant metastasis (excludes peritoneal metastasis) |

**pTNM Pathologic Classification.** The pT, pN, and pM categories correspond to the T, N, and M categories.

### ANATOMIC STAGE/PROGNOSTIC GROUPS

| Stage I | T1 | N0 | M0 |
|---|---|---|---|
| Stage IA | T1a | N0 | M0 |
| Stage IB | T1b | N0 | M0 |
| Stage IC | T1c | N0 | M0 |
| Stage II | T2 | N0 | M0 |
| Stage IIA | T2a | N0 | M0 |
| Stage IIB | T2b | N0 | M0 |
| Stage IIC | T2c | N0 | M0 |
| Stage III | T3 | N0 | M0 |
| Stage IIIA | T3a | N0 | M0 |
| Stage IIIB | T3b | N0 | M0 |
| Stage IIIC | T3c | N0 | M0 |
| | Any T | N1 | M0 |
| Stage IV | Any T | Any N | M1 |

**37**

## PROGNOSTIC FACTORS (SITE-SPECIFIC FACTORS)
### (Recommended for Collection)

| | |
|---|---|
| Required for staging | None |
| Clinically significant | FIGO stage<br>Preoperative CA 125<br>Gross residual tumor after primary cyto-reductive surgery (present, absent, unknown, "y" meaning patient received chemotherapy prior to surgery)<br>Residual tumor volume after primary cyto-reductive surgery (no gross, ≤1cm, >1cm, unknown, "y" meaning patient received chemotherapy prior to surgery)<br>Residual tumor location following primary cyto-reductive surgery ("y" indicates patient received chemotherapy prior to surgery)<br>Malignant ascites volume |

## HISTOLOGIC GRADE (G)

GX     Grade cannot be assessed
GB     Borderline malignancy
G1     Well differentiated
G2     Moderately differentiated
G3–4   Poorly differentiated or undifferentiated

## HISTOPATHOLOGIC TYPE

The American Joint Committee on Cancer (AJCC) endorses the histologic typing of malignant ovarian tumors as endorsed by the World Health Organization (WHO) and recommends that all ovarian epithelial tumors be subdivided according to a simplified version of this classification. The three main histologic types, which include nearly all ovarian cancers, are epithelial tumors, sex-cord stromal tumors, and germ cell tumors. Nonepithelial primary ovarian cancers may be staged using this classification but should be reported separately.

I. Epithelial tumors
   a. Serous tumors
      1. Benign serous cystadenoma
      2. Of borderline malignancy: Serous cystadenoma with proliferating activity of the epithelial cells and nuclear abnormalities, but with no infiltrative destructive growth (carcinomas of low potential malignancy)
      3. Serous cystadenocarcinoma

b. Mucinous tumors
   1. Benign mucinous cystadenoma
   2. Of borderline malignancy: Mucinous cystadenoma with proliferating activity of the epithelial cells and nuclear abnormalities, but with no infiltrative destructive growth (carcinomas of low potential malignancy)
   3. Mucinous cystadenocarcinoma
c. Endometrioid tumors
   1. Benign endometrioid cystadenoma
   2. Endometrioid tumors with proliferating activity of the epithelial cells and nuclear abnormalities, but with no infiltrative destructive growth (carcinomas of low potential malignancy)
   3. Endometrioid adenocarcinoma
d. Clear cell tumors
   1. Benign clear cell tumors
   2. Clear cell tumors with proliferating activity of the epithelial cells and nuclear abnormalities, but with no infiltrative destructive growth (low potential malignancy)
   3. Clear cell cystadenocarcinoma
e. Brenner (transitional cell tumors)
   1. Benign Brenner
   2. Borderline malignancy
   3. Malignant
   4. Transitional cell
f. Squamous cell tumor
g. Undifferentiated carcinoma
   1. A malignant tumor of epithelial structure that is too poorly differentiated to be placed in any other group
h. Mixed epithelial tumor
   1. Tumors composed of two or more of the five major cell types of common epithelial tumors (types should be specified)

Cases with intraperitoneal carcinoma in which the ovaries appear to be incidentally involved and not the primary origin should be labeled as extraovarian peritoneal carcinoma. They are usually staged with the ovarian staging classification. Because the peritoneum is essentially always involved throughout the abdomen, the peritoneal tumors are usually within the Stage III (T3) or Stage IV (M1) categories.

**37**

## OUTCOMES RESULTS

Epithelial carcinoma accounts for approximately 80% of all patients with cancer of the ovary. Because of the difficulty of diagnosing this cancer at an early stage, the overall prognosis of women with epithelial ovarian cancer is poor, despite the fact that patients with early stage disease have a favorable outlook. The prognostic significance of stage is shown in Figure 37.1.

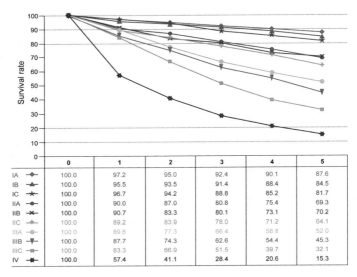

| | | 0 | 1 | 2 | 3 | 4 | 5 |
|---|---|---|---|---|---|---|---|
| IA | ◆ | 100.0 | 97.2 | 95.0 | 92.4 | 90.1 | 87.6 |
| IB | ▲ | 100.0 | 95.5 | 93.5 | 91.4 | 88.4 | 84.5 |
| IC | ★ | 100.0 | 96.7 | 94.2 | 88.8 | 85.2 | 81.7 |
| IIA | ● | 100.0 | 90.0 | 87.0 | 80.8 | 75.4 | 69.3 |
| IIB | ✕ | 100.0 | 90.7 | 83.3 | 80.1 | 73.1 | 70.2 |
| IIC | ▲ | 100.0 | 89.2 | 83.9 | 78.0 | 71.2 | 64.1 |
| IIIA | ⊙ | 100.0 | 89.6 | 77.3 | 66.4 | 58.8 | 52.0 |
| IIIB | ▼ | 100.0 | 87.7 | 74.3 | 62.6 | 54.4 | 45.3 |
| IIIC | ■ | 100.0 | 83.3 | 66.9 | 51.5 | 39.7 | 32.1 |
| IV | ✱ | 100.0 | 57.4 | 41.1 | 28.4 | 20.6 | 15.3 |

Years from diagnosis

**FIGURE 37.1.** Observed survival rates for 11,738 cases with primary ovarian epithelial cancer. Data from the National Cancer Data Base (Commission on Cancer of the American College of Surgeons and the American Cancer Society) diagnosed in years 1998–2002. Stage 0 includes 60 patients; Stage IA, 1,415; Stage IB, 160; Stage IC, 878; Stage IIA 211; Stage IIB, 304; Stage IIC, 473; Stage IIIA, 284; Stage IIIB, 425; Stage IIIC, 3,815; and Stage IV, 3,773.

## BIBLIOGRAPHY

Friedlander ML. Prognostic factors in ovarian cancer. Semin Oncol. 1998;25: 305–14.

Heintz APM, Odicino F, Maisonneuve P, et al. Carcinoma of the ovary. FIGO Annual Report. J Epidemiol Biostat. 2001;6:107–38.

Leblanc E, Querleu D, Narducci F, et al. Surgical staging of early invasive epithelial ovarian tumors. Semin Surg Oncol. 2000;19:36–41.

Manek S, Wells M. Pathology of borderline ovarian tumours. Clin Oncol. 1999;11:73–7.

Silverberg SG. Histopathologic grading of ovarian carcinoma: a review and proposal. Intl J Gynecol Pathol. 2000;19:7–15.

Trope C. Prognostic factors in ovarian cancer. Cancer Treat Res. 1998;95: 287–352.

# Fallopian Tube

## *At-A-Glance*

---

**SUMMARY OF CHANGES**

- The definition of TNM and the Stage Grouping for this chapter have not changed from the Sixth Edition

---

| ANATOMIC STAGE/PROGNOSTIC GROUPS | | | |
|---|---|---|---|
| Stage 0* | Tis | N0 | M0 |
| Stage I | T1 | N0 | M0 |
| Stage IA | T1a | N0 | M0 |
| Stage IB | T1b | N0 | M0 |
| Stage IC | T1c | N0 | M0 |
| Stage II | T2 | N0 | M0 |
| Stage IIA | T2a | N0 | M0 |
| Stage IIB | T2b | N0 | M0 |
| Stage IIC | T2c | N0 | M0 |
| Stage III | T3 | N0 | M0 |
| Stage IIIA | T3a | N0 | M0 |
| Stage IIIB | T3b | N0 | M0 |
| Stage IIIC | T3c | N0 | M0 |
| | Any T | N1 | M0 |
| Stage IV | Any T | Any N | M1 |

ICD-O-3
TOPOGRAPHY
CODES
C57.0    Fallopian tube

ICD-O-3 HISTOLOGY
CODE RANGES
8000–8576, 8940–8950,
8980–8981

*Note*: FIGO no longer includes Stage 0 (Tis).

## ANATOMY

**Primary Site.** The fallopian tube extends from the posterior superior aspect of the uterine fundus laterally and anteriorly to the ovary. Its length is approximately 10 cm. The medial end arises in the cornual portion of the uterine cavity, and the lateral end opens to the peritoneal cavity.

Carcinoma of the fallopian tube is almost always an adenocarcinoma arising from an in situ lesion of the tubal mucosa. It invades locally into the muscular wall of the tube and then into the peritubal soft tissue or adjacent organs such as the uterus or ovary, or through the serosa of the tube into

**38**

the peritoneal cavity. Metastatic tumor implants can be found throughout the peritoneal cavity. The tumor may obstruct the tubal lumen and present as a ruptured or unruptured hydrosalpinx or hematosalpinx.

**Regional Nodes.** Carcinoma of the fallopian tube can also metastasize to the regional lymph nodes, which include the following:

Common iliac
External iliac
Internal iliac (hypogastric)
Obturator
Paraaortic
Inguinal
Pelvic lymph nodes, NOS

Adequate evaluation of the regional lymph nodes usually includes aortic and pelvic nodes.

**Distant Metastases.** Surface implants within the pelvic cavity and the abdominal cavity are common, but these are classified as T2 and T3 disease, respectively. Parenchymal liver metastases and extraperitoneal sites, including lung and skeletal metastases, are M1.

## RULES FOR CLASSIFICATION

There should be histologic confirmation of primary disease with complete evaluation of the abdomen and pelvis as outlined in the staging of ovarian malignancy (see Chap. 37). In many patients, the diagnosis may be unsuspected until the fallopian tube is examined histopathologically. Tumors may involve one or both fallopian tubes, and complete assessment of both adnexal areas affects the staging of the disease.

**Clinical Staging.** Perioperative imaging studies, including chest X-ray, computerized tomography scans, and magnetic resonance imaging, may identify distant metastases. Staging may be modified by imaging studies or clinical findings obtained prior to the initiation of treatment.

**Pathologic Staging.** Laparotomy or laparoscopy with resection of tubal masses, usually including hysterectomy and bilateral oophorectomy, form the basis for the operative management of fallopian tube carcinoma. Widespread intra-abdominal disease is common; therefore, adequate evaluation of potentially early stage lesions requires multiple biopsies of commonly involved sites, such as omentum, pelvic peritoneum, mesentery, bowel serosa, diaphragm, and regional nodes, in order to rule out microscopic metastases to any of these sites.

Cytologic studies of ascites (if present) or of pelvic and abdominal peritoneal washings (if no ascites are present) should be included in the staging. The surgical-pathologic findings form the basis for staging. Staging is based on the findings at the time the abdomen is opened, not on the residual disease after debulking.

It may be preferable to classify a patient as TX (primary tumor cannot be assessed) if inadequate staging biopsies and/or a lack of peritoneal cytology make it inaccurate to classify the patient with confidence as early stage (Stage T3a/IIIA has not been excluded by adequate staging biopsies).

## PROGNOSTIC FEATURES

The surgical-pathologic stage is the most significant prognostic characteristic. Tumor differentiation is an important prognostic characteristic in all stages of disease. In patients with localized tumors, depth of invasion into the tubal musculature and rupture of the tube have prognostic importance. With advanced disease, the volume of residual tumor after surgical debulking appears to be related to prognosis.

## DEFINITIONS OF TNM

### Primary Tumor (T)

| TNM Categories | FIGO Stages | |
|---|---|---|
| TX | | Primary tumor cannot be assessed |
| T0 | | No evidence of primary tumor |
| Tis* | | Carcinoma in situ (limited to tubal mucosa) |
| T1 | I | Tumor limited to the fallopian tube(s) |
| T1a | IA | Tumor limited to one tube, without penetrating the serosal surface; no ascites |
| T1b | IB | Tumor limited to both tubes, without penetrating the serosal surface; no ascites |
| T1c | IC | Tumor limited to one or both tubes with extension onto or through the tubal serosa, or with malignant cells in ascites or peritoneal washings |
| T2 | II | Tumor involves one or both fallopian tubes with pelvic extension |
| T2a | IIA | Extension and/or metastasis to the uterus and/or ovaries |
| T2b | IIB | Extension to other pelvic structures |
| T2c | IIC | Pelvic extension with malignant cells in ascites or peritoneal washings |
| T3 | III | Tumor involves one or both fallopian tubes, with peritoneal implants outside the pelvis |
| T3a | IIIA | Microscopic peritoneal metastasis outside the pelvis |
| T3b | IIIB | Macroscopic peritoneal metastasis outside the pelvis 2 cm or less in greatest dimension |
| T3c | IIIC | Peritoneal metastasis outside the pelvis and more than 2 cm in diameter |

*Note: FIGO no longer includes Stage 0 (Tis).

Note: Liver capsule metastasis is T3/Stage III; liver parenchymal metastasis is M1/Stage IV. Pleural effusion must have positive cytology for M1/Stage IV.

**38**

### Regional Lymph Nodes (N)

| TNM Categories | FIGO Stages | |
|---|---|---|
| NX | | Regional lymph nodes cannot be assessed |
| N0 | | No regional lymph node metastasis |
| N1 | IIIC | Regional lymph node metastasis |

### Distant Metastasis (M)

| TNM Categories | FIGO Stages | |
|---|---|---|
| M0 | | No distant metastasis |
| M1 | IV | Distant metastasis (excludes metastasis within the peritoneal cavity) |

### ANATOMIC STAGE/PROGNOSTIC GROUPS

| Stage 0* | Tis | N0 | M0 |
|---|---|---|---|
| Stage I | T1 | N0 | M0 |
| Stage IA | T1a | N0 | M0 |
| Stage IB | T1b | N0 | M0 |
| Stage IC | T1c | N0 | M0 |
| Stage II | T2 | N0 | M0 |
| Stage IIA | T2a | N0 | M0 |
| Stage IIB | T2b | N0 | M0 |
| Stage IIC | T2c | N0 | M0 |
| Stage III | T3 | N0 | M0 |
| Stage IIIA | T3a | N0 | M0 |
| Stage IIIB | T3b | N0 | M0 |
| Stage IIIC | T3c | N0 | M0 |
| | Any T | N1 | M0 |
| Stage IV | Any T | Any N | M1 |

*Note: FIGO no longer includes Stage 0 (Tis).

### PROGNOSTIC FACTORS (SITE-SPECIFIC FACTORS)
### (Recommended for Collection)

| Required for staging | None |
|---|---|
| Clinically significant | FIGO Stage |
| | Tumor location, involvement of fimbria |
| | Pelvic nodal status and method of assessment |

### HISTOLOGIC GRADE (G)

Grade is reported in registry systems by the grade value. A two-grade, three-grade, or four-grade system may be used. If a grading system is not specified, generally the following system is used:

| GX | Grade cannot be assessed |
|----|--------------------------|
| G1 | Well differentiated |
| G2 | Moderately differentiated |
| G3 | Poorly differentiated |
| G4 | Undifferentiated |

## HISTOPATHOLOGIC TYPES

Adenocarcinoma is the most frequently seen histology.

## OUTCOMES RESULTS

This is a very uncommon tumor. It is usually treated with surgery followed by chemotherapy. The 5-year survival in early disease is approximately 70%, but surgical staging is often inadequate. At 5 years, the overall survival for patients with advanced disease is about 20% (Figure 38.1).

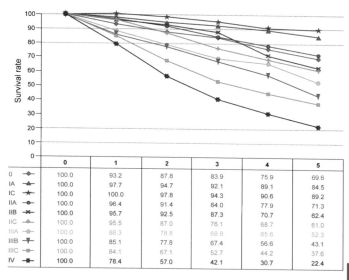

| | | 0 | 1 | 2 | 3 | 4 | 5 |
|-----|---|-------|-------|-------|------|------|------|
| 0 | ◆ | 100.0 | 93.2 | 87.8 | 83.9 | 75.9 | 69.6 |
| IA | ▲ | 100.0 | 97.7 | 94.7 | 92.1 | 89.1 | 84.5 |
| IC | ★ | 100.0 | 100.0 | 97.8 | 94.3 | 90.6 | 89.2 |
| IIA | ● | 100.0 | 96.4 | 91.4 | 84.0 | 77.9 | 71.3 |
| IIB | ✻ | 100.0 | 95.7 | 92.5 | 87.3 | 70.7 | 62.4 |
| IIC | ▲ | 100.0 | 95.5 | 87.0 | 76.1 | 68.7 | 61.0 |
| IIIA | ● | 100.0 | 88.3 | 78.8 | 68.9 | 65.6 | 52.3 |
| IIIB | ▼ | 100.0 | 85.1 | 77.8 | 67.4 | 56.6 | 43.1 |
| IIIC | ■ | 100.0 | 84.1 | 67.1 | 52.7 | 44.2 | 37.6 |
| IV | ✳ | 100.0 | 78.4 | 57.0 | 42.1 | 30.7 | 22.4 |

Years from diagnosis

**FIGURE 38.1.** Observed survival rates for 1,456 cases with carcinoma of the fallopian tube. Data from the National Cancer Data Base (Commission on Cancer of the American College of Surgeons and the American Cancer Society) diagnosed in years 1998–2002. Stage 0 includes 60 patients; Stage IA, 319; Stage IC, 99; Stage IIA 87; Stage IIB, 76; Stage IIC, 75; Stage IIIA, 37; Stage IIIB, 48; Stage IIIC, 405; and Stage IV, 222. Stage IB is omitted because of the small number of Stage IB patients (28).

38

## BIBLIOGRAPHY

Alvarado-Cabrero I, Young RH, Vamvakas EC, et al. Carcinoma of the fallopian tube: a clinicopathological study of 105 cases with observations on staging and prognostic factors. Gynecol Oncol. 1999;72:367–79.

Baekelandt M, Nesbakken AJ, Kristensen GB, et al. Carcinoma of the fallopian tube: clinicopathologic study of 151 patients treated at the Norwegian Radium Hospital. Cancer. 2000;89:2076–84.

Heintz APM, Odicino F, Maisonneuve P, et al. Carcinoma of the fallopian tube. FIGO annual report. J Epidemiol Biostat. 2001;6:87–103.

Nikrui N, Duska LR. Fallopian tube carcinoma. Surg Oncol Clin North Am. 1998;7:363–73.

# Gestational Trophoblastic Tumors

## *At-A-Glance*

**ANATOMIC STAGE/PROGNOSTIC GROUPS**

| Group | T | M | Risk Factors |
|---|---|---|---|
| Stage I | T1 | M0 | Unknown |
| Stage IA | T1 | M0 | Low risk |
| Stage IB | T1 | M0 | High risk |
| Stage II | T2 | M0 | Unknown |
| Stage IIA | T2 | M0 | Low risk |
| Stage IIB | T2 | M0 | High risk |
| Stage III | Any T | M1a | Unknown |
| Stage IIIA | Any T | M1a | Low risk |
| Stage IIIB | Any T | M1a | High risk |
| Stage IV | Any T | M1b | Unknown |
| Stage IVA | Any T | M1b | Low risk |
| Stage IVB | Any T | M1b | High risk |

ICD-O-3
TOPOGRAPHY
CODES

C58.9    Placenta

ICD-O-3 HISTOLOGY
CODE RANGES
9100–9105

## INTRODUCTION

Gestational trophoblastic tumors are uncommon (1 in 1,000 pregnancies) malignancies that arise from the placenta. Usually as a result of a genetic accident in the developing egg, the maternal chromosomes are lost, and the paternal chromosomes duplicate (46xx). The resulting tumor is known as a *complete* hydatidiform mole: There are no fetal parts; the tumor is composed of dilated, avascular, "grape-like" vesicles that may grow as large as, or larger than, the normal pregnancy that it replaces. There is obviously no heartbeat detected, and the patient may have vaginal bleeding similar to a miscarriage. Many times, the diagnosis is not made until a dilatation and curettage is done and the tissue is examined pathologically. In some patients, fetal parts will be found in association with mild proliferative

**39**

trophoblastic (placental) tissue. Such patients have a *partial* hydatidiform mole, which has a 69xxx or 69xxy chromosomal complement resulting from twice the normal number of paternal chromosomes. Both of these tumors usually follow a benign course, resolving completely after evacuation by dilatation and suction or curettage, but approximately 20% of complete moles and 5% of partial moles persist locally or metastasize and thus require chemotherapy.

Much less frequently (about 1 in 20,000 pregnancies in the USA), a highly malignant, rapidly growing metastatic form of gestational trophoblastic disease called choriocarcinoma is encountered. This solid, anaplastic, vascular, and aggressively proliferative tumor is easily recognized microscopically and may present with symptoms of vaginal bleeding (as with a hydatidiform mole). However, metastatic lesions may be the first sign of this lesion, which can follow any pregnancy event, including an incomplete abortion or a full-term pregnancy.

The trophoblastic tissue that makes up these tumors produces a serum tumor marker, beta-human chorionic gonadotropin ($\beta$-hCG), which is very helpful in the diagnosis and monitoring of therapy in these patients. Gestational trophoblastic tumors are very responsive to chemotherapy, with cure rates approaching 100%.


## ANATOMY

Because of the responsiveness of this tumor to treatment and the accuracy of the serum tumor marker hCG in reflecting the status of disease, the traditional anatomic staging system used in most solid tumors has little prognostic significance. Trophoblastic tumors not associated with pregnancy (ovarian teratomas) are not included in this classification.

**Primary Site.** By definition, gestational trophoblastic tumors arise from placental tissue in the uterus. Although most of these tumors are noninvasive and are removed by dilatation and suction evacuation, local invasion of the myometrium can occur. When this is diagnosed on a hysterectomy specimen (rarely done these days), it may be reported as an *invasive* hydatidiform mole.

**Regional Lymph Nodes.** Nodal involvement in gestational trophoblastic tumors is rare but has a very poor prognosis when diagnosed. There is no regional nodal designation in the staging of these tumors. Nodal metastases should be classified as metastatic (M1) disease.

**Metastatic Sites.** This is a highly vascular tumor that results in frequent, widespread metastases when these lesions become malignant. The cervix and vagina are common pelvic sites of metastases (T2), and the lungs are often involved by distant metastases (M1a). Other, less frequently encountered metastatic sites include kidney, gastrointestinal tract, and spleen (M1b). The liver and brain are occasionally involved and may harbor metastatic sites that are difficult to treat with chemotherapy.

## RULES FOR CLASSIFICATION

Gestational trophoblastic tumors have a very high cure rate, and as a result, the ultimate goal of staging is to identify patients who are likely to respond to less intensive chemotherapeutic protocols and distinguish these individuals from patients who will require more intensive chemotherapy in order to achieve remission. In 1991, the International Federation of Gynecology and Obstetrics (FIGO) added nonanatomic risk factors to the traditional staging system. Further modifications have been made in an attempt to merge several prognostic classification systems. The current staging classification is still evolving.

**Indications for Treatment.** The following criteria are suggested for the diagnosis of trophoblastic tumors requiring chemotherapy:

- Three or more values of hCG showing no significant change (a plateau) over 4 weeks, *or*
- Rise of hCG of 10% or greater for 2 values over 3 weeks or longer, *or*
- Persistence of elevated hCG 6 months after evacuation of molar pregnancy, *or*
- Histologic diagnosis of choriocarcinoma

### Diagnosis of Metastasis

- For the diagnosis of lung metastasis, chest X-ray is appropriate and should be used to count metastases for risk scoring. Lung CT scan may be used.
- For the diagnosis of intra-abdominal metastasis, CT scanning is preferred, although many institutions still use ultrasound to detect liver metastasis.
- For the diagnosis of brain metastasis, MRI is superior to CT scan, even with 1-cm cuts.

**Prognostic Index Scores.** The score on the Prognostic Scoring Index is used to substage patients (Table 39.1). Each stage is anatomically defined, but substage A (low risk) and B (high risk) are assigned on the basis of a nonanatomic risk factor scoring system. The prognostic scores are 0, 1, 2, and 4 for the individual risk factors. The current prognostic scoring system eliminates the ABO blood group risk factors that were featured in the WHO scoring system and upgrades the risk factor for liver metastasis from 2 to 4, the highest category. Low risk is a score of 7 or less, and high risk is a score of 8 or greater.

## PROGNOSTIC FEATURES

**Outcomes Results.** Gestational trophoblastic tumors may require only uterine evacuation for treatment, but even when chemotherapy is required, cure rates approach 100%. Prognostic factors are listed in the

**39**

**TABLE 39.1.** Prognostic scoring index for gestational trophoblastic tumors

| Prognostic factor | Risk score | | | |
|---|---|---|---|---|
| | 0 | 1 | 2 | 4 |
| Age | <40 | ≥40 | | |
| Antecedent pregnancy | Hydatidiform mole | Abortion | Term pregnancy | |
| Interval months from index pregnancy | <4 | 4–6 | 7–12 | >12 |
| Pretreatment hCG (IU/ml) | $<10^3$ | $10^3$ to $<10^4$ | $10^4$ to $<10^5$ | $\geq10^5$ |
| Largest tumor size, including uterus | <3 cm | 3–5 cm | >5 cm | |
| Site of metastases | Lung | Spleen, kidney | Gastrointestinal tract | Brain, liver |
| Number of metastases identified | | 1–4 | 5–8 | >8 |
| Previous failed chemotherapy | | | Single drug | Two or more drugs |
| Total Score | | | | |

Low risk is a score of 6 or less. High risk is a score of 7 or greater.

Prognostic Scoring Index. Patients with low-risk disease are usually treated with single-agent chemotherapy, whereas combined, multiple-agent chemotherapy usually results in a cure for high-risk patients.

## DEFINITIONS OF TNM

### Primary Tumor (T)

| TNM Categories | FIGO Stages | |
|---|---|---|
| TX | | Primary tumor cannot be assessed |
| T0 | | No evidence of primary tumor |
| T1 | I | Tumor confined to uterus |
| T2 | II | Tumor extends to other genital structures (ovary, tube, vagina, broad ligaments) by metastasis or direct extension |

### Distant Metastasis (M)

| TNM Categories | FIGO Stages | |
|---|---|---|
| M0 | | No distant metastasis |
| M1 | | Distant metastasis |
| M1a | III | Lung metastasis |
| M1b | IV | All other distant metastasis |

### ANATOMIC STAGE/PROGNOSTIC GROUPS

| Group | T | M | Risk Factors |
|---|---|---|---|
| Stage I | T1 | M0 | Unknown |
| Stage IA | T1 | M0 | Low risk |
| Stage IB | T1 | M0 | High risk |
| Stage II | T2 | M0 | Unknown |
| Stage IIA | T2 | M0 | Low risk |
| Stage IIB | T2 | M0 | High risk |
| Stage III | Any T | M1a | Unknown |
| Stage IIIA | Any T | M1a | Low risk |
| Stage IIIB | Any T | M1a | High risk |
| Stage IV | Any T | M1b | Unknown |
| Stage IVA | Any T | M1b | Low risk |
| Stage IVB | Any T | M1b | High risk |

39

## PROGNOSTIC FACTORS (SITE-SPECIFIC FACTORS)
**(Recommended for Collection)**

Required for staging     Risk factors (Table 39.1)

Clinically significant     FIGO Stage

## HISTOLOGIC GRADE (G)

Grade is reported in registry systems by the grade value. A two-grade, three-grade, or four-grade system may be used. If a grading system is not specified, generally the following system is used:

GX     Grade cannot be assessed
G1     Well differentiated
G2     Moderately differentiated
G3     Poorly differentiated
G4     Undifferentiated

## HISTOPATHOLOGIC TYPE

Hydatidiform mole
    Complete
    Partial
Invasive hydatidiform mole
Choriocarcinoma
Placental site trophoblastic tumors

## BIBLIOGRAPHY

Horn LC, Bilek K. Histologic classification and staging of gestational tropho-blastic disease. Gen Diagn Pathol. 1997;143:87–101.

Lage JM. Protocol for the examination of specimens from patients with gestational trophoblastic malignancies: a basis for checklists. Cancer Committee, College of American Pathologists. Arch Pathol Lab Med. 1999;123:50–4.

Ngan HYS, Odicino F, Maisonneuve P, et al. Gestational trophoblastic diseases. FIGO annual report. J Epidemiol Biostat. 2001;6:175–84.

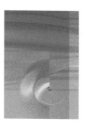

# PART IX
# Genitourinary Sites

# Penis

*(Primary urethral carcinomas and melanomas
are not included)*

## At-A-Glance

### SUMMARY OF CHANGES

The following changes in the definition of TNM and the Stage Grouping for this chapter have been made since the Sixth Edition

* T1 has been subdivided into T1a and T1b based on the presence or absence of lymphovascular invasion or poorly differentiated cancers

* T3 category is limited to urethral invasion and prostatic invasion is now considered T4

* Nodal staging is divided into both clinical and pathologic categories

* The distinction between superficial and deep inguinal lymph nodes has been eliminated

* Stage II grouping includes T1b N0M0 as well as T2-3 N0M0

**ANATOMIC STAGE/PROGNOSTIC GROUPS**

| Stage 0 | Tis | N0 | M0 |
|---------|-----|-----|-----|
|         | Ta  | N0 | M0 |
| Stage I | T1a | N0 | M0 |
| Stage II | T1b | N0 | M0 |
|          | T2  | N0 | M0 |
|          | T3  | N0 | M0 |
| Stage IIIa | T1-3 | N1 | M0 |
| Stage IIIb | T1-3 | N2 | M0 |
| Stage IV | T4 | Any N | M0 |
|          | Any T | N3 | M0 |
|          | Any T | Any N | M1 |

ICD-O-3
TOPOGRAPHY
CODES

| C60.0 | Prepuce |
| C60.1 | Glans penis |
| C60.2 | Body of penis |
| C60.8 | Overlapping lesion of penis |
| C60.9 | Penis, NOS |

ICD-O-3 HISTOLOGY
CODE RANGES
8000–8246, 8248–8576,
8940–8950, 8980–8981

## INTRODUCTION

**Incidence and Histology.**   Cancers of the penis are rare in the USA, although the incidence varies in different countries of the world. Most are squamous cell carcinomas that arise in the skin of the penile shaft or on the glans penis. Prognosis is favorable provided that the regional lymph nodes are not involved. Melanomas can also occur. The staging classification, however, applies to carcinomas. Melanoma staging is discussed in Chap. 31. Sarcomas of the penis have also been reported but are quite rare and staged according to Soft Tissue Sarcoma criteria in Chap. 28. Some squamous cancers of the penis may be described as distinct clinicopathologic entities such as verrucous carcinoma, which is well differentiated, has an expansile border, and is essentially nonmetastatic. In contrast, basaloid tumors are recognized as a poorly differentiated subtype of squamous carcinoma that is infiltrative and frequently metastasizes to the inguinal lymph nodes. These are included under this classification. An in situ lesion is also included and by definition should be coded as an in situ carcinoma of the penis.

## ANATOMY

**Primary Site.**   The penis is composed of three cylindrical masses of cavernous tissue bound together by fibrous tissue. Two masses are lateral and are known as the corpora cavernosa penis. The corpus spongiosum penis is a median mass and contains the greater part of the urethra. The distal expansion of the corpus spongoiusum forms the glans penis. The penis is attached to the front and the sides of the pubic arch. The skin covering the penis is thin and loosely connected with the deeper parts of the organ. This skin at the root of the penis is continuous with that over the scrotum and perineum. Distally, the skin becomes folded upon itself to form the prepuce, or foreskin. Circumcision has been associated with a decreased incidence of cancer of the penis.

**Regional Lymph Nodes.**   The regional lymph nodes are as follows:

> Superficial and deep inguinal (femoral)
> External iliac
> Internal iliac (hypogastric)
> Pelvic nodes, NOS

**Metastatic Sites.**   Lung, liver, and bone are most often involved.

## RULES FOR CLASSIFICATION

The anatomic extent of the primary tumor plays an important role in clinical decision making with respect to management of the primary tumor and the likelihood of inguinal lymph node metastasis. Superficial tumors including stages Tis, Ta, and T1 are often managed using organ preserving strategies whereas stage T2–T4 tumors often require amputative approaches. However, T1 tumor substratification has been adopted based on the impact of lymphovascular invasion and its associated increased risk of lymph node metastasis that should prompt more aggressive care. Patients with direct extension into the prostate from the penile shaft have extensive tumors involving an adjacent organ (i.e., stage T4) with an accompanying poor prognosis. Thus, prostatic involvement is now appropriately staged as T4. Beyond management of the primary tumor clinicians must decide if the inguinal region is at risk for metastases from the primary tumor as the incidence and extent of metastases are the most important factors determining survival.

There is general consensus that in patients with palpable adenopathy there is a higher likelihood of finding metastasis, a lower survival, and thus lymphadenectomy is justified. There is also evolving consensus in the literature that among patients without palpable inguinal adenopathy with stage T2–3 tumors as well as those exhibiting lymphovascular invasion (LVI) or poorly differentiated tumors (without invasion of the corpora cavernosum or spongiousum) should still also undergo inguinal staging procedures.

However, there is also significant agreement that in patients with stage Tis, Ta, and T1 tumors without LVI, without poorly differentiated disease and with the absence of palpable adenopathy that careful surveillance without immediate lymphadenectomy is a rational strategy as the incidence of metastasis is less than 10% under these conditions. Patients identified with pathologic extranodal extension of cancer, clinically bulky inguinal masses, or pelvic adenopathy have an ominous prognosis with a 5-year survival of 5–15% when treated with surgery alone. *Patients with minimal nodal metastases exhibit the best disease free survival. In contrast, those with extranodal extension of cancer and pelvic lymph node metastases are rarely cured with surgery alone.* Patients with multiple unilateral or bilateral nodes that do not exhibit extranodal extension or pelvic disease form an intermediate prognosis group (N2). Thus, clinical and pathologic staging information not only determines prognosis but forms the basis of integrating systemic chemotherapy or radiation into the treatment regimen for select patients with more advanced disease.

Lymphatic invasion and vascular embolism have been shown to be independent predictors of node involvement (Table 40.1).

**TABLE 40.1.** Lymphatic and vascular embolizations are independent predictive variables of inguinal lymph node involvement in patients with squamous cell carcinoma of the penis

| Variable | HR | 95% CI | P value |
| --- | --- | --- | --- |
| Tumor thickness (5 mm vs. >5 mm) | 1.435 | 0.538–3.833 | 0.47 |
| Pathologic tumor classification (pTa/pT1 vs. pT2 vs. > pT2)[a] | 2.288 | 1.118–4.684 | 0.02 |
| Histologic grade (Grade 1 vs. Grade 2–3) | 4.268 | 1.278–14.364 | 0.01 |
| Venous embolization (absent vs. present) | 5.240 | 1.139–24.101 | 0.03 |
| Lymphatic embolization (absent vs. present) | 6.941 | 1.967–24.498 | 0.003 |

*HR* hazard ratio; *95% CI* 95% confidence interval.

From Ficarra V, Zattoni F, Cunico SC, et al. Lymphatic and vascular embolizations are independent predictive variables of inguinal lymph node involvement in patients with squamous cell carcinoma of the penis: Gruppo Uro-Oncologico del Nord Est (Northeast Uro-Oncological Group) Penile Cancer data base data. Cancer. 2005;103:2507–6, with permission of Wiley.

[a] According to the 1997 classification TNM system.

The multiple variables in addition to anatomic stage that have been proposed as prognostic in penile carcinoma have been recently evaluated using an outcomes prediction nomogram tool to define lymph node involvement by Ficarra et al. Their group has proposed the prediction tool shown in Table 40.1 and which was designed and validated in 175 patients from 11 centers in Italy. This tool may serve as a clinically useful adjunct to standard anatomic staging enabling physicians to counsel patients regarding the selection of therapeutic interventions based on risk of clinical recurrence. This model will need to be validated in larger groups of patients prior to widespread implementation.

### Clinical Staging

*Primary Tumor.* Clinical examination by palpation should be performed. Penile imaging studies may occasionally be useful. Histologic confirmation provided by an adequate excisional-incisional biopsy to determine the extent of anatomic invasion, tumor grade, and the presence of lymphovascular invasion is required.

**Regional Lymph Nodes.** Clinical examination by palpation of the inguinal region is required. Computed tomography is a useful adjunct to palpation in patients with palpable inguinal adenopathy or those in whom palpation is unreliable (i.e., obese, prior inguinal surgery)

**Distant Metastasis.** Clinical examination along with cross-sectional imaging and chest radiography should be performed as appropriate.

**Pathologic Staging.** Complete resection of the primary site with appropriate margins is required. Lymphadenectomy is performed in those patients felt to be at significant risk for metastasis by virtue of palpable adenopathy or histopathologic features of the primary tumor. Pathologic confirmation can also be achieved via lymph node biopsy of clinically suspicious lymph nodes. The definitions of primary tumor (T) for Ta, T1, T2, T3, and T4 are illustrated in Figures 40.1–40.5.

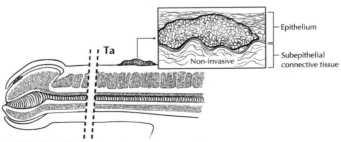

**FIGURE 40.1.** Ta: Noninvasive verrucous carcinoma.

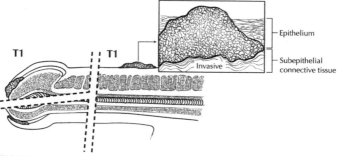

**FIGURE 40.2.** T1: Tumor invading subepithelial connective tissue; T1a: no vascular invasion and not poorly differentiated; and T1b: high grade and/or poorly differentiated.

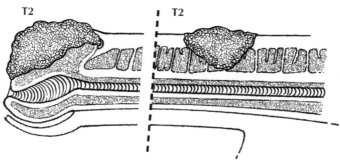

**FIGURE 40.3.** T2: Tumor invading corpus spongiosum or cavernosum.

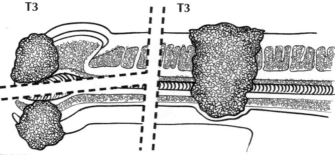

**FIGURE 40.4.** T3: Tumor invading urethra.

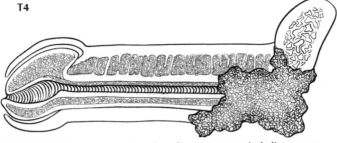

**FIGURE 40.5.** T4: Tumor invading other adjacent structures including prostate.

## DEFINITIONS OF TNM

*Primary Tumor (T)*

| | |
|---|---|
| TX | Primary tumor cannot be assessed |
| T0 | No evidence of primary tumor |
| Tis | Carcinoma in situ |
| Ta | Noninvasive verrucous carcinoma* |
| T1a | Tumor invades subepithelial connective tissue without lymph vascular invasion and is not poorly differentiated (i.e., grade 3–4) |
| T1b | Tumor invades subepithelial connective tissue with lymph vascular invasion or is poorly differentiated |
| T2 | Tumor invades corpus spongiosum or cavernosum |
| T3 | Tumor invades urethra |
| T4 | Tumor invades other adjacent structures |

*Note: Broad pushing penetration (invasion) is permitted; destructive invasion is against this diagnosis.

*Regional Lymph Nodes (N)*

*Clinical Stage Definition\**

| | |
|---|---|
| cNX | Regional lymph nodes cannot be assessed |
| cN0 | No palpable or visibly enlarged inguinal lymph nodes |
| cN1 | Palpable mobile unilateral inguinal lymph node |
| cN2 | Palpable mobile multiple or bilateral inguinal lymph nodes |
| cN3 | Palpable fixed inguinal nodal mass or pelvic lymphadenopathy unilateral or bilateral |

*Note: Clinical stage definition based on palpation, imaging.

*Pathologic Stage Definition\**

| | |
|---|---|
| pNX | Regional lymph nodes cannot be assessed |
| pN0 | No regional lymph node metastasis |
| pN1 | Metastasis in a single inguinal lymph node |
| pN2 | Metastasis in multiple or bilateral inguinal lymph nodes |
| pN3 | Extranodal extension of lymph node metastasis or pelvic lymph node(s) unilateral or bilateral |

*Note: Pathologic stage definition based on biopsy or surgical excision.

*Distant Metastasis (M)*

M0   No distant metastasis

M1   Distant metastasis*

*Note*: Lymph node metastasis outside of the true pelvis in addition to visceral or bone sites.

**Additional Descriptor.**   The m suffix indicates the presence of multiple primary tumors and is recorded in parentheses – e.g., pTa (m) N0M0.

## ANATOMIC STAGE/PROGNOSTIC GROUPS

| Stage | T | N | M |
|---|---|---|---|
| Stage 0 | Tis | N0 | M0 |
|  | Ta | N0 | M0 |
| Stage I | T1a | N0 | M0 |
| Stage II | T1b | N0 | M0 |
|  | T2 | N0 | M0 |
|  | T3 | N0 | M0 |
| Stage IIIa | T1-3 | N1 | M0 |
| Stage IIIb | T1-3 | N2 | M0 |
| Stage IV | T4 | Any N | M0 |
|  | Any T | N3 | M0 |
|  | Any T | Any N | M1 |

## PROGNOSTIC FACTORS (SITE-SPECIFIC FACTORS)
### (Recommended for Collection)

| | |
|---|---|
| Required for staging | None |
| Clinically significant | Involvement of corpus spongiosum |
|  | Involvement of corpus cavernosum |
|  | Percent of tumor that is poorly differentiated |
|  | Verrucous carcinoma depth of invasion |
|  | Size of largest lymph node metastasis |
|  | Extranodal/extracapsular extension |
|  | HPV status |

## HISTOLOGIC GRADE (G)

Grade is reported in registry systems by the grade value. A two-grade, three-grade, or four-grade system may be used. If a grading system is not specified, generally the following system is used:

GX   Grade cannot be assessed

G1   Well differentiated

G2   Moderately differentiated

G3   Poorly differentiated

G4   Undifferentiated

## HISTOPATHOLOGIC TYPE

Cell types are limited to carcinomas.
Squamous cell carcinoma, not otherwise specified
Verrucous carcinoma
Papillary squamous carcinoma
Warty squamous carcinoma
Basaloid carcinoma

## BIBLIOGRAPHY

Aynaud O, Ionesco M, Barrasso R. Penile intraepithelial neoplasia: specific clinical features correlate with histologic and virologic findings. Cancer. 1994;74: 1762–7.

Clemente CD. Anatomy: a regional atlas of the human body. Philadelphia, PA: Lea & Fibiger; 1975.

Cubilla AL, Reuter VE, Gregoire L, et al. Basaloid squamous cell carcinoma: a distinctive human papilloma virus-related penile neoplasm. Am J Surg Pathol. 1998;22:755–61.

Cubilla AL, Reuter V, Velasquez E, Piris A, Saito S, Young RH. Histologic classification of penile carcinoma and its relation to outcome in 61 patients with primary resection. Int J Surg Pathol. 2001;9(2):111–20.

Ficarra V, Zattoni F, Artibani W, et al. G.U.O.N.E. Penile Cancer Project members: nomogram predictive of pathological inguinal lymph node involvement in patients with squamous cell carcinoma of the penis. J Urol. 2006;175:1700–5.

Fraley EE, Zhang G, Manivel C, Niehans GA. The role of ilioinguinal lymphadenectomy and significance of histological differentiation in treatment of carcinoma of the penis. J Urol. 1989;142:1478.

Horenblas S, van Tinteren H. Squamous cell carcinoma of the penis. IV. Prognostic factors of survival: analysis of tumors, nodes and metastasis classification system. J Urol. 1994;151:1239–43.

Horenblas S, van Tinteren H, Delemarre JFM, Moonen LMF, Lustig V, Kroger R. Squamous cell carcinoma of the penis: accuracy of tumor, nodes and metastasis classification system, and role of lymphangiography, computerized tomography scan and fine needle aspiration cytology. J Urol. 1991;146: 1279–83.

Kattan MW, Ficarra V, Artibani W, Cunico SC, Fandella A, Martignoni G, et al. GUONE Penile Cancer Project members: nomogram predictive of cancer specific survival in patients undergoing partial or total amputation for squamous cell carcinoma of the penis. J Urol. 2006;175:2103–8.

Lont AP, Besnard APE, Gallee MPW, van Tinteren H, Horenblas S. A comparison of physical examination and imaging in determining the extent of primary penile carcinoma. BJU Int. 2003;91:493–5.

Lopes A, Hidalgo GS, Kowalski LP, et al. Prognostic factors in carcinoma of the penis: multivariate analysis of 145 patients treated with amputation and lymphadenectomy. J Urol. 1996;156:1637–42.

McDougal WS, Kirchner FKJ, Edwards RH, Killion LT. Treatment of carcinoma of the penis in a case of primary lymphadenectomy. J Urol. 1986;136:38.

Pettaway CA, Lynch DF, Davis JW. Campbell's urology. In: Kavoussi LR, Novick AC, Partin AW, Peters CA, Wein AJ, editors. 9th ed. Tumors of the penis. Philadelphia, PA: Saunders Elsevier; 2007. Chapter 31, p. 959–92.

Ravi R. Correlation between the extent of nodal involvement and survival following groin dissection for carcinoma of the penis. Br J Urol. 1993;72(5 Part 2):817–9.

Slaton JW, Morgenstern N, Levy DA, Santos MW Jr, Tamboli P, Ro JY, Ayala AG, Pettaway CA. Tumor stage, vascular invasion, and the percentage of poorly differentiated cancer: independent prognosticators for inguinal lymph node metastasis in penile squamous. J Urol. 2001;165:1138–42.

Solsona E, Algaba F, Horenblas S, Pizzocaro G, Windahl T. EAU guidelines on penile cancer. Eur Urol. 2004;46:1–8.

Srinivas V, Morse MJ, Herr HW, Sogani PC, Whitmore WF. Penile cancer:-relation of extent of nodal metastasis to survival. J Urol. 1987;137:880–2.

# Prostate

*(Sarcomas and transitional cell carcinomas are
not included)*

## *At-A-Glance*

### SUMMARY OF CHANGES

- Extraprostatic invasion with microscopic bladder neck invasion (T4) is included with T3a

- Gleason Score now recognized as the preferred grading system

- Prognostic factors have been incorporated in the Anatomic Stage/Prognostic Groups

  - Gleason Score

  - Preoperative prostate-specific antigen (PSA)

### ANATOMIC STAGE/PROGNOSTIC GROUPS*

| Group | T | N | M | PSA | Gleason |
|---|---|---|---|---|---|
| I | T1a – c | N0 | M0 | PSA < 10 | Gleason ≤ 6 |
| | T2a | N0 | M0 | PSA < 10 | Gleason ≤ 6 |
| | T1 – 2a | N0 | M0 | PSA X | Gleason X |
| IIA | T1a – c | N0 | M0 | PSA < 20 | Gleason 7 |
| | T1a – c | N0 | M0 | PSA ≥ 10 < 20 | Gleason ≤ 6 |
| | T2a | N0 | M0 | PSA < 20 | Gleason ≤ 7 |
| | T2b | N0 | M0 | PSA < 20 | Gleason ≤ 7 |
| | T2b | N0 | M0 | PSA X | Gleason X |
| IIB | T2c | N0 | M0 | Any PSA | Any Gleason |
| | T1 – 2 | N0 | M0 | PSA ≥ 20 | Any Gleason |
| | T1 – 2 | N0 | M0 | Any PSA | Gleason ≥ 8 |
| III | T3a – b | N0 | M0 | Any PSA | Any Gleason |
| IV | T4 | N0 | M0 | Any PSA | Any Gleason |
| | Any T | N1 | M0 | Any PSA | Any Gleason |
| | Any T | Any N | M1 | Any PSA | Any Gleason |

*When either PSA or Gleason is not available, grouping should be determined by T stage and/or either PSA or Gleason as available.

ICD-O-3
TOPOGRAPHY
CODES
C61.9    Prostate gland

ICD-O-3 HISTOLOGY
CODE RANGES
8000–8110, 8140–8576,
8940–8950, 8980–8981

## INTRODUCTION

Prostate cancer is the most common noncutaneous cancer in men, with increasing incidence in older age groups. Prostate cancer has a tendency to metastasize to bone. Earlier detection is possible with a blood test, prostate-specific antigen (PSA), and the diagnosis is generally made using transrectal ultrasound (TRUS) guided biopsy.

The incidence of both clinical and latent carcinoma increases with age. However, this cancer is rarely diagnosed clinically in men under 40 years of age. There are substantial limitations in the ability of both digital rectal examination (DRE) and TRUS to precisely define the size or local extent of disease; DRE is currently the most common modality used to define the local stage. Heterogeneity within the T1c category resulting from inherent limitations of either DRE or imaging to quantify the cancer may be balanced by the inclusion of other prognostic factors, such as histologic grade, PSA level, and possibly extent of cancer on needle biopsies that contain cancer. Diagnosis of clinically suspicious areas of the prostate can be confirmed histologically by needle biopsy. Less commonly, prostate cancer may be diagnosed by inspection of the resected tissue from a transurethral resection of the prostate (TURP) for obstructive voiding symptoms.

In the seventh edition of AJCC staging for prostate cancer, a few major changes have been made. The stage classification of true bladder neck invasion in prostate cancer has been an issue of controversy due to its uncommon occurrence and less well-defined clinical course. In the sixth edition (2002) of AJCC staging it was assigned to stage pT4. Several recent studies have demonstrated that bladder neck invasion is not an independent prognostic factor and that clinical outcome is likely to be better than in cases with seminal vesicle invasion, thus underscoring the necessity of classifying bladder neck invasion as pT3a disease rather than pT4 disease.

In the sixth edition of AJCC staging, the subclassification of pT2 was reverted to the scheme utilized in the fourth edition. Several recent studies including very large cohorts of patients have failed to demonstrate a significant prognostic difference between substages of pT2a vs. pT2b; some studies also show conflicting data on the prognostic significance of pT2c disease. For the seventh edition we have opted to retain the same schemata as the sixth edition to allow for accumulation of more data to address this issue. For the cT2 staging there are limited data in radiation-treated patients that justify maintaining the stratification as proposed currently.

TNM staging, particularly for organ-confined prostate cancers, had limitations. The sixth edition Stage Groups encompassed a wide variety of patients in this heterogenous disease process. Several prognostic parameters including preoperative PSA levels, tumor volume (number of positive biopsy cores and length or percentage of cancer), and Gleason score have been incorporated into predictive nomograms and integrated algorithms. These tables and tools play an important role in patient counseling and attempt to individualize patient prognosis based on a number of data points. For this seventh edition of AJCC staging, we have maintained the core paradigm of TNM staging and have modified prognostic grouping categories based on clinical tumor stage, pretreatment serum PSA, and Gleason score. Major professional groups already employ PSA and Gleason score to define treatment for patients with T1 and T2, organ confined disease, as evidenced by the treatment guidelines of the National Comprehensive Cancer Network (NCCN) and the American Urological Association (AUA).

## ANATOMY

**Primary Site.** Adenocarcinoma of the prostate most commonly arises within the peripheral zone of the gland, where it may be amenable to detection by DRE. A less common site of origin is the anteromedial prostate, the transition zone, which is remote from the rectal surface and is the site of origin of benign nodular hyperplasia. The central zone, which makes up most of the base of the prostate, seldom is the source of cancer but is often invaded by the spread of larger cancers. Pathologically, cancers of the prostate are often multifocal; 80–85% arise from peripheral zone, 10–15% from transitional zone, and 5–10% from central zone.

The histologic grade of the prostate cancer is important for prognosis. The histopathologic grading of these tumors can be complex because of the morphologic heterogeneity of prostate cancer and its inherent tendency to be multifocal. There have been many grading schemes proposed for prostate cancer. However, the scoring system for assessing this histologic pattern or prostate cancer with the highest reproducibility and best validation in relation to outcome is the Gleason score. This is now considered the grading scheme of choice and should be utilized in assessing all cases of prostate cancer.

**Regional Lymph Nodes.** The regional lymph nodes are the nodes of the true pelvis, which essentially are the pelvic nodes below the bifurcation of the common iliac arteries. They include the following groups:

Pelvic, NOS
Hypogastric
Obturator
Iliac (internal, external, or NOS)
Sacral (lateral, presacral, promontory [Gerota's], or NOS)

Laterality does not affect the N classification.

**Distant Lymph Nodes.** Distant lymph nodes lie outside the confines of the true pelvis. They can be imaged using ultrasound, computed tomography, magnetic resonance imaging, or lymphangiography. Although enlarged lymph nodes can occasionally be visualized on radiographic imaging, fewer patients are initially discovered with clinically evident metastatic disease. In lower risk patients, imaging tests have proven unhelpful. In lieu of imaging, risk tables are many times used to determine individual patient risk of nodal involvement prior to therapy. Involvement of distant lymph nodes is classified as M1a. The distant lymph nodes include the following:

Aortic (para-aortic lumbar)
Common iliac
Inguinal, deep
Superficial inguinal (femoral)

Supraclavicular
Cervical
Scalene
Retroperitoneal, NOS

**Metastatic Sites.** Osteoblastic metastases are the most common nonnodal site of prostate cancer metastasis. In addition, this tumor can spread to distant lymph nodes. Lung and liver metastases are usually identified late in the course of the disease.

## RULES FOR CLASSIFICATION

**Clinical Staging.** Primary tumor assessment includes digital rectal examination of the prostate and histologic or cytologic confirmation of prostate carcinoma. All information available before the first definitive treatment may be used for clinical staging. Imaging techniques may be valuable in some cases; TRUS is the most commonly used imaging tool, but it has a poor ability to identify tumor location and extent. Tumor that is found in one or both lobes by needle biopsy, but is not palpable or visible by imaging, is classified as T1c. Considerable uncertainty exists about the ability of imaging to define the extent of a nonpalpable lesion (see the definition of T1c below). For research purposes, investigators should specify whether clinical staging into the T1c category is based on DRE only or on DRE plus TRUS. In general, most patients diagnosed in an environment of ubiquitous PSA screening will be at a low risk of positive nodes or metastases, and the risk of false-positive imaging studies in asymptomatic patients has exceeded the frequency of true-positive or true-negative studies in several reports. For this reason, in patients with Gleason scores less than 7 and PSA values <20 ng/ml, imaging studies will oftentimes not be helpful in staging and should not be routinely performed.

If either the DRE or PSA test suggests neoplasm, a transrectal ultrasound-guided needle biopsy of the prostate gland is usually performed in healthy men suspected of as having prostate cancer. Alternatively, prostate cancer may be found in the tissue obtained during a transurethral resection of the prostate (TURP), although this procedure is becoming less common. Recent studies, however, support the notion that there are few clinical differences in outcome for patients with T1c compared to T2a. The major value of maintaining the category defined as T1c appears to be that it helps to define the clinical circumstances that resulted in a diagnosis being made (i.e., screening) and the lack of palpable disease. The distinction between T1c by palpation and T2a based on imaging is problematic however, because of (1) inconsistent use of imaging as a clinical staging tool, (2) interobserver variability of imaging modalities, and (3) the lack of sensitivity and specificity of imaging technologies.

The digital rectal examination (DRE) is still considered the "gold standard" for staging although it is insensitive for detecting extracapsular tumor extension. Although imaging could one day potentially improve clinical staging accuracy, interobserver reproducibility, problems with patient selection and contradictory results have limited the utility of imaging in clinical staging, and imaging alone cannot replace the DRE as the clinical staging standard. Transrectal ultrasound (TRUS) has not been proven to be satisfactory for predicting extracapsular extension. Color Doppler and power Doppler identify increased vascularity but have not yet been shown to improve staging accuracy. Similarly, contrast-enhanced and 3D US has not yet been tested or shown to improve the delineation of the cancer and prostate capsule. Endorectal coil magnetic resonance imaging MRI (erMRI) provides high spatial resolution. Three major techniques that have been used to stage prostate cancer with MRI are T2 weighted MRI, MR spectroscopic imaging (MRSI), and dynamic contrast-enhanced MRI (DCE-MRI). None of these approaches have been proven to be consistently helpful in staging attempts. Since the significant weight of the clinical data utilizes DRE, it remains the critical component of clinical staging.

**Pathologic Staging.** Documenting and reporting pathologic staging parameters in radical prostatectomy specimens is a key component in providing optimal management for patients.

In general, total prostatectomy including regional lymph node dissection with full histologic evaluation is required for complete pathologic classification. However, under certain circumstances, pathologic T classification can be determined with other means. For example, (1) positive biopsy of the rectum permits a pT4 classification without prostatectomy, and (2) a biopsy revealing carcinoma in extraprostatic soft tissue permits a pT3 classification, as does a biopsy revealing adenocarcinoma infiltrating the seminal vesicles. There is no pT1 category because there is insufficient tissue to assess the highest pT category.

In addition to pathologic stage, independent prognostic factors for survival have been identified for prostate cancer. These include number of positive biopsy cores, comorbid illnesses, Gleason score, serum PSA, and surgical margin status.

It is of relevance to review studies assessing the practicality and prognostic significance of previous versions of the AJCC system with respect to prostate cancer particularly in terms of the clinical and pathological sub staging of pT2, pT3, and pT4 subgroups.

*pT2.* The sixth edition of the AJCC TNM staging system subdivides pT2 disease into three categories pT2a, pT2b, pT2c as determined by involvement of one half of one side, more than one half of one side, and involvement of both sides of the prostate gland. This system has been relied upon as a broad surrogate to describe cancer volume, which can be correlated to risk of clinical relapse. Several retrospective outcome data analyses have challenged the utility of this subdivision and these data sets were reviewed during the creation of the seventh edition of the AJCC pathologic staging system. Insufficient evidence was found to justify collapsing pT2a and pT2b stages into a single stage, and in fact conflicting results exist in the currently available literature. No data exist to allow correlation of PT2 stage subgroupings with survival in localized prostate cancer due to the indolent and prolonged clinical course of the disease. Continued follow-up and analysis of large multi-institutional data sets and central cancer registry data is encouraged to allow resolution of this question in future versions of the TNM system.

***pT3.*** The sixth edition of the AJCC TNM staging system subdivides pT3 disease into two categories pT3a and pT3b as determined by the presence of extracapsular invasion in any location and presence of seminal vesical invasion with or without extracapsular invasion. The 1992 version of the AJCC TNM system (fifth edition) subdivided patients with extracapsular extension into either unilateral or bilateral and separated seminal vesicle involvement. Several retrospective outcome data analyses have challenged the utility of eliminating this subdivision in the subsequent sixth edition. A thorough review of these analyses has revealed conflicting evidence regarding the correlation of subdividing unilateral and bilateral extracapsular extension and biochemical recurrence rates following surgery. Again, definitive data do not exist to allow correlation of particular pT3 stage subgroupings with survival in localized prostate cancer, and a reversion to the previous subdividing classification was not made. Data continue to be accumulated in the NCDB and other institutional databases to help determine the pT3 staging system.

***pT4.*** In the sixth edition of the AJCC TNM system pathologic T4 substage included patients with microscopic finding of bladder invasion. Four large retrospective analyses have addressed this issue, and each series has revealed that microscopic involvement of the bladder neck tissue by prostate cancer does not independently predict a significantly worse prognosis than extracapsular extension in general. Therefore, microscopic bladder neck invasion will now be considered within the category of pT3a.

**Surgical Margin Status.** Perhaps one of the more extensively debated aspects of pathologic staging and risk stratification is one that is technically not an element of the current AJCC TNM staging system, namely the status of surgical resection margins in radical prostatectomy specimens. There is controversy regarding the "parameters or elements" to be reported in the case of identifying positive surgical margins in resected glands. While most agree that the pT stage regardless of the margin status needs to be documented, there is no consensus on what aspects of surgical margin involvement are important to report. Although the status of surgical margins per se is not an element, the prognostic importance of the phenomenon including its potential impact for further postsurgical treatment and outcome is an important prognostic factor. In reporting pathologic results of prostatectomy specimens pT stage should be reported along with margin status and a positive surgical margin should be indicated by an R1 descriptor (residual microscopic disease) as is currently the case.

## PROGNOSTIC FEATURES

An increasing number of proposed molecular markers (such as ploidy, p53, and bcl-2) as well as other clinical features have been identified that may predict stage at diagnosis and outcomes following therapy. A number of algorithms have been published that enable the merging of these data to predict local stage, risk of positive nodes, or risk of treatment failure. Each of these predictive tools employ common as well as unique variables and vary in their evaluation technique. Within the confines of the TNM staging, the clinical predictors of serum prostate-specific antigen, Gleason score, and tumor stage all have a clear, recognized, and significant impact on prognosis.

Recent studies have demonstrated that Gleason score provides extremely important information about prognosis. In an analysis, conducted by the Radiation Therapy Oncology Group (RTOG), of nearly 1,500 men treated on prospective randomized trials, Gleason score was the single most important predictor of death from prostate cancer. Combined with the AJCC stage, investigators demonstrated that four prognostic subgroups could be identified that allowed disease-specific survival to be predicted at 5, 10, and 15 years. Additional studies conducted by the RTOG also demonstrated that a pretreatment PSA > 20 ng/ml predicts a greater likelihood of distant failure and a greater need for hormonal therapy. A recent validation study confirmed that a PSA > 20 ng/ml was associated with a greater risk of prostate cancer death.

Thus, in addition to the AJCC clinical stage, pretreatment PSA and Gleason score provide important prognostic information that might affect decisions regarding therapy. In an attempt to better stratify these patients compared to the previous Stage groups and avoid the large number of patients previously placed in stage group 1, the seventh edition includes a new prognostic staging for clinically localized (T1 and T2) disease that include these clinically based variables. Any type of grouping scheme such as this will not apply equally well to every individual patient situation, and this grouping still is primarily based on anatomic clinical T staging, the crux of the TNM staging historically. Other clinical features as well as pathologic features postprostatectomy, such as the number/percentage of positive biopsies and surgical margin status, likely provide additional prognostic information, and other prognostic tools that go well beyond the TNM structure may be more accurate for an individual patient. As a result, data continue to be collected in the National Cancer Database Registry by registrars to provide long-term confirmatory data on the independent impact of multiple variables on prognosis.

## OUTCOMES BY STAGE, GRADE, AND PSA

A number of endpoints are useful in assessing disease outcomes following therapy. Because the vast majority of patients diagnosed with prostate cancer are diagnosed with clinically localized disease, similar to pretreatment tools, multiple predictive models for clinical outcome have been proposed posttherapy. Biochemical (or PSA)-free recurrence indicates the likelihood that a patient treated for prostate cancer remains free of recurrent disease as manifested by a rising PSA. Prostate cancer-specific survival and overall survival are key endpoints that many studies do not evaluate due to the length of follow-up required. Biochemical failure can be a useful surrogate endpoint to predict risk of death from prostate cancer in patients with a prolonged expected survival; however, the natural history of biochemical failure progressing to clinical disease recurrence is highly variable and may depend on multiple variables including TNM characteristics as well as PSA and PSA kinetics, Gleason sum, treatment modality, and timing of biochemical recurrence. Studies continue to evaluate predictors of ultimate outcome for patients following different therapies.

## DEFINITIONS OF TNM

### Primary Tumor (T)

*Clinical*

| | |
|---|---|
| TX | Primary tumor cannot be assessed |
| T0 | No evidence of primary tumor |
| T1 | Clinically inapparent tumor neither palpable nor visible by imaging |
| T1a | Tumor incidental histologic finding in 5% or less of tissue resected |
| T1b | Tumor incidental histologic finding in more than 5% of tissue resected |
| T1c | Tumor identified by needle biopsy (e.g., because of elevated PSA) |
| T2 | Tumor confined within prostate* |
| T2a | Tumor involves one-half of one lobe or less |
| T2b | Tumor involves more than one-half of one lobe but not both lobes |
| T2c | Tumor involves both lobes |
| T3 | Tumor extends through the prostate capsule** |
| T3a | Extracapsular extension (unilateral or bilateral) |
| T3b | Tumor invades seminal vesicle(s) |
| T4 | Tumor is fixed or invades adjacent structures other than seminal vesicles such as external sphincter, rectum, bladder, levator muscles, and/or pelvic wall (Figure 41.1) |

*Note: Tumor found in one or both lobes by needle biopsy, but not palpable or reliably visible by imaging, is classified as T1c.

**Note: Invasion into the prostatic apex or into (but not beyond) the prostatic capsule is classified not as T3 but as T2.

### Pathologic (pT)*

| | |
|---|---|
| pT2 | Organ confined |
| pT2a | Unilateral, one-half of one side or less |
| pT2b | Unilateral, involving more than one-half of side but not both sides |
| pT2c | Bilateral disease |
| pT3 | Extraprostatic extension |
| pT3a | Extraprostatic extension or microscopic invasion of bladder neck** |
| pT3b | Seminal vesicle invasion |
| pT4 | Invasion of rectum, levator muscles, and /or pelvic wall |

*Note: There is no pathologic T1 classification.

**Note: Positive surgical margin should be indicated by an R1 descriptor (residual microscopic disease).

**T4**

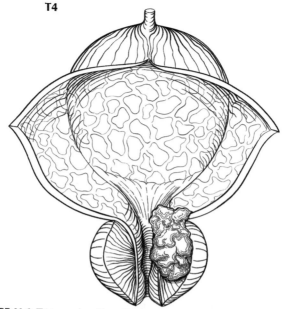

**FIGURE 41.1.** T4 tumor invading adjacent structures other than seminal vesicles, such as bladder, rectum, levator muscles, and/or pelvic wall.

### Regional Lymph Nodes (N)

*Clinical*

| | |
|---|---|
| NX | Regional lymph nodes were not assessed |
| N0 | No regional lymph node metastasis |
| N1 | Metastasis in regional lymph node(s) |

*Pathologic*

| | |
|---|---|
| pNX | Regional nodes not sampled |
| pN0 | No positive regional nodes |
| pN1 | Metastases in regional node(s) |

### Distant Metastasis (M)*

| | |
|---|---|
| M0 | No distant metastasis |
| M1 | Distant metastasis |
| M1a | Nonregional lymph node(s) |
| M1b | Bone(s) |
| M1c | Other site(s) with or without bone disease |

*Note: When more than one site of metastasis is present, the most advanced category is used. pM1c is most advanced.

## ANATOMIC STAGE/PROGNOSTIC GROUPS*

| Group | T | N | M | PSA | Gleason |
|---|---|---|---|---|---|
| I | T1a – c | N0 | M0 | PSA < 10 | Gleason ≤ 6 |
| | T2a | N0 | M0 | PSA < 10 | Gleason ≤ 6 |
| | T1 – 2a | N0 | M0 | PSA X | Gleason X |
| IIA | T1a – c | N0 | M0 | PSA < 20 | Gleason 7 |
| | T1a – c | N0 | M0 | PSA ≥ 10 < 20 | Gleason ≤ 6 |
| | T2a | N0 | M0 | PSA < 20 | Gleason ≤ 7 |
| | T2b | N0 | M0 | PSA < 20 | Gleason ≤ 7 |
| | T2b | N0 | M0 | PSA X | Gleason X |
| IIB | T2c | N0 | M0 | Any PSA | Any Gleason |
| | T1 – 2 | N0 | M0 | PSA ≥ 20 | Any Gleason |
| | T1 – 2 | N0 | M0 | Any PSA | Gleason ≥ 8 |
| III | T3a – b | N0 | M0 | Any PSA | Any Gleason |
| IV | T4 | N0 | M0 | Any PSA | Any Gleason |
| | Any T | N1 | M0 | Any PSA | Any Gleason |
| | Any T | Any N | M1 | Any PSA | Any Gleason |

*When either PSA or Gleason is not available, grouping should be determined by T stage and/or either PSA or Gleason as available.

## PROGNOSTIC FACTORS (SITE-SPECIFIC FACTORS)
### (Recommended for Collection)

| | |
|---|---|
| Required for staging | Prostate-specific antigen |
| | Gleason score |
| Clinically significant | Gleason primary and secondary patterns |
| | Gleason tertiary pattern |
| | Clinical staging procedures performed |
| | Number of biopsy cores examined |
| | Number of biopsy cores positive for cancer |

## HISTOLOGIC GRADE (G)

Gleason score is recommended because as the grading system of choice, it takes into account the inherent morphologic heterogeneity of prostate cancer, and several studies have clearly established its prognostic value. A primary and a secondary pattern (the range of each is 1–5) are assigned and them summed to yield a total score. Scores of 2–10 are thus theoretically possible. The vast majority of newly diagnosed needle biopsy detected prostate cancers are graded Gleason score 6 or above. (If a single pattern of disease is seen, it should be reported as both grades. For example, if a single focus of Gleason pattern 3 disease is seen, it is reported as Gleason score 3 + 3 = 6.) In a radical prostatectomy, if a tertiary pattern is present, it is commented upon but not reflected in the Gleason score. It is recommended that radical prostatectomy specimens should be processed in an organized fashion where a determination can be made of a dominant nodule or separate tumor nodules. If a dominant nodule/s is present, the Gleason score of this nodule should be separately mentioned as this nodule is often the focus with highest grade and/or stage of disease.

| | |
|---|---|
| Gleason X | Gleason score cannot be processed |
| Gleason ≤6 | Well differentiated (slight anaplasia) |
| Gleason 7 | Moderately differentiated (moderate anaplasia) |
| Gleason 8–10 | Poorly differentiated/undifferentiated (marked anaplasia) |

**41**

## HISTOPATHOLOGIC TYPE

This classification applies to adenocarcinomas and squamous carcinomas, but not to sarcoma or transitional cell (urothelial) carcinoma of the prostate. Adjectives used to describe histologic variants of adenocarcinomas of prostate include mucinous, signet ring cell, ductal, and neuroendocrine including small cell carcinoma. Transitional cell (urothelial) carcinoma of the prostate is classified as a urethral tumor (see Chap. 46). There should be histologic confirmation of the disease.

## BIBLIOGRAPHY

Aihara M, Wheeler TM, Ohori M, et al. Heterogeneity of prostate cancer in radical prostatectomy specimens. Urology. 1994;43:60–7.

Albertsen PC, Fryback DG, Storer BE, et al. Long-term survival among men with conservatively treated localized prostate cancer. JAMA. 1995;274:626–31.

Albertsen PC, Hanley JA, Gleason DF, Barry MJ. Competing risk analysis of men aged 55 to 74 years at diagnosis managed conservatively for clinically localized prostate cancer. JAMA. 1998;280(11):975–80.

Albertsen PC, Hanley JA, Harlan LC, Gilliland FD, Hamilton A, Liff JM, et al. The positive yield of imaging studies in the evaluation of men with newly diagnosed prostate cancer: a population-based analysis. J Urol. 2000;163(4): 1138–43.

Armatys SA, Koch MO, Bihrle R, Gardner TA, Cheng L. Is it necessary to separate clinical stage T1c from T2 prostate adenocarcinoma? BJU Int. 2005;96(6): 777–80.

Bahnson RR, Hanks GE, Huben RP, et al. NCCN practice guidelines for prostate cancer. Oncology. 2000;14:111–9.

Bazinet M, Meshref AW, Trudel C, Aronson S, et al. Prospective evaluation of prostate-specific antigen density and systematic biopsies for early detection of prostatic carcinoma. Urology. 1994;43:44–52.

Billis A, et al. Prostate cancer with bladder neck involvement: pathologic findings with application of a new practical method for tumor extent evaluation and recurrence-free survival after radical prostatectomy. Int Urol Nephrol. 2004;36(3):363–8.

Blute ML, Bergstralh EJ, Partin AW, et al. Validation of Partin tables for predicting pathological stage of clinically localized prostate cancer. J Urol. 2000;64(5): 1591–5.

Bostwick DG. Staging prostate cancer – 1997: current methods and limitations. Eur Urol. 1997;32 Suppl 3:2–14.

Cagiannos I, Graefen M, Karakiewicz PI, et al. Analysis of clinical stage T2 prostate cancer: do current subclassifications represent an improvement? J Clin Oncol. 2002;20(8):2025–30.

Campbell T, Blasko J, Crawford ED, et al. Clinical staging of prostate cancer: reproducibility and clarification of issues. Int J Cancer. 2001;96(3):198–209.

Carroll P, Coley C, McLeod D, Schellhammer P, Sweat G, Wasson J, Zietman A, Thompson I. Prostate-specific antigen best practice policy. Part II: prostate cancer staging and posttreatment follow-up. Urology. 2001;57:225–9.

Carvalhal GF, Smith DS, Mager DE, Ramos C, Catalona WJ. Digital rectal examination for detecting prostate cancer at prostate-specific antigen levels of 4 ng/ml or less. J Urol. 1999;161(3):835–9.

Carver BS, Bianco FJ Jr, Scardino PT, Eastham JA. Long-term outcome following radical prostatectomy in men with clinical stage T3 prostate cancer. J Urol. 2006;176(2):564–8.

Catalona WJ, Smith DS. Cancer recurrence and survival rates after anatomic radical retropubic prostatectomy for prostate cancer: intermediate-term results. J Urol. 1998;160(6, Part 2):2428–34.

Catalona WJ, Hudson MA, Scardino PT, et al. Selection of optimal prostate-specific antigen cutoffs for early detection of prostate cancer: receiver operating characteristic curves. J Urol. 1994;152:2037–42.

Chodak GW, Thisted RA, Gerber GS, et al. Results of conservative management of clinically localized prostate cancer. N Engl J Med. 1994;330:242–8.

Chuang AY, et al. The significance of positive surgical margin in areas of capsular incision in otherwise organ confined disease at radical prostatectomy. J Urol. 2007;178(4):1306–10.

Chun FK, Briganti A, Lebeau T, Fradet V, Steuber T, Walz J, Schlomm T, Eichelberg C, Haese A, Erbersdobler A, McCormack M, Perrotte P, Graefen M, Huland H, Karakiewicz PI. The 2002 AJCC pT2 substages confer no prognostic information on the rate of biochemical recurrence after radical prostatectomy. Eur Urol. 2006;49(2):273–8; discussion 278–9.

D'Amico AV. Combined-modality staging for localized adenocarcinoma of the prostate. Oncology. 2001;15:1049–59; discussion 1060–2, 1064–5, 1069–70, 1073–5.

Dash A, Sanda MG, Yu M, Taylor JM, Fecko A, Rubin MA. Prostate cancer involving the bladder neck: recurrence-free survival and implications for AJCC staging modification. American Joint Committee on Cancer. Urology. 2002;60(2):276–80.

Epstein JI, Pizov G, Walsh PC. Correlation of pathologic findings with progression after radical retropubic prostatectomy. Cancer. 1993;71:3582–93.

Epstein JI, Partin AW, Sauvageot J, Walsh PC. Prediction of progression following radical prostatectomy: a multivariate analysis of 721 men with long-term follow-up. Am J Surg Path. 1996;20:286.

Epstein JI, Chan DW, Sokoll LJ, Walsh PC, Cox JL, Rittenhouse H, et al. Nonpalpable stage T1c prostate cancer: prediction of insignificant disease using free/total prostate-specific antigen levels and needle biopsy findings. J Urol. 1998;160(6, Part 2):2407–11.

Ferguson JK, Bostwick DG, Suman V, et al. Prostate-specific antigen detected prostate cancer: pathological characteristics of ultrasound visible versus ultrasound invisible tumors. Eur Urol. 1995;27:8–12.

Freedland SJ, et al. Should a positive surgical margin following radical prostatectomy be pathological stage T2 or T3? Results from the SEARCH database. J Urol. 2003;169(6):2142–6.

Freedland SJ, Partin AW, Epstein JI, Walsh PC. Biochemical failure after radical prostatectomy in men with pathologic organ-confined disease: pT2a versus pT2b. Cancer. 2004;100(8):1646–9.

Ghavamian R, Blute ML, Bergstralh EJ, Slezak J, Zincke H. Comparison of clinically nonpalpable prostate-specific antigen-detected (cT1c) versus palpable (cT2) prostate cancers in patients undergoing radical retropubic prostatectomy. Urology. 1999;54(1):105–10.

Grignon DJ, Hammond EH. College of American Pathologists Conference XXVI on clinical relevance of prognostic markers in solid tumors. Arch Pathol Lab Med. 1995;119:1115–21.

Grignon DJ, Sakr WA. Pathologic staging of prostate carcinoma. What are the issues? Cancer. 1996;78(2):337–40.

Han M, Walsh PC, Partin AW, Rodriguez R. Ability of the 1992 and 1997 American Joint Committee on Cancer staging systems for prostate cancer to predict progression-free survival after radical prostatectomy for Stage T2 disease. J Urol. 2000;164(1):89–92.

Henson DE, Hutter RV, Farrow G. Practice protocol for the examination of specimens removed from patients with carcinoma of the prostate gland. Arch Pathol Lab Med. 1994;118:779–83.

Humphrey PA, Frazier HA, Vollmer RT, et al. Stratification of pathologic features in radical prostatectomy specimens that are predictive of elevated initial postoperative serum prostate-specific antigen levels. Cancer. 1992;71:1822–7.

Iyer RV, Hanlon AL, Pinover WH, Hanks GE. Outcome evaluation of the 1997 American Joint Committee on Cancer staging system for prostate carcinoma treated by radiation therapy. Cancer. 1999;85(8):1816–21.

Kausik SJ, et al. Prognostic significance of positive surgical margins in patients with extraprostatic carcinoma after radical prostatectomy. Cancer. 2002;95(6): 1215–9.

May F, Hartung R, Breul J. The ability of the American Joint Committee on Cancer Staging system to predict progression-free survival after radical prostatectomy. BJU Int. 2001;88(7):702–7.

McNeal JE, Villers AA, Redwine EA, et al. Histologic differentiation, cancer volume, and pelvic lymph node metastasis in adenocarcinoma of the prostate. Cancer. 1990;66:1225–33.

Miller GJ. New developments in grading prostate cancer. Semin Urol. 1990;8:9–18.

Montie JE. Staging of prostate cancer: current TNM classifications and future prospects for prognostic factors. Cancer Suppl. 1995;75:1814–18.

Obek C, et al. Positive surgical margins with radical retropubic prostatectomy: anatomic site-specific pathologic analysis and impact on prognosis. Urology. 1999;54(4):682–9.

Optenberg SA, Clark JY, Brawer MK, Thompson IM, Stein CR, Friedrichs P. Development of a decision-making tool to predict risk of prostate cancer: the cancer of the prostate risk index (CAPRI) test. Urology. 1997;50:665–72.

Partin AW, Oesterling JE. The clinical usefulness of prostate-specific antigen: update 1994. J Urol. 1994;152:1358–68.

Pinover WH, Hanlon A, Lee WR, et al. Prostate carcinoma patients upstaged by imaging and treated with irradiation—an outcome-based analysis. Cancer. 1996;77(7):1334–41.

Poulos CK, et al. Bladder neck invasion is an independent predictor of prostate-specific antigen recurrence. Cancer. 2004;101(7):1563–8.

Pound CR, Partin AW, Eisenberger MA, Chan DW, Pearson JD, Walsh PC. Natural history of progression after PSA elevation following radical prostatectomy. JAMA. 1999;281(17):1591–7.

Ramos CG, Carvalhal GF, Smith DS, Mager DE, Catalona WJ. Clinical and pathological characteristics, and recurrence rates of Stage T1c versus T2a or T2b prostate cancer. J Urol. 1999;161(5):1525–9.

Ravery V, Boccon-Gibod L. T3 prostate cancer: how reliable is clinical staging? Semin Urol Oncol. 1997;15(4):202–6.

Rifkin MD, Zerhouni EA, Gatsonis CA, Quint LE, et al. Comparison of magnetic resonance imaging and ultrasonography in staging early prostate cancer: results of a multi-institutional cooperative trial. N Engl J Med. 1990;323:621–5.

Roach M 3rd, Weinberg V, Sandler H, et al. Staging for prostate cancer: time to incorporate pretreatment prostate-specific antigen and Gleason score? Cancer. 2007;109:213–20.

Simon R, Altman DG. Statistical aspects of prognostic factor studies in oncology. Br J Cancer. 1994;69:979–85.

---

Smith DS, Catalona WJ. Interexaminer variability of digital rectal examination in detecting prostate cancer. Urology. 1995;45:70–4.

Southwick PC, Catalona WJ, Partin AW, et al. Prediction of post-radical prostatectomy pathological outcome for Stage T1c prostate cancer with percent free prostate specific antigen: a prospective multicenter clinical trial. J Urol. 1999;162(4):1346–51.

Steuber T, Erbersdobler A, Graefen M, Haese A, Huland H, Karakiewicz PI. Comparative assessment of the 1992 and 2002 pathologic T3 substages for the prediction of biochemical recurrence after radical prostatectomy. Cancer. 2006;06(4):775–82.

Swindle P, et al. Do margins matter? The prognostic significance of positive surgical margins in radical prostatectomy specimens. J Urol. 2005;174(3): 903–7.

Terris MK, McNeal JE, Freiha FS, et al. Efficacy of transrectal ultrasound-guided seminal vesicle biopsies in the detection of seminal vesicle invasion by prostate cancer. J Urol. 1993;149:1035–9.

Thompson I, Thrasher JB, Aus G, et al. Guideline for the management of clinically localized prostate cancer: 2007 update. J Urol. 2007;177:2106–31.

van der Kwast TH, et al. Impact of pathology review of stage and margin status of radical prostatectomy specimens (EORTC trial 22911). Virchows Arch. 2006;449(4):428–34.

Yossepowitch O, Engelstein D, Konichezky M, et al. Bladder neck involvement at radical prostatectomy: positive margins or advanced T4 disease? Urology. 2000;56:448–52.

Yossepowitch O, Sircar K, Scardino PT, Ohori M, Kattan MW, Wheeler TM, et al. Bladder neck involvement in pathological stage pT4 radical prostatectomy specimens is not an independent prognostic factor. J Urol. 2002;168(5): 2011–5.

Zagars GK, von Eschenbach AC. Prostate-specific antigen—an important marker for prostate cancer treated by external beam radiation therapy. Cancer. 1993;72:538–48.

Zincke H, Bergstrahl EJ, Blute ML, et al. Radical prostatectomy for clinically localized prostate cancer: long-term results of 1, 143 patients from a single institution. J Clin Oncol. 1994;12:2254–63.

*At-A-Glance*

---

### SUMMARY OF CHANGES

- The definition of TNM and the Stage Grouping for this chapter have not changed from the Sixth Edition

---

### ANATOMIC STAGE/PROGNOSTIC GROUPS

| Group | T | N | M | S (Serum Tumor Markers) |
|-------|---|---|---|-------------------------|
| Stage 0 | pTis | N0 | M0 | S0 |
| Stage I | pT1–4 | N0 | M0 | SX |
| Stage IA | pT1 | N0 | M0 | S0 |
| Stage IB | pT2 | N0 | M0 | S0 |
| | pT3 | N0 | M0 | S0 |
| | pT4 | N0 | M0 | S0 |
| Stage IS | Any pT/Tx | N0 | M0 | S1–3 (measured post orchiectomy) |
| Stage II | Any pT/Tx | N1–3 | M0 | SX |
| Stage IIA | Any pT/Tx | N1 | M0 | S0 |
| | Any pT/Tx | N1 | M0 | S1 |
| Stage IIB | Any pT/Tx | N2 | M0 | S0 |
| | Any pT/Tx | N2 | M0 | S1 |
| Stage IIC | Any pT/Tx | N3 | M0 | S0 |
| | Any pT/Tx | N3 | M0 | S1 |
| Stage III | Any pT/Tx | Any N | M1 | SX |
| Stage IIIA | Any pT/Tx | Any N | M1a | S0 |
| | Any pT/Tx | Any N | M1a | S1 |
| Stage IIIB | Any pT/Tx | N1–3 | M0 | S2 |
| | Any pT/Tx | Any N | M1a | S2 |
| Stage IIIC | Any pT/Tx | N1–3 | M0 | S3 |
| | Any pT/Tx | Any N | M1a | S3 |
| | Any pT/Tx | Any N | M1b | Any S |

**ICD-O-3 TOPOGRAPHY CODES**

| C62.0 | Undescended testis |
| C62.1 | Descended testis |
| C62.9 | Testis, NOS |

**ICD-O-3 HISTOLOGY CODE RANGES**

8000–8576, 8590–8670, 8940–8950, 8980–8981, 9060–9090, 9100–9105

## INTRODUCTION

Cancers of the testis are usually found in young adults and account for less than 1% of all malignancies in males. However, during the twentieth century, the incidence has more than doubled. Cryptorchidism is a predisposing condition, and other associations include atypical germ cells and multiple atypical nevi. Germ cell tumors of the testis are categorized into two main histologic types: seminomas and nonseminomas. The latter group is composed of either individual or combinations of histologic subtypes, including embryonal carcinoma, teratoma, choriocarcinoma, and yolk sac tumor. The presence of elevation in serum tumor markers, including alpha-fetoprotein (AFP), human chorionic gonadotropin (hCG), and lactate dehydrogenase (LDH), is frequent in this disease. Staging and prognostication are based on determination of the extent of disease and assessment of serum tumor markers. The TNM staging system for male germ cell tumors incorporates serum tumor maker elevation as a separate category of staging information. Cancer of the testis is highly curable, even in cases with advanced, metastatic disease.

Since the sixth edition of the *AJCC Cancer Staging Manual,* there are no changes in anatomic or tumor marker staging that require a change in the AJCC staging for testis cancer.

## ANATOMY

**Primary Site.** The testes are composed of convoluted seminiferous tubules with a stroma containing functional endocrine interstitial cells. Both are encased in a dense capsule, the tunica albuginea, with fibrous septa extending into the testis and separating them into lobules. The tubules converge and exit at the mediastinum of the testis into the rete testis and efferent ducts, which join a single duct. This duct – the epididymis – coils outside the upper and lower poles of the testicle and then joins the vas deferens, a muscular conduit that accompanies the vessels and lymphatic channels of the spermatic cord. The major route for local extension of cancer is through the lymphatic channels. The tumor emerges from the mediastinum of the testis and courses through the spermatic cord. Occasionally, the epididymis is invaded early, and then the external iliac nodes may become involved. If there has been previous scrotal or inguinal surgery or if invasion of the scrotal wall is found (though this is rare), then the lymphatic spread may be to inguinal nodes.

**Regional Lymph Nodes.** The following nodes are considered regional:

    Interaortocaval
    Para-aortic (periaortic)
    Paracaval
    Preaortic
    Precaval
    Retroaortic
    Retrocaval

The left and right testicles demonstrate different patterns of primary drainage that mirror the differences in venous drainage. The left testicle primarily drains to the paraaortic lymph nodes and the right testicle primarily drains to the interaortocaval lymph nodes. The intrapelvic, external iliac, and inguinal nodes are considered regional only after scrotal or inguinal surgery prior to the presentation of the testis tumor. All nodes outside the regional nodes are distant. Nodes along the spermatic vein are considered regional.

**Metastatic Sites.** Distant spread of testicular tumors occurs most commonly to the lymph nodes, followed by metastases to the lung, liver, bone, and other visceral sites. Stage is dependent on the extent of disease and on the determination of serum tumor markers. Extent of disease includes assessment for involvement and size of regional lymph nodes, evidence of disease in nonregional lymph nodes, and metastases to pulmonary and nonpulmonary visceral sites. The stage is subdivided on the basis of the presence and degree of elevation of serum tumor markers. Serum tumor markers are measured immediately after orchiectomy and, if elevated, should be measured serially after orchiectomy to determine whether normal decay curves are followed. The physiological half-life of AFP is 5–7 days, and the half-life of HCG is 24–48 h. The presence of prolonged half-life times implies the presence of residual disease after orchiectomy. It should be noted that in some cases, tumor marker release may occur (e.g., in response to chemotherapy or handling of a primary tumor intraoperatively) and may cause artificial elevation of circulating tumor marker levels. The serum level of LDH has prognostic value in patients with metastatic disease and is included for staging.

## RULES FOR CLASSIFICATION

**Clinical Staging.** Staging of testis tumors includes determination of the T, N, M, and S categories. Clinical examination and histologic assessment are required for clinical staging. Radiographic assessment of the chest, abdomen, and pelvis is necessary to determine the N and M status of disease. Serum tumor markers, including AFP, hCG, and LDH, should be obtained prior to orchiectomy to complete the status of the serum tumor markers (S). The only exception is for stage grouping classification of Stage IS in which persistent elevation of serum tumor markers following orchiectomy is required.

**Pathologic Staging.** Histologic evaluation of the radical orchiectomy specimen must be used for the pT classification. The gross size of the tumor should be recorded. Careful gross examination should determine whether the tumor is intra- or extratesticular. If intratesticular, it should be determined whether the tumor extends through the tunica albuginea and whether it invades the epididymis and/or spermatic cord. Tissue sections should document these findings. The tumor should be sampled extensively, including all grossly diverse areas (hemorrhagic, mucoid, solid, cystic, etc.).

The junction of tumor and nonneoplastic testis and at least one section remote from the tumor should be obtained to determine whether intratubular germ cell neoplasia (carcinoma in situ) is present. These sections will allow assessment of either the presence or absence of vascular invasion. If possible, most tissue sections should include overlying tunica albuginea. Small tumors (2 cm or less) may be submitted in toto. In larger tumors, a sufficient amount of tissue should be sampled, perhaps one section for each 1 or 2 cm of maximum tumor diameter.

The specimens from a defined node-bearing area (such as retroperitoneal lymph node dissection) must be used for the pN classification. Retroperitoneal lymph node dissection should be oriented by the surgeon. All lymph nodes should be dissected, and the diameters of the largest nodes should be recorded, along with the number of lymph nodes involved by tumor. Extranodal soft tissue extension of disease should be noted, if present. It is important to examine carefully and liberally sample the specimen, including cystic, fibrotic, hemorrhagic, necrotic, and solid areas. Laterality does not affect the N classification. In posttreatment specimens, it may be difficult to distinguish individual lymph nodes. The definitions for primary tumor (T) for pT2 and pT3 are illustrated in Figures 42.1 and 42.2.

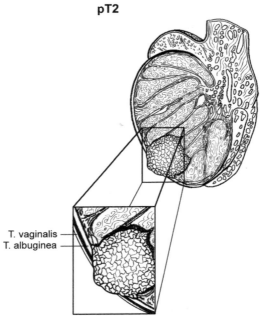

**pT2**

T. vaginalis
T. albuginea

**FIGURE 42.1.** pT2 Tumor extending through the tunica albuginea with involvement of the tunica vaginalis.

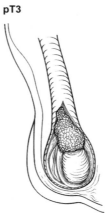

**pT3**

**FIGURE 42.2.** pT3 Tumor invades the spermatic cord.

## DEFINITIONS OF TNM

### *Primary Tumor (T)**

The extent of primary tumor is usually classified after radical orchiectomy, and for this reason, a *pathologic* stage is assigned.

pTX     Primary tumor cannot be assessed

pT0     No evidence of primary tumor (e.g., histologic scar in testis)

pTis     Intratubular germ cell neoplasia (carcinoma in situ)

pT1     Tumor limited to the testis and epididymis without vascular/lymphatic invasion; tumor may invade into the tunica albuginea but not the tunica vaginalis

pT2     Tumor limited to the testis and epididymis with vascular/lymphatic invasion, or tumor extending through the tunica albuginea with involvement of the tunica vaginalis

pT3     Tumor invades the spermatic cord with or without vascular/lymphatic invasion

pT4     Tumor invades the scrotum with or without vascular/lymphatic invasion

*Note*: Except for pTis and pT4, extent of primary tumor is classified by radical orchiectomy. TX may be used for other categories in the absence of radical orchiectomy.

### *Regional Lymph Nodes (N)*

*Clinical*

NX     Regional lymph nodes cannot be assessed

N0     No regional lymph node metastasis

N1     Metastasis with a lymph node mass 2 cm or less in greatest dimension; or multiple lymph nodes, none more than 2 cm in greatest dimension

### Regional Lymph Nodes (N) (continued)

N2   Metastasis with a lymph node mass more than 2 cm but not more than 5 cm in greatest dimension; or multiple lymph nodes, any one mass greater than 2 cm but not more than 5 cm in greatest dimension

N3   Metastasis with a lymph node mass more than 5 cm in greatest dimension

*Pathologic (pN)*

pNX   Regional lymph nodes cannot be assessed

pN0   No regional lymph node metastasis

pN1   Metastasis with a lymph node mass 2 cm or less in greatest dimension and less than or equal to five nodes positive, none more than 2 cm in greatest dimension

pN2   Metastasis with a lymph node mass more than 2 cm but not more than 5 cm in greatest dimension; or more than five nodes positive, none more than 5 cm; or evidence of extranodal extension of tumor

pN3   Metastasis with a lymph node mass more than 5 cm in greatest dimension

### Distant Metastasis (M)

M0    No distant metastasis

M1    Distant metastasis

M1a   Nonregional nodal or pulmonary metastasis

M1b   Distant metastasis other than to nonregional lymph nodes and lung

### ANATOMIC STAGE/PROGNOSTIC GROUPS

| Group | T | N | M | S (Serum Tumor Markers) |
|---|---|---|---|---|
| Stage 0 | pTis | N0 | M0 | S0 |
| Stage I | pT1–4 | N0 | M0 | SX |
| Stage IA | pT1 | N0 | M0 | S0 |
| Stage IB | pT2 | N0 | M0 | S0 |
| | pT3 | N0 | M0 | S0 |
| | pT4 | N0 | M0 | S0 |
| Stage IS | Any pT/Tx | N0 | M0 | S1–3 (measured post orchiectomy) |
| Stage II | Any pT/Tx | N1–3 | M0 | SX |
| Stage IIA | Any pT/Tx | N1 | M0 | S0 |
| | Any pT/Tx | N1 | M0 | S1 |
| Stage IIB | Any pT/Tx | N2 | M0 | S0 |
| | Any pT/Tx | N2 | M0 | S1 |
| Stage IIC | Any pT/Tx | N3 | M0 | S0 |
| | Any pT/Tx | N3 | M0 | S1 |

| Stage III | Any pT/Tx | Any N | M1 | SX |
|-----------|-----------|-------|-----|-----|
| Stage IIIA | Any pT/Tx | Any N | M1a | S0 |
| | Any pT/Tx | Any N | M1a | S1 |
| Stage IIIB | Any pT/Tx | N1–3 | M0 | S2 |
| | Any pT/Tx | Any N | M1a | S2 |
| Stage IIIC | Any pT/Tx | N1–3 | M0 | S3 |
| | Any pT/Tx | Any N | M1a | S3 |
| | Any pT/Tx | Any N | M1b | Any S |

**42**

## PROGNOSTIC FACTORS (SITE-SPECIFIC FACTORS)
### (Recommended for Collection)

Required for staging    Serum tumor markers (S)

SX    Marker studies not available or not performed

S0    Marker study levels within normal limits

S1    LDH $< 1.5 \times N^*$ *and* hCG (mIu/ml) $<5{,}000$ *and* AFP (ng/ml) $<1{,}000$

S2    LDH $1.5{-}10 \times N$ *or* hCG (mIu/ml) $5{,}000{-}50{,}000$ *or* AFP (ng/ml) $1{,}000{-}10{,}000$

S3    LDH $> 10 \times N$ *or* hCG (mIu/ml) $> 50{,}000$ *or* AFP (ng/ml) $> 10{,}000$

*N indicates the upper limit of normal for the LDH assay.

Serum tumor marker levels should be measured prior to orchiectomy for assignment of S category. The only exception is for stage grouping classification of Stage IS in which persistent elevation of serum tumor markers following orchiectomy is required.

The Serum Tumor Markers (S) category comprises the following:

- Alpha fetoprotein (AFP)
- Human chorionic gonadotropin (hCG)
- Lactate dehydrogenase (LDH)

Clinically significant    Size of largest metastases in lymph nodes
                          Radical orchiectomy performed

## HISTOPATHOLOGIC TYPE

Following the guidelines of the *World Health Organization Histological Classification of Tumours,* germ cell tumors may be either seminomatous or nonseminomatous. Seminomas may be classic type or with syncytiotrophoblasts. A distinct variant is spermatocytic seminoma, which is characteristically found in older patients, is often associated with intratumoral calcification, and tends not to metastasize. The presence of an elevated AFP level in a patient with pure seminoma found at orchiectomy should be classified as having nonseminomatous germ cell tumor. Nonseminomatous germ cell tumors may be pure (embryonal carcinoma, yolk sac tumor, teratoma, choriocarcinoma) or mixed. Mixtures of these types (including seminoma) should be noted, starting with the most prevalent component and ending with the least represented. Similarly, gonadal stromal tumors should be classified according to the *World Health Organization Histological Classification of Tumours.*

## BIBLIOGRAPHY

Bajorin D, Katz A, Chan E, et al. Comparison of criteria for assigning germ cell tumor patients to "good risk" and "poor risk" studies. J Clin Oncol. 1986;4:786–92.

Birch R, Williams S, Cone A, et al. Prognostic factors for favorable outcome in disseminated germ cell tumors. J Clin Oncol. 1986;4:400–7.

Boyer M, Raghavan D. Toxicity of treatment of germ cell tumors. Semin Oncol. 1992;19:128–42.

Einhorn LH. Testicular cancer as a model for a curable neoplasm: the Richard and Hinda Rosenthal Foundation Award Lecture. Cancer Res. 1981;41: 3274–80.

Freedman LS, Parkinson MC, Jones WG, et al. Histopathology in the prediction of relapse of patients with Stage I testicular teratoma treated by orchiectomy alone. Lancet. 1987;2:294–8.

Hoskin P, Dilly S, Easton D, et al. Prognostic factors in Stage I non-seminomatous germ cell tumors managed by orchiectomy and surveillance: implications for adjuvant chemotherapy. J Clin Oncol. 1986;4:1031–6.

International Germ Cell Cancer Collaborative Group. International germ cell consensus classification: a prognostic factor–based staging system for metastatic germ cell cancers. J Clin Oncol. 1997;15:594–603.

McKiernan JM, Goluboff ET, Liberson GL, Golden R, Fisch H. Rising risk of testicular cancer by birth cohort in the United States from 1973 to 1995. J Urol. 1999; 162:361–3.

Mead GM, Stenning SP, Parkinson MC, et al. The Second Medical Research Council study of prognostic factors in nonseminomatous germ cell tumors. J Clin Oncol. 1992;10:85–94.

Peckham MJ, Barrett A, McElwain TJ, et al. Nonseminoma germ cell tumours (malignant teratoma) of the testis: results of treatment and an analysis of prognostic factors. Br J Urol. 1981;53:162–72.

Raghavan D, Colls B, Levi J, et al. Surveillance for Stage I non-seminomatous germ cell tumours of the testis: the optimal protocol has not yet been defined. Br J Urol. 1988;61:522–6.

Williams SD, Birch R, Einhorn LH, et al. Treatment of disseminated germ-cell tumors with cisplatin, bleomycin and either vinblastine or etoposide. N Engl J Med. 1987;317:1433–8.

## At-A-Glance

### SUMMARY OF CHANGES

- The following changes in the definition of TNM and the Stage Grouping for this chapter have been made since the Sixth Edition

- T2 lesions have been divided into T2a (greater than 7 cm but less than or equal to 10 cm) and T2b (>10 cm)

- Ipsilateral adrenal involvement is reclassified as T4 if contiguous invasion and M1 if not contiguous

- Renal vein involvement is reclassified as T3a

- Nodal involvement is simplified to N0 vs. N1

### ANATOMIC STAGE/PROGNOSTIC GROUPS

| Stage | T | N | M |
|---|---|---|---|
| Stage I | T1 | N0 | M0 |
| Stage II | T2 | N0 | M0 |
| Stage III | T1 or T2 | N1 | M0 |
| | T3 | N0 or N1 | M0 |
| Stage IV | T4 | Any N | M0 |
| | Any T | Any N | M1 |

ICD-O-3 TOPOGRAPHY CODES

C64.9    Kidney, NOS

ICD-O-3 HISTOLOGY CODE RANGES
8000–8576, 8940–8950, 8980–8981

## INTRODUCTION

Cancers of the kidney account for 3% of all malignancies and are amongst the most lethal of the urologic cancers. Nearly all malignant tumors are carcinomas arising from the renal tubular epithelium or, less frequently, from the renal pelvis (see Chap. 44). These tumors are more common in males by a 3/2 ratio. Most are sporadic, but 2–3% are hereditary. Pain and hematuria are potential presenting signs and 3–5% of patients may present with evidence of vascular tumor thrombus. The majority of kidney tumors are now being detected incidentally in asymptomatic individuals. Common sites of metastasis include the lungs, lymph nodes, liver, bone, and brain. Staging depends on the size of the primary tumor, invasion of adjacent structures, and vascular extension.

Since publication of the sixth edition of the *AJCC Cancer Staging Manual* compelling evidence has accumulated that supports division of T2 tumors and reclassification of the T3a and N categories. The rationale for division of T2 into T2a (>7 cm but not more than 10 cm) and T2b

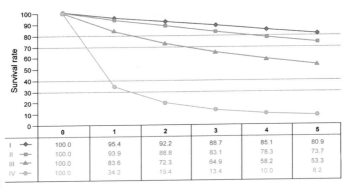

| | 0 | 1 | 2 | 3 | 4 | 5 |
|---|---|---|---|---|---|---|
| I ◆ | 100.0 | 95.4 | 92.2 | 88.7 | 85.1 | 80.9 |
| II ■ | 100.0 | 93.9 | 88.8 | 83.1 | 78.3 | 73.7 |
| III ▲ | 100.0 | 83.6 | 72.3 | 64.9 | 58.2 | 53.3 |
| IV ● | 100.0 | 34.2 | 19.4 | 13.4 | 10.0 | 8.2 |

Years from diagnosis

**FIGURE 43.1.** Observed survival rates for 37,166 patients with kidney cancer classified by the current AJCC staging classification. Data taken from the National Cancer Data Base (Commission on Cancer of the American College of Surgeons and the American Cancer Society) for the years 2001–2002. Stage I includes 18,912 patients; Stage II, 4,443; Stage III, 5,952; and Stage IV, 7,859.

(>10 cm) is based on large retrospective cohort studies with extended follow-up that demonstrate substantially different outcomes for these subgroups. These differences in outcomes were also observed in the National Cancer Data Base as outcomes were examined from patients undergoing nephrectomy for renal cell carcinoma (RCC) (Figure 43.1). The National Cancer Data Base (NCDB) findings were confirmed regarding impact of size on T2 category on cancer-specific and observed survival (Table 43.1).

Multiple studies have documented a poor prognosis for patients with ipsilateral adrenal involvement similar to patients with T4 or M1 disease, and these tumors are now reclassified to reflect current concepts about likely mechanisms of spread.

In contrast, tumors with isolated renal vein thrombus are known to have a relatively favorable prognosis and are now staged as T3a rather

**TABLE 43.1.** The National Cancer Data Base findings regarding impact of size on T2 category on cancer-specific and observed survival

| Size (cm) | Dx | 1 Year | 2 Years | 3 Years | 4 Years | 5 Years |
|---|---|---|---|---|---|---|
| ≤4.0 | 100 | 93.7 | 88.8 | 84.5 | 79.8 | 75.4 |
| 95% CI | | | | | | 74.6–76.1 |
| 4.1–7.0 | 100 | 90.6 | 83.6 | 77.6 | 72.5 | 67.9 |
| 95% CI | | | | | | 67.0–68.7 |
| 7.1–10.0 | 100 | 84.9 | 75.0 | 68.1 | 62.5 | 57.0 |
| 95% CI | | | | | | 55.9–58.1 |
| >10.0 | 100 | 78.7 | 66.3 | 58.8 | 52.5 | 47.5 |
| 95% CI | | | | | | 46.1–48.9 |

Data from the National Cancer Data Base (http://www.facs.org/cancer/ncdb/index.html).

than T3b. Finally, nodal involvement is now consolidated as N1 since most studies suggest a relatively poor prognosis with any extent of nodal involvement.

Recent data also demonstrate that multiple adverse features can act in a collaborative manner to further worsen the prognosis and emerging algorithms are incorporating all of these parameters. These adverse features include perirenal fat invasion, tumor size as a continuous variable, size of the largest involved lymph node, and extranodal extension. In addition, there are a number of potential molecular prognostic factors including genetic variables, proliferative markers, angiogenic parameters, growth factors and receptor, and adhesion molecules. Most have not been formally validated and are best still considered experimental. Ideally future staging protocols would capture this information to facilitate individualized counseling and foster further progress in this field. Specific factors to be examined include degree of invasion, the presence/level of venous involvement, the presence and type of adrenal gland involvement, the type of grading system employed and grade determined, the presence/absence of sarcomatoid features, the presence/absence of lymphovascular invasion, and the presence/absence of necrosis.

## ANATOMY

**Primary Site.** Encased by a fibrous capsule and surrounded by perirenal fat, the kidney consists of the cortex (glomeruli, convoluted tubules) and the medulla (Henle's loops, collecting ducts, and pyramids of converging tubules). Each papilla opens in the minor calices; these in turn unite in the major calices and drain into the renal pelvis. At the hilus are the pelvis, ureter, and renal artery and vein. Gerota's fascia overlies the psoas and quadratus lumborum muscles. The anatomic sites and subsites of the kidney are illustrated in Figure 43.2.

**Regional Lymph Nodes.** The regional lymph nodes, illustrated in Figure 43.3, are as follows:

Renal hilar
Caval (paracaval, precaval, and retrocaval)
Interaortocaval
Aortic (paraaortic, preaortic, and retroaortic)

The primary landing zone for right sided tumors is the interaortocaval zone and for left sided tumors the aortic region. The more extended landing zones for RCC are analogous to those for right and left testicular tumors, respectively, although patterns of spread are somewhat more unpredictable. Lymph nodes outside of these templates should be considered distal (metastatic) rather than regional.

**Metastatic Sites.** Common metastatic sites include the bone, liver, lung, brain, and distant lymph nodes.

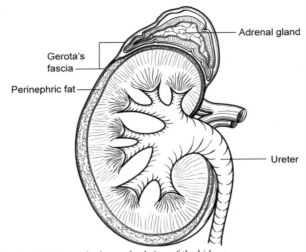

**FIGURE 43.2.** Anatomic sites and subsites of the kidney.

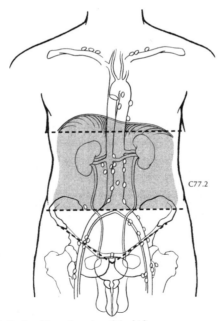

**FIGURE 43.3.** Regional lymph nodes of the kidney.

## RULES FOR CLASSIFICATION

This classification applies only to renal cell carcinomas. Adenoma is excluded. There should be histologic confirmation of disease.

**Clinical Staging.** Clinical examination, abdominal computed tomography scanning, and other appropriate imaging techniques are required for assessment of the primary tumor and its extensions, both local and distant. Evaluation for distant metastasis should be done by laboratory biochemical studies, chest radiographs, and if clinically indicated, additional studies.

**Pathologic Staging.** Histologic examination and confirmation of extent required. Resection of the primary tumor, overlying Gerota's fascia, and overlying perinephric fat is recommended. Careful assessment of the adrenal gland and regional lymph nodes is recommended with resection on a selective basis. Partial nephrectomy is an acceptable treatment for localized tumors amenable to this approach and is the preferred form of management when preservation of renal function is at issue. For staging purposes pathologic tumor size is preferred.

**Specimen Handling.** The pathologic specimen should be processed in such a fashion as to allow for full pathologic assessment. Perinephric and perisinus fat should be left intact and sectioned in such a manner that allows for careful evaluation of these regions and they should be defined independently. Recent studies suggest a worse prognosis with perisinus fat invasion that may be related to increased access to lymphatic and vascular structures. For specimens for partial nephrectomy, the margins should be evaluated from at least two sections and should include the renal sinus for central tumors. For patients with familial RCC or for whom multiple tumors are suspected, thin sections will be needed (0.5–1.0 cm).

## PROGNOSTIC FEATURES AND INTEGRATED ALGORITHMS

Established prognostic factors for various subgroups of patients with RCC include tumor-related factors, patient-related factors, and laboratory biochemical tests. *Integrated algorithms* that incorporate these factors have been validated and have been shown to improve prognostication over anatomic tumor stage alone. The use of these instruments for estimating prognosis and patient counseling can aid in decision-making.

### Prognostic Features for RCC

- Tumor related: Stage, tumor size, tumor grade, histologic type, histologic tumor necrosis, sarcomatoid transformation
- Patient related: Asymptomatic vs. local symptoms vs. systemic symptoms, performance status, substantial weight loss, presence of well-defined paraneoplastic syndrome, metastasis free interval, history of prior nephrectomy
- Laboratory biochemical tests: Elevated LDH levels, hypercalcemia, anemia, thrombocytosis, elevated ESR or CRP

These prognostic and predictive algorithms may be useful in guiding patient counseling and therapy (Table 43.2). However, caution should be exercised

**TABLE 43.2.** Predictive algorithms for renal cell carcinoma

| Institution | Year | Extent of disease | Tumor subtype | Prognostic indicators | Prognostic information | Presentation |
|---|---|---|---|---|---|---|
| | | | | *Preoperative* | | |
| Cleveland Clinic | 2007 | Localized | All | Tumor size, symptoms, age, gender, smoking history | Pathology | Nomogram |
| Many Institutions | 2007 | Localized | All | Tumor size, symptoms, performance status, age, gender, comorbidity, radiographic lymphadenopathy, necrosis | Recurrence | Nomogram |
| | | | | *Postoperative* | | |
| MSKCC | 2001 | Localized | All | TNM stage, tumor size, histology, symptoms | Recurrence | Nomogram |
| MSKCC | 2004 | Metastatic | All | Anemia, corrected calcium level, performance status | Survival | Algorithm |
| MSKCC | 2005 | Localized | Clear cell | TNM stage, tumor size, nuclear grade, histological necrosis, microvascular invasion, symptoms | Recurrence | Nomogram |
| UCLA | 2001 | Localized | All | TNM stage, nuclear grade, performance status | Survival | Algorithm, decision boxes |
| UCLA | 2002 | Localized, metastatic | All | TNM stage, nuclear grade, performance status, metastasis | Survival | Algorithm, decision boxes |
| UCLA | 2003 | Metastatic | All | Lymph node status, constitutional symptoms, metastasis location, histology, TSH level | Survival | Algorithm |
| Mayo Clinic | 2002 | Localized, metastatic | Clear cell | TNM stage, tumor size, nuclear grade, histological necrosis | Survival | Algorithm |
| Mayo Clinic | 2005 | Metastatic | Clear cell | Symptoms; location, number of sites and complete resection of metastases; IVC thrombus level; nuclear grade; histological necrosis | Survival | Algorithm |

*MSKCC* Memorial Sloan-Kettering Cancer Center. http://www.mskcc.org/mskcc/html/6156.cfm, with permission of Memorial Sloan-Kettering Cancer Center.

if used for this purpose as the extent to which the utility of each algorithm has been validated varies. Each used different data sets for development, and the specifics of the data elements used in their application must be precise. In addition, new factors and predictors continue to be discovered and studied. To promote broader use, transparency, and applicability, we hope that future algorithms will utilize the core anatomic elements as specified in the AJCC Staging System.

## DEFINITIONS OF TNM

### Primary Tumor (T)

| | |
|---|---|
| TX | Primary tumor cannot be assessed |
| T0 | No evidence of primary tumor |
| T1 | Tumor 7 cm or less in greatest dimension, limited to the kidney |
| T1a | Tumor 4 cm or less in greatest dimension, limited to the kidney (Figure 43.4A) |
| T1b | Tumor more than 4 cm but not more than 7 cm in greatest dimension limited to the kidney (Figure 43.4B) |
| T2 | Tumor more than 7 cm in greatest dimension, limited to the kidney (Figure 43.5) |
| T2a | Tumor more than 7 cm but less than or equal to 10 cm in greatest dimension, limited to the kidney |
| T2b | Tumor more than 10 cm, limited to the kidney |
| T3 | Tumor extends into major veins or perinephric tissues but not into the ipsilateral adrenal gland and not beyond Gerota's fascia |
| T3a | Tumor grossly extends into the renal vein or its segmental (muscle containing) branches, or tumor invades perirenal and/or renal sinus fat but not beyond Gerota's fascia (Figure 43.6A) |
| T3b | Tumor grossly extends into the vena cava below the diaphragm (Figure 43.6B) |
| T3c | Tumor grossly extends into the vena cava above the diaphragm or invades the wall of the vena cava (Figure 43.6C) |
| T4 | Tumor invades beyond Gerota's fascia (Figure 43.7A) (including contiguous extension into the ipsilateral adrenal gland) (Figure 43.7B) |

### Regional Lymph Nodes (N)

| | |
|---|---|
| NX | Regional lymph nodes cannot be assessed |
| N0 | No regional lymph node metastasis |
| N1 | Metastasis in regional lymph node(s) (Figure 43.8) |

### Distant Metastasis (M)

| | |
|---|---|
| M0 | No distant metastasis |
| M1 | Distant metastasis |

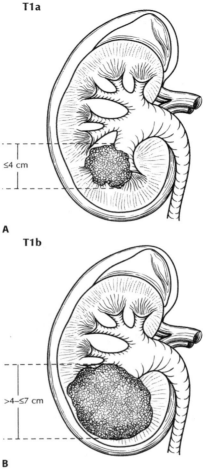

**T1a**

≤4 cm

**A**

**T1b**

>4–≤7 cm

**B**

**FIGURE 43.4.** (**A**) T1a: Tumor 4 cm or less in greatest dimension, limited to the kidney. (**B**) T1b: Tumor more than 4 cm but not more than 7 cm in greatest dimension, limited to the kidney.

| ANATOMIC STAGE/PROGNOSTIC GROUPS | | | |
|---|---|---|---|
| Stage I | T1 | N0 | M0 |
| Stage IIII | T2 | N0 | M0 |
| Stage III | T1 or T2 | N1 | M0 |
| | T3 | N0 or N1 | M0 |
| StageIV | T4 | any N | M0 |
| | Any T | Any N | M1 |

**T2a**

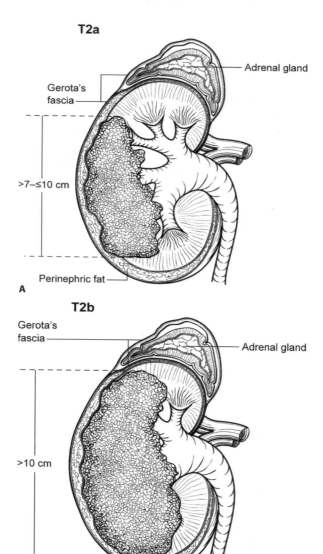

Adrenal gland

Gerota's fascia

>7–≤10 cm

Perinephric fat

**A**

**43**

**T2b**

Gerota's fascia

Adrenal gland

>10 cm

Perinephric fat

**B**

**FIGURE 43.5.** (**A**) T2a: Tumor more than 7 cm in greatest dimension but less than or equal to 10 cm, limited to the kidney. (**B**) T2b tumors are greater than 10 cm.

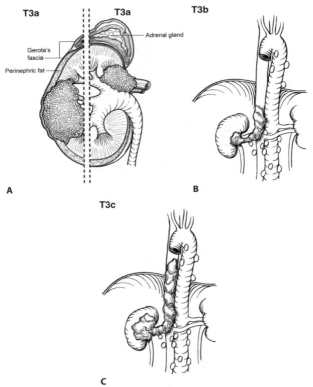

**FIGURE 43.6.** (**A**) (*Left*) T3a: Invasion into perirenal and/or renal sinus fat but not beyond Gerota's fascia. (*Right*) T3a: In addition to perirenal and/or renal sinus fat, tumor grossly invades into the renal vein. (**B**) T3b: Tumor grossly extends into the renal vein or its segmental (muscle-containing) branches, or vena cava below the diaphragm. (**C**) T3c: Tumor grossly extends into vena cava above diaphragm or invades the wall of the vena cava.

## PROGNOSTIC FACTORS (SITE-SPECIFIC FACTORS)
### (Recommended for Collection)

| | |
|---|---|
| Required for staging | None |
| Clinically significant | Invasion beyond capsule into fat or peri-sinus tissues |
| | Venous involvement |
| | Adrenal extension |
| | Fuhrman grade |
| | Sarcomatoid features |
| | Histologic tumor necrosis |
| | Extranodal extension |
| | Size of metastasis in lymph nodes |
| | Presence or absence of extranodal extension |
| | Size of the largest tumor deposit in the lymph nodes |

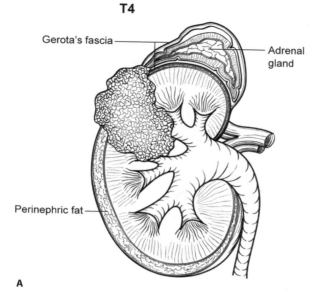

**T4**

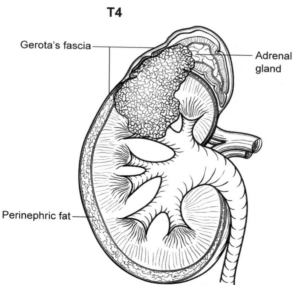

**FIGURE 43.7.** (**A**) T4: Invasion beyond Gerota's fascia. (**B**) T4: Invasion into ipsilateral adrenal gland.

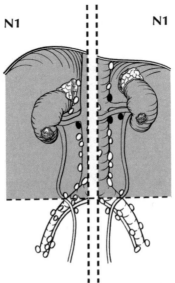

**FIGURE 43.8.** N1 disease is defined as a single or multiple regional lymph node involvement.

## HISTOLOGIC GRADE

A four-tier classification system for nuclear grade is preferred and the protocol used should be specified.

GX    Grade cannot be assessed
G1    Well differentiated
G2    Moderately differentiated
G3    Poorly differentiated
G4    Undifferentiated

## HISTOPATHOLOGIC TYPE

Classification should be based on the WHO 2004 recommendations. Each of the more common histopathologic types of renal cell carcinoma have distinct molecular characteristics and are associated with prognostic or predictive significance, as reflected by their integration in predictive algorithms for renal cell carcinoma. The main categories are as follows:

Clear cell (conventional) renal carcinoma
Papillary renal cell carcinoma
Chromophobe renal cell carcinoma
Collecting duct carcinoma and renal medullary carcinoma
Unclassified renal cell carcinoma
Others

# BIBLIOGRAPHY

Campbell SC, Novick AC, Bukowski RM. Renal tumors. In: Wein AJ, Kavoussi LR, Novick AC, Partin AW, Peters CA, editors. Campbell-Walsh urology. 9th ed. Philadelphia, PA: Elsevier; 2006. Chapter 46, p. 1567–637.

Cindolo L, Patard JJ, Chiodini P, et al. Comparison of predictive accuracy of four prognostic models for nonmetastatic renal cell carcinoma after nephrectomy. Cancer. 2005;104:1362.

Dimashkieh H, Lohse C, Blute M, Kwon E, Leibovich B, Cheville J. Extranodal extension in regional lymph nodes is associated with outcome in patients with renal cell carcinoma. J Urol. 2006;176:1978–83.

Frank I, Blute ML, Cheville JC, Lohse CM, Weaver AL, Zincke H. An outcome prediction model for patients with clear cell renal cell carcinoma treated with radical nephrectomy based on tumor stage, size, grade and necrosis: the SSIGN score. J Urol. 2002;168(6):2395–400.

Han KR, Bui MH, Pantuck AJ, et al. TNM T3a renal cell carcinoma: adrenal gland involvement is not the same as renal fat invasion. J Urol. 2003;169(3):899–903; discussion 904.

Igor F, Blute M, Leibovich B, Cheville J, Lohse C, Kwon E, Zincke H. pT2 Classification for renal cell carcinoma. Can its accuracy be improved? J Urol. 2005;173: 380–4.

Kattan MW, Reuter V, Motzer RJ, Katz J, Russo P. A postoperative prognostic nomogram for renal cel carcinoma. J Urol. 2001;166(1):63–7.

Kim H, Seligson D, Liu X, Janzen N, Bui M, Yu H, et al. Using tumor markers to predict the survival of patients with metastatic renal cell carcinoma. J Urol. 2005;173:1496–501.

Klatte T, Patard JJ, Goel RH, et al. Prognostic impact of tumor size on pT2 RCC: An international multicenter experience. J Urol. 2007;178:35–40.

Kontak JA, Campbell SC. Prognostic factors in renal cell carcinoma. Urol Clin North Am. 2003;30(3):467–80.

Lam JS, Patard JJ, Leppert JT, et al. Prognostic significance of T3a renal cell carcinoma with adrenal gland involvement: an international multicenter experience. J Urol. 2005;173:269.

Lane BR, Kattan MW. Predicting outcomes in renal cell carcinoma. Curr Opin Urol. 2005;15(5):289–97.

Lane BR, Kattan M, Novick A. Prediction models of renal cell carcinoma. AUA update series. Vol. 25, Lesson 7; 2006.

Lane BR, Babineau D, Kattan MW, et al. A preoperative prognostic nomogram for solid enhancing renal tumors 7 cm or less amenable to partial nephrectomy. J Urol. 2007;178(2):429–34.

Leibovich BC, Han KR, Bui MH, et al. Scoring algorithm to predict survival after nephrectomy and immunotherapy in patients with metastatic renal cell carcinoma: a stratification tool for prospective clinical trials. Cancer. 2003;98: 2566–75.

Leibovich BC, Cheville J, Lohse C, et al. Cancer specific survival for patients with pT3 renal cell carcinoma: can the 2002 primary tumor classification be improved? J Urol. 2005a;173:716–9.

Leibovich BC, Cheville JC, Lohse CM, et al. A scoring algorithm to predict survival for patients with metastatic clear cell renal cell carcinoma: a stratification tool for prospective clinical trials. J Urol. 2005b;174:1759–63.

Moinzadeh A, Libertino J. Prognostic significance of tumor thrombus level in patients with renal cell carcinoma and venous tumor thrombus extension. Is all T3b the same? J Urol. 2004;171:598–601.

Motzer RJ, Mazumdar M, Bacik J, et al. Survival and prognostic stiatification of 670 patients with advanced renal cell carcinoma. J Clin Oncol. 1999;17: 2530–40.

**43**

Motzer RJ, Bacik J, Mariani T, Russo P, Mazumdar M, Reuter V. Treatment outcome and survival associated with metastatic renal cell carcinoma of non-clear-cell histology. J Clin Oncol. 2002;20(9):2376–81.

Motzer RJ, Bacik J, Schwartz LH, et al. Prognostic factors for survival in previously treated patients with metastatic renal cell carcinoma. J Clin Oncol. 2004;22:454–63.

Nguyen C, Campbell SC. Staging of renal cell carcinoma: past, present, and future. Clin Genitourin Cancer. 2006;5:190–7.

Pantuck AJ, Zisman A, Dorey F, et al. Renal cell carcinoma with retroperitoneal lymph nodes. Impact on survival and benefits of immunotherapy. Cancer. 2003;97(12):2995–3002.

Patard JJ, Leray E, Cindolo L, et al. Multi-institutional validation of a symptom based classification for renal cell carcinoma. J Urol. 2004a;172(3):858–62.

Patard JJ, Kim HL, Lam JS, et al. Use of University of California Los Angeles integrated staging system to predict survival in renal cell carcinoma: an international multicenter study. J Clin Oncol. 2004b;22(16):3316–22.

Paul R, Mordhorst J, Leyh H, Hartung R. Incidence and outcome of patients with adrenal metastases of renal cell cancer. Urology. 2001;57(5):878–82.

Phillips CK, Taneja SS. The role of lymphadenectomy in the surgical management of renal cell carcinoma. Urol Oncol. 2004;22(3):214–23; discussion 23–4.

Sagalowsky AL, Kadesky KT, Ewalt DM, Kennedy TJ. Factors influencing adrenal metastasis in renal cell carcinomas. J Urol. 1994;151(5):1181–4.

Sandock DS, Seftel AD, Resnick MI. Adrenal metastases from renal cell carcinoma: role of ipsilateral adrenalectomy and definition of stage. Urology. 1997;49(1):28–31.

Siemer S, Lehmann J, Loch A, et al. Current TNM classification of renal cell carcinoma evaluated: revising stage T3a. J Urol. 2005;173(1):33–7.

Sorbellini M, Kattan MW, Snyder ME. A postoperative prognostic nomogram predicting recurrence for patients with conventional clear cell renal cell carcinoma. J Urol. 2005;173:48–51.

Thompson R, Cheville J, Lohse C, Webster W, Zincke H, Dwon E, et al. Reclassification of patients with pT3 and pT4 renal cell carcinoma improves prognostic accuracy. Cancer. 2005a;104(1):53–60.

Thompson R, Leibovich B, Cheville J, Lohse C, Frank I, Kwon E, et al. Should direct ipsilateral adrenal invasion from renal cell carcinoma be classified as pT3a. J Urol. 2005b;173:918–21.

von Knobloch R, Varga Z, Schrader AJ, Hofmann R. All patients with adrenal metastasis from RCC will eventually die in tumor progression: there is no cure or benefit from simultaneous adrenalectomy. J Urol. 2004;171(4S):15.

Zisman A, Pantuck AJ, Figlin RA, Belldegrun AS. Validation of the UCLA integrated staging system for patients with renal cell carcinoma (comment). J Clin Oncol. 2001a;19(17):3792–3.

Zisman A, Pantuck AJ, Dorey F, et al. Improved prognostication of renal cell carcinoma using an integrated staging system. J Clin Oncol. 2001b;19:1649–57.

Zisman A, Pantuck AJ, Wieder J, et al. Risk group assessment and clinical outcome algorithm to predict the natural history of patients with surgically resected renal cell carcinoma. J Clin Oncol. 2002;20:4559–66.

# Renal Pelvis and Ureter

## At-A-Glance

---

### SUMMARY OF CHANGES

- The definition of TNM and the Stage Grouping for this chapter have not changed from the Sixth Edition

- Grading: a low- and high-grade designation will replace previous four-grade system to match current World Health Organization/International Society of Urologic Pathology (WHO/ISUP) recommended grading system

---

| ANATOMIC STAGE/PROGNOSTIC GROUPS | | | |
|---|---|---|---|
| Stage 0a | Ta | N0 | M0 |
| Stage 0is | Tis | N0 | M0 |
| Stage I | T1 | N0 | M0 |
| Stage II | T2 | N0 | M0 |
| Stage III | T3 | N0 | M0 |
| Stage IV | T4 | N0 | M0 |
| | Any T | N1 | M0 |
| | Any T | N2 | M0 |
| | Any T | N3 | M0 |
| | Any T | Any N | M1 |

ICD-O-3 TOPOGRAPHY CODES
C65.9    Renal pelvis
C66.9    Ureter

ICD-O-3 HISTOLOGY CODE RANGES
8000–8576, 8940–8950, 8980–8981

## INTRODUCTION

Urothelial (transitional cell) carcinoma may occur at any site within the upper urinary collecting system from the renal calyx to the ureterovesical junction. The tumors occur most commonly in adults and are rare before 40 years of age. There is a two- to threefold increase in incidence in men than in women. The lesions are often multiple and are more common in patients with a history of urothelial carcinoma of the bladder. In addition to cigarette smoking a number of analgesics (such as phenacetin) have also been associated with this disease. Local staging depends on the depth of invasion. A common staging system is used regardless of tumor location within the upper urinary collecting system, except for category T3, which differs between the pelvis or calyceal system and the ureter.

## ANATOMY

**Primary Site.**   The renal pelvis and ureter form a single unit that is continuous with the collecting ducts of the renal pyramids and comprises the minor and major calyces, which are continuous with the renal pelvis.

---

The ureteropelvic junction is variable in position and location but serves as a "landmark" that separates the renal pelvis and the ureter, which continues caudad and traverses the wall of the urinary bladder as the intramural ureter opening in the trigone of the bladder at the ureteral orifice. The renal pelvis and ureter are composed of the following layers: epithelium, subepithelial connective tissue, and muscularis, which is continuous with a connective tissue adventitial layer. It is in this outer layer that the major blood supply and lymphatics are found.

The intrarenal portion of the renal pelvis is surrounded by renal parenchyma; the extrarenal pelvis, by perihilar fat. The ureter courses through the retroperitoneum adjacent to the parietal peritoneum and rests on the retroperitoneal musculature above the pelvic vessels. As it crosses the vessels and enters the deep pelvis, the ureter is surrounded by pelvic fat until it traverses the bladder wall.

**Regional Lymph Nodes.** The regional lymph nodes for the renal pelvis are as follows:

> Renal hilar
> Paracaval
> Aortic
> Retroperitoneal, NOS

The regional lymph nodes for the ureter are as follows:

> Renal hilar
> Iliac (common, internal [hypogastric], external)
> Paracaval
> Periureteral
> Pelvic, NOS

Any amount of regional lymph node metastasis is a poor prognostic finding, and outcome is minimally influenced by the number, size, or location of the regional nodes that are involved.

**Metastatic Sites.** Distant spread is most commonly to lung, lymph nodes, bone, or liver.

## RULES FOR CLASSIFICATION

**Clinical Staging.** Primary tumor assessment includes radiographic imaging, usually by intravenous and/or retrograde pyelography. Computerized tomography scanning can be used to assess regional nodes. Ureteroscopic visualization of the tumor is desirable, and tissue biopsy through the ureteroscope may be performed if feasible. Urine cytology may help determine tumor grade if tissue is not available. Staging of tumors of the renal pelvis and ureter is not influenced by the presence of any concomitant bladder tumors that may be identified, although it may not be possible to identify the true source of the primary tumor in the presence of metastases if both upper- and lower-tract tumors are present. In that situation, the tumor of highest grade and/or stage is most likely to have contributed to the nodal or metastatic spread.

**Pathologic Staging.** Pathologic staging depends on histologic determination of the extent of invasion by the primary tumor. Treatment frequently requires resection of the entire kidney, ureter, and a cuff of bladder surrounding the ureteral orifice. Appropriate regional nodes may be sampled. A more conservative surgical resection may be performed, especially with distal ureteral tumors or in the presence of compromised renal function.

Endoscopic resection through a ureteroscope or a percutaneous approach may be used in some circumstances. Submitted tissue may be insufficient for accurate histologic examination and will often be insufficient for adequate pathologic staging. Laser or electrocautery coagulation or vaporization of the tumor may be performed, especially if the visible appearance is consistent with a low-grade and low-stage tumor. Under these circumstances, there may be no material available for histologic review. Figures 44.1 and 44.2 illustrate the primary tumor (T) definition for Ta, T1, T2, and T3.

## DEFINITIONS OF TNM

44

*Primary Tumor (T)*

| | |
|---|---|
| TX | Primary tumor cannot be assessed |
| T0 | No evidence of primary tumor |
| Ta | Papillary noninvasive carcinoma |
| Tis | Carcinoma in situ |
| T1 | Tumor invades subepithelial connective tissue |
| T2 | Tumor invades the muscularis |
| T3 | (For renal pelvis only) Tumor invades beyond muscularis into peripelvic fat or the renal parenchyma T3. (For ureter only) Tumor invades beyond muscularis into periureteric fat |
| T4 | Tumor invades adjacent organs, or through the kidney into the perinephric fat. |

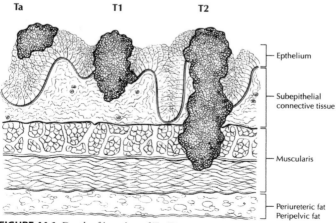

**FIGURE 44.1.** Depth of invasion of Ta–T2 tumors.

**T3**

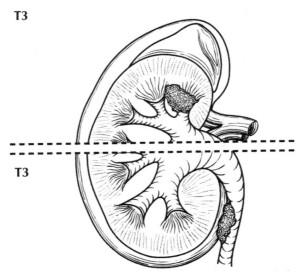

**FIGURE 44.2.** T3 (for renal pelvis only, *top of diagram*): tumor invades beyond muscularis into peripelvic fat or the renal parenchyma. T3 (for ureter only, *bottom of diagram*): tumor invades beyond muscularis into periureteric fat.

### Regional Lymph Nodes (N)*

| | |
|---|---|
| NX | Regional lymph nodes cannot be assessed |
| N0 | No regional lymph node metastasis |
| N1 | Metastasis in a single lymph node, 2 cm or less in greatest dimension |
| N2 | Metastasis in a single lymph node, more than 2 cm but not more than 5 cm in greatest dimension; or multiple lymph nodes, none more than 5 cm in greatest dimension |
| N3 | Metastasis in a lymph node, more than 5 cm in greatest dimension |

*Note: Laterality does not affect the N classification.

### Distant Metastasis (M)

| | |
|---|---|
| M0 | No distant metastasis |
| M1 | Distant metastasis |

### ANATOMIC STAGE/PROGNOSTIC GROUPS

| | | | |
|---|---|---|---|
| Stage 0a | Ta | N0 | M0 |
| Stage 0is | Tis | N0 | M0 |
| Stage I | T1 | N0 | M0 |
| Stage II | T2 | N0 | M0 |
| Stage III | T3 | N0 | M0 |

| Stage IV | T4 | N0 | M0 |
| | Any T | N1 | M0 |
| | Any T | N2 | M0 |
| | Any T | N3 | M0 |
| | Any T | Any N | M1 |

## PROGNOSTIC FACTORS (SITE-SPECIFIC FACTORS)
### (Recommended for Collection)

| | |
|---|---|
| Required for staging | None |
| Clinically significant | Renal parenchymal invasion |
| | World Health Organization/International Society of Urologic Pathology (WHO/ISUP) grade |

## HISTOLOGIC GRADE (G)

**44**

Grade is reported in registry systems by the grade value. For urothelial histologies, a low- and high-grade designation is used to match the current World Health Organization/International Society of Urologic Pathology (WHO/ISUP) recommended grading system:

| | |
|---|---|
| LG | Low grade |
| HG | High grade |

If a grading system is not specified, generally the following system is used:

| | |
|---|---|
| GX | Grade cannot be assessed |
| G1 | Well differentiated |
| G2 | Moderately differentiated |
| G3 | Poorly differentiated |
| G4 | Undifferentiated |

## HISTOPATHOLOGIC TYPE

The histologic types are as follows:

Urothelial (transitional cell) carcinoma
  In situ
    Papillary
    Flat
    With squamous differentiation
    With glandular differentiation
    With squamous and glandular differentiation
Squamous cell carcinoma
Adenocarcinoma
Undifferentiated carcinoma

The predominant cancer is urothelial (transitional cell) carcinoma. Histologic variants include micropapillary and nested subtypes.

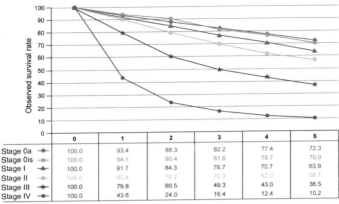

| | 0 | 1 | 2 | 3 | 4 | 5 |
|---|---|---|---|---|---|---|
| Stage 0a | 100.0 | 93.4 | 88.3 | 82.2 | 77.4 | 72.3 |
| Stage 0is | 100.0 | 94.1 | 90.4 | 81.6 | 76.7 | 70.0 |
| Stage I | 100.0 | 91.7 | 84.3 | 76.7 | 70.7 | 63.9 |
| Stage II | 100.0 | 90.4 | 79.2 | 70.3 | 62.0 | 56.7 |
| Stage III | 100.0 | 79.8 | 60.5 | 49.3 | 43.0 | 36.5 |
| Stage IV | 100.0 | 43.6 | 24.0 | 16.4 | 12.4 | 10.2 |

Years from diagnosis

**FIGURE 44.3.** Observed overall survival rates for 6,174 patients with renal pelvis and ureter cancer classified by the current AJCC staging classification. Data taken from the National Cancer Data Base (Commission on Cancer of the American College of Surgeons and the American Cancer Society) for the years 2000 to 2002. Stage 0a includes 1,434 patients; Stage 0is, 263; Stage I, 1,472; Stage II, 669; Stage III, 1,198; Stage IV, 1,138.

## OUTCOMES RESULTS

Observed survival rates for 6,174 patients with renal pelvis and ureter cancer classified by the current AJCC staging classification from 2000 to 2002 are shown in Figure 44.3.

## BIBLIOGRAPHY

al-Abadi H, Nagel R. Transitional cell carcinoma of the renal pelvis and ureter: prognostic relevance of nuclear deoxyribonucleic acid ploidy studied by slide cytometry: an 8-year survival time study. J Urol. 1992;148(l):31–7.

Anderstrom C, Johansson SL, Pettersson S, et al. Carcinoma of the ureter: a clinicopathologic study of 49 cases. J Urol. 1989;142(2 Part 1):280–3.

Balaji KC, McGuire M, Grotas J, et al. Upper tract recurrences following radical cystectomy: an analysis of prognostic factors, recurrence pattern and stage at presentation. J Urol. 1999;162:1603–6.

Borgmann V, al-Abadi H, Nagel R. Prognostic relevance of DNA ploidy and proliferative activity in urothelial carcinoma of the renal pelvis and ureter: a study on a follow-up period of 6 years. Urol Int. 1991;47(l):7–11.

Corrado F, Ferri C, Mannini D, et al. Transitional cell carcinoma of the upper urinary tract: evaluation of prognostic factors by histopathology and flow cytometric analysis. J Urol. 1991;145(6):1159–63.

Grasso M, Fraiman M, Levine M. Ureteropyeloscopic diagnosis and treatment of upper urinary tract urothelial malignancies. Urology. 1999;54:240–6.

Hall MC, Womack S, Sagalowsky AI, et al. Prognostic factors, recurrence, and survival in transitional cell carcinoma of the upper urinary tract: a 30-year experience in 252 patients. Urology. 1998;52:594–601.

Herr HW. Extravesical tumor relapse in patients with superficial bladder tumors. J Clin Oncol. 1998;16:1099–102.

Hisataki T, Miyao N, Masumori N, et al. Risk factors for the development of bladder cancer after upper tract urothelial cancer. Urology. 2000;55:663–7.

Huben RP, Mounzer AM, Murphy GP. Tumor grade and stage as prognostic variables in upper urothelial tumors. Cancer. 1988;62(9):2016–20.

Hurle R, Losa A, Manzetti A, Lembo A. Upper urinary tract tumors developing after treatment of superficial bladder cancer: 7-year follow-up of 591 consecutive patients. Urology. 1999;53:1144–8.

Jabbour ME, Desgrandchamps F, Cazin S, et al. Percutaneous management of grade II upper urinary tract transitional cell carcinoma: the long-term outcome. J Urol. 2000;163:1105–7.

Jinza S, Iki M, Noguchi S, et al. Nucleolar organizer regions: a new prognostic factor for upper tract urothelial cancer. J Urol. 1995;154(5):1688–92.

Millan-Rodriguez F, Chechile-Toniolo G, Salvador-Bayarri J, et al. Upper urinary tract tumors after primary superficial bladder tumors: prognostic factors and risk groups. J Urol. 2000;164:1183–7.

Scolieri MJ, Paik ML, Brown SL, Resnick MI. Limitations of computed tomography in the preoperative staging of upper tract urothelial carcinoma. Urology. 2000;56:930.

Williams RD. Tumors of the kidney, ureter, and bladder. West J Med. 1992;56(5):523–34.

44

# 45

# Urinary Bladder

## *At-A-Glance*

---

### SUMMARY OF CHANGES

- Primary staging: T4 disease defined as including prostatic stromal invasion directly from bladder cancer. Subepithelial invasion of prostatic urethra will not constitute T4 staging status

- Grading: a low and high grade designation will replace previous 4 grade system to match current World Health Organization/International Society of Urologic Pathology (WHO/ISUP) recommended grading system

- Nodal classification

  - Common iliac nodes defined as secondary drainage region as regional nodes and not as metastatic disease

  - N staging system change

    - N1: single positive node in primary drainage regions

    - N2: multiple positive nodes in primary drainage regions

    - N3: common iliac node involvement

---

**45**

| ANATOMIC STAGE/PROGNOSTIC GROUPS | | | |
|---|---|---|---|
| Stage 0a | Ta | N0 | M0 |
| Stage 0is | Tis | N0 | M0 |
| Stage I | T1 | N0 | M0 |
| Stage II | T2a | N0 | M0 |
| | T2b | N0 | M0 |
| Stage III | T3a | N0 | M0 |
| | T3b | N0 | M0 |
| | T4a | N0 | M0 |
| Stage IV | T4b | N0 | M0 |
| | Any T | N1-3 | M0 |
| | Any T | Any N | M1 |

ICD-O-3
TOPOGRAPHY
CODES

| | |
|---|---|
| C67.0 | Trigone of bladder |
| C67.1 | Dome of bladder |
| C67.2 | Lateral wall of bladder |
| C67.3 | Anterior wall of bladder |
| C67.4 | Posterior wall of bladder |
| C67.5 | Bladder neck |
| C67.6 | Ureteric orifice |
| C67.7 | Urachus |
| C67.8 | Overlapping lesion of bladder |
| C67.9 | Bladder, NOS |

ICD-O-3 HISTOLOGY
CODE RANGES
8000–8576, 8940–8950,
8980–8981

---

# INTRODUCTION

Bladder cancer is one of the most common malignancies in Western society, and it occurs more commonly in males. Predisposing factors include smoking, exposure to chemicals such as phenacetin and dyes, and schistosomiasis. It has also been suggested that the incidence of this disease correlates inversely with fluid intake. Hematuria is the most common presenting feature. Bladder cancer can present as a low or high-grade papillary lesion, as a high-grade in situ lesion that can occupy large areas of the mucosal surface, or as an infiltrative cancer that invades the bladder wall and progresses into the perivesical tissues, regional lymph nodes and can thereafter metastasize. Noninvasive papillary lesions have a relatively low risk for progression to invasive disease; however, this risk is dependent on the grade of the lesion (i.e., high vs. low grade). High-grade papillary and in situ lesions may be associated with a malignant course, including invasion of the bladder wall and the subsequent development of regional and/or distant metastases. The most common histologic variant is urothelial (transitional cell) carcinoma, although this may exhibit features of glandular or squamous differentiation. In less than 10% of cases, pure adenocarcinoma or squamous carcinoma of the bladder may occur, and less frequently, sarcoma, lymphoma, small cell anaplastic carcinoma, pheochromocytoma, or choriocarcinoma. Squamous carcinoma is associated with schistosomiasis, inflammation, and smoking.

# ANATOMY

**Primary Site.** The urinary bladder consists of three layers: the epithelium and the subepithelial connective tissue (also referred to as lamina propria), the muscularis propria, and the perivesical fat (peritoneum covering the superior surface and upper part). In the male, the bladder adjoins the rectum and seminal vesicle posteriorly, the prostate inferiorly, and the pubis and peritoneum anteriorly. In the female, the vagina is located posteriorly and the uterus superiorly. The bladder is located extraperitoneally.

**Regional Lymph Nodes.** The regional lymph nodes draining the bladder include primary and secondary nodal drainage regions. Primary lymph nodes include the external iliac, hypogastric and obturator basins. The presacral lymph nodes are classified as a primary drainage region; however, mapping studies have found this area to be a less frequent site of primary regional metastases. Primary nodal regions drain into the common iliac nodes, which constitute a secondary drainage region. Regional lymph node staging is of significant prognostic importance given the negative impact on recurrence after treatment and long-term survival. The relevant information from regional lymph node staging is obtained from the extent of disease within the nodes (number of positive nodes, extranodal extension) not in whether metastases are unilateral or contralateral. Overall 5-year survival in node positive bladder cancer following definitive local therapy is approximately 33%; however, patients with a greater node burden may be expected to do significantly worse.

Regional nodes include the following:

Primary Drainage
    Hypogastric
    Obturator
    Iliac (internal, external, NOS)
    Perivesical Pelvic, NOS
    Sacral (lateral, sacral promontory [Gerota's])
    Presacral
Secondary Drainage
    Common iliac

The common iliac nodes are considered sites of secondary regionally lymphatic involvement.

**Metastatic Sites.** Distant spread is most commonly to retroperitoneal lymph nodes, lung, bone, and liver.

## RULES FOR CLASSIFICATION

**Clinical Staging.** Primary tumor assessment includes bimanual examination under anesthesia before and after endoscopic surgery (biopsy or transurethral resection) and histologic verification of the presence or absence of tumor when indicated. Bimanual examination following endoscopic surgery is an indicator of clinical stage. The finding of bladder wall thickening, a mobile mass, or a fixed mass suggests the presence of T3 and/or T4 disease, respectively. The suffix "m" is added to denote multiple tumors. The suffix "is" is added to any T to indicate associated carcinoma in situ. Appropriate imaging techniques for extravesical extension of the primary tumor and lymph node evaluation should be incorporated into clinical staging. Care should be taken when interpreting postbiopsy scans as biopsy-induced inflammatory changes may lead to overstaging. When indicated, evaluation for distant metastases includes imaging of the chest, biochemical studies, and isotopic studies to detect common metastatic sites. Computed tomography, MRI, or other modalities may be used to supply information concerning minimal requirements for staging. As yet, the role of positron emission tomography (PET) scanning using current standard isotopes (FDG-glucose) in the staging and management of bladder cancer has not been defined. The primary tumor may be noninvasive or invasive and can be partially or totally resected with sufficient tissue from the tumor base for evaluation of full depth of tumor invasion. Repeat resection of early invasive tumors (T1) can provide optimal staging information, and multiple biopsies can be taken from other suspicious sites to rule out a field effect; urinary cytology and upper tract imaging are important. It should be recalled that bladder cancer may occur in association with malignancies of the ureters, renal pelvis, or urethra. The definitions for Primary Tumor (T) are illustrated in Figure 45.1.

**Pathologic Staging.** Pathologic staging is based on the histologic review of the radical or partial cystectomy specimen. Microscopic examination and

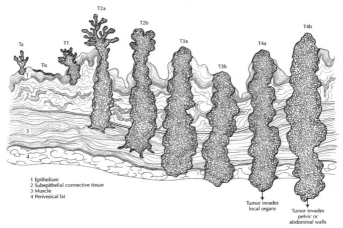

**FIGURE 45.1.** Extent of primary bladder cancer.

confirmation of extent are required. Total cystectomy and lymph node dissection generally are required for this staging; however, a pathologic staging classification should be given for partial cystectomy specimens. Laterality does not affect the N classification. Pathologic staging should include the findings of the cystectomy specimen following surgery and should be assigned independent of previous clinical or biopsy information that is used for clinical stage assignment.

Adequate nodal staging requires removal of the primary lymph node regions that include the left and right external iliac, hypogastric and obturator nodes. Skip metastases to secondary drainage sites (common iliac nodes) are uncommon. Based on contemporary mapping studies in which standard techniques were used to evaluate the pathologic specimen, excision of the primary nodal regions should result in an average of >12 lymph nodes. Evaluation of the National Cancer Database revealed a significant difference in survival in those patients who had fewer than four lymph nodes removed compared with those who had more than four lymph nodes removed, even in patients with node negative (N0) disease. This should serve as a guide for the number of lymph nodes to be evaluated for optimized staging after radical cystectomy. However, the lymph nodes examined may vary dependent on previous patient treatment, body habitus, and pathologic technique.

The number of lymph nodes examined from the operative specimen and the number of positive lymph nodes have been reported to be associated with survival. In addition, the size of the largest tumor deposit and presence of extranodal extension may independently impact survival. A pN status should be assessed regardless of the number of nodes examined. If no lymph nodes are evaluated pNX status should be assigned.

## PROGNOSTIC FEATURES

Prognostic features for bladder cancer include a variety of pathologic, clinical, and molecular characteristics. Primary tumor stage and grade are important independent predictors of tumor progression and outcome. More recently morphologic prognostic features including lymphovascular invasion and variants of the pattern of tumor growth, such as micropapillary and nested variants, have been found to portend an adverse outcome. Lymph node status has a profound effect on the risk of tumor recurrence and patient survival. Various lymph node parameters demonstrating prognostic significance include the total number of excised lymph nodes, the number of positive lymph nodes, extranodal tumor extension, and the ratio of number of positive lymph nodes to total number of lymph nodes evaluated.

Several molecular factors with prognostic importance have been identified for bladder cancer. These markers are involved in the regulation of the cell cycle, programmed cell death, growth factor signaling, and angiogenesis. Two distinct molecular pathways for bladder tumor progression have been established. Noninvasive tumors appear to progress through a pathway that involves the frequent alteration to chromosome 9, specifically 9q deletions. In contrast high-grade tumors are associated with a loss of heterozygosity of chromosome 17p, 14q, 5q, 3p. Alterations to the TP53 and RB pathways play a central role in the progression of high-grade bladder cancer. Additional regulatory proteins including p21/WAF1, p16, p14ARF, and MDM2 have also been implicated in the dysregulation of cell growth via both TP53/RB-dependent and -independent pathways. Overexpression of tyrosine-kinase receptors that effect signaling of many growth factors including epidermal growth factor (EGF), vascular endothelial growth factor (VEGF), and HER2/neu have been identified as prognostically relevant alterations in bladder cancer.

Ploidy has been investigated as a prognostic factor. In superficial disease, an aneuploid DNA content is associated with shorter disease-free survival and with an increased chance of progression to a higher stage; however, in invasive and metastatic disease, the majority of cases are aneuploid, thus reducing the role of aneuploid DNA content as a discriminant of outcome. In the setting of advanced disease, patient performance status, the presence of visceral metastases, and elevated levels of alkaline phosphatase are important predictors of response to systemic therapy and patient survival.

## DEFINITIONS OF TNM

*Primary Tumor (T)*

| | |
|---|---|
| TX | Primary tumor cannot be assessed |
| T0 | No evidence of primary tumor |
| Ta | Noninvasive papillary carcinoma |
| Tis | Carcinoma in situ: "flat tumor" |
| T1 | Tumor invades subepithelial connective tissue |
| T2 | Tumor invades muscularis propria |
| pT2a | Tumor invades superficial muscularis propria (inner half) |
| pT2b | Tumor invades deep muscularis propria (outer half) |
| T3 | Tumor invades perivesical tissue |

45

### Primary Tumor (T) (continued)

pT3a Microscopically

pT3b Macroscopically (extravesical mass)

T4 Tumor invades any of the following: prostatic stroma, seminal vesicles, uterus, vagina, pelvic wall, abdominal wall

T4a Tumor invades prostatic stroma, uterus, vagina

T4b Tumor invades pelvic wall, abdominal wall

### Regional Lymph Nodes (N)

Regional lymph nodes include both primary and secondary drainage regions. All other nodes above the aortic bifurcation are considered distant lymph nodes.

NX Lymph nodes cannot be assessed

N0 No lymph node metastasis

N1 Single regional lymph node metastasis in the true pelvis (hypogastric, obturator, external iliac, or presacral lymph node)

N2 Multiple regional lymph node metastasis in the true pelvis (hypogastric, obturator, external iliac, or presacral lymph node metastasis)

N3 Lymph node metastasis to the common iliac lymph nodes

### Distant Metastasis (M)

M0 No distant metastasis

M1 Distant metastasis

### ANATOMIC STAGE/PROGNOSTIC GROUPS

| Stage 0a | Ta | N0 | M0 |
|---|---|---|---|
| Stage 0is | Tis | N0 | M0 |
| Stage I | T1 | N0 | M0 |
| Stage II | T2a | N0 | M0 |
| | T2b | N0 | M0 |
| Stage III | T3a | N0 | M0 |
| | T3b | N0 | M0 |
| | T4a | N0 | M0 |
| Stage IV | T4b | N0 | M0 |
| | Any T | N1-3 | M0 |
| | Any T | Any N | M1 |

### PROGNOSTIC FACTORS (SITE-SPECIFIC FACTORS)
### (Recommended for Collection)

Required for staging    None

Clinically significant    Presence or absence of extranodal extension
Size of the largest tumor deposit in the lymph nodes
World Health Organization/International Society of Urologic Pathology (WHO/ISUP) grade

## HISTOLOGIC GRADE (G)

Grade is reported in registry systems by the grade value. For urothelial histologies, a low- and high-grade designation is used to match the current World Health Organization/International Society of Urologic Pathology (WHO/ISUP) recommended grading system:

LG    Low grade
HG    High grade

If a grading system is not specified, generally the following system is used:

GX    Grade cannot be assessed
G1    Well differentiated
G2    Moderately differentiated
G3    Poorly differentiated
G4    Undifferentiated

## HISTOPATHOLOGIC TYPE

The histologic types are as follows:

Urothelial (transitional cell) carcinoma
    In situ
        Papillary
        Flat
        With squamous differentiation
        With glandular differentiation
        With squamous and glandular differentiation
Squamous cell carcinoma
Adenocarcinoma
Undifferentiated carcinoma

The predominant cancer is urothelial (transitional cell) carcinoma.
    Histologic variants include micropapillary and nested subtypes.

45

## BIBLIOGRAPHY

Barentsz JO, Jager GJ, Witjes JA, Ruijs JH. Primary staging of urinary bladder carcinoma: the role of MRI and a comparison with CT. Eur Radiol. 1996;6(2):129–33.

Bochner BH, Cho D, Herr HW, et al. Prospectively packaged lymph node dissections with radical cystectomy: evaluation of node count variability and node mapping. J Urol. 2004;172:1286.

Bochner BH, Kattan MW, Vora KC. Postoperative nomogram predicting risk of recurrence after radical cystectomy for bladder cancer. J Clin Oncol. 2006;24:3967.

Brown JL, Russell PJ, Philips J, Wotherspoon J, Raghavan D. Clonal analysis of a bladder cancer cell line: an experimental model of tumour heterogeneity. Br J Cancer. 1990;61:369–76.

deVere White RW, Olsson CA, Deitch AD. Flow cytometry: role in monitoring transitional cell carcinoma of bladder. Urology. 1986;28:15–20.

Epstein JI, Amin MB, Reuter VR, Mostofi FK. The World Health Organization/International Society of Urological Pathology consensus classification of urothelial (transitional cell) neoplasms of the urinary bladder. Am J Surg Pathol. 1998;22:1435.

Esrig D, Elmajian D, Groshen S, et al. Accumulation of nuclear p53 and tumor progression in bladder cancer. N Engl J Med. 1994;331:1259–64.

Fleischmann A, Thalmann GN, Markwalder R, et al. Extracapsular extension of pelvic lymph node metastases from urothelial carcinoma of the bladder is an independent prognostic factor. J Clin Oncol. 2005;23:2358.

Geller NL, Sternberg CN, Penenberg D, Scher H, Yagoda A. Prognostic factors for survival of patients with advanced urothelial tumors treated with methotrexate, vinblastine, doxorubicin, and cisplatin chemotherapy. Cancer. 1991;67: 1525–31.

Greenlee RT, Hill-Harmon MB, Taylor M, Thun M. Cancer Statistics, 2001. CA Cancer J Clin. 2001;51:15–36.

Herr HW. Staging invasive bladder tumors. J Surg Oncol. 1992;51:217–20.

Jewett HJ, Strong GH. Infiltrating carcinoma of the bladder: relation of depth of penetration of the bladder wall to incidence of local extension and metastasis. J Urol. 1946;55:366–72.

Johansson SL, Anderstrom CR. Primary adenocarcinoma of the urinary bladder and urachus. In: Raghavan D, Brecher MI, Johnson DH, Meropol NJ, Moots PJ, Thigpen JT, editors. Textbook of uncommon cancer. Chichester, UK: Wiley-Liss; 1999. p. 29–43.

Kamat AM, Dinney CP, Gee JR, et al. Micropapillary bladder cancer: a review of the University of Texas M. D. Anderson Cancer Center experience with 100 consecutive patients. Cancer. 2007;110:62.

Koppie TM, Vickers AJ, Vora K, et al. Standardization of pelvic lymphadenectomy performed at radical cystectomy: can we establish a minimum number of lymph nodes that should be removed? Cancer. 2006;107:2368.

Koss LG. Tumors of the urinary bladder. In: Atlas of tumor pathology. 2nd series, fascicle 11. Washington, DC: Armed Forces Institute of Pathology; 1975.

Lacombe L, Orlow I, Silver D, Gerald W, Fair WR, Reuter VE, et al. Analysis of p21WAF1/CIP1 in primary bladder tumors. Oncol Res. 1997;8:409–14.

Leissner J, Ghoneim MA, Abol-Enein H, et al. Extended radical lymphadenectomy in patients with urothelial bladder cancer: results of a prospective multicenter study. J Urol. 2004;171:139.

Loehrer PJ, Einhorn LH, Elson PJ, et al. A randomized comparison of cisplatin alone or in combination with methotrexate, vinblastine, and doxorubicin in patients with metastatic urothelial carcinoma: a cooperative group study. J Clin Oncol. 1992;10:1066–73.

Lu ML, Wikman F, Orntoft TF, et al. Impact of alterations affecting the p53 pathway in bladder cancer on clinical outcome, assessed by conventional and array-based methods. Clin Cancer Res. 2002;8:171.

Michaud DS, Spiegelman D, Clinton SK, et al. Fluid intake and the risk of bladder cancer in men. New Engl J Med. 1999;340:1390–7.

Neal DE, Marsh C, Bennett MK, et al. Epidermal-growth-factor receptors in human bladder cancer: comparison of invasive and superficial tumours. Lancet. 1985;1:366–8.

Pagano F, Guazzieri S, Artibani W, et al. Prognosis of bladder cancer. III. The value of radical cystectomy in the management of invasive bladder cancer. Eur Urol. 1988;15:166–70.

Pagano F, Bassi P, Ferrante GL, et al. Is stage pT4 (D1) reliable in assessing transitional cell carcinoma involvement of the prostate in patients with a concurrent bladder cancer? A necessary distinction for contiguous or noncontiguous involvement. J Urol. 1996;155:244–7.

Raghavan D, Shipley WU, Garnick MB, et al. Biology and management of bladder cancer. N Engl J Med. 1990;322:1129–33.

Sarkis AS, Dalbagni G, Cordon-Cardo C, et al. Association of p53 nuclear over-expression and tumor progression in carcinoma *in situ* of the bladder. J Urol. 1994;152:388–92.

Saxman SB, Propert K, Einhorn LH, et al. Long-term follow-up of phase III intergroup study of cisplatin alone or in combination with methotrexate, vinblastine, and doxorubicin in patients with metastatic urothelial carcinoma: a cooperative group study. J Clin Oncol. 1997;15:2564–9.

Shipley WU, Prout GR Jr, Kaufman DS, Peronne TL. Invasive bladder carcinoma: the importance of initial transurethral surgery and other significant prognostic factors for improved survival with full-dose irradiation. Cancer. 1987;60:514.

Siemiatycki J, Dewar R, Nadon L, et al. Occupational risk factors for bladder cancer: results from a case-control study in Montréal, Québec, Canada. Am J Epidemiol. 1994;140:1061–80.

Spruck CH III, Ohneseit PF, Gonzalez-Zulueta M, et al. Two molecular pathways to transitional cell carcinoma of the bladder. Cancer Res. 1994;54:784–8.

Sternberg CN, Swanson DA. Non-transitional cell bladder cancer. In: Raghavan D, Scher HI, Leibel SA, Lange PH, editors. Principles and practice of genitourinary oncology. Philadelphia, PA: Lippincott-Raven; 315. p. 330–1997.

Torti FM, Lum BL, Astron D, et al. Superficial bladder cancer: the primacy of grade in the development of invasive disease. J Clin Oncol. 1987;5:125.

Wishnow KI, Levinson AK, Johnson DE. Stage B (P2/3aN0) transitional cell carcinoma of the bladder highly curable by radical cystectomy. Urology. 1992;39:12–6.

**45**

# 46

# Urethra

## *At-A-Glance*

**SUMMARY OF CHANGES**

* For urothelial (transitional cell) carcinoma of the prostate, T1 category is defined as tumors invading subepithelial connective tissue

| ANATOMIC STAGE/PROGNOSTIC GROUPS | | | |
|---|---|---|---|
| Stage 0a | Ta | N0 | M0 |
| Stage 0is | Tis | N0 | M0 |
| | Tis pu | N0 | M0 |
| | Tis pd | N0 | M0 |
| Stage I | T1 | N0 | M0 |
| Stage II | T2 | N0 | M0 |
| Stage III | T1 | N1 | M0 |
| | T2 | N1 | M0 |
| | T3 | N0 | M0 |
| | T3 | N1 | M0 |
| Stage IV | T4 | N0 | M0 |
| | T4 | N1 | M0 |
| | Any T | N2 | M0 |
| | Any T | Any N | M1 |

ICD-O-3
TOPOGRAPHY
CODES
C68.0    Urethra

ICD-O-3 HISTOLOGY
CODE RANGES
8000–8576, 8940–8950,
8980–8981

## INTRODUCTION

Cancer of the urethra is a rare neoplasia that is found in both sexes but more common in females. The cancer may be associated in males with chronic stricture disease and in females with urethral diverticula. Tumors of the urethra may be of primary origin from the urethral epithelium or ducts, or they may be associated with multifocal urothelial neoplasia. Histologically, these tumors may represent the spectrum of epithelial neoplasms, including squamous, glandular (adenocarcinoma), or urothelial (transitional cell) carcinoma. Prostatic urethral neoplasms arising from the prostatic urethral epithelium or from the periurethral portion of the prostatic ducts are considered urethral neoplasms as distinct from those arising elsewhere in the prostate (see Chap. 41). These tumors will be staged in conjunction with bladder staging for urothelial neoplasms to differentiate them from primary urethral cancers.

## ANATOMY

**Primary Site.** The male penile urethra consists of mucosa, submucosal stroma, and the surrounding corpus spongiosum. Histologically, the meatal and parameatal urethra are lined with squamous epithelium; the penile and bulbomembranous urethra with pseudostratified or stratified columnar epithelium, and the prostatic urethra with urothelium (transitional epithelium). There are scattered islands of stratified squamous epithelium and glands of Littré liberally situated throughout the entire urethra distal to the prostate portion.

The epithelium of the female urethra is supported on subepithelial connective tissue. The periurethral glands of Skene are concentrated near the meatus but extend along the entire urethra. The urethra is surrounded by a longitudinal layer of smooth muscle continuous with the bladder. The urethra is contiguous to the vaginal wall. The distal two-thirds of the urethra is lined with squamous epithelium, the proximal one-third with urothelium (transitional epithelium). The periurethral glands are lined with pseudostratified and stratified columnar epithelium.

**Regional Lymph Nodes.** The regional lymph nodes are as follows:

Inguinal (superficial or deep)
Iliac (common, internal [hypogastric], obturator, external)
Presacral
Sacral, NOS
Pelvic, NOS

The significance of regional lymph node metastasis in staging urethral cancer lies in the number and size, not in whether unilateral or bilateral.

**Metastatic Sites.** Distant spread is most commonly to lung, liver, or bone.

## RULES FOR CLASSIFICATION

**Clinical Staging.** Radiographic imaging, cystourethroscopy, palpation, and biopsy or cytology of the tumor prior to definitive treatment are desirable. The site of origin should be confirmed to exclude metastatic disease.

**Pathologic Staging.** The assignment of stage for nonprostatic urethral tumors is based on depth of invasion. Prostatic urethral tumor may arise from the prostatic epithelium or from the distal portions of the prostatic ducts and will be classified as prostatic urethral neoplasms. Other prostatic malignancies will be classified under prostate.

Figures 46.1 and 46.2 illustrate Primary Tumor (T) definitions for urethral malignancies and urothelial (transitional cell) carcinoma of the prostate.

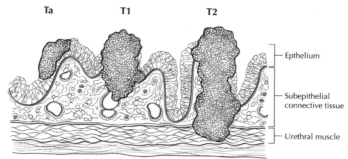

**FIGURE 46.1.** Definition of primary tumor (T) for Ta, T1, and T2 with depth of invasion ranging from the epithelium to the urogenital diaphragm.

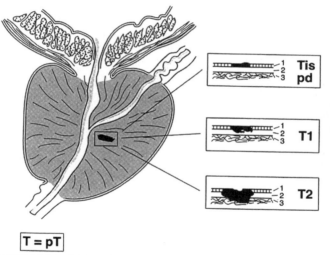

**FIGURE 46.2.** Definition of primary tumor (T) for urothelial (transitional cell) carcinoma of the prostate. 1, Epithelium; 2, subepithelial connective tissue; 3, prostatic stroma.

## DEFINITIONS OF TNM

| *Primary Tumor (T) (Male and Female)* | |
|---|---|
| TX | Primary tumor cannot be assessed |
| T0 | No evidence of primary tumor |
| Ta | Noninvasive papillary, polypoid, or verrucous carcinoma |
| Tis | Carcinoma in situ |
| T1 | Tumor invades subepithelial connective tissue |
| T2 | Tumor invades any of the following: corpus spongiosum, prostate, periurethral muscle |

## Primary Tumor (T) (Male and Female) (continued)

T3    Tumor invades any of the following: corpus cavernosum, beyond prostatic capsule, anterior vagina, bladder neck

T4    Tumor invades other adjacent organs

*Urothelial (Transitional Cell) Carcinoma of the Prostate*

Tis pu    Carcinoma in situ, involvement of the prostatic urethra

Tis pd    Carcinoma in situ, involvement of the prostatic ducts

T1    Tumor invades urethral subepithelial connective tissue

T2    Tumor invades any of the following: prostatic stroma, corpus spongiosum, periurethral muscle

T3    Tumor invades any of the following: corpus cavernosum, beyond prostatic capsule, bladder neck (extraprostatic extension)

T4    Tumor invades other adjacent organs (invasion of the bladder)

## Regional Lymph Nodes (N)

NX    Regional lymph nodes cannot be assessed

N0    No regional lymph node metastasis

N1    Metastasis in a single lymph node 2 cm or less in greatest dimension

N2    Metastasis in a single node more than 2 cm in greatest dimension, or in multiple nodes

## Distant Metastasis (M)

M0    No distant metastasis

M1    Distant metastasis

## ANATOMIC STAGE/PROGNOSTIC GROUPS

| Stage | T | N | M |
|---|---|---|---|
| Stage 0a | Ta | N0 | M0 |
| Stage 0is | Tis | N0 | M0 |
|  | Tis pu | N0 | M0 |
|  | Tis pd | N0 | M0 |
| Stage I | T1 | N0 | M0 |
| Stage II | T2 | N0 | M0 |
| Stage III | T1 | N1 | M0 |
|  | T2 | N1 | M0 |
|  | T3 | N0 | M0 |
|  | T3 | N1 | M0 |
| Stage IV | T4 | N0 | M0 |
|  | T4 | N1 | M0 |
|  | Any T | N2 | M0 |
|  | Any T | Any N | M1 |

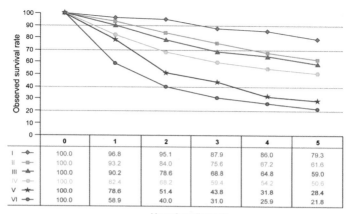

| | | 0 | 1 | 2 | 3 | 4 | 5 |
|---|---|---|---|---|---|---|---|
| I | ◆ | 100.0 | 96.8 | 95.1 | 87.9 | 86.0 | 79.3 |
| II | ■ | 100.0 | 93.2 | 84.0 | 75.6 | 67.2 | 61.6 |
| III | ▲ | 100.0 | 90.2 | 78.6 | 68.8 | 64.8 | 59.0 |
| IV | ● | 100.0 | 82.4 | 68.2 | 59.4 | 54.2 | 50.6 |
| V | ★ | 100.0 | 78.6 | 51.4 | 43.8 | 31.8 | 28.4 |
| VI | ● | 100.0 | 58.9 | 40.0 | 31.0 | 25.9 | 21.8 |

Years from diagnosis

**FIGURE 46.3.** Observed and overall survival rates for 1,278 patients with urethral cancer classified by the current AJCC staging classification. Data taken from the National Cancer Data Base (Commission on Cancer of the American College of Surgeons and the American Cancer Society) for the years 1998–2002. Stage 0a includes 129 patients; Stage 0is, 170; Stage I, 243; Stage II, 193; Stage III, 250; and Stage IV, 293.

## PROGNOSTIC FACTORS (SITE-SPECIFIC FACTORS)
### (Recommended for Collection)

Required for staging     None

Clinically significant     World Health Organization/International Society of Urologic Pathology (WHO/ISUP) grade

Figure 46.3 shows observed and overall survival rates for 1,278 patients with urethral cancer classified by the current AJCC staging classification for the years 1998–2002.

## HISTOLOGIC GRADE (G)

Grade is reported in registry systems by the grade value. For urothelial histologies, a low- and high-grade designation is used to match the current World Health Organization/International Society of Urologic Pathology (WHO/ISUP) recommended grading system:

LG     Low grade
HG     High grade

If a grading system is not specified, generally the following system is used:

GX     Grade cannot be assessed
G1     Well differentiated
G2     Moderately differentiated
G3     Poorly differentiated
G4     Undifferentiated

## HISTOPATHOLOGIC TYPE

The classification applies to urothelial (transitional cell), squamous, and glandular carcinomas of the urethra and to urothelial (transitional cell) carcinomas of the prostate and prostatic urethra. There should be histologic or cytologic confirmation of the disease.

## BIBLIOGRAPHY

Amin MB, Young RH. Primary carcinomas of the urethra. Semin Diagn Pathol. 1997;14(2):147–60.

Dalbagni G, Zhang ZF, Lacombe L, Herr HW. Female urethral carcinoma: an analysis of treatment outcome and a plea for a standardized management strategy. Br J Urol. 1998;82(6):835–41.

Dalbagni G, Zhang ZF, Lacombe L, Herr HW. Male urethral carcinoma: analysis of treatment outcome. Urology. 1999;53(6):1126–32.

Davis JW, Schellhammer PF, Schlossberg SM. Conservative surgical therapy for penile and urethral carcinoma. Urology. 1999;53(2):386–92.

Gheiler EL, Tefilli MV, Tiguert R, de Oliveira JG, Pontes JE, Wood DP Jr. Management of primary urethral cancer. Urology. 1998;52(3):487–93.

Grigsby PW. Carcinoma of the urethra in women. Int J Radiat Oncol Biol Phys. 1998;41(3):535–41.

Krieg R, Hoffman R. Current management of unusual genitourinary cancers. Part 2: urethral cancer. Oncology. 1999;13(11):1511–20.

Levine RL. Urethral cancer. Cancer. 1980;45:1965–72.

Matzkin H, Soloway MS, Hardeman S. Transitional cell carcinoma of the prostate. J Urol. 1991;146:1207–12.

Micaily B, Dzeda MF, Miyamoto CT, Brady LW. Brachytherapy for cancer of the female urethra. Semin Surg Oncol. 1997;13(3):208–14.

Milosevic MF, Warde PR, Banerjee D, et al. Urethral carcinoma in women: results of treatment with primary radiotherapy. Radiother Oncol. 2000;56(1):29–35.

Rogers RE, Burns B. Carcinoma of the female urethra. Obstet Gynecol. 1969; 33:54–7.

Steele GS, Fielding JR, Renshaw A, Loughlin KR. Transitional cell carcinoma of the fossa navicularis. Urology. 1997;50(5):792–5 (review).

Vernon HK, Wilkins RD. Primary carcinoma of the male urethra. Br J Urol. 1950;21:232–5.

Wishnow KI, Ro JY. Importance of early treatment of transitional cell carcinoma of the bladder. J Urol. 1988;140:289.

**47**

# Adrenal

## *At-A-Glance*

| SUMMARY OF CHANGES |
|---|
| • The definition of TNM and the Stage Grouping for this chapter has been created for the first time for the Seventh Edition |

**ANATOMIC STAGE/PROGNOSTIC GROUPS**

| Stage I | T1 | N0 | M0 |
|---|---|---|---|
| Stage II | T2 | N0 | M0 |
| Stage III | T1 | N1 | M0 |
| | T2 | N1 | M0 |
| | T3 | N0 | M0 |
| Stage IV | T3 | N1 | M0 |
| | T4 | N0 | M0 |
| | T4 | N1 | M0 |
| | Any T | Any N | M1 |

**ICD-O-3 TOPOGRAPHY CODES**

C74.0 Cortex of adrenal gland
C74.9 Adrenal gland, NOS

**ICD-O-3 HISTOLOGY CODE**
8010 (C74.0 only), 8140 (C74.0 only), 8370

## INTRODUCTION

The adrenal gland can be thought of as two distinct organs embryologically and functionally: the adrenal cortex, which produces the steroid hormones – aldosterone, cortisol, and testosterone – and the adrenal medulla, which produces catecholamines. Tumors of the adrenal gland are relatively uncommon, with a dearth of information available for staging purposes. A staging system for adrenal cortical cancers has not previously been promoted by the AJCC. This new staging system is limited to the adrenal cortex and only addresses adrenal cortical carcinoma. This staging system does not include tumors of the adrenal medullary compartment such as pheochromocytoma or other unusual tumors such a neuroblastic tumors of the adrenal gland, which are primarily tumors of the pediatric population. The staging system is based on information and data primarily from adult populations. The currently proposed staging system uses the anatomic known prognostic features such as size of the primary tumor, local invasion, and the presence or absence of invasion into adjacent organs. In the future vascular invasion may be incorporated into the staging system. However, currently there are insufficient outcome data to establish staging based on this putative factor. The presence or absence of vascular invasion will be collected as an investigational *site-specific factor* so that such outcome data may be collected. Additionally, with more advanced imaging techniques adrenal cortical neoplasms are being discovered at much smaller limits, and often are incidentally discovered. As more information becomes available on these incidentally detected tumors the staging system may need to be modified. Because of the rarity of adrenal cortical carcinoma validation and publication of additional results from multi-institutional collaborative efforts and population registries is encouraged.

## ANATOMY

**Primary Site.** The adrenal glands sit in a supra renal location (retroperitoneal) surrounded by connective tissue and a layer of adipose tissue. They are intimately associated with the kidneys and are enclosed within the renal fascia (Gerota's). Each gland has an outer cortex, which is lipid rich and on gross examination appears bright yellow surrounding an inner "gray-white" medullary compartment composed of chromaffin cells. There is a rich vascular supply derived from the aorta, inferior phrenic arteries, and renal arteries. Veins emerge from the hilus of the glands. The shorter right central vein opens into the inferior vena cava and the left central vein opens into the renal vein.

**Regional Lymph Nodes.** The regional lymph nodes are as follows:

Aortic (para-aortic, peri-aortic)
Retroperitoneal, NOS

**Metastatic Sites.** Common metastatic sites include liver, lung, and retroperitoneum. Metastases to brain and skin are uncommon although cutaneous involvement of the scalp can simulate angiosarcoma.

## RULES FOR CLASSIFICATION

The classification applies only to adrenal cortical carcinoma. Adenoma is excluded as well as pheochromocytoma and neuroblastic tumors. The currently proposed staging system is based on information from studies of adult adrenal cortical carcinoma. Adrenal cortical carcinoma in the pediatric population appears to have a better prognosis overall than pathologically identical tumors in the adult population. The staging system for pediatric adrenal cortical carcinoma used by most pediatric oncology groups, however, is based on the same data, and the stage of disease appears to be the most relevant prognostic factor in this group of patients. A separate staging system based on tumor weight (less than or greater than 200 g) has also been proposed.

**Clinical Staging.** Clinical examination and radiographic imaging are required to assess the size of the primary tumor and the extent of disease, both local and distant. Biochemical studies should be performed to evaluate the functional status of the tumor.

**Pathologic Staging.** Resection of the primary tumor and examination for lymph node involvement and extent of disease (including vascular invasion) should be performed. Tumor size and *weight* should be recorded accurately in every case. Histologic examination and confirmation of extent of disease are required. Disease free and overall survival rates appear to correlate strongly with stage of adrenal cortical carcinoma.

## DEFINITIONS OF TNM

### Primary Tumor (T)

TX     Primary tumor cannot be assessed
T0     No evidence of primary tumor
T1     Tumor 5 cm or less in greatest dimension, no extra-adrenal invasion (Figure 47.1)
T2     Tumor greater than 5 cm, no extra-adrenal invasion (Figure 47.2)
T3     Tumor of any size with local invasion, but not invading adjacent organs* (Figure 47.3)
T4     Tumor of any size with invasion of adjacent organs* (Figure 47.4)

*Note*: Adjacent organs include kidney, diaphragm, great vessels, pancreas, spleen, and liver.

### Regional Lymph Nodes (N)

NX     Regional lymph nodes cannot be assessed
N0     No regional lymph node metastasis
N1     Metastasis in regional lymph node(s)

**47**

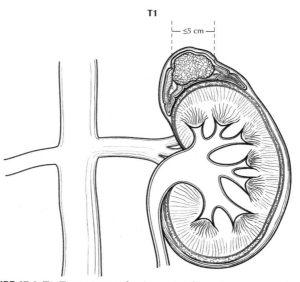

**FIGURE 47.1.** T1: Tumor 5 cm or less in greatest dimension, no extra-adrenal invasion.

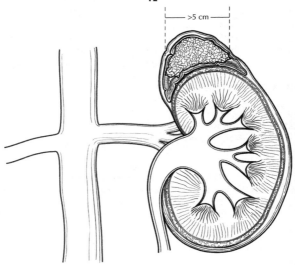

**FIGURE 47.2.** T2: Tumor greater than 5 cm, no extra-adrenal invasion.

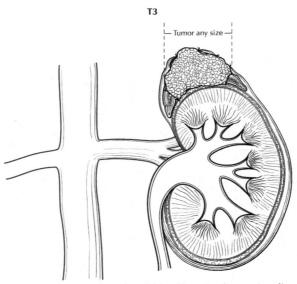

**FIGURE 47.3.** T3: Tumor of any size with local invasion, but not invading adjacent organs.

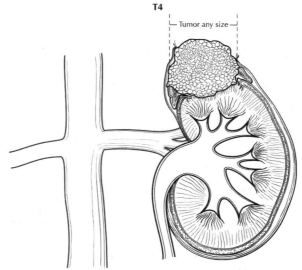

**FIGURE 47.4.** T4: Tumor of any size with invasion of adjacent organs.

| *Distant Metastasis (M)* | | | |
|---|---|---|---|
| M0 | No distance metastasis | | |
| M1 | Distance metastasis | | |

**ANATOMIC STAGE/PROGNOSTIC GROUPS**

| Stage I | T1 | N0 | M0 |
|---|---|---|---|
| Stage II | T2 | N0 | M0 |
| Stage III | T1 | N1 | M0 |
| | T2 | N1 | M0 |
| | T3 | N0 | M0 |
| Stage IV | T3 | N1 | M0 |
| | T4 | N0 | M0 |
| | T4 | N1 | M0 |
| | Any T | Any N | M1 |

## PROGNOSTIC FACTORS (SITE-SPECIFIC FACTORS)
### (Recommended for Collection)

| Required for staging | None |
|---|---|
| Clinically significant | Tumor weight in grams |
| | Vascular invasion |

47

## BIBLIOGRAPHY

Cagle PT, Hough AJ, Pysher J, et al. Comparison of adrenal cortical tumors in children and adults. Cancer. 1986;57:2235–7.

Grumbach MM, Biller BMK, Braunstein GD, et al. Management of the clinically inapparent adrenal mass ("incidentaloma"). Ann Intern Med. 2003;138: 424–9.

Henley DJ, van Heerden JA, Grant CS, et al. Adrenal cortical carcinoma—a continuing challenge. Surgery. 1983;94(6):926–31.

Lack EE. Tumors of the adrenal gland and extra-adrenal paraganglia. In: Rosai J, Sobin LH, editors. Atlas of tumor pathology, third series fascicle. Washington, DC: Armed Forces Institute of Pathology; 1997. p. 144–5.

Lack EE, Mulivihil JJ, Travis WD, et al. Adrenocortical neoplasms in the pediatric and adolescent age group. Clinicopathologic study of 30 cases with emphasis on epidemiologic and prognostic factors. 1992;27:1–53.

Lack EE, Askin FB, Dehner LP, et al. Recommendations for reporting of tumors of the adrenal cortex and medulla. Hum Pathol. 1999;30:887–90.

Macfarlane DA. Cancer of the adrenal cortex. The natural history, prognosis and treatment in a study of 55 cases. Ann Roy Coll Surg. 1958;23:155–86.

Melvin M, et al. NIH state-of-the-science statement on management of the clinically inapparent adrenal mass ("incidentaloma"). NIH Consensus State Sci Statements. 2002;19:1–25.

Meyer A, Niemann U, Behrend M. Experience with the surgical treatment of adrenal cortical carcinoma. EJSO. 2004;30:444–9.

Michalkiewicz E, Sandrini R, Figueiredo B, et al. Clincial and outcome characteristics of children with adrenocortical tumors: a report from the international pediatric adrenocortical tumor registry. J Clin Oncol. 2004;22:838–45.

Sandrini R, Ribeiro RC, DeLacerda L. Childhood adrenocortical tumors. J Clin Endocrinol Metab. 1997;82:2027–31.

Sullivan M, Boileau M, Hodges CV. Adrenal cortical carcinoma. J Urol. 1978;120:660–5.

Tucci A, Martins ACP, Suaid HJ, et al. The impact of tumor stage on prognosis in children with adrenocortical carcinoma. J Urol. 2005;174(6):2338–42.

Wajchenberg BL, Albergaria Pereira MA, Medonca BB, et al. Adrenocortical carcinoma. Clinical and laboratory observations. Cancer. 2000;88:711–36.

Wieneke JA, Thompson LDR, Heffess CS. Adrenal cortical neoplasms in the pediatric population. A clinicopathologic and immunophenotypic analysis of 83 patients. Am J Surg Pathol. 2003;77:867–81.

Wooten MD, King DK. Adrenal cortical carcinoma. Cancer. 1993;72:3145–55.

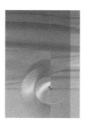

# PART X
# Ophthalmic Sites

# Carcinoma of the Eyelid

## *At-A-Glance*

| ANATOMIC STAGE/PROGNOSTIC GROUPS | | | |
|---|---|---|---|
| Stage 0 | Tis | N0 | M0 |
| Stage IA | T1 | N0 | M0 |
| Stage IB | T2a | N0 | M0 |
| Stage IC | T2b | N0 | M0 |
| Stage II | T3a | N0 | M0 |
| Stage IIIA | T3b | N0 | M0 |
| Stage IIIB | Any T | N1 | M0 |
| Stage IIIC | T4 | Any N | M0 |
| Stage IV | Any T | Any N | M1 |

ICD-O-3
TOPOGRAPHY
CODES
C:44.1    Eyelid

ICD-O-3 HISTOLOGY
CODE RANGES
8000–8576, 8940–8950,
8980–8981

## INTRODUCTION

The tumor biology of primary eyelid carcinoma encompasses a broad spectrum of behaviors, from indolent low-grade nodular tumors to highly aggressive sebaceous and Merkel cell carcinomas. Primary carcinoma of the eyelid can be categorized into four staging groups: (1) localized eyelid disease, (2) resectable adjacent structure infiltration, (3) regional lymph node infiltration, enucleation, exenteration, or nonresectable tumor, and (4) metastatic spread.

The staging system presented here is to be used for eyelid tumors of all histologic types. During the development of this edition of the *AJCC Cancer Staging Manual*, both the Ophthalmic and the non-Melanoma Skin Cancer Task Forces proposed staging systems for eyelid squamous cell carcinomas. The Editorial Board made the decision to assign eyelid SCC to the

Ophthalmic staging system. However, it was also decided to recommend collection of the prognostic and site specific factors recommended for all cutaneous squamous cell carcinomas by the nonmelanoma skin cancer task force (see Chap. 29).

## ANATOMY

**Primary Site.** The eyelid is composed of anterior and posterior lamellae, which divide along the mucocutaneous lid margin. From anterior to posterior, the eyelid is composed of skin, orbicularis muscle, tarsus and conjunctiva. The levator aponeurosis and Müller's muscle are attached at the superior aspect of the tarsus, with similar retractors of the lower eyelid. There is a rich supply of sebaceous, eccrine, apocrine, and neuroendocrine glandular elements diffused within the eyelid, caruncle and periorbital tissues. Sebaceous glands are concentrated in the tarsus, the eyelash margin, and within smaller pilo-sebaceous units that cover the eyelid and caruncle. Glandular elements and skin are the precursor cell-types for carcinoma of the eyelid.

**Local Invasion.** Carcinoma of the eyelid may extend directly into adjacent structures through mechanisms of direct infiltration, perineural or perivascular spread, and mucosal invasion. Sites of local invasion include orbital soft tissue and bone, the globe, face, nasal cavity and paranasal sinuses, orbital apex, base of the skull, and the central nervous system.

**Regional Lymph Nodes.** The eyelids and ocular adnexa are supplied with lymphatics that drain into the pre-auricular, parotid, and infra-auricular (cervical, submandibular, and supraclavicular lymph node basins).

**Lymph Node Staging.** With exception of a rare infiltrative basal cell carcinoma, the remaining eyelid carcinomas have progressive capacity for lymph node metastasis. The risk benefit ratio for lymph node surgical evaluation is based upon tumor size, histopathologic type, and tumor grade.

We have gained considerable understanding of lymph node staging in eyelid carcinoma, through the tumor experience of head and neck squamous cell carcinoma (HNSCC), Merkel cell and sebaceous carcinoma. In HNSCC lymph node metastasis is a vital independent prognostic factor. A clinically positive N1 lymph node should be biopsied for confirmation and patient care planning. Clinical and imaging assessment can fail to detect lymph node metastasis in up to 25% of cases of HNSCC and 32% of head and neck Merkel cell carcinomas. However, complete lymph node dissection carries its own morbidity and surgical risk.

Technetium (Tc-99m) sentinel lymph node (SLN) biopsy has emerged as a useful tool that allows for sampling first order lymph nodes draining the tumor bed, with less morbidity than a full lymph node dissection. A positive SLN provides critical staging information and can help select patients who may benefit from additional treatments.

Tc-99m lymphoscintigraphy with SLN biopsy requires modest adaptation for eyelid carcinoma. The volume of radioactive isotope is reduced, to match the reduced thickness of the eyelid tissues. Step serial sectioning with immunohistochemical staining improves the sensitivity of this sampling technique. As with any patient care or surgical tool, the decision to perform sentinel lymph node biopsy is weighed as a risk benefit ratio for each patient. The decision is highly dependent upon the tumor biology aggressiveness of the underlying carcinoma.

**Metastatic Sites.** Metastatic potential is highly dependent upon histopathologic type and grade. It is widely believed that eyelid carcinomas metastasize via the cascade of lymphatic channels and less frequently hematogenous spread. Distant sites include lung, liver, other viscera, and brain.

## RULES FOR CLASSIFICATION

**Clinical Staging.** Staging of eyelid carcinoma begins with a comprehensive ophthalmic, orbital, and periorbital clinical examination. This approach includes a slit lamp or equivalent biomicroscopy evaluation, neuro-ophthalmic examination for evidence of perineural invasion, and regional assessment of the head and neck to include lymphatic drainage basins. Preoperative photography of the extent of disease is recommended. The requirement for imaging modalities including computed tomography, magnetic resonance imaging, and ultrasonography is highly dependent upon the histopathology type and clinical findings.

**Pathologic Staging.** The surgical nature of the histopathology specimen should be noted including incisional biopsy, excisional biopsy, wide local excision, radical excision including exenteration. The specimen should be carefully oriented and inked for margin evaluation. Pathologic classification is based on the specific tumor type, its differentiation (grade), and the extent of removal. In excisional specimens, greatest tumor dimension and evaluation of the surgical specimen margins are mandatory.

**48**

## DEFINITIONS OF TNM

The following definitions apply to clinical and pathologic staging.

| *Primary Tumor (T)* | |
|---|---|
| TX | Primary tumor cannot be assessed |
| T0 | No evidence of primary tumor |
| Tis | Carcinoma in situ |
| T1 | Tumor 5 mm or less in greatest dimension |
| | Not invading the tarsal plate or eyelid margin |
| T2a | Tumor more than 5 mm, but not more than 10 mm in greatest dimension |
| | Or, any tumor that invades the tarsal plate or eyelid margin |
| T2b | Tumor more than 10 mm, but not more than 20 mm in greatest dimension |
| | Or, involves full thickness eyelid |

### Primary Tumor (T) (continued)

| | |
|---|---|
| T3a | Tumor more than 20 mm in greatest dimension |
| | Or, any tumor that invades adjacent ocular or orbital structures |
| | Any T with perineural tumor invasion |
| T3b | Complete tumor resection requires enucleation, exenteration, or bone resection |
| T4 | Tumor is not resectable due to extensive invasion of ocular, orbital, craniofacial structures, or brain |

### Regional Lymph Nodes (N)

| | |
|---|---|
| NX | Regional lymph nodes cannot be assessed |
| cN0 | No regional lymph node metastasis, based upon clinical evaluation or imaging |
| pN0 | No regional lymph node metastasis, based upon lymph node biopsy |
| N1 | Regional lymph node metastasis |

### Distant Metastasis (M)

| | |
|---|---|
| M0 | No distant metastasis |
| M1 | Distant metastasis |

### ANATOMIC STAGE/PROGNOSTIC GROUPS

| | | | |
|---|---|---|---|
| Stage 0 | Tis | N0 | M0 |
| Stage IA | T1 | N0 | M0 |
| Stage B | T2a | N0 | M0 |
| Stage IC | T2b | N0 | M0 |
| Stage II | T3a | N0 | M0 |
| Stage IIIA | T3b | N0 | M0 |
| Stage IIIB | Any T | N1 | M0 |
| Stage IIIC | T4 | Any N | M0 |
| Stage IV | Any T | Any N | M1 |

## PROGNOSTIC FACTORS (SITE-SPECIFIC FACTORS)
### (Recommended for Collection)

| | |
|---|---|
| Required for staging | None |
| Clinically significant | Sentinel lymph node biopsy (SLNB) results |
| | Regional nodes identified on clinical or radiographic examination |
| | Perineural invasion |
| | Tumor necrosis |
| | Pagetoid spread |
| | More than 3 Mohs micrographic surgical layers required |
| | Immunosuppression – patient has HIV |

Immunosuppression – history of solid organ transplant or leukemia
Prior radiation to the tumor field
Excluding skin cancer, patient has history of two or more carcinomas
Patient has Muir-Torre syndrome
Patient has Xeroderma pigmentosa

For eyelid cutaneous squamous cell carcinoma only (see "Cutaneous Squamous Cell Carcinoma," Chap. 29):

| | |
|---|---|
| Required for staging | Tumor thickness (in mm) |
| | Clark's level |
| | Presence/absence of perineural invasion |
| | Primary site location on ear or hair-bearing lip |
| | Histologic grade |
| | Size of largest lymph node metastasis |
| Clinically significant | No additional factors |

## HISTOLOGIC GRADE (G)

Grade is reported in registry systems by the grade value. A two-grade, three-grade, or four-grade system may be used. If a grading system is not specified, generally the following system is used:

| | |
|---|---|
| GX | Grade cannot be assessed |
| G1 | Well differentiated |
| G2 | Moderately differentiated |
| G3 | Poorly differentiated |
| G4 | Undifferentiated |

## HISTOPATHOLOGIC TYPE

The primary eyelid carcinoma tumors include the following group and list of histologies:

Basal cell carcinoma
Squamous cell carcinoma
Mucoepidermoid carcinoma
Sebaceous carcinoma
Primary eccrine adenocarcinoma
Primary apocrine adenocarcinoma
Adenoid cystic carcinoma
Merkel cell carcinoma

## BIBLIOGRAPHY

Allen PJ, Bowne WB, Jaques DP, et al. Merkel cell carcinoma: prognosis and treatment of patients from a single institution. J Clin Oncol. 2005;23:2300–9.
Barta RS, Kelley LC. A risk scale for predicting extensive subclinical spread of nonmelanoma skin cancer. Dermatol Surg. 2002;28(2):107–12.

Betis F, Hofman V, Lagier J, et al. Primary signet ring cell carcinoma of the Eccrine sweat gland in the eyelid. Immunohistochemical and ultrastructural study of a case. J Fr Ophthalmol. 2002;25(5):547–51.

Dequanter D, Lothaire P, Bourgeois P, et al. Sentinel lymph node evaluation in squamous cell carcinoma of the head and neck cancer: preliminary results. Acta Chir Belg. 2006;106:519–22.

Ducasse A, Pluot M, Gotzamanis A, et al. Factors of recurrence of basal cell carcinomas of the eyelid. J Fr Ophthalmol. 2002;25(5):512–16.

El-Domeiri AA, Brasfield RD, Huvos AG, et al. Sweat gland carcinoma: a clinicopathologic study of 83 patients. Ann Surg. 1971;173;270–74.

Esmaeli B, Naderi A, Hidaji L, et al. Merkel cell carcinoma of the eyelid with a positive sentinel node. Arch Ophthalmol. 2002;120:650–2.

Faustina M, Diba R, Ahmadi MA, Esmaeli B. Patterns of regional and distant metastasis in patients with eyelid and periocular squamous cell carcinoma. Ophthalmology. 2004;111(10):1930–32.

Gupta SG, Wang LC, Peñas PF, et al. Sentinel lymph node biopsy for evaluation and treatment of patients with Merkel cell carcinoma. Arch Dermatol. 2006;142:685–90.

Nijhawan N, Ross MI, Diba R, et al. Experience with sentinel lymph node biopsy for the eyelid and conjunctival malignancies at a cancer center. Ophthal Plastic Reconstr Surg. 2004;20(4):291–5.

Rao NA, Hidayat AA, McLean IW, Zimmerman LE. Sebaceous carcinomas of the ocular adnexa: a clincopathologic study of 104 cases, with five year follow-up data. Hum Pathol. 1982;13:113–22.

Ross GL, Shoaib T, Soutar DS, et al. The first international conference on sentinel node biopsy in mucosal head and neck cancer and adoption of a multicenter trial protocol. J Surg Oncol. 2002;94(4):406–10.

Soysal HG, Markoc F. Invasive squamous cell carcinoma of the eyelids and periorbital region. Br J Ophthalmol. 2007;91(3):325–9.

Yiengpruksawan A, Coit DG, Thaler HT, Urmacher C, Knapper WK. Merkel cell carcinoma. Prognosis and management. Arch Surg. 1991;126:1514–9.

# Carcinoma of the Conjunctiva

## *At-A-Glance*

---

### SUMMARY OF CHANGES

- A listing of site-specific categories is included in T3
- Sebaceous gland carcinoma with pagetoid conjunctival spread was added under histopathologic type

---

### ANATOMIC STAGE/PROGNOSTIC GROUPS

No stage grouping is presently recommended

ICD-O-3
TOPOGRAPHY
CODES
C69.0     Conjunctiva

ICD-O-3 HISTOLOGY
CODE RANGES
8000–8576, 8940–8950,
8980–8981

## INTRODUCTION

This classification only applies to carcinoma of the conjunctiva. Other tumors of the conjunctiva are not classified using this schema. The differential diagnoses include nonpigmented primary conjunctival tumors and pseudotumors (e.g., leukemia infiltrates, ligneous conjunctivitis, myxoma, non-Hodgkin's lymphoma) as well as secondary conjunctival tumors (e.g., intraocular tumors extending through the sclera into the conjunctiva such as nonpigmented uveal melanoma or uveal non-Hodgkin's lymphoma and orbital tumors extending into the conjunctiva such as rhabdomyosarcoma).

**49**

## ANATOMY

**Primary Site.**   The conjunctiva consists of stratified epithelium that contains mucus-secreting goblet cells; these cells are most numerous in the fornices. Palpebral conjunctiva lines the eyelid; bulbar conjunctiva covers the eyeball. Conjunctival epithelium merges with that of the cornea at the limbus. It is at this exposed site, particularly at the temporal limbus, that carcinoma is most likely to arise. Conjunctival intraepithelial neoplasia (CIN) embraces all forms of intraepithelial dysplasia, including in situ squamous cell carcinoma.

---

**Regional Lymph Nodes.** The regional lymph nodes are as follows:

Preauricular (parotid)
Submandibular
Cervical

For pN, histologic examination of a regional lymphadenectomy specimen, if performed, will include one or more regional lymph nodes.

**Metastatic Sites.** Tumors of the conjunctiva, in addition to spreading by way of regional lymphatics, may also metastasize hematogenously. Additionally, these tumors may directly invade the eyelid, the eye, orbit, adjacent paranasal sinus structures, and brain.

## RULES FOR CLASSIFICATION

**Clinical Staging.** The assessment of cancer is based on inspection, slit-lamp examination, and palpation of the regional lymph nodes. All conjunctival surfaces are inspected and photographed with eversion of the upper eyelid. High-frequency ultrasound (UBM) imaging should be performed when the tumor is found to be affixed to the globe and when intraocular invasion is suspected. Low-frequency ultrasound may also be used to evaluate the sclera, eye, and orbit. Radiologic examinations (computed axial tomography, magnetic resonance imaging, and PET/CT imaging) can be used to examine regional lymph nodes, paranasal sinuses, the orbit, brain, and chest. There are ongoing studies to clarify the role of sentinel lymph node involvement and sentinel lymph node biopsy.

Conjunctival carcinoma has been particularly associated with AIDS, neurodermatitis (atopic keratoconjunctivitis), other forms of immunosuppression (including iatrogenic), UV radiation, and human papillomavirus (HPV 16 and 18).

**Pathologic Staging.** Complete resection of the primary site is indicated (if possible). Cryotherapy and/or topical chemotherapy (mitomycin, 5-fluoruracil, and/or interferon alpha-2b) may be considered as adjunctive therapies. Extensive tumor involvement of orbital soft tissues may require exenteration with or without adjuvant external beam radiation therapy.

The specimen should be thoroughly sampled for histologic study of surgical margins, type of tumor, and grade of malignancy.

## DEFINITIONS OF TNM

These definitions apply to both clinical and pathologic staging.

| *Primary Tumor (T)* | |
|---|---|
| TX | Primary tumor cannot be assessed |
| T0 | No evidence of primary tumor |
| Tis | Carcinoma in situ |
| T1 | Tumor 5 mm or less in greatest dimension* |
| T2 | Tumor more than 5 mm in greatest dimension, without invasion of adjacent structures** |

| T3 | Tumor invades adjacent structures** (excluding the orbit) |
| T4 | Tumor invades the orbit with or without further extension |
| T4a | Tumor invades orbital soft tissues, without bone invasion |
| T4b | Tumor invades bone |
| T4c | Tumor invades adjacent paranasal sinuses |
| T4d | Tumor invades brain |

*Note: Tumors occur most commonly in the bulbar limbal conjunctiva.

**Note: Adjacent structures include the cornea (3, 6, 9, or 12 clock hours), intraocular compartments, forniceal conjunctiva (lower and/or upper), palpebral conjunctiva (lower and/or upper), tarsal conjunctiva (lower and/or upper), lacrimal punctum and canaliculi (lower and/or upper), plica, caruncle, posterior eyelid lamella, anterior eyelid lamella, and/or eyelid margin (lower and/or upper).

### Regional Lymph Nodes (N)
| NX | Regional lymph nodes cannot be assessed |
| N0 | No regional lymph node metastasis |
| N1 | Regional lymph node metastasis |

### Distant Metastasis (M)
| M0 | No distant metastasis |
| M1 | Distant metastasis |

### ANATOMIC STAGE/PROGNOSTIC GROUPS
No stage grouping is presently recommended.

### PROGNOSTIC FACTORS (SITE-SPECIFIC FACTORS)
### (Recommended for Collection)

Required for staging    None

Clinically significant    Ki-67 growth fraction

49

### HISTOPATHOLOGIC TYPE

The classification applies only to carcinoma of the conjunctiva.

Conjunctival intraepithelial neoplasia (CIN) including in situ squamous cell carcinoma
Squamous cell carcinoma
Mucoepidermoid carcinoma
Spindle cell carcinoma
Sebaceous gland carcinoma including pagetoid (conjunctival) spread
Basal cell carcinoma

## HISTOLOGIC GRADE (G)

Grade is reported in registry systems by the grade value. A two-grade, three-grade, or four-grade system may be used. If a grading system is not specified, generally the following system is used:

GX    Grade cannot be assessed
G1    Well differentiated
G2    Moderately differentiated
G3    Poorly differentiated
G4    Undifferentiated

## BIBLIOGRAPHY

Brownstein S. Mucoepidermoid carcinoma of the conjunctiva with intraocular invasion. Ophthalmology. 1981;88:1226–30.

Buus DR, Tse DT, Folberg R. Microscopically controlled excision of conjunctival squamous cell carcinoma. Am J Ophthalmol. 1994;117:97–102.

Campbell RJ. Tumors of eyelid, conjunctiva and cornea. In: Garner A, Klintworth GK, editors. Pathobiology of ocular disease: a dynamic approach, Part A. 2nd ed. New York: Marcel Dekker; 1367. p. 1403–994.

Cohen BH, Green WR, Iliff NT, et al. Spindle cell carcinoma of the conjunctiva. Arch Ophthal. 1980;98:1809–13.

Cursiefen C, Holbach LM, Lafaut B, Heimann K, Kirchner T, Naumann GOH. Oculocerebral non-Hodgkin's lymphoma with uveal involvement: development of an epibulbar tumor after vitrectomy. Arch Ophthalmol. 2000;118:1437–40.

Finger PT. Guest editorial: topical mitomycin chemotherapy for malignant conjunctival and corneal neoplasia. Br J Ophthalmol. 2006;90:807–9.

Finger PT, Tran HV, Turbin RE, Perry HD, Abramson DH, Chin K, et al. High-frequency ultrasonographic evaluation of conjunctival intraepithelial neoplasia and squamous cell carcinoma. Arch Ophthalmol. 2003;121:168–72.

Grossniklaus HE, Green WR, Luckenbach M, Chan CC. Conjunctival lesions in adults. A clinical and histopathologic review. Cornea. 1987;6:78–116.

Grossniklaus HE, Martin DF, Solomon AR. Invasive conjunctival tumor with keratoacanthoma features. Am J Ophthalmol. 1990;109:736–8.

Husain SE, Patrinely JR, Zimmermann LE, et al. Primary basal cell carcinoma of the limbal conjunctiva. Ophthalmology. 1993;100:1720–2.

Jakobiec FA, Folberg R, Iwamoto T. Clinicopathologic characteristics of premalignant and malignant melanocytic lesions of the conjunctiva. Ophthalmology. 1989;96:147–66.

Johnson TE, Tabbara KF, Weatherhead RG, et al. Secondary squamous cell carcinoma of the orbit. Arch Ophthalmol. 1997;115:75–8.

Karcioglu ZA, Issa TM. Human papillomavirus (HPV) in neoplastic and non-neoplastic conditions of the external eye. Br J Ophthalmol. 1997;81:595–8.

Lee GA, Hirst LW. Ocular surface squamous neoplasia. Surv Ophthalmol. 1995;39:429–50.

McKelvie PA, Daniell M, McNab A, Loughnan M, Santamaria JD. Squamous cell carcinoma of the conjunctiva: a series of 26 cases. Br J Ophthalmol. 2002;86:168–73.

McLean IW, Burnier MN, Zimmermann LE, et al. Tumors of the conjunctiva. In: Rosai J, editor. Atlas of tumor pathology: tumors of the eye and ocular adnexa, third series, fascicle 12. Washington, DC: Armed Forces Institute of Pathology; 1994. p. 49–95.

Rao NA, Font RL. Mucoepidermoid carcinoma of the conjunctiva: a clinico-pathologic study of five cases. Cancer. 1976;38:1699–709.

Seitz B, Fischer M, Holbach LM, Naumann GOH. Differential diagnosis and prognosis of 112 excised epibulbar epithelial tumors. Klin Monatsbl Augenheilk. 1995;207:239–46.

Shields CL, Naseripour M, Shields JA. Topical mitomycin C for extensive, recurrent conjuncitval-corneal squamous cell carcinoma. Am J Ophthalmol. 2002;133:601–6.

Shields JA, Demirci H, Marr BP, Eagle RC, Stefanyszyn M, Shields CL. Conjunctival epithelial involvement by eyelid sebaceous carcinoma. Ophthal Plast Reconstr Surg. 2005;21:92–6.

Tunc M, Erbilen E. Topical cyclosporine -A (0.05%) combined with mitomycin C (0.01%) for conjunctival and corneal squamous cell carcinoma. Am J Ophthalmol. 2006;142:673–75.

Wilson MW, Fleming JC, Fleming RM, Haik BG. Sentinel node biopsy for orbital and ocular adnexal tumors. Ophthal Plast Reconstr Surg. 2001a;17:338–44.

Wilson MW, Czechonska G, Finger PT, Rausen A, Hooper ME, Haik BG. Chemotherapy for eye cancer. Surv Ophthalmol. 2001b;45:416–44.

**49**

# Malignant Melanoma of the Conjunctiva

## At-A-Glance

---

### SUMMARY OF CHANGES

- Definitions of T classification have changed to describe location (bulbar, noncaruncular, caruncular)

- Definitions of N category have changed to describe whether a biopsy was performed

- Definitions of pT status have changed to describe local invasion and tumor thickness

- Definition of T(is) or melanoma *in situ* when tumor is limited to the epithelium

- Definitions of "Histologic Grade" were changed to describe cases of synchronous PAM with atypia and conjunctival melanoma (G3 and G4)

---

**ANATOMIC STAGE/PROGNOSTIC GROUP**

No stage grouping is presently recommended

ICD-O-3
TOPOGRAPHY
CODES
C69.0    Conjunctiva

ICD-O-3 HISTOLOGY
CODE RANGES
8720–8790

## ANATOMY

**Primary Site.** Melanocytes have been known to exist in the basal layer of the conjunctival epithelium. These melanocytes can be the source of acquired melanosis, malignant melanoma, junctional and compound nevi. Melanocytic conjunctival tumors range from melanocytic hypertrophy and melanoma in situ to invasive malignant melanoma. Local clinically relevant classifications divide these tumors by conjunctival location, uni- or multi-focality, and tumor thickness. Factors that influence both treatment and prognosis include local invasion, nodal spread, and distant metastasis.

**Regional Lymph Nodes.** Regional lymph nodes are as follows:

Preauricular
Submandibular
Cervical

---

The pN histological examination of a regional lymphadenectomy specimen will ordinarily include one or more regional lymph nodes.

**Metastatic Sites.** In addition to spread by the lymphatics and the bloodstream, direct extension into the eye, eyelids, nasolacrimal system, sinuses, orbit, and central nervous system occurs.

## RULES FOR CLASSIFICATION

**Clinical Staging.** The classification applies only to conjunctival melanoma and primary acquired melanosis with atypia. In general, there should be a histologic evaluation of the tumor.

The clinical assessment of a melanocytic conjunctival tumor is based on inspection, slit-lamp examination, and palpation of the regional lymph nodes. All conjunctival surfaces should be inspected and photographed (including eversion of the upper eyelid).

Tumor photography should pay particular attention to its margins, evidence of pagetoid spread, and involvement of the punctum. Inspection of the ipsilateral sinuses is indicated (particularly if punctal involvement has been noted). Impression or exfoliative cytology may be obtained in the clinical setting.

Radiological evaluation to stage local disease may include computed tomography, magnetic resonance imaging, and/or ultrasonography of the eye, orbits, and sinuses. Metastatic surveys typically include a physical examination as well as hematology screening and radiological evaluations of the head, chest, and abdomen. Radionuclide-based bone scans may be employed.

**Pathologic Staging.** Complete resection of the primary site is indicated. Cryotherapy, topical chemotherapy (mitomycin, 5-fluorouracil, and interferon), and radiation therapy (both teletherapy and brachytherapy) have been employed when complete resection is not possible or as an adjunctive treatment. Histopathologic evaluation for negative peripheral and deep margins should be performed. To best judge the depth of penetration of the tumor, sections should be made perpendicular to the epithelial surface. Perpendicular sections can be facilitated if the surgeon places the specimen epithelial side superior on a moist filter paper. The role of sentinel node biopsy is presently being investigated.

## DEFINITIONS OF TNM

### Clinical

| *Primary Tumor (T)* | |
|---|---|
| TX | Primary tumor cannot be assessed |
| T0 | No evidence of primary tumor |
| T(is) | Melanoma confined to the conjunctival epithelium |

*Malignant conjunctival melanoma of the bulbar conjunctiva*
*T1*

| | |
|---|---|
| T1a | Less than or equal to 1 quadrant* |
| T1b | More than 1 but less than or equal to 2 quadrants |
| T1c | More than 2 but less than or equal to 3 quadrants |
| T1d | Greater than 3 quadrants |

*Malignant conjunctival melanoma of the nonbulbar (palpebral, forniceal caruncular)*
*T2*

| | |
|---|---|
| T2a | No caruncular, less than or equal to 1 quadrant |
| T2b | No caruncular, greater than 1 quadrant |
| T2c | Any caruncular, with less than or equal to 1 quadrant |
| T2d | Any caruncular, with greater than 1 quadrant |

*Any malignant conjunctival melanoma with local invasion*
*T3*

| | |
|---|---|
| T3a | Globe |
| T3b | Eyelid |
| T3c | Orbit |
| T3d | Sinus |
| T4 | Tumor invades the central nervous system |

*Note: Quadrants are defined by clock hour, starting at the limbus (e.g., 6, 9, 12, 3) extending from the central cornea, to and beyond the eyelid margins. This will bisect the caruncle.

### Regional Lymph Node (N)

| | |
|---|---|
| NX | Regional lymph nodes cannot be assessed |
| N0a (biopsied) | No regional lymph node metastasis, biopsy performed |
| N0b (not biopsied) | No regional lymph node metastasis, biopsy not performed |
| N1 | Regional lymph node metastasis |

### Metastasis (M)

| | |
|---|---|
| M0 | No distant metastasis |
| M1 | Distant metastasis |

### ANATOMIC STAGE/PROGNOSTIC GROUP

No stage grouping is presently recommended

**50**

### Pathologic

### Primary Tumor (pT)

| | |
|---|---|
| pTX | Primary tumor cannot be assessed |
| pT0 | No evidence of primary tumor |
| pT(is) | Melanoma of the conjunctiva confined to the epithelium* |

## Primary Tumor (pT) (continued)

| | |
|---|---|
| pT1a | Melanoma of the bulbar conjunctiva not more than 0.5 mm in thickness with invasion of the substantia propria |
| pT1b | Melanoma of the bulbar conjunctiva more than 0.5 mm but not more than 1.5 mm in thickness with invasion of the substantia propria |
| pT1c | Melanoma of the bulbar conjunctiva greater than 1.5 mm in thickness with invasion of the substantia propria |
| pT2a | Melanoma of the palpebral, forniceal, or caruncular conjunctiva not more than 0.5 mm in thickness with invasion of the substantia propria |
| pT2b | Melanoma more than 0.5 but not greater than 1.5 mm in thickness with invasion of the substantia propria |
| pT2c | Melanoma of the palpebral, forniceal, or caruncular conjunctiva greater than 1.5 mm in thickness with invasion of the substantia propria |
| pT3 | Melanoma invades the eye, eyelid, nasolacrimal system, sinuses, or orbit |
| pT4 | Melanoma invades the central nervous system |

*Note: pT(is) melanoma in situ (includes the term primary acquired melanosis) with atypia replacing greater than 75% of the normal epithelial thickness, with cytologic features of epithelioid cells, including abundant cytoplasm, vesicular nuclei or prominent nucleoli, and/or presence of intraepithelial nests of atypical cells.

## Regional Lymph Nodes (pN)

| | |
|---|---|
| pNX | Regional lymph nodes cannot be assessed |
| pN0 | No regional lymph node metastasis |
| pN1 | Regional lymph node metastasis present |

## Distant Metastasis (pM)

| | |
|---|---|
| cM0 | No distant metastasis |
| pM1 | Distant metastasis |

## ANATOMIC STAGE/PROGNOSTIC GROUP

No stage grouping is presently recommended

## PROGNOSTIC FACTORS (SITE-SPECIFIC FACTORS)
### (Recommended for Collection)

| | |
|---|---|
| Required for staging | None |
| Clinically significant | Measured thickness (depth) |

## HISTOPATHOLOGIC TYPE

This categorization applies only to melanoma of the conjunctiva.

## HISTOLOGIC GRADE (G)

Histologic grade represents the origin of the primary tumor.

GX    Origin cannot be assessed
G0    Primary acquired melanosis without cellular atypia
G1    Conjunctival nevus
G2    Primary acquired melanosis with cellular atypia (epithelial disease only)
G3    Primary acquired melanosis with epithelial cellular atypia and invasive melanoma
G4    De novo malignant melanoma

## BIBLIOGRAPHY

Anastassiou G, Heiligenhaus A, Bechrakis N, Bader E, Bornfeld N, Steuhl KP. Prognostic value of clinical and histopathological parameters in conjunctival melanomas: a retrospective study. Br J Ophthalmol. 2002;86: 163–7.

Damato B, Coupland SE. An audit of conjunctival melanoma treatment in Liverpool. Eye. 2008b. doi:10.1038/eye.2008.154.

Damato B, Coupland SE. Clinical mapping of conjunctival melanomas. Br J Ophthalmol. 2008a;92(11):1545–9.

Damato B, Coupland SE. Conjunctival melanoma and melanosis: a reappraisal of terminology, classification and staging. Clin Exper Ophthalmol. 2008;36:786–95.

Finger PT, Tran HV, Turbin RE, Perry HD, Abramson DH, Chin K, et al. High-frequency ultrasonographic evaluation of conjunctival intraepithelial neoplasia and squamous cell carcinoma. Arch Ophthalmol. 2003;121: 168–72.

Kurli M, Finger PT. Melanocytic conjunctival tumors. Ophthalmol Clin North Am. 2005;18:15–24.

Kurli M, Chin K, Finger PT. Whole-body 18 FDG PET/CT imaging for lymph node and metastatic staging of conjunctival melanoma. Br J Ophthalmol. 2008;92:479–82.

Missotten GS, Keijser S, De Keizer RJ, De Wolff-Rouendaal D. Conjunctival melanoma in the Netherlands: a nationwide study. Invest Ophthalmol Vis Sci. 2005;46:75–82.

Seregard S. Conjunctival melanoma. Surv Ophthalmol. 1998;42:321–50.

Sugiura M, Colby KA, Mihm MC, Zembowicz A. Low-risk and high-risk histologic features in conjunctival primary acquired melanosis with atypia: clinicopathologic analysis of 29 cases. Am J Surg Pathol. 2007;31(2): 185–92.

Tuomaala S, Kivela T. Metastatic pattern and survival in disseminated conjunctival melanoma: implications for sentinel lymph node biopsy. Ophthalmology. 2004;111:816–21.

Tuomaala S, Eskelin S, Tarkkanen A, Kivela T. Population-based assessment of clinical characteristics predicting outcome of conjunctival melanoma in whites. Invest Ophthalmol Vis Sci. 2002;43:3399–408.

**50**

Werschnik C, Lommatzsch P. Long-term follow-up of patients with conjunctival melanoma. Am J Clin Oncol. 2002;25:248–55.

Wilson MW, Fleming JC, Fleming RM, Haik BG. Sentinel node biopsy fororbital and ocular adnexal tumors. Ophthal Plast Reconstr Surg. 2001a;17:338–44.

Wilson MW, Czechonska G, Finger PT, Rausen A, Hooper ME, Haik BG. Chemotherapy for eye cancer. Surv Ophthalmol. 2001b;45:416–44.

Yu GP, Hu DN, McCormick S, Finger PT. Conjunctival melanoma: is it increasing in the United States? Am J Ophthalmol. 2003;135:800–6.

# Malignant Melanoma
# of the Uvea

## *At-A-Glance*

---

### SUMMARY OF CHANGES

**Iris**

- T4 is subdivided according to the size of extrascleral extension

**Ciliary Body and Choroid**

- The definitions of T1-T4 lesions have been modified

- The definitions of T1a-c, T2a-c, and T3a have been modified, and T1-T3 has been divided into T1a-d, T2a-d, and T3a-d

- T4 has been divided into T4a-e

- T1 through T4 are defined as tumors representing tabulated combinations of largest basal tumor diameter and tumor thickness (height)

- T1a, T2a, T3a, and T4a are defined as tumors without ciliary body involvement and without extrascleral extension

- T1b, T2b, T3b, and T4b are defined as tumors with ciliary body involvement but without extrascleral extension

- T1c, T2c, T3c, and T4c are defined as tumors without ciliary body involvement but with extrascleral extension equal to or less than 5 mm

- T1d, T2d, T3d, and T4d are defined as tumors with ciliary body involvement and with extrascleral extension equal to or less than 5 mm

- T4e is defined as tumor of any size with an extrascleral extension greater than 5 mm in diameter

---

### ANATOMIC STAGE/PROGNOSTIC GROUPS

| Stage | T | N | M |
|-------|-----|-----|-----|
| Stage I | T1a | N0 | M0 |
| Stage IIA | T1b-d | N0 | M0 |
| | T2a | N0 | M0 |
| Stage IIB | T2b | N0 | M0 |
| | T3a | N0 | M0 |
| Stage IIIA | T2c-d | N0 | M0 |
| | T3b-c | N0 | M0 |
| | T4a | N0 | M0 |
| Stage IIIB | T3d | N0 | M0 |
| | T4b-c | N0 | M0 |
| Stage IIIC | T4d-e | N0 | M0 |
| Stage IV | Any T | N1 | M0 |
| | Any T | Any N | M1a-c |

**ICD-O-3 TOPOGRAPHY CODES**

C69.3   Choroid
C69.4   Ciliary body
        and iris

**ICD-O-3 HISTOLOGY CODE RANGES**
8720–8790

**51**

---

## ANATOMY

**Primary Site.** The uvea (uveal tract) is the middle layer of the eye, situated between the sclera externally and the retina and its analogous neuroepithelial tissues internally. The uveal tract is divided into three regions – the iris, ciliary body, and choroid. It is a highly vascular structure, which comprises blood vessels and intervening stroma. The stroma contains variable numbers of melanocytes of neural crest origin, from which uveal melanomas are believed to arise. Because there are no lymphatic channels within the eye and orbit, uveal melanomas metastasize almost exclusively hematogenously to the liver and other visceral organs. In the rare event that uveal melanomas metastasize to the regional lymph nodes, it is after extraocular spread and invasion of conjunctival or adnexal lymphatics. Many uveal melanomas are slowly growing tumors, so that clinical metastases may appear decades after successful treatment of the primary tumor.

Uveal melanomas arise most commonly in the choroid, less frequently in the ciliary body, and least often in the iris. Choroidal melanomas extend commonly through Bruch's membrane into the subretinal space, retina and vitreous, less commonly through the sclera into the orbit and to the conjunctiva, and rarely into the optic nerve.

The size of uveal melanoma and the presence of extrascleral extension are strongly associated with a patient's risk for metastasis. Intraocular location of a uveal melanoma also affects this risk. Tumors confined to the iris carry the most favorable prognosis, followed by those confined in the choroid; ciliary body involvement carries the least favorable prognosis. The size and location of uveal melanoma are interrelated: melanomas of the iris tend to be small and those arising from or extending to the ciliary body typically are large.

Even though it is generally accepted that largest basal tumor diameter is the predominant predictor of prognosis, tumor thickness is an independent clinical prognostic indicator, even when ciliary body involvement and extraocular extension are simultaneously taken into account.

The large randomized Collaborative Ocular Melanoma Study has shown that clinical diagnosis of medium-sized and large choroidal melanomas is 99% accurate.

It is currently impossible to distinguish clinically between a nevus and a small uveal melanoma. Clinical findings of Tumor thickness greater than 2 mm, subretinal Fluid, visual Symptoms, Orange pigment, and tumor Margin touching the optic disk are more commonly associated with growing than stationary melanocytic tumors and may help to identify small uveal melanomas (mnemonic: To Find Small Ocular Melanomas). Degenerative drusen over a small melanocytic tumor suggest slow or no growth, thus favoring the diagnosis of a nevus. Small uveal melanocytic lesions are frequently observed for growth prior to being clinically defined as uveal melanomas.

Pigmented iris tumors that demonstrate intrinsic vascularity measure greater than 3 clock hours, are greater than 1 mm in thickness, are associated with sector cataract, dispersion of melanocytic tumor cells, secondary glaucoma and extrascleral extension, are more likely to be iris melanomas than benign melanocytic proliferations.

**Regional Lymph Nodes.** This category applies only to uveal melanomas with extrascleral extension and conjunctival invasion. Regional lymphadenectomy will ordinarily include six or more regional lymph nodes. The regional lymph nodes include the following:

- Preauricular (parotid)
- Submandibular
- Cervical

**Metastatic Sites.** Uveal melanomas may metastasize hematogenously to various visceral organs. The liver is the most common initial site – over 90% of patients – and often the only site of clinically detectable metastasis. It is increasingly common to examine patients one to two times per year with liver imaging (e.g., magnetic resonance imaging, computed radiographic tomography, and ultrasound). Less common sites of metastasis include the lung, subcutaneous tissues, bone, and brain, which usually are involved later in the course of dissemination.

## RULES FOR CLASSIFICATION

**Clinical Staging.** Up to the 1997 edition of the uveal melanoma staging system, size thresholds for choroidal melanoma were based on definitions in one particular epidemiological study, and ciliary body melanomas were categorized according to the extent of invasion of adjacent ocular tissues. All uveal melanomas with extraocular extension were assigned to T4.

The 2003 edition introduced for ciliary body and choroidal melanoma common size thresholds, which were modified from the Collaborative Ocular Melanoma Study (COMS). No distinction was made between melanomas confined in the choroid and those involving the ciliary body. The T1 and T2 categories included melanomas with extraocular extension, but tumors that corresponded to T3 in size were defined as T4 if they had extraocular extension. In these two systems, the largest basal tumor diameter and tumor thickness did not always fit in the same category, in which case the largest basal diameter was used for classification.

For the present edition, T categories were derived empirically from a collaborative database of over 7,000 patients with uveal melanoma. The secondary criterion for T staging is the anatomical extent of the tumor based on involvement of the ciliary body and extrascleral tissues – the two predominant and independent predictors of prognosis of uveal melanoma in addition to tumor size identified both in world literature and in the data set used to model the T categories. Because rectangular T categories based on largest tumor basal diameter and tumor thickness will lead to inclusion in each T category of tumors that appreciably differ in prognosis from the majority of tumors in any particular T category, the category thresholds were defined in a nonrectangular, tabular format (Figure 51.1).

Ten-year survival rates for the four size categories T1–T4 were 90%, 78%, 58%, and 40%, respectively, among 7,585 uveal melanoma patients.

Enough empirical data to propose major changes to T categories of iris melanomas were not available. T4 was subdivided according to the size of

**51**

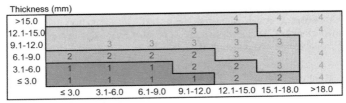

**FIGURE 51.1.** Classification for ciliary body and choroid uveal melanoma based on thickness and diameter.

extrascleral extension, analogous with the ciliary body and choroidal melanoma subcategories.

The assessment of the tumor is based on clinical examination, including slit-lamp examination, direct and indirect ophthalmoscopy, and ultrasonography. Additional methods, such as high-frequency ultrasonography, ultrasound biomicroscopy, fundus photography, fluorescein and indocyanine green angiography, positron emission tomography (PET), and magnetic resonance imaging may enhance the accuracy of appraisal, especially in atypical cases.

Systemic metastases are found in only 1–4% of patients at the time of diagnosis of the intraocular tumor. In addition to physical examination, liver imaging and chest radiogram are recommended to exclude both hepatic metastasis and a primary tumor elsewhere. Some centers are using total body PET/CT imaging for initial staging and for follow-up (high-risk patients). Liver enzyme tests may be useful to exclude diffuse hepatic metastasis.

M1 was divided into three subcategories based on the largest diameter of the largest metastasis, a measure that has been shown to correlate strongly with survival after diagnosis of metastases. Divisions were based on a collaborative data set of over 200 patients with metastatic uveal melanoma. Median survival times for the subcategories M1a to M1c were 17 months, 9 months, and 4.5 months, respectively, among 239 uveal melanoma patients.

Stages I–III are confined to uveal melanoma patients who have no evidence of metastases, either at regional or distant sites, based on clinical, radiological, and laboratory evaluation. Stage IV uveal melanoma patients are those with clinical or radiological evidence of regional or systemic metastases. Because of the rarity of regional lymph node metastasis, sentinel lymph node biopsy is not practiced. Because staging of metastatic uveal melanoma is evolving and depends on several factors additional to diameter of the largest metastasis, e.g., liver enzyme levels and performance status, no sub staging is yet proposed.

Ten-year survival rates for the seven stages I, IIA–B, IIIA–C, and IV were 88%, 80%, 68%, 45%, 26%, 21%, and 0%, respectively, among 5,470 uveal melanoma patients with data on ciliary body involvement and extraocular extension in addition to tumor dimensions.

**Pathologic Staging.**  Resection of the primary tumor by iridectomy, iridocyclectomy, local resection, or enucleation is needed for complete pathologic staging. Assessment of the extent of the tumor, measured in clock hours of involvement, basal dimensions, tumor thickness, and margins of resection, is necessary. It is also possible to pursue a needle aspiration biopsy or use a vitreous cutter for biopsy purposes, but a negative report will not exclude the possibility of uveal melanoma because of potential sampling or technical error.

Suspected orbital invasion, regional lymph node involvement, and systemic metastasis are confirmed by needle biopsy or resection.

Uveal melanomas exhibit marked variation in cytological composition. They exhibit a spectrum of cell types ranging from spindle cells through plump spindle cells to epithelioid cells. Many tumors contain some admixture of these different cells. Spindle cells have ovoid nuclei and tend to grow in a compact cohesive fashion. Epithelioid cells are larger, more irregularly contoured, pleomorphic cells with abundant typically acidophilic cytoplasm. Their nuclei and nucleoli are larger and they grow less cohesively than spindle cells. No consensus has been reached regarding which proportion of epithelioid cells qualifies a uveal melanoma as being of mixed and epithelioid type. Some ophthalmic pathologists now record the presence or absence of epithelioid cells and do not classify tumors into mixed and epithelioid type.

Monosomy 3 and defined abnormalities of chromosomes 6 and 8 have consistently been associated with metastatic death in choroidal and ciliary body melanoma. The strongest single predictor of prognosis is loss of heterozygosity detected in chromosome 3; because of the possibility of isochromosome, some of these patients falsely appear to be disomic, e.g., in fluorescent *in situ* hybridization (FISH) analysis. Recent studies suggest that genetic profiling is a more accurate way than karyotyping to differentiate uveal melanoma patients with favorable and adverse prognosis.

In addition to cell type, mitotic count, mean diameter of the ten largest nucleoli (measured, e.g., from silver-stained sections), presence of defined extravascular matrix patterns (e.g., closed loops and networks detected with periodic acid-Schiff staining or clinically with confocal angiography), microvascular density (determined from areas of dense vascularization after staining with antibodies to vascular endothelial cells), high numbers of tumor-infiltrating lymphocytes and macrophages, and low level of HLA Class I and high level of insulin-like growth factor 1 receptor expression (detected, e.g., by immunohistochemistry) have been shown to be independent predictors of subsequent survival in more than one study.

## PROGNOSTIC FEATURES

There are a number of key prognostic factors that are important to collect in malignant melanoma of the uvea, even though they are not included in staging algorithms. These include the following:

1. Chromosomal alterations
   a. Chromosome 3 status (loss or no loss; complete or partial)
   b. Chromosome 6p status (gain or no gain)
   c. Chromosome 8q status (gain or no gain)
      Indicate:
      • Technique used for assessing chromosome status (e.g., karyotyping, fluorescent in situ hybridization (FISH), comparative genomic

51

hybridization (CGH), loss of heterozygosity using DNA polymorphism analysis (e.g., SNP, microsatellite), or other (describe)).

- How specimen was obtained (e.g., enucleation, local resection, biopsy, fine needle aspiration biopsy).
- For needle biopsies, whether cytopathologic evaluation was performed to confirm the presence of tumor cells.

2. Gene expression profile: class 1 or class 2
   Indicate:
   - Technique used for gene expression profiling (e.g., microarray, PCR).
   - How specimen was obtained (e.g., enucleation, local resection, biopsy, fine needle aspiration biopsy)
   - For needle biopsies, whether cytopathologic evaluation was performed to confirm the presence of tumor cells.

1. Clinical
   a. Positron emission tomography/computed tomography (PET/CT)
      - 18-Fluorine-labelled 2-deoxy-2-fluoro-D-glucose standardized uptake values (higher values in primary tumor may be associated with shorter survival)
   b. Confocal indocyanine green angiography
      - Identification of complex monocirculatory patterns (loops, networks, arcs with branching, parallel with cross-linking or a combination thereof may be associated with shorter survival)

2. Histopathologic
   a. Mitotic count
      - Number of mitotic figures per 40 high-power fields (typical field area 0.15–0.19 mm$^2$, higher counts are associated with shorter survival)
   b. Mean diameter of the ten largest nucleoli (MLN)
      - MLN is measured along a central 5-mm long strip, e.g., after silver staining (larger values are associated with shorter survival)
   c. Presence of extravascular matrix patterns
      - Loops
        – Absent
        – Present (shorter survival)
      - Loops forming networks
        – Absent
        – Present (shorter survival)
      - Other complex patterns (arcs with branching, parallel with cross-linking: absent or present)
        The patterns are assessed with light microscopy under a dark green filter after staining with periodic-acid Schiff without counterstain
   d. Microvascular density (MVD)
      - Number of immunopositive elements labeled with markers for vascular endothelial cells (e.g., CD34 epitope, factor VIII-related antigen) in areas of densest vascularization (typical field area 0.31 mm$^2$, higher counts are associated with shorter survival)
   e. Insulin-like growth factor 1 receptor (IGF1-R)
      - Percentage of immunopositive tumor cells (high expression is associated with shorter survival)

f. Tumor-infiltrating lymphocytes
- Few (longest survival)
- Moderate numbers
- Many (shortest survival)

g. Tumor-infiltrating macrophages
- Few (longest survival)
- Moderate numbers
- Many (shortest survival)

  The number can be compared with standard photographs in Mäkitie et al. Invest Ophthalmol Vis Sci. 2001;42:1414–21.

h. HLA Class I expression
- Percentage of immunopositive tumor cells (low expression is associated with longer survival)

## DEFINITIONS OF TNM

These definitions apply to both clinical* and pathologic** staging.

### Primary Tumor

*All Uveal Melanomas*

| | |
|---|---|
| TX | Primary tumor cannot be assessed |
| T0 | No evidence of primary tumor |

*Iris*\*\*\*

| | |
|---|---|
| T1 | Tumor limited to the iris |
| T1a | Tumor limited to the iris not more than 3 clock hours in size |
| T1b | Tumor limited to the iris more than 3 clock hours in size |
| T1c | Tumor limited to the iris with secondary glaucoma |
| T2 | Tumor confluent with or extending into the ciliary body, choroid, or both |
| T2a | Tumor confluent with or extending into the ciliary body, choroid, or both, with secondary glaucoma |
| T3 | Tumor confluent with or extending into the ciliary body, choroid, or both, with scleral extension |
| T3a | Tumor confluent with or extending into the ciliary body, choroid, or both, with scleral extension and secondary glaucoma |
| T4 | Tumor with extrascleral extension |
| T4a | Tumor with extrascleral extension less than or equal to 5 mm in diameter |
| T4b | Tumor with extrascleral extension more than 5 mm in diameter |

*Note: In clinical practice, the largest tumor basal diameter may be estimated in optic disc diameters (dd, average: 1 dd=1.5 mm). Tumor thickness may be estimated in diopters (average: 2.5 diopters=1 mm). However, techniques such as ultrasonography and fundus photography are used to provide more accurate measurements. Ciliary body involvement can be evaluated by the slit-lamp, ophthalmoscopy, gonioscopy, and transillumination. However, high-frequency ultrasonography (ultrasound biomicroscopy) is used for more accurate assessment. Extension through the sclera is evaluated visually before and during surgery, and with ultrasonography, computed tomography, or magnetic resonance imaging.

**51**

### Primary Tumor (continued)

**Note*: When histopathologic measurements are recorded after fixation, tumor diameter and thickness may be underestimated because of tissue shrinkage.

***Note*: Iris melanomas originate from, and are predominantly located in, this region of the uvea. If less than half of t-he tumor volume is located within the iris, the tumor may have originated in the ciliary body and consideration should be given to classifying it accordingly.

*Ciliary Body and Choroid*
Primary ciliary body and choroidal melanomas, as defined in Figure 51.1, are classified according to the four tumor size categories below:

| | |
|------|--------------------------------------------------------------------------------------------------------|
| T1 | Tumor size category 1 |
| T1a | Tumor size category 1 without ciliary body involvement and extraocular extension |
| T1b | Tumor size category 1 with ciliary body involvement |
| T1c | Tumor size category 1 without ciliary body involvement but with extraocular extension less than or equal to 5 mm in diameter |
| T1d | Tumor size category 1 with ciliary body involvement and extraocular extension less than or equal to 5 mm in diameter |
| T2 | Tumor size category 2 |
| T2a | Tumor size category 2 without ciliary body involvement and extraocular extension |
| T2b | Tumor size category 2 with ciliary body involvement |
| T2c | Tumor size category 2 without ciliary body involvement but with extraocular extension less than or equal to 5 mm in diameter |
| T2d | Tumor size category 2 with ciliary body involvement and extraocular extension less than or equal to 5 mm in diameter |
| T3 | Tumor size category 3 |
| T3a | Tumor size category 3 without ciliary body involvement and extraocular extension |
| T3b | Tumor size category 3 with ciliary body involvement |
| T3c | Tumor size category 3 without ciliary body involvement but with extraocular extension less than or equal to 5 mm in diameter |
| T3d | Tumor size category 3 with ciliary body involvement and extraocular extension less than or equal to 5 mm in diameter |
| T4 | Tumor size category 4 |
| T4a | Tumor size category 4 without ciliary body involvement and extraocular extension |
| T4b | Tumor size category 4 with ciliary body involvement |
| T4c | Tumor size category 4 without ciliary body involvement but with extraocular extension less than or equal to 5 mm in diameter |
| T4d | Tumor size category 4 with ciliary body involvement and extraocular extension less than or equal to 5 mm in diameter |
| T4e | Any tumor size category with extraocular extension more than 5 mm in diameter |

### Regional Lymph Nodes (N)

NX     Regional lymph nodes cannot be assessed
N0     No regional lymph node metastasis
N1     Regional lymph node metastasis

### Distant Metastasis (M)

M0     No distant metastasis
M1     Distant metastasis
M1a    Largest diameter of the largest metastasis 3 cm or less
M1b    Largest diameter of the largest metastasis 3.1–8.0 cm
M1c    Largest diameter of the largest metastasis 8 cm or more

### ANATOMIC STAGE/PROGNOSTIC GROUPS

| Stage | T | N | M |
|---|---|---|---|
| Stage I | T1a | N0 | M0 |
| Stage IIA | T1b-d | N0 | M0 |
| | T2a | N0 | M0 |
| Stage IIB | T2b | N0 | M0 |
| | T3a | N0 | M0 |
| Stage IIIA | T2c-d | N0 | M0 |
| | T3b-c | N0 | M0 |
| | T4a | N0 | M0 |
| Stage IIIB | T3d | N0 | M0 |
| | T4b-c | N0 | M0 |
| Stage IIIC | T4d-e | N0 | M0 |
| Stage IV | Any T | N1 | M0 |
| | Any T | Any N | M1a-c |

## PROGNOSTIC FACTORS (SITE-SPECIFIC FACTORS)
### (Recommended for Collection)

| | |
|---|---|
| Required for staging | Height |
| | Largest tumor diameter |
| Clinically significant | Measured thickness (height) |
| | Chromosomal alterations |
| | Gene expression profile |
| | Positron emission tomography/computed tomography |
| | Mitotic count per 40 high power fields (HPF) |
| | Mean diameter of the ten largest nucleoli (MLN) |
| | Presence of extravascular matrix patterns |
| | Microvascular density (MVD) |

**51**

## HISTOPATHOLOGIC TYPE

The histopathologic types are as follows:

Spindle cell melanoma (greater than 90% spindle cells)
Mixed cell melanoma (>10% epithelioid cells and <90% spindle cells)
Epithelioid cell melanoma (greater than 90% epithelioid cells)

## HISTOLOGIC GRADE (G)*

GX     Grade cannot be assessed
G1     Spindle cell melanoma
G2     Mixed cell melanoma
G3     Epithelioid cell melanoma

*Note: Because of general lack of agreement regarding which proportion of epithelioid cells classifies a tumor as mixed and epithelioid in type, some ophthalmic pathologists currently combine grades 2 and 3 (nonspindle, epithelioid cells detected) and contrast them with grade 1 (spindle, no epithelioid cells detected).

## BIBLIOGRAPHY

Al Jamal RT, Kivelä T. KI-67 immunopositivity in choroidal and ciliary body melanoma with respect to nucleolar diameter and other prognostic factors. Curr Eye Res. 2006;31:57–67.

All-Ericsson C, Girnita L, Seregard S, Bartolazzi A, Jager MJ, Larsson O. Insulin-like growth factor-1 receptor in uveal melanoma: a predictor for metastatic disease and a potential therapeutic target. Invest Ophthalmol Vis Sci. 2002;43:1–8.

Blanco G. Diagnosis and treatment of orbital invasion in uveal melanoma. Can J Ophthalmol. 2004;39:388–96.

Blom DJ, Luyten GP, Mooy C, Kerkvliet S, Zwinderman AH, Jager MJ. Human leukocyte antigen class I expression. Marker of poor prognosis in uveal melanoma. Invest Ophthalmol Vis Sci. 1997;38:1865–72.

The Collaborative Ocular Melanoma Study Group. Accuracy of diagnosis of choroidal melanomas in the Collaborative Ocular Melanoma Study. COMS report no. 1. Arch Ophthalmol. 1990;108:1268–73.

The Collaborative Ocular Melanoma Study Group. Comparison of clinical, echographic, and histopathological measurements from eyes with medium-sized choroidal melanoma in the collaborative ocular melanoma study: COMS report no. 21. Arch Ophthalmol. 2003;121:1163–71.

The Collaborative Ocular Melanoma Study Group. Factors predictive of growth and treatment of small choroidal melanoma: COMS report no. 5. Arch Ophthalmol. 1997a;115:1537–44.

The Collaborative Ocular Melanoma Study Group. Mortality in patients with small choroidal melanoma. COMS report no. 4. Arch Ophthalmol. 1997b;115:886–93.

The Collaborative Ocular Melanoma Study Group. The COMS randomized trial of iodine 125 brachytherapy for choroidal melanoma: V. Twelve-year mortality rates and prognostic factors: COMS report no. 28. Arch Ophthalmol. 2006;124:1684–93.

Damato B, Duke C, Coupland SE, Hiscott P, Smith PA, Campbell I, et al. Cytogenetics of uveal melanoma: a 7-year clinical experience. Ophthalmology. 2007;114:1925–31.

Diener-West M, Reynolds SM, Agugliaro DJ, Caldwell R, Cumming K, Earle JD, Hawkins BS, Hayman JA, Jaiyesimi I, Jampol LM, Kirkwood JM, Koh WJ, Robertson DM, Shaw JM, Straatsma BR, Thoma J. Development of metastatic disease after enrollment in the COMS trials for treatment of choroidal melanoma: Collaborative Ocular Melanoma Study Group report no. 26. Arch Ophthalmol. 2005;123:1639–43.

Durie FH, Campbell AM, Lee WR, Damato BE. Analysis of lymphocytic infiltration in uveal melanoma. Invest Ophthalmol Vis Sci. 1990;31:2106–10.

Eskelin S, Pyrhönen S, Summanen P, Prause JU, Kivelä T. Screening for metastatic malignant melanoma of the uvea revisited. Cancer. 1999;85:1151–9.

Eskelin S, Pyrhönen S, Hahka-Kemppinen M, Tuomaala S, Kivelä T. A prognostic model and staging for metastatic uveal melanoma. Cancer. 2003;97: 465–75.

Finger PT, Kurli M, Reddy S, Tena LB, Pavlick AC. Whole body PET/CT for initial staging of choroidal melanoma. Br J Ophthalmol. 2005a;89(10):1270–4.

Finger PT, Latkany P, Kurli M, Iacob C. The Finger iridectomy technique: small incision biopsy of anterior segment tumors. Br J Ophthalmol. 2005b;89: 946–9.

Finger PT, Chin K, Iacob CE. 18-Fluorine-labelled 2-deoxy-2-fluoro-D-glucose positron emission tomography/computed tomography standardised uptake values: a non-invasive biomarker for the risk of metastasis from choroidal melanoma. Br J Ophthalmol. 2006;90:1263–6.

Folberg R, Rummelt V, Parys-Van Ginderdeuren R, Hwang T, Woolson RF, Pe'er J, et al. The prognostic value of tumor blood vessel morphology in primary uveal melanoma. Ophthalmology. 1993;100:1389–98.

Foss AJ, Alexander RA, Jefferies LW, Hungerford JL, Harris AL, Lightman S. Microvessel count predicts survival in uveal melanoma. Cancer Res. 1996;56: 2900–3.

Hawkins BS. The Collaborative Ocular Melanoma Study (COMS) randomized trial of pre-enucleation radiation of large choroidal melanoma: IV. Ten-year mortality findings and prognostic factors. COMS report number 24. Am J Ophthalmol. 2004;138:936–51.

Hughes S, Damato BE, Giddings I, Hiscott PS, Humphreys J, Houlston RS. Microarray comparative genomic hybridisation analysis of intraocular uveal melanomas identifies distinctive imbalances associated with loss of chromosome 3. Br J Cancer. 2005;93:1191–6.

Jager MJ, Hurks HM, Levitskaya J, Kiessling R. HLA expression in uveal melanoma: there is no rule without some exception. Hum Immunol. 2002;63: 444–51.

Kivelä T, Eskelin S, Kujala E. Metastatic uveal melanoma. Int Ophthalmol Clin. 2006;46:133–49.

Kujala E, Mäkitie T, Kivelä T. Very long-term prognosis of patients with malignant uveal melanoma. Invest Ophthalmol Vis Sci. 2003;44:4651–9.

Kurli M, Reddy S, Tena LB, Pavlick AC, Finger PT. Whole body positron emission tomography/computed tomography staging of metastatic choroidal melanoma. Am J Ophthalmol. 2005;104(2):193–9.

Mäkitie T, Summanen P, Tarkkanen A, Kivelä T. Microvascular density in predicting survival of patients with choroidal and ciliary body melanoma. Invest Ophthalmol Vis Sci. 1999a;40:2471–80.

Mäkitie T, Summanen P, Tarkkanen A, Kivelä T. Microvascular loops and networks as prognostic indicators in choroidal and ciliary body melanomas. J Natl Cancer Inst. 1999b;91:359–67.

Mäkitie T, Summanen P, Tarkkanen A, Kivelä T. Tumor-infiltrating macrophages (CD68(+) cells) and prognosis in malignant uveal melanoma. Invest Ophthalmol Vis Sci. 2001;42:1414–21.

51

McLean IW, Zimmerman LE, Evans RM. Reappraisal of Callender's spindle a type of malignant melanoma of choroid and ciliary body. Am J Ophthalmol. 1978;86:557–64.

McLean IW, Foster WD, Zimmerman LE, Gamel JW. Modifications of Callender's classification of uveal melanoma at the Armed Forces Institute of Pathology. Am J Ophthalmol. 1983;96:502–9.

Mueller AJ, Freeman WR, Schaller UC, Kampik A, Folberg R. Complex microcirculation patterns detected by confocal indocyanine green angiography predict time to growth of small choroidal melanocytic tumors: MuSIC Report II. Ophthalmology. 2002;109:2207–14.

Onken MD, Worley LA, Person E, Char DH, Bowcock AM, Harbour JW. Loss of heterozygosity of chromosome 3 detected with single nucleotide polymorphisms is superior to monosomy 3 for predicting metastasis in uveal melanoma. Clin Cancer Res. 2007;13:2923–7.

Pach JM, Robertson DM, Taney BS, Martin JA, Campbell RJ, O'Brien PC. Prognostic factors in choroidal and ciliary body melanomas with extrascleral extension. Am J Ophthalmol. 1986;101:325–31.

Petrausch U, Martus P, Tonnies H, Bechrakis NE, Lenze D, Wansel S, Hummel M, Bornfeld N, Thiel E, Foerster MH, Keilholz U. Significance of gene expression analysis in uveal melanoma in comparison to standard risk factors for risk assessment of subsequent metastases. Eye. 2008;22:997–1007.

Prescher G, Bornfeld N, Hirche H, Horsthemke B, Jockel KH, Becher R. Prognostic implications of monosomy 3 in uveal melanoma. Lancet. 1996;347:1222–5.

Reddy S, Kurli M, Tena LB, Finger PT. PET/CT imaging: detection of choroidal melanoma. Br J Ophthalmol. 2005;89(10):1270–4.

Shields CL, Shields JA. Clinical features of small choroidal melanoma. Curr Opin Ophthalmol. 2002;13:135–41.

Tschentscher F, Husing J, Holter T, Kruse E, Dresen IG, Jockel KH, et al. Tumor classification based on gene expression profiling shows that uveal melanomas with and without monosomy 3 represent two distinct entities. Cancer Res. 2003;63:2578–84.

Worley LA, Onken MD, Person E, Robirds D, Branson J, Char DH, et al. Transcriptomic versus chromosomal prognostic markers and clinical outcome in uveal melanoma. Clin Cancer Res. 2007;13:1466–71.

# Retinoblastoma

## *At-A-Glance*

---

### SUMMARY OF CHANGES

**Clinical Classification**

* The definitions of T1–T4 were modified
* The definitions for M1 were modified

**Pathologic Classification**

* Minor modifications were made to the definitions for pT2–pT4
* Definition of choroidal invasion, focal versus massive
* The definitions for pM1 were modified

**Other**

* A description of proper processing of the enucleated retinoblastoma globe for pathological examination was added

---

**ANATOMIC STAGE/PROGNOSTIC GROUPS**

No stage grouping applies

ICD-O-3
TOPOGRAPHY
CODES
C69.2    Retina

ICD-O-3 HISTOLOGY
CODE RANGES
9510–9514

## ANATOMY

**Primary Site.** The retina is composed of neurons and glial cells. The precursors of the neuronal elements give rise to retinoblastoma, whereas the glial cells give rise to astrocytomas, which are benign and extremely rare in the retina. The retina is limited internally by a membrane that separates it from the vitreous cavity. Externally, it is limited by the retinal pigment epithelium (RPE) and Bruch's membrane, which separate it from the choroid and act as natural barriers to extension of retinal tumors into the choroid. The continuation of the retina with the optic nerve allows direct extension of retinoblastomas into the optic nerve and then to the subarachnoid space. Because the retina has no lymphatics, spread of retinal tumors is either by direct extension into adjacent structures or by distant metastasis through hematogenous routes.

52

---

**Regional Lymph Nodes.** Because there are no intraocular lymphatics, this category of staging applies only to anterior extrascleral extension. The regional lymph nodes are preauricular (parotid), submandibular, and cervical.

**Local Extension.** Local extension anteriorly can result in soft tissue involvement of the face or a mass protruding from between the lids. Posterior extension results in retinoblastoma extending into the orbit, paranasal sinuses, and/or brain.

**Metastatic Sites.** Retinoblastoma can metastasize through hematogenous routes to various sites, most notably the bone marrow, skull, long bones, and brain.

## RULES FOR CLASSIFICATION

**Choroidal Invasion.** The presence and the extent (focal vs. massive) of choroidal invasion by tumor should be stated. Differentiation should be made between true choroidal invasion and artifactual invasion due to seeding of fresh tumor cells during postenucleation retrieval of tumor tissue and/or gross sectioning.

*Artifactual invasion* is identified when there are groups of tumor cells present in the open spaces between intraocular structures, extraocular tissues, and/or subarachnoid space.

*True invasion* is defined as one or more solid nests of tumor cells that fills or replaces the choroid and has pushing borders. Note: Invasion of the sub-RPE space, where tumor cells are present under the RPE (but not beyond Bruch's membrane into the choroid) is not choroidal invasion.

*Focal choroidal invasion* is defined as a solid nest of tumor that measures less than 3 mm in maximum diameter (width or thickness).

*Massive choroidal invasion* is defined as a solid tumor nest 3 mm or more in maximum diameter (width or thickness).

**Clinical Staging.** All suspected cases of retinoblastoma should have a neural imaging scan. If it is possible to obtain only one imaging study, computerized tomography (CT) is recommended because detection of calcium in the eye on CT confirms the clinical suspicion of retinoblastoma. The request should include cuts through the pineal region of the brain. Magnetic resonance imaging is particularly useful if extension into either the extraocular space or the optic nerve is suspected or if there is a concern about the possible presence of a primitive neuroectodermal tumor (PNET) in the pineal region (trilateral retinoblastoma).

A staging examination under anesthesia should include ocular ultrasound and retinal drawings of each eye, with each identifiable tumor measured and numbered. Digital images of the retina may be very helpful. In bilateral cases, each eye must be classified separately. Tumor size or the distance from the tumor to the disc or fovea is recorded in millimeters. These millimeter distances are measured by ultrasound, estimated by comparison with a normalized optic disc (1.5 mm), or deduced from the fact that the field of a 28-diopter condensing lens has a retinal diameter of 13 mm.

**Pathologic Staging.** If one eye is enucleated, pathologic staging of that eye provides information supplemental to the clinical staging. First, the pathology should provide histologic verification of the disease. All clinical and pathologic data from the resected specimen are to be used.

*Processing the Enucleated Retinoblastoma Globe.* In certain situations fresh tumor material may be needed from the enucleated globe for research purposes or genetic testing. In these cases the globe should be moved to a sterile area in the Operating Room away from the operative field. After collecting the specimen, the surgeon should change his/her gloves before reentering the operative field.

*Processing With Tumor Sampling.* To collect the tumor specimen, the optic nerve should be removed before opening the globe to prevent the optic nerve from accidentally becoming contaminated with artifactual clumps of tumor cells (so-called floaters). The surgeon should first ink the surgical margin of the optic nerve, then cut the optic nerve stump off from the sclera with a sharp razor about 2 mm behind the globe. The optic nerve stump should be placed into a jar of 10% buffered formaldehyde that will be kept separate from the globe. Then, a sample of tumor should be obtained by opening a small sclero-choroidal window adjacent to the tumor near the equator with a 6–8 mm corneal trephine. Once the opening into the vitreous chamber is established, tumor tissue should be gently removed with forceps and scissors. It is best to leave a hinge on one side of the scleral flap so that it can be closed with one or two suture(s) following the removal of tumor sample. This is done in an attempt to maintain the overall spherical architecture of the specimen during fixation. The globe should be placed in a second jar of formalin (separate from the optic nerve stump) and be allowed to fix for at least 24–48 h.

*Processing Without Tumor Sampling.* If there is no need for fresh tissue sampling, the enucleated globe should simply be fixed in 10% buffered formaldehyde for at least 24 and preferably 48 h. When the fixed globe is examined by the pathologist, if the optic nerve was not previously amputated in the operative room, that should be performed first as described previously. The surgical margin of the nerve stump should be embedded face down in paraffin for sectioning (i.e., thereby obtaining cross-sections of the nerve, starting at the surgical margin). Then, the eye itself is sectioned. First, a section should be made that extends from pupil through the optic nerve (the "P-O" section), which contains the center of the optic nerve with all the optic nerve structures (optic nerve head, lamina cribrosa, and postlaminar optic nerve). Preferably this plane should bisect the largest dimension of the tumor, previously identified by transillumination and during clinical examination. When possible, the plane should avoid the scleral opening if one was made for fresh tumor sampling. This section is critical for evaluation of the optic nerve for tumor invasion. The P-O section and minor calottes are then embedded in paraffin. The embedded P-O calotte is then sectioned every 100–150 μm (each section being about 5 μm thick), for a total of about 10–20 sections. Additional sections should also be made anterior-posteriorly in a bread loaf fashion through the minor

**52**

calottes if they contain visible tumor. These segments should be submitted in one cassette per calotte on edge to evaluate the choroid for invasion. Three levels of this block are usually sufficient for examination. In total, four cassettes are submitted: the optic nerve stump, the P-O section, and the two minor calottes (unless one or both of these has no visible tumor).

## PROGNOSTIC FEATURES

There are a number of key prognostic factors that are important to collect in retinoblastoma even though they are not required for staging algorithms. These include the presence or absence of an RB gene mutation, a family history of retinoblastoma, and whether the primary globe-sparing treatment failed, and the greatest extent of choroid involved by choroidal tumor invasion.

## DEFINITIONS OF TNM

### Clinical Classification (cTNM)

| *Primary Tumor (T)* | |
|---|---|
| TX | Primary tumor cannot be assessed |
| T0 | No evidence of primary tumor |
| T1 | Tumors no more than 2/3 the volume of the eye with no vitreous or subretinal seeding |
| T1a | No tumor in either eye is greater than 3 mm in largest dimension or located closer than 1.5 mm to the optic nerve or fovea |
| T1b | At least one tumor is greater than 3 mm in largest dimension or located closer than 1.5 mm to the optic nerve or fovea. No retinal detachment or subretinal fluid beyond 5 mm from the base of the tumor |
| T1c | At least one tumor is greater than 3 mm in largest dimension or located closer than 1.5 mm to the optic nerve or fovea, with retinal detachment or subretinal fluid beyond 5 mm from the base of the tumor |
| T2 | Tumors no more than 2/3 the volume of the eye with vitreous or subretinal seeding. Can have retinal detachment |
| T2a | Focal vitreous and/or subretinal seeding of fine aggregates of tumor cells is present, but no large clumps or "snowballs" of tumor cells |
| T2b | Massive vitreous and/or subretinal seeding is present, defined as diffuse clumps or "snowballs" of tumor cells |
| T3 | Severe intraocular disease |
| T3a | Tumor fills more than 2/3 of the eye |
| T3b | One or more complications present, which may include tumor-associated neovascular or angle closure glaucoma, tumor extension into the anterior segment, hyphema, vitreous hemorrhage, or orbital cellulitis |
| T4 | Extraocular disease detected by imaging studies |
| T4a | Invasion of optic nerve |
| T4b | Invasion into the orbit |
| T4c | Intracranial extension not past chiasm |
| T4d | Intracranial extension past chiasm |

### Regional Lymph Nodes (N)

| | |
|---|---|
| NX | Regional lymph nodes cannot be assessed |
| N0 | No regional lymph node involvement |
| N1 | Regional lymph node involvement (preauricular, cervical, submandibular) |
| N2 | Distant lymph node involvement |

### Metastasis (M)

| | |
|---|---|
| M0 | No metastasis |
| M1 | Systemic metastasis |
| M1a | Single lesion to sites other than CNS |
| M1b | Multiple lesions to sites other than CNS |
| M1c | Prechiasmatic CNS lesion(s) |
| M1d | Postchiasmatic CNS lesion(s) |
| M1e | Leptomeningeal and/or CSF involvement |

## Pathologic Classification (pTNM)

### Primary Tumor (pT)

| | |
|---|---|
| pTX | Primary tumor cannot be assessed |
| pT0 | No evidence of primary tumor |
| pT1 | Tumor confined to eye with no optic nerve or choroidal invasion |
| pT2 | Tumor with minimal optic nerve and/or choroidal invasion: |
| pT2a | Tumor superficially invades optic nerve head but does not extend past lamina cribrosa *or* tumor exhibits focal choroidal invasion |
| pT2b | Tumor superficially invades optic nerve head but does not extend past lamina cribrosa *and* exhibits focal choroidal invasion |
| pT3 | Tumor with significant optic nerve and/or choroidal invasion: |
| pT3a | Tumor invades optic nerve past lamina cribrosa but not to surgical resection line *or* tumor exhibits massive choroidal invasion |
| pT3b | Tumor invades optic nerve past lamina cribrosa but not to surgical resection line *and* exhibits massive choroidal invasion |
| pT4 | Tumor invades optic nerve to resection line or exhibits extra-ocular extension elsewhere |
| pT4a | Tumor invades optic nerve to resection line but no extra-ocular extension identified |
| pT4b | Tumor invades optic nerve to resection line and extra-ocular extension identified |

### Regional Lymph Nodes (pN)

| | |
|---|---|
| pNX | Regional lymph nodes cannot be assessed |
| pN0 | No regional lymph node involvement |
| pN1 | Regional lymph node involvement (preauricular, cervical) |
| N2 | Distant lymph node involvement |

**52**

## Metastasis (pM)

cM0   No metastasis
pM1   Metastasis to sites other than CNS
pM1a   Single lesion
pM1b   Multiple lesions
pM1c   CNS metastasis
pM1d   Discrete mass(es) without leptomeningeal and/or CSF involvement
pM1e   Leptomeningeal and/or CSF involvement

## ANATOMIC STAGE/PROGNOSTIC GROUPS

No stage grouping applies

## PROGNOSTIC FACTORS (SITE-SPECIFIC FACTORS)
## (Recommended for Collection)

Required for staging    None

Clinically significant    Extension evaluated at enucleation
RB gene mutation
Positive family history of retinoblastoma
Primary globe-sparing treatment failure
Greatest linear extent of choroid involved by choroidal tumor invasion

## HISTOLOGIC GRADE (G)

Grade is reported in registry systems by the grade value. A two-grade, three-grade, or four-grade system may be used. If a grading system is not specified, generally the following system is used:

GX   Grade cannot be assessed
G1   Well differentiated
G2   Moderately differentiated
G3   Poorly differentiated
G4   Undifferentiated

## HISTOPATHOLOGIC TYPE

This classification applies only to retinoblastoma.

## BIBLIOGRAPHY

Chantada G, Doz F, Antoneli CB, Grundy R, Clare Stannard FF, Dunkel IJ, et al. A proposal for an international retinoblastoma staging system. Pediatr Blood Cancer. 2006;47:801–5.

Chantada GL, Doz F, Orjuela M, Qaddoumi I, Sitorus RS, Kepak T, Furmanchuk A, Castellanos M, Sharma T, Chevez-Barrios P, Rodriguez-Galindo C; on behalf of the International Retinoblastoma Staging Working Group. World disparities in risk definition and management of retinoblastoma: a report from the International Retinoblastoma Staging Working Group. Pediatr Blood Cancer. 2008;50:692–4.

Cohen MD, Bugaieski EM, Haliloglu M, Faught P, Siddiqui AR. Visual presentation of the staging of pediatric solid tumors. Radiographics. 1996;16:523–45.

Dagher R, Helman L. Rhabdomyosarcoma: an overview. Oncologist. 1999;4:34–44.

Ellsworth RM. The practical management of retinoblastoma. Trans Am Ophthalmol Soc. 1969;67:462–534.

Fleming ID. Staging of pediatric cancers: problems in the development of a national system. Semin Surg Oncol. 1992;8:94–7.

Warrier RP, Regueira O. Wilms' tumor. Pediatr Nephrol. 1992;6:358–64.

# Carcinoma of the Lacrimal Gland

## *At-A-Glance*

---

### SUMMARY OF CHANGES

The staging system for lacrimal gland carcinomas has been made consistent with that for salivary gland carcinomas by:

- Proposing changes in the size cutoffs between T1, T2, and T3
- By subdividing T4
- By expanding the histologic categories to those used for salivary gland malignancies, since all of these have been reported in the lacrimal gland
- Lacrimal sac tumors have been removed from this section

---

### ANATOMIC STAGE/PROGNOSTIC GROUPS

No stage grouping is presently recommended

ICD-O-3
TOPOGRAPHY
CODES
C69.5    Lacrimal gland
         (excluding
         lacrimal sac)

ICD-O-3 HISTOLOGY
CODE RANGES
8000–8576, 8940–8950,
8980–8982

## INTRODUCTION

The retrospective study of 265 epithelial tumors of the lacrimal gland conducted by the Armed Forces Institute of Pathology (AFIP) improved our understanding of the histologic classification and clinical behavior of epithelial tumors of the lacrimal gland. The historic works of Forrest (1954) and Zimmerman (1962) alleviated confusion by applying to epithelial tumors of the lacrimal gland the histopathologic classification of salivary gland tumors. The histologic classification used herein is a modification of the World Health Organization (WHO) classification of salivary gland tumors and is similar to that used in the most recent AFIP fascicle on Tumors of the Eye and Ocular Adnexa (2006).

## ANATOMY

**Primary Site.**   In the normal, fully developed orbit, the lacrimal gland is clinically impalpable and is situated in the lacrimal fossa posterior to the superotemporal orbital rim. The gland is not truly encapsulated and

---

is divided into the deep orbital and the superficial palpebral lobes by the levator aponeurosis.

**Regional Lymph Nodes.**  The regional lymph nodes include the following:

Preauricular (parotid)
Submandibular
Cervical

For pN, histologic examination of a regional lymphadenectomy specimen, if performed, will include one or more regional lymph nodes.

**Metastatic Sites.**  The lung is the most common metastatic site, followed by bone and remote viscera.

## RULES FOR CLASSIFICATION

**Clinical Staging.**  This includes a complete history (with emphasis on duration of symptoms, pain, or dysesthesia) and physical examination (including globe displacement or distortion, palpation, and sensory and motor examination). Imaging of the orbit should be performed. Computed tomography and/or magnetic resonance imaging can provide critical diagnostic and staging data. Orbital imaging should evaluate size, shape, extent, and invasion of adjacent structures, including the bone, skull base, and periorbital areas. The lateral orbital wall and roof are often involved with adenoid cystic carcinoma of the lacrimal gland; thus, en-bloc excision of these orbital walls may be indicated when the bony walls look either clinically (intraoperatively) or radiographically involved. Evaluation of the cervical lymph nodes, the lungs, and bone should be included to stage disease.

**Pathologic Staging.**  Complete resection of the mass is indicated. The specimen should be thoroughly sampled for evaluation of histologic type and grade of tumor, size, possible presence of a preexistent pleomorphic adenoma, and surgical margins (including the periosteum). Perineural spread, most characteristic of adenoid cystic carcinoma, can result in a clinical underestimation of the true anatomic extent of disease. Any bone removed during surgical treatment should be fully examined pathologically for evidence of involvement by carcinoma.

## DEFINITIONS OF TNM

This classification applies to both clinical and pathologic staging of lacrimal gland carcinomas.

| Primary Tumor (T) | |
| --- | --- |
| TX | Primary tumor cannot be assessed |
| T0 | No evidence of primary tumor |
| T1 | Tumor 2 cm or less in greatest dimension, with or without extra-glandular extension into the orbital soft tissue |
| T2 | Tumor more than 2 cm but not more than 4 cm in greatest dimension* |

| T3 | Tumor more than 4 cm in greatest dimension* |
| T4 | Tumor invades periosteum or orbital bone or adjacent structures |
| T4a | Tumor invades periosteum |
| T4b | Tumor invades orbital bone |
| T4c | Tumor invades adjacent structures (brain, sinus, pterygoid fossa, temporal fossa) |

*Note: As the maximum size of the lacrimal gland is 2 cm, T2 and greater tumors will usually extend into the orbital soft tissue.

### Regional Lymph Nodes (N)
| NX | Regional lymph nodes cannot be assessed |
| N0 | No regional lymph node metastasis |
| N1 | Regional lymph node metastasis |

### Distant Metastasis (M)
| M0 | No distant metastasis |
| M1 | Distant metastasis |

## ANATOMIC STAGE/PROGNOSTIC GROUPS

No stage grouping is presently recommended.

## PROGNOSTIC FACTORS (SITE-SPECIFIC FACTORS)
### (Recommended for Collection)

Required for staging     None

Clinically significant     Ki-67 growth fraction
Nuclear NM23 staining

### Pathology Related

Greatest diameter of the tumor
Regional lymph node involvement present by any modality of evaluation
Perineural invasion present on pathologic examination
Level of invasion for carcinoma ex pleomorphic adenoma
For adenoid cystic carcinoma, basaloid pattern present on pathologic examination
For mucoepidermoid carcinoma, tumor is low or high grade on pathologic examination

### Treatment Related

Globe-sparing surgery performed
Exenteration performed
Orbital bone removed
Bone involved by carcinoma
Postoperative radiotherapy

Preoperative chemotherapy
Postoperative chemotherapy

## HISTOLOGIC GRADE (G)

In most cases, the histology defines the grade of malignancy in lacrimal gland carcinomas as in salivary gland carcinomas.

GX    Grade cannot be assessed
G1    Well differentiated
G2    Moderately differentiated: includes adenoid cystic carcinoma without basaloid (solid) pattern
G3    Poorly differentiated: includes adenoid cystic carcinoma with basaloid (solid) pattern
G4    Undifferentiated

## HISTOPATHOLOGIC TYPE

The major malignant primary epithelial tumors include the following:

### Low Grade

Carcinoma ex pleomorphic adenoma [where the carcinoma is noninvasive or minimally invasive as defined by the WHO classification (extension <1.5 mm beyond the capsule – into surrounding tissue)]
Polymorphous low-grade carcinoma
Mucoepidermoid carcinoma, grades 1 and 2
Epithelial-myoepithelial carcinoma
Cystadenocarcinoma and papillary cystadenocarcinoma
Acinic cell carcinoma
Basal cell adenocarcinoma
Mucinous adenocarcinoma

### High Grade

Carcinoma ex pleomorphic adenoma (malignant mixed tumor) that includes adenocarcinoma and adenoid cystic carcinoma arising in a pleomorphic adenoma [where the carcinoma is invasive as defined by the WHO classification (extension >1.5 mm beyond the capsule – into surrounding tissue)]
Adenoid cystic carcinoma, not otherwise specified
Adenocarcinoma, not otherwise specified
Mucoepidermoid carcinoma, grade 3
Ductal adenocarcinoma
Squamous cell carcinoma
Sebaceous adenocarcinoma
Myoepithelial carcinoma
Lymphoepithelial carcinoma

Other Rare and Unclassifiable Carcinomas

## BIBLIOGRAPHY

Cheuk W, Chan JKC. Advances in salivary gland pathology. Histopathology. 2007;51: 1–20.

Font RL, Gamel JW. Epithelial tumors of the lacrimal gland: an analysis of 265 cases. In: Jakobiec FA, editor. Ocular and adnexal tumors. Birmingham, AL: Aesculapius; 1978. Chapter 53.

Font RL, Croxatto JO, Rao NA. Tumors of the lacrimal gland. In: Silverberg SG, Sobin LH, editors. AFIP atlas of tumor pathology: tumors of the eye and ocular adnexa, series 4, fascicle 5. Washington, DC: American Registry of Pathology and Armed Forces Institute of Pathology; 2006. p. 223–46.

Forrest AW. Epithelial lacrimal gland tumors: pathology as a guide to prognosis. Trans Am Acad Ophthalmol Otolaryngol. 1954;58(6):848–66.

Henderson JW. Orbital tumors. 3rd ed. New York: Raven; 1994.

Jakobiec FA, Bilyk JR, Font RL. Lacrimal gland tumors. In: Spencer WH, editor. Ophthalmic pathology: an atlas and textbook, vol. 4. 4th ed. Philadelphia, PA: Saunders; 1996. p. 2485–2525.

Luukaa H, Klemi P, Leivo I, et al. Prognostic significance of Ki-67 and p53 as tumor markers in salivary gland malignancies in Finland: An evaluation of 212 cases. Acta Oncol. 2006;45:669–75.

Tellado MV, McLean IW, Specht CS, et al. Adenoid cystic carcinomas of the lacrimal gland in childhood and adolescence. Ophthalmology. 1997;104:1622–5.

Vangveeravong S, Katz SE, Rootman J, et al. Tumors arising in the palpebral lobe of the lacrimal gland. Ophthalmology. 1996;103:1606–12.

Weis E, Rootman J, Joly TJ, et al. Epithelial lacrimal gland tumors: pathologic classification and current understanding. Arch Ophthalmol. 2009;127:1016–1028.

World Health Organization Classification of Tumours. Pathology and genetics of head and neck tumours. Lyon: IARC; 2005.

Zimmerman LE, Sanders TE, Ackerman LV. Epithelial tumors of the lacrimal gland: prognostic and therapeutic significance of histologic types. In: Zimmerman LE, editor. Tumors of the eye and adnexa, international ophthalmology clinics. Boston, MA: Little, Brown; 1962. p. 337–67.

# Sarcoma of the Orbit

## *At-A-Glance*

---

### SUMMARY OF CHANGES

- A listing of site-specific categories is now included in T4
- The anatomy description was expanded
- Regional lymph nodes were defined

---

**ANATOMIC STAGE/PROGNOSTIC GROUPS**

No stage grouping is presently recommended

ICD-O-3
TOPOGRAPHY
CODES
C69.6    Orbit, NOS
C69.8    Overlapping
           lesion of eye
           and adnexa

ICD-O-3 HISTOLOGY
CODE RANGES
8800–9136, 9142–9582,
9751–9758

## INTRODUCTION

The commonly encountered primary malignant neoplasms of the orbit include soft tissue sarcomas (rhabdomyosarcoma, osteogenic sarcoma, leiomyosarcoma, etc.), lymphoproliferative tumors (lymphoma, plasma cell tumors, etc.), and melanocytic tumors.

## ANATOMY

The orbit is a cone-shaped bony structure with a volume of 30 ml in which the 7-ml globe is positioned centrally and anteriorly. All the support systems of the globe, including the optic nerve and its meninges, lacrimal gland and lymphoid tissue, extraocular muscles, fibroadipose tissue, peripheral nerves, ganglionic tissue, and blood vessels are designed to be confined within approximately 25 ml of space surrounding the eyeball. Many types of tissues are crowded in this limited space and give origin to a variety of primary carcinomatous, sarcomatous, lymphoid and melanocytic tumors. Secondary neoplasia (from adjacent structures such as paranasal sinuses, conjunctiva, globe, etc.) as well as metastatic tumors from distant organs are encountered in the orbit. Also, and because of their immediate proximity, the orbital primary tumors often present invasions into CNS, nasal cavity, and paranasal sinuses. Orbit has two unique histopathological features that may have some influence on tumor dissemination to and from this location. Orbit does not contain a lymphatic vascular network and its venous channels do not have valves.

**Primary Site.** Orbital sarcomas originate from fat (liposarcoma), striated muscle (rhabdomyosarcoma), smooth muscle (leiomyosarcoma), cartilage (chondrosarcoma), bone (osteogenic sarcoma), fibroconnective tissue (fibrosarcoma, fibrous histiocytoma), vascular tissues (angiosarcoma, hemangiopericytoma), peripheral nerve (Schwannoma, paraganglioma), and optic nerve tissues (glioma, meningioma) as well as from primitive mesenchymal cells within the orbit.

**Regional Lymph Nodes.** Although there is no organized lymphatic network behind the orbital septum, the drainage of the orbit is into the submandibular, parotid, and cervical lymph nodes through vascular anastamosis. The venous drainage of the orbit is primarily into the cavernous sinus. Preauricular, submandibular, and cervical nodes may receive drainage secondarily from orbit via the lymphatics of conjunctiva and eyelids. For pN, the examination of a regional lymphadenectomy specimen would ordinarily include one or more lymph node(s).

The regional lymph nodes include the following:

Preauricular (parotid)
Submandibular
Cervical

**Local Invasion.** The malignancy of the orbit may directly extend into adjacent structures. Therefore, local tumor invasion (T4) would include extension to involve the eyelid, globe, temporal fossa, nasal cavity and paranasal sinuses, and central nervous system.

**Metastatic Sites.** Metastatic spread occurs by the bloodstream and lymphatics.

## RULES FOR CLASSIFICATION

**Clinical Staging.** Clinical classification should be based on the symptoms and signs related to loss of vision and visual field, degree of global displacement and loss of extraocular motility, and degree of compressive optic neuropathy. Diagnostic tests should include perimetry, ultrasonography, computed tomography, magnetic resonance imaging, and other imaging procedures when indicated.

**Pathologic Staging.** The nature of the histopathology specimen (fine-needle aspiration biopsy, excisional biopsy, lumpectomy, or total excision) should be noted. Pathologic classification is based on the specific histopathology of the tumor, its differentiation (grade), and the extent of removal (evaluation of its excisional margins). In total excision specimens, evaluation of the surgical margins is mandatory.

## DEFINITIONS OF TNM

This classification applies to both clinical and pathologic staging of sarcomas of the orbit.

### Primary Tumor (T)

| | |
|---|---|
| TX | Primary tumor cannot be assessed |
| T0 | No evidence of primary tumor |
| T1 | Tumor 15 mm or less in greatest dimension |
| T2 | Tumor more than 15 mm in greatest dimension without invasion of globe or bony wall |
| T3 | Tumor of any size with invasion of orbital tissues and/or bony walls |
| T4 | Tumor invasion of globe or periorbital structure, such as eyelids, temporal fossa, nasal cavity and paranasal sinuses, and/or central nervous system |

### Regional Lymph Nodes (N)

| | |
|---|---|
| NX | Regional lymph nodes cannot be assessed |
| N0 | No regional lymph node metastasis |
| N1 | Regional lymph node metastasis |

### Distant Metastasis (M)

| | |
|---|---|
| M0 | No distant metastasis |
| M1 | Distant metastasis |

### ANATOMIC STAGE/PROGNOSTIC GROUPS

No stage grouping is presently recommended

## PROGNOSTIC FACTORS (SITE-SPECIFIC FACTORS)
### (Recommended for Collection)

| | |
|---|---|
| Required for staging | None |
| Clinically significant | None |

## HISTOLOGIC GRADE (G)

Grade is reported in registry systems by the grade value. A two-grade, three-grade, or four-grade system may be used. If a grading system is not specified, generally the following system is used:

| | |
|---|---|
| GX | Grade cannot be assessed |
| G1 | Well differentiated |
| G2 | Moderately differentiated |
| G3 | Poorly differentiated |
| G4 | Undifferentiated |

## HISTOPATHOLOGIC TYPE

Malignancies of the orbit primarily include a broad spectrum of malignant soft tissue tumors.

## BIBLIOGRAPHY

Collaco L, Goncalves M, Gomes L, Miranda R. Orbital Kaposi's sarcoma in acquired immunodeficiency syndrome. Eur J Ophthalmol. 2000;10:88–90.

Karcioglu ZA. Orbital tumors: diagnosis and treatment. New York: Springer; 2005.

Karcioglu ZA, Hadjistilianou D, Rozans M, DeFrancesco S. Diagnosis and management of orbital rhabdomyosarcoma. Cancer Control. 2004;11:328–33.

Khan AO, Burke MJ. Alveolar soft-part sarcoma of the orbit. J Pediatr Ophthalmol Strabismus. 2004;41:245–6.

Miettinen M. Diagnostic soft tissue pathology. New York: Churchill/Livingston; 2000.

Pang NK, Bartley GB, Giannini C. Primary Ewing sarcoma of the orbit in an adult. Ophthal Plast Reconstr Surg. 2007;23:153–4.

Rootman J. Diseases of the orbit: a multidisciplinary approach. 2nd ed. Philadelphia, PA: Lippincott; 2002.

Rootman J. Desmoplastic inflammatory disorders affecting the orbit. Ophthal Plast Reconstr Surg. 2006;22:161–2.

Saeed P, Rootman J, Nugent RA, et al. Optic nerve sheath meningiomas. Ophthalmology. 2003;110:2019–30.

Selva D, White VA, O'Connell JX, Rootman J. Primary bone tumors of the orbit. Surv Ophthalmol. 2004;49:328–42.

Weiss S. Enzinger and Weiss's soft tissue tumors. Philadelphia, PA: Mosby; 2001.

# Ocular Adnexal Lymphoma

## *At-A-Glance*

**SUMMARY OF CHANGES**

• This is an entirely new chapter

**ANATOMIC STAGE/PROGNOSTIC GROUPS**

No stage grouping is presently recommended

ICD-O-3
TOPOGRAPHY
CODES

| | |
|---|---|
| C44.1 | Eyelid |
| C69.0 | Conjunctiva |
| C69.5 | Lacrimal gland |
| C69.6 | Orbit, NOS |

ICD-O-3 HISTOLOGY
CODE RANGES
9590–9699, 9702–9738,
9811–9818, 9820–9837

## INTRODUCTION

Ocular adnexal lymphomas (OAL) originate in conjunctiva, eyelids, lacrimal gland, lacrimal drainage apparatus, and other orbital tissues surrounding the eye. Almost all are extranodal non-Hodgkin lymphomas (NHL), typically comprising extranodal marginal zone B-cell lymphoma (EMZL) of MALT type, according to the WHO lymphoma classification.[1–5] Although rare, T/NK-cell lymphomas also arise in the ocular adnexa.[6,7]

The Ann Arbor system[8,9] is widely used for clinical staging of lymphomas but is not ideally suited to extranodal disease.[10,11] For example, in OALs, eyelid lymphomas have a worse prognosis than conjunctival lymphomas, but both are categorized as Stage I.[5,12–15] The following TNM staging system for OALs addresses these limitations. It must be emphasized that this system should not be used for secondary lymphomatous involvement of ocular adnexa or for any intraocular lymphomas.

## ANATOMY

### Primary Sites

*Eyelid.* The eyelids consist of 8 layers: skin, subcutaneous connective tissue, orbicularis oculi muscle, orbital septum, levator muscle, tarsal plate, Müller's muscle, and conjunctiva. Accessory eyelid structures include the plica semilunaris and the caruncle. OAL is defined as involving eyelid if the

OAL infiltrates preseptal tissues such as dermis or orbicularis muscle of the anterior eyelid skin.[16]

*Conjunctiva.* The conjunctiva lines the posterior eyelid surface and the anterior surface of the eye, with these two areas meeting at the fornix. It is a mucous membrane overlying substantia propria, which contains a sparse population of lymphoid cells.

*Orbit.* The orbit is a bony cavity containing the eye, lacrimal gland, lacrimal sac, nasolacrimal duct, extraocular muscles, fat, arteries, veins, and nerves, but no lymphatics. The orbit is adjacent to the ethmoid sinuses medially, the frontal sinus and cranial cavity superiorly and posteriorly, the maxillary sinus inferiorly, and the temporalis fossa laterally.

*Lacrimal Gland.* The lacrimal gland is situated immediately posterior to the superotemporal orbital rim. It is an exocrine gland secreting tears containing IgA and other protective agents. Several tiny accessory glands of Krause and Wolfring are located in the region of the fornices. The lacrimal drainage system comprises the upper and lower canaliculi, the lacrimal sac, and the nasolacrimal duct.

The arterial blood supply is provided by branches of the internal and external carotid arteries. Venous drainage from pretarsal tissues is via the angular vein medially and the superficial temporal vein laterally. Posttarsal tissue drainage is into the orbital veins and the deeper branches of the anterior facial vein and pterygoid plexus. Lymphatic drainage from medial conjunctiva and medial eyelids is to submandibular nodes with lateral areas of these tissues draining to preauricular lymph nodes and then into the deeper cervical nodes.

**Regional Lymph Nodes.** The regional lymph nodes of the ocular adnexa include the submandibular, preauricular, and cervical lymph nodes. Distant nodes include "central" nodes, located in the trunk (e.g., mediastinal and para-aortic nodes) and "peripheral" nodes at other distant sites not draining the ocular adnexa (e.g., popliteal lymph nodes).

**Metastatic Sites.** The most common metastatic sites of OAL are other extranodal tissues that are noncontiguous with the ocular adnexa. These include organs such as the salivary glands, gastrointestinal tract, lung, and the liver.

**Bone Marrow.** Bone marrow infiltration can be micronodular, paratrabecular, or diffuse interstitial.


## RULES FOR CLASSIFICATION

**Clinical Staging.** This includes a complete history and ophthalmic examination including but not limited to exophthalmometry, color vision testing, inspection and palpation of the eyelids and orbit, evaluation of ocular motility, and examination of the entire conjunctiva (with eversion of the upper eyelids). Intraocular pressure measurements and findings on dilated ophthalmoscopy may indicate compressive ocular disease. Ultrasonography can be used in the clinical setting to evaluate the orbit. Systemic physical examination should be performed as well as radiographic imaging of both orbits and sinuses, chest, abdomen, and pelvis. This can be performed using computer tomography (CT) and/or magnetic resonance imaging (MRI). Some centers now use whole-body positron emission tomography/computed tomography (PET/CT) for staging patients with OAL.

**Pathologic Staging.** An incisional biopsy should be performed, providing a sufficient specimen for pathological staging and subtyping of the lymphoma on the basis of morphology, immunophenotype and, if possible, the genotype. If feasible, suspected lymph node or extranodal involvement should be confirmed histopathologically [e.g., by fine needle aspiration biopsy (FNAB) or incisional biopsy]. Bone marrow biopsy should be performed for complete staging.

**Descriptors for the Proposed System.** As defined by the AJCC/IUCC,[17,18] prefix descriptors "m," "r," or "a" can be used, these respectively indicating multiple tumors in one ocular adnexal structure, recurrent disease, and autopsy. For example, mT1*a* indicates multiple bulbar conjunctival (extralimbal) tumors in one eye. The *prefix* "b" indicates bilateral lymphomas in ocular adnexal structures: this can be applied at all T stages. For example, bT2*b* indicates bilateral lacrimal gland involvement.

## PROGNOSTIC FEATURES

The proposed TNM classification of OAL defines the anatomic extent of disease in greater detail. This has been considered of prognostic value in the literature. Similar to nodal lymphomas, the International Prognostic Index (IPI)[19] should be applied to subdivide patients with primary diffuse large B-cell lymphomas of the ocular adnexa according to prognosis, thereby enhancing individual patient care. Similarly, the Follicular Lymphoma International Prognostic Index (FLIPI),[20] which includes age, Ann Arbor stage, number of nodal sites, serum lactate dehydrogenase level, and hemoglobin level to build a three-category index, should be applied in patients with primary ocular adnexal follicular lymphomas, e.g., see Table 57.2 in Chap. 57 of Lymphoid Neoplasms (Part XII).

**Tumor Cell Growth Fraction (Ki-67, MIB-1).** This should be assessed by counting the number of tumor cells with clear nuclear positivity for Ki-67 per $5 \times 100$ tumor cells using the 40× objective. A percentage value is therefore obtained, e.g., a Ki-67 tumor cell growth fraction of 15%. Reactive cells should not be included where possible. For example, the germinal centre in MALT lymphomas should NOT be included in the assessment.

**Serum Lactate Dehydrogenase.** The serum lactate dehydrogenase (LDH) value should be assessed at the time of diagnosis.

## DEFINITIONS OF TNM

This classification applies to both clinical and pathologic staging of ocular adnexal lymphomas.

### Primary Tumor (T)

| | |
|---|---|
| TX | Lymphoma extent not specified |
| T0 | No evidence of lymphoma |
| T1 | Lymphoma involving the conjunctiva alone without orbital involvement |
| T1a | Bulbar conjunctiva only |
| T1b | Palpebral conjunctiva +/− fornix +/− caruncle |
| T1c | Extensive conjunctival involvement |
| T2 | Lymphoma with orbital involvement +/− any conjunctival involvement |
| T2a | Anterior orbital involvement (+/− conjunctival involvement) |
| T2b | Anterior orbital involvement (+/− conjunctival involvement + lacrimal involvement) |
| T2c | Posterior orbital involvement (+/− conjunctival involvement +/− anterior involvement and +/− any extraocular muscle involvement) |
| T2d | Nasolacrimal drainage system involvement (+/− conjunctival involvement but not including nasopharynx) |
| T3 | Lymphoma with preseptal eyelid involvement (defined above)[16] +/− orbital involvement +/− any conjunctival involvement |
| T4 | Orbital adnexal lymphoma extending beyond orbit to adjacent structures such as bone and brain |
| T4a | Involvement of nasopharynx |
| T4b | Osseous involvement (including periosteum) |
| T4c | Involvement of maxillofacial, ethmoidal, and/or frontal sinuses |
| T4d | Intracranial spread |

### Regional Lymph Node (N)

| | |
|---|---|
| NX | Involvement of lymph nodes not assessed |
| N0 | No evidence of lymph node involvement |
| N1 | Involvement of ipsilateral regional lymph nodes* |
| N2 | Involvement of contra lateral or bilateral regional lymph nodes* |
| N3 | Involvement of peripheral lymph nodes not draining ocular adnexal region |
| N4 | Involvement of central lymph nodes |

*Note: The regional lymph nodes include preauricular (parotid), submandibular, and cervical.

### Distant Metastasis (M)

| | |
|---|---|
| M0 | No evidence of involvement of other extranodal sites |
| M1a | Noncontiguous involvement of tissues or organs external to the ocular adnexa (e.g., parotid glands, submandibular gland, lung, liver, spleen, kidney, breast, etc.) |
| M1b | Lymphomatous involvement of the bone marrow |
| M1c | Both M1a and M1b involvement |

No stage grouping is presently recommended

## PROGNOSTIC FACTORS (SITE-SPECIFIC FACTORS)
### (Recommended for Collection)

| | |
|---|---|
| Required for staging | None |
| Clinically significant | Tumor cell growth fraction (Ki-67, MIB-1) |
| | Serum lactate dehydrogenase (LDH) at diagnosis |
| | History of rheumatoid arthritis |
| | History of Sjögren's syndrome |
| | History of connective tissue disease |
| | History of recurrent dry eye syndrome (sicca syndrome) |
| | Any evidence of a viral infection (e.g., hepatitis C or HIV) |
| | Any evidence of a bacterial infection (e.g., *Helicobacter pylori*) |
| | Any evidence of an infection caused by other microorganisms (e.g., *Chlamydia psittaci*) |

**55**

## HISTOLOGIC GRADE (G)

Grades are given only to *follicular lymphomas* as described by the 2002 WHO classification[21] for malignant lymphomas as follows:

| | |
|---|---|
| G1 | 1–5 centroblasts per 10 high power field |
| G2 | Between 5 and 15 centroblasts per 10 high power fields |
| G3a | More than 15 centroblasts per 10 high power fields but with admixed centrocytes |
| G3b | More than 15 centroblasts per 10 high power fields but without centrocytes |

## HISTOPATHOLOGIC TYPE

The lymphomas arising as *primary tumors* in the ocular adnexa are subtyped according to the WHO Lymphoma classification.[21] The main ocular adnexal lymphoma subtypes include the following:

Extranodal marginal zone B-cell lymphoma (MALT lymphoma)
Diffuse large B-cell lymphoma
Follicular lymphoma
Mantle cell lymphoma
Lymphoplasmacytic lymphoma
Plasmacytoma
Burkitt lymphoma
Peripheral T-cell lymphoma, unspecified
Mycosis fungoides
Extranodal NK/T-cell lymphoma, nasal type
Anaplastic large cell lymphoma

# REFERENCES

1. Coupland SE, Krause L, Delecluse HJ, et al. Lymphoproliferative lesions of the ocular adnexa. Analysis of 112 cases. Ophthalmology. 1998;105:1430–41.
2. Jenkins C, Rose GE, Bunce C, et al. Histological features of ocular adnexal lymphoma (REAL classification) and their association with patient morbidity and survival. Br J Ophthalmol. 2000;84:907–13.
3. Decaudin D, de Cremoux P, Vincent-Salomon A, Dendale R, Lumbroso-Le Rouic L. Ocular adnexal lymphoma. Blood. 2006;108:1451–60.
4. Ferry JA, Fung CY, Zukerberg L, Lucarelli MJ, Hasserjian R, Preffer FI, et al. Lymphoma of the ocular adnexa: a study of 353 cases. Am J Surg Pathol. 2007;31:170–84.
5. Jakobiec FA. Ocular adnexal lymphoid tumors: progress in need of clarification. Am J Ophthalmol. 2008;145:941–50.
6. Coupland SE, Foss HD, Assaf C, Auw-Haedrich C, Anastassiou G, Anagnostopoulos I, et al. T-cell and T/natural killer-cell lymphomas involving ocular and ocular adnexal tissues: a clinicopathologic, immunohistochemical, and molecular study of seven cases. Ophthalmology. 1999;106: 2109–20.
7. Woog JJ, Kim YD, Yeatts RP, Kim S, Esmaeli B, Kikkawa D, et al. Natural killer/T-cell lymphoma with ocular and adnexal involvement. Ophthalmology. 2006;113:140–7.
8. Carbone PP, Kaplan HS, Musshoff K, Smithers DW, Tubiana M. Report of the committee on Hodgkin's disease staging classification. Cancer Res. 1971;31:1860–1.
9. Musshoff K. Clinical staging classification of non-Hodgkin's lymphomas (author's transl). Strahlentherapie. 1977;153:218–21.
10. Ruskone-Fourmestraux A, Dragosics B, Morgner A, Wotherspoon AC, de Jong D. Paris staging system for primary gastrointestinal lymphomas. Gut. 2003;52:912–6.
11. Kim YH, Willemze R, Pimpinelli N, Whittaker S, Olsen EA, Ranki A, et al. EORTC Iat: TNM classification system for primary cutaneous lymphomas other than mycosis fungoides and Sezary syndrome: a proposal of the International Society for Cutaneous Lymphomas (ISCL) and the Cutaneous Lymphoma Task Force of the European Organization of Research and Treatment of Cancer (EORTC). Blood. 2007;110:479–84.
12. Auw-Haedrich C, Coupland SE, Kapp A, et al. Long term outcome of ocular adnexal lymphoma subtyped according to the REAL classification. Revised European and American lymphoma. Br J Ophthalmol. 2001;85: 63–9.
13. Johnson TE, Tse DT, Byrne GE Jr, et al. Ocular-adnexal lymphoid tumors: a clinicopathologic and molecular genetic study of 77 patients. Ophthal Plast Reconstr Surg. 1999;15:171–9.
14. Knowles DM, Jakobiec FA, McNally L, Burke JS. Lymphoid hyperplasia and malignant lymphoma occurring in the ocular adnexa (orbit, conjunctiva, and eyelids): a prospective multiparametric analysis of 108 cases during 1977 to 1987. Hum Pathol. 1990;21:959–73.
15. White WA, Ferry JA, Harris NL, Grove AS. Ocular adnexal lymphoma. A clinicopathologic study with identification of lymphomas of mucosa-associated lymphoid tissue type. Ophthalmology. 1995;102:1994–2006.
16. Knowles DM. Neoplastic hematopathology. Philadelphia, PA: Lippincott Williams and Wilkins; 2000. p. 1303–49.
17. UICC. TNM classification of malignant tumors. New York: Wiley-Liss; 2002.
18. Sobin LH, Wittekind Ch. AJCC cancer staging manual. New York: Springer; 2002.

19. TIN-HsLPF P. A predictive model for aggressive non-Hodgkin's lymphoma. The International Non-Hodgkin's Lymphoma Prognostic Factors Project. N Engl J Med. 1993;329:987–94.
20. Solal-Céligny P, Roy P, Colombat P, et al. Follicular lymphoma international prognostic index. Blood. 2004;104:1258–65.
21. Jaffe ES, Harris NL, Stein H, Vardiman JW. World Health Organization classification of tumours. Tumours of haematopoietic and lymphoid tissues. Pathology and genetics. IARC: Lyon; 2001.

55

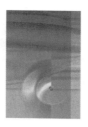

# PART XI
# Central Nervous System

# Brain and Spinal Cord

## *At-A-Glance*

**ANATOMIC STAGE/PROGNOSTIC GROUP**

No stage grouping applies

| ICD-O-3 TOPOGRAPHY CODES | | | | ICD-O-3 HISTOLOGY CODE RANGES |
|---|---|---|---|---|
| | | C71.9 | Brain NOS | 8000, 8680–9136, |
| | | C72.0 | Spinal cord | 9141–9582 |
| C70.0 | Cerebral meninges | C72.1 | Cauda equina | |
| | | C72.2 | Olfactory nerve | |
| C70.1 | Spinal meninges | C72.3 | Optic nerve | |
| | | C72.4 | Acoustic/ vestibular nerve | |
| C70.9 | Meninges, NOS | C72.5 | Cranial nerve, NOS | |
| C71.0 | Cerebrum | | | |
| C71.1 | Frontal lobe | C72.8 | Overlapping lesion of brain and central nervous system | |
| C71.2 | Temporal lobe | | | |
| C71.3 | Parietal lobe | | | |
| C71.4 | Occipital lobe | | | |
| C71.5 | Ventricle NOS | C72.9 | Nervous system, NOS | |
| C71.6 | Cerebellum NOS | | | |
| | | C75.1 | Pituitary gland | |
| C71.7 | Brain stem | C75.2 | Craniopharyngeal duct | |
| C71.8 | Overlapping lesion of brain | C75.3 | Pineal gland | |

## INTRODUCTION

Attempts at developing a TNM-based classification and staging system for tumors of the central nervous system (CNS) have not been successful. Previous editions of this manual had proposed a system that was used with poor compliance and proved not to be particularly useful as a predictor of outcome in clinical trials for the management of patients with primary CNS tumors. The reasons for this are several. (1) Tumor size is significantly less relevant than tumor histology and location of the tumor, so the T classification is less pertinent than the biologic nature of the tumor itself.

(2) Because the brain and spinal cord have no lymphatics, the N classification does not apply, as there are no lymph nodes that can be identified in either classification or staging. (3) An M classification is not pertinent to the majority of neoplasms that affect the central nervous system, because of the inherent biology favoring local recurrence, and the fact that most patients with tumors of the central nervous system do not live long enough to develop metastatic disease (except for some pediatric tumors that tend to "seed" through the cerebrospinal fluid spaces).

Many important studies have been done regarding the most common tumors affecting the brain and spinal cord, and a variety of prognostic factors have been identified. Unfortunately, these factors do not easily fall into the usual categories that have traditionally been part of the American Joint Committee on Cancer (AJCC) TNM system.

For those reasons, it continues to be the recommendation of the CNS Tumor Task Force that a formal classification and staging system not be attempted. This chapter, however, attempts to highlight what is known about prognostic factors in tumors of the central nervous system (Table 56.1).

**TABLE 56.1.** Prognostic factors in CNS tumors

| |
| --- |
| Histology |
|     Pathologic grade and accuracy of diagnosis |
|     Presence and extent of necrosis |
|     Presence of gemistocytes |
|     Proliferative fraction (Ki-67; MIB-1) |
|     Presence of oligodendroglial component |
|     Presence or absence of cells in mitosis, endothelial proliferation |
| Age of patient |
| Functional neurologic status |
|     Karnofsky Performance Score |
| Symptom presentation and duration before diagnosis |
|     Presentation with seizure, long duration are favorable prognostic factors |
| Location of tumor |
|     Unifocal or multifocal |
| Primary or recurrent tumor |
| Extent of resection |
|     Biopsy, subtotal, radical removal |
| Metastatic spread |
|     CNS or extraneural |
| Patterns of enhancement on imaging studies |
| Molecular aspects |
|     1 p, 19 q definitions |
|     MGMT methylation |

## PROGNOSTIC FEATURES

**Tumor Histology.** The histology of tumors that affect the brain and spinal cord is by far the most important variable affecting prognosis, and in many cases it determines the treatment modalities that are employed. The latest World Health Organization (WHO) classification system has combined tumor nomenclature with an associated grading system, so that the actual histologic diagnosis directly correlates with the histologic grade of the tumor. This helps to clarify some of the inconsistencies that existed in the past when a number of different grading systems, each slightly different from the others, were used. The most common histologies for brain and spinal cord tumors are given in Tables 56.2 and 56.3, along with the tumor grade for each different diagnostic category. Note: The histologic grade code used for staging purposes is *not* the same code that is assigned as the differentiation code in the sixth digit of the ICD-O morphology code.

**56**

**TABLE 56.2.** WHO classification of tumors of the central nervous system (2007)

| *Tumors of neuroepithelial tissue* | | Ependymoma | 9391/3 |
|---|---|---|---|
| **Astrocytic tumors** | | Cellular | 9391/3 |
| Pilocytic astrocytoma | 9421/1[a] | Papillary | 9393/3 |
| Pilomyxoid astrocytoma | *9425/3*[b] | Clear cell | 9391/3 |
| Subependymal giant cell astrocytoma | 9384/1 | Tanycytic | 9391/3 |
| | | Anaplastic ependymoma | 9392/3 |
| Pleomorphic xanthoastrocytoma | 9424/3 | **Choroid plexus tumors** | |
| Diffuse astrocytoma | 9400/3 | Choroid plexus papilloma | 9390/0 |
| Fibrillary astrocytoma | 9420/3 | Atypical choroid plexus papilloma | *9390/1*[b] |
| Gemistocytic astrocytoma | 9411/3 | Choroid plexus carcinoma | 9390/3 |
| Protoplasmic astrocytoma | 9410/3 | **Other neuroepithelial tumors** | |
| Anaplastic astrocytoma | 9401/3 | Astroblastoma | 9430/3 |
| Glioblastoma | 9440/3 | Chordoid glioma of the third ventricle | 9444/1 |
| Giant cell glioblastoma | 9441/3 | Angiocentric glioma | *9431/1*[b] |
| Gliosarcoma | 9442/3 | **Neuronal and mixed neuronal-glial tumors** | |
| Gliomatosis cerebri | 9381/3 | | |
| **Oligodendroglial tumors** | | Dysplastic gangliocytoma of cerebellum (Lhermitte-Duclos) | 9493/0 |
| Oligodendroglioma | 9450/3 | Desmoplastic infantile astrocytoma/ganglioglioma | 9412/1 |
| Anaplastic oligodendroglioma | 9451/3 | Dysembryoplastic neuroepithelial tumor | 9413/0 |
| **Oligoastrocytic tumors** | | Gangliocytoma | 9492/0 |
| Oligoastrocytoma | 9382/3 | Ganglioglioma | 9505/1 |
| Anaplastic oligoastrocytoma | 9382/3 | Anaplastic ganglioglioma | 9505/3 |
| **Ependymal tumors** | | Central neurocytoma | 9506/1 |
| Subependymoma | 9383/1 | | |
| Myxopapillary ependymoma | 9394/1 | | *continued* |

| Neuronal and mixed neuronal-glial tumors (cont.) | | |
|---|---|---|
| Extraventricular neurocytoma | 9506/1[b] | |
| Cerebellar liponeurocytoma | 9506/1[b] | |
| Papillary glioneuronal tumor | 9509/1[b] | |
| Rosette-forming glioneuronal tumor of the fourth ventricle | 9509/1[b] | |
| Paraganglioma | 8680/1 | |
| **Tumors of the pineal region** | | |
| Pineocytoma | 9361/1 | |
| Pineal parenchymal tumor of intermediate differentiation | 9362/3 | |
| Pineoblastoma | 9362/3 | |
| Papillary tumor of the pineal region | 9395/3[b] | |
| **Embryonal tumors** | | |
| Medulloblastoma | 9470/3 | |
| Desmoplastic/nodular medulloblastoma | 9471/3 | |
| Medulloblastoma with extensive nodularity | 9471/3[b] | |
| Anaplastic medulloblastoma | 9474/3[b] | |
| Large cell medulloblastoma | 9474/3 | |
| CNS primitive neuroectodermal tumor | 9473/3 | |
| CNS Neuroblastoma | 9500/3 | |
| CNS Ganglioneuroblastoma | 9490/3 | |
| Medulloepithelioma | 9501/3 | |
| Ependymoblastoma | 9392/3 | |
| Atypical teratoid/rhabdoid tumor | 9508/3 | |
| *Tumors of cranial and paraspinal nerves* | | |
| **Schwannoma** (neurilemoma, neurinoma) | 9560/0 | |
| Cellular | 9560/0 | |
| Plexiform | 9560/0 | |
| Melanotic | 9560/0 | |
| **Neurofibroma** | 9540/0 | |
| Plexiform | 9550/0 | |

| Perineurioma | | |
|---|---|---|
| Perineurioma, NOS | 9571/0 | |
| Malignant perineurioma | 9571/3 | |
| **Malignant peripheral nerve sheath tumor (MPNST)** | | |
| Epithelioid MPNST | 9540/3 | |
| MPNST with mesenchymal differentiation | 9540/3 | |
| Melanotic MPNST | 9540/3 | |
| MPNST with glandular differentiation | 9540/3 | |
| *Tumors of the meninges* | | |
| **Tumors of meningothelial cells** | | |
| Meningioma | 9530/0 | |
| Meningothelial | 9531/0 | |
| Fibrous (fibroblastic) | 9532/0 | |
| Transitional (mixed) | 9537/0 | |
| Psammomatous | 9533/0 | |
| Angiomatous | 9534/0 | |
| Microcystic | 9530/0 | |
| Secretory | 9530/0 | |
| Lymphoplasmacyte-rich | 9530/0 | |
| Metaplastic | 9530/0 | |
| Chordoid | 9538/1 | |
| Clear cell | 9538/1 | |
| Atypical | 9539/1 | |
| Papillary | 9538/3 | |
| Rhabdoid | 9538/3 | |
| Anaplastic (malignant) | 9530/3 | |
| **Mesenchymal tumors** | | |
| Lipoma | 8850/0 | |
| Angiolipoma | 8861/0 | |
| Hibernoma | 8880/0 | |
| Liposarcoma | 8850/3 | |
| Solitary fibrous tumor | 8815/0 | |
| Fibrosarcoma | 8810/3 | |
| Malignant fibrous histiocytoma | 8830/3 | |
| Leiomyoma | 8890/0 | |
| Leiomyosarcoma | 8890/3 | |
| Rhabdomyoma | 8900/0 |

*continued*

**TABLE 56.2.** WHO classification of tumors of the central nervous system (2007) (continued)

| Mesenchymal tumors (cont.) | | Lymphomas and hematopoietic neoplasms | |
|---|---|---|---|
| Rhabdomyosarcoma | 8900/3 | | |
| Chondroma | 9220/0 | Malignant lymphomas | 9590/3 |
| Chondrosarcoma | 9220/3 | Plasmacytoma | 9731/3 |
| Osteoma | 9180/0 | Granulocytic sarcoma | 9930/3 |
| Osteosarcoma | 9180/3 | *Germ cell tumors* | |
| Osteochondroma | 9210/0 | Germinoma | 9064/3 |
| Hemangioma | 9120/0 | Embryonal carcinoma | 9070/3 |
| Epithelioid hemangioendothelioma | 9133/1 | Yolk sac tumor | 9071/3 |
| | | Choriocarcinoma | 9100/3 |
| Hemangiopericytoma | 9150/1 | Teratoma | 9080/1 |
| Anaplastic hemangiopericytoma | 9150/3 | Mature | 9080/0 |
| | | Immature | 9080/3 |
| Angiosarcoma | 9120/3 | Teratoma with malignant transformation | 9084/3 |
| Kaposi sarcoma | 9140/3 | | |
| Ewing sarcoma – PNET | 9364/3 | Mixed germ cell tumor | 9085/3 |
| **Primary melanocytic lesions** | | *Tumors of the sellar region* | |
| Diffuse melanocytosis | 8728/0 | Craniopharyngioma | 9350/1 |
| Melanocytoma | 8728/1 | Adamantinomatous | 9351/1 |
| Malignant melanoma | 8720/3 | Papillary | 9352/1 |
| Meningeal melanomatosis | 8728/3 | Granular cell tumor | 9582/0 |
| **Other neoplasms related to the meninges** | | Pituicytoma | 9432/1[b] |
| Hemangioblastoma | 9161/1 | Spindle cell oncocytoma of the adenohypophysis | 8291/0[b] |

From World Health Organization (http://www.who.int/en/), with permission.

[a] Morphology code of the International Classification of Diseases for Oncology (ICO-O) (614A) and the Systematized Nomenclature of Medicine (http://snomed.org). Behavior is coded /0 for benign tumors, /3 for malignant tumors, and /1 for borderline or uncertain behavior.

[b] The italicized numbers are provisional codes proposed for the 4th edition of ICD-O. While they are expected to be incorporated into the next ICD-O edition, they currently remain subject to change.

**Age of the Patient.** Most retrospective outcome studies of brain tumor therapy show that the age of the patient at the time of diagnosis is one of the most powerful predictors of outcome. This fact holds true for the gliomas, which are the most common primary brain tumors, and for most other tumors that affect the adult population, including most metastatic tumors to the brain. There are, however, some childhood tumors that have a very poor prognosis, are inherently high grade, and rapidly progress to a fatal outcome. Some metastatic tumors, such as melanoma, occur in younger patients and also violate this general statement with regard to the specific effect of age on prognosis.

**Extent of Tumor Resection.** In patients who are treated surgically for tumors of the central nervous system, the extent of resection is often directly correlated with the outcome. This is a less powerful predictor than tumor

**TABLE 56.3.** WHO grades of CNS tumors

| | I | II | III | IV |
|---|:---:|:---:|:---:|:---:|
| **Astrocytic tumors** | | | | |
| Subependymal giant cell astrocytoma | • | | | |
| Pilocytic astrocytoma | • | | | |
| Pilomyxoid astrocytoma | | • | | |
| Diffuse astrocytoma | | • | | |
| Pleomorphic xanthoastrocytoma | | • | | |
| Anaplastic astrocytoma | | | • | |
| Glioblastoma | | | | • |
| Giant cell glioblastoma | | | | • |
| Gliosarcoma | | | | • |
| **Oligodendroglial tumors** | | | | |
| Oligodendroglioma | | • | | |
| Anaplastic oligodendroglioma | | | • | |
| **Oligoastrocytic tumors** | | | | |
| Oligoastrocytoma | | • | | |
| Anaplastic oligoastrocytoma | | | • | |
| **Ependymal tumors** | | | | |
| Subependymoma | • | | | |
| Myxopapillary ependymoma · | • | | | |
| Ependymoma | | • | | |
| Anaplastic ependymoma | | | • | |
| **Choroid plexus tumors** | | | | |
| Choroid plexus papilloma | • | | | |
| Atypical choroid plexus papilloma | | • | | |
| Choroid plexus carcinoma | | | • | |
| **Other neuroepithelial tumors** | | | | |
| Angiocentric glioma | • | | | |
| Chordoid glioma of the third ventricle | | • | | |
| **Neuronal and mixed neuronal-glial tumors** | | | | |
| Gangliocytoma | • | | | |
| Ganglioglioma | • | | | |
| Anaplastic ganglioglioma | | | • | |
| Desmoplastic infantile astrocytoma and ganglioglioma | • | | | |
| Dysembryoplastic neuroepithelial tumor | • | | | |
| Central neurocytoma | | • | | |
| Extraventricular neurocytoma | | • | | |
| Cerebellar liponeurocytoma · | | • | | |
| Paraganglioma of the spinal cord | • | | | |
| Papillary glioneuronal tumor | • | | | |
| Rosette-forming glioneuronal tumor of the fourth ventricle | • | | | |

*continued*

**TABLE 56.3.** WHO grades of CNS tumors (continued)

| | I | II | III | IV |
|---|---|---|---|---|
| **Pineal tumors** | | | | |
| Pineocytoma | • | | | |
| Pineal parenchymal tumor of intermediate differentiation | | • | • | |
| Pineoblastoma | | | | • |
| Papillary tumor of the pineal region | | • | • | |
| **Embryonal tumors** | | | | |
| Medulloblastoma | | | | • |
| CNS primitive neuroectodermal tumor (PNET) | | | | • |
| Atypical teratoid/rhabdoid tumor | | | | • |
| **Tumors of the cranial and paraspinal nerves** | | | | |
| Schwannoma | • | | | |
| Neurofibroma | • | | | |
| Perineurioma | • | • | • | |
| Malignant peripheral nerve sheath tumor (MPNST) | | • | • | • |
| **Meningeal tumors** | | | | |
| Meningioma | • | | | |
| Atypical meningioma | | • | | |
| Anaplastic/malignant meningioma | | | • | |
| Hemangiopericytoma | | • | | |
| Anaplastic hemangiopericytoma | | | • | |
| Hemangioblastoma | • | | | |
| **Tumors of the sellar region** | | | | |
| Craniopharyngioma | • | | | |
| Granular cell tumor of the neurohypophysis | • | | | |
| Pituicytoma | • | | | |
| **Spindle cell oncocytoma of the adenohypophysis** | • | | | |

From World Health Organization (http://www.who.int/en/), with permission.

histology or age, but most retrospective studies confirm that extent of removal is positively correlated with survival. For this reason, documentation of whether a surgical tumor removal is "gross total," "subtotal," or "biopsy only" is useful in determining future therapy and prognosis and ideally is accompanied by MRI-based quantitative assessment. Any staging system to be developed for CNS tumors should take into account, in a systematic and clearly documented fashion, the extent of removal and residual tumor.

**Tumor Location.** Because of the differential importance of various areas of the brain, the location of a given tumor affecting the brain can have a major impact on the functional outcome, survival, and nature of therapy. The location codes available for tumors affecting the central nervous system in the ICD-O and ICD-10 manuals are generally satisfactory, and they offer the advantage of consistency to the records of patients with CNS tumors.

**Functional Neurologic Status.** Another important prognostic factor in most retrospective studies of CNS tumors is the functional neurologic status of the patient at the time of diagnosis. This has been estimated traditionally using the Karnofsky Performance Scale, which is reproducible, is well known by most investigators, and is in common use for stratification of patients entering clinical trials for the treatment of brain tumors. The outcome and prognosis of patients correlate fairly well with functional neurologic status, and once again, any staging system should include a validated and reliable measure of this parameter. Other measures of outcome, both cognitive and functional, are increasingly used in studies of CNS tumors.

**Metastatic Spread.** Tumors affecting the central nervous system rarely develop extraneural metastases, probably because of inherent biologic characteristics of these tumors, and also because the brain does not have a well-developed lymphatic drainage system. In addition, many patients with tumors of the central nervous system have a short life expectancy, which further limits the likelihood of metastatic spread. Certain tumors do spread through cerebrospinal fluid (CSF) pathways, and such spread has a major impact on survival. Dissemination through the CSF pathway is a hallmark of certain childhood tumors, e.g., primitive neuroectodermal tumors, many of which carry a poor prognosis; this phenomenon, however, is rarely seen in adult patients with the more common CNS tumors. Primary lymphomas of the central nervous system may spread along the craniospinal axis and sometimes exhibit intraocular dissemination. Although metastatic spread is of importance in certain instances, its overall impact in staging is relatively minor. The M category, however, should be part of any classification and staging system that is developed in the future for CNS tumors, and it should differentiate between extraneural metastasis and metastasis within the CNS and CSF pathways.

## BRAIN TUMOR SURVIVAL DATA

Data are available from the SEER program for current survival statistics for "brain tumors," a category that includes malignant primary brain tumors (gliomas). For this relatively ill-defined group of patients, there were 17,200 new cases estimated for 2001. Five-year survivals are 30% in adults and 64% in children.

Excellent observational insight and patterns of care data for surgically treated malignant gliomas [glioblastomas and malignant (grade 3) gliomas] are available from the Glioma Outcome Project, which evaluated 788 patients accrued from 1997 to 2000. The median survival for glioblastoma multiforme (GBM) was 10.6 months, and the 96-week survival was 10%. For grade 3 gliomas, 70% had survived 96 weeks. Approximately 11% of the patients were enrolled in clinical trials.

For the most common adult primary CNS malignancy, glioblastoma multiforme (GBM), a recent randomized trial of concurrent chemotherapy with temozolomide and radiation followed by 6 months of adjuvant chemotherapy reported that the median survival was about 15 months. This strategy is now considered the standard treatment for newly diagnosed GBM.

**TABLE 56.4.** Prognostic biogenetic markers (under investigation)

| |
|---|
| Proliferation index – Ki-67(MIB-1), PCNA, bcl-2 expression, cyclin-D1 expression |
| DNA studies – flow cytometry, DNA index, BrdULI, comparative genomic hybridization |
| Activation of cellular oncogenes – ras, N-myc, C-myc, pescadillo |
| Inactivation of tumor suppressor genes – p53, p16(CDKN2A), Rb, PTEN, DMBT1, MDM2, NF2 |
| Allelic loss / loss of heterozygosity (LOH) – chromosomes 10, 22q, 19q, 17p |
| Cytokine dysregulation – CDK4, EGFR, VEGF, PKC |
| Chromosomal aberrations – chromosomes 1, 9, 10, 11, 17, 19, and 22 |
| Other molecular observations – telomerase activity and hTERT expression, DNA methyltransferase, double minutes, AgNOR instability, MGMT methylation |

## PROGNOSTIC BIOGENETIC MARKERS (UNDER CONTINUED INVESTIGATION)

The field of molecular neuropathology has provided us with a number of potential biogenetic markers that may be useful in staging CNS tumors and in making recommendations for therapy. The discovery of the pivotal role of oncogenes and of the loss of tumor suppressor genes in the tumorigenesis of CNS tumors has led to a flurry of activity that may prove quite fruitful in providing valid biologic markers in these difficult tumors. One of the most promising is the codeletion of 1p 19q in anaplastic oligodendroglioma and its prognostic value. In addition to biogenetic markers, signaling pathway abnormalities are being evaluated in primary CNS tumors. Methylation of MGMT, an important DNA repair enzyme, is an important factor in the effectiveness of temozolomide. Table 56.4 provides a glimpse of some of the current markers and techniques under investigation. It is hoped that ways will be found to apply these methods of scientific analysis of tumor growth potential to predict survival more effectively than is possible today.

## PROGNOSTIC FACTORS (SITE-SPECIFIC FACTORS)
### (Recommended for Collection)

| | |
|---|---|
| Required for staging | None |
| Clinically significant | Functional neurologic status (KPS) |
| | Location of tumor |
| | Unifocal or multifocal |
| | Primary or recurrent tumor |
| | Extent of resection |
| | Metastatic spread (CNS or extraneural) |
| | Proliferative fraction (Ki-67, M1B-1) |
| | Gene deletions (1p, 19q) |
| | MGMT methylation |

## HISTOLOGIC GRADE (G)

Grade is reported in registry systems by the grade value. A two-grade, three-grade, or four-grade system may be used. If a grading system is not specified, generally the following system is used:

GX     Grade cannot be assessed
G1     Well differentiated
G2     Moderately differentiated
G3     Poorly differentiated
G4     Undifferentiated

## BIBLIOGRAPHY

Aldape K, Simmons M, Davis RL, et al. Discrepancies in diagnoses of neuroepithelial neoplasms: the San Francisco Bay Area Gliomas Study. Cancer. 2000;88:2342–9.

Anderson FA, et al. The Glioma Outcomes Project: a resource for measuring and improving glioma outcomes. Neurosurg Focus. 1998;4:1–5.

Avgeropoulos NG, Batchelor TT. New treatment strategies for malignant gliomas. The Oncologist. 1999;4:209–24.

Cairncross G, Berkey B, Shaw E, Jenkins R, Scheithauer B, Brachman D, et al. Phase III trial of chemotherapy plus radiotherapy compared with radiotherapy alone for pure and mixed anaplastic oligodendroglioma: Intergroup Radiation Therapy Oncology Group Trial 9402. J Clin Oncol. 2006;24(18):2707–14.

Curran WJ, Scott CB, Horton J, et al. Recursive partitioning analysis of prognostic factors in three Radiation Therapy Oncology Group malignant glioma trials. J Natl Cancer Inst. 1993;85:704–10.

Guthrie BL, Laws ER Jr. Prognostic factors in patients with brain tumors. In: Morantz RA, Walsh JW, editors. Brain tumors. New York: Marcel Dekker; 1994. p. 799–808.

Jelsma R, Bucy PC. Glioblastoma multiforme: its treatment and some factors affecting survival. Arch Neurol. 1969;20:161–71.

Kaye AH, Laws ER Jr. Brain Tumors. 2nd ed. London: Churchill Livingstone; 2001.

Louis DN, Ohgaki H, Wiestler OD, Cavenee WK, editors. WHO classification of tumours of the central nervous system. Geneva: WHO Press; 2007.

Salcman M. Survival in glioblastoma: historical perspective. Neurosurgery. 1980;7:435–9.

Scanlon PW, Taylor WF. Radiotherapy of intracranial astrocytomas: analysis of 417 cases treated from 1960 through 1969. Neurosurgery. 1979;5:301–8.

Stupp R, Mason WP, van den Bent MJ, Weller M, Fisher B, Taphoorn MJ, et al. Radiotherapy plus concomitant and adjuvant temozolomide for glioblastoma. N Engl J Med. 2005;352(10):987–96.

van den Bent MJ, Carpentier AF, Brandes AA, Sanson M, Taphoorn MJ, Bernsen HJ, et al. Adjuvant procarbazine, lomustine, and vincristine improves progression-free survival but not overall survival in newly diagnosed anaplastic oligodendrogliomas and oligoastrocytomas: a randomized European Organisation for Research and Treatment of Cancer phase III trial. J Clin Oncol. 2006;24(18):2715–22.

VandenBerg SR. Current diagnostic concepts of astrocytic tumors. J Neuropathol Exp Neurol. 1992;51:644–57.

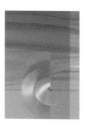

# PART XII
# Lymphoid Neoplasms

## INTRODUCTION

Lymphoid malignancies are a diverse group of disorders. These malignancies share derivation from B-cells, T-cells, and NK-cells, but they have a wide range of presentations, clinical course, and response to therapy. The incidence of lymphoid malignancies is significant and increasing. Non-Hodgkin lymphomas occur in more than 63,000 new individuals each year and have been increasing in incidence over the past several decades. Hodgkin lymphoma occurs in approximately 8,000 new individuals each year in the USA and seems stable in incidence. Approximately 20,000 new cases of multiple myeloma and more than 20,000 new cases of lymphoid leukemias occur annually in the USA (Figure 1).

## PATHOLOGY

Lymphoid neoplasms are malignancies of B-cells, T-cells, and NK (natural killer) cells. They include Hodgkin lymphoma (Hodgkin disease), non-Hodgkin lymphoma, multiple myeloma, and lymphoid leukemias. Traditionally, classifications have distinguished between "lymphomas" – i.e., neoplasms that typically present with an obvious tumor or mass of lymph nodes or extranodal sites – and "leukemias" – i.e., neoplasms that typically involve the bone marrow and peripheral blood, without tumor masses. However, we now know that many B- and T/NK-cell neoplasms may have both tissue masses *and* circulating cells. Thus, it is artificial to call them different diseases, when in fact they are just different presentations of the same disease. For this reason, we now refer to these diseases as lymphoid neoplasms rather than as lymphomas or leukemias, reserving the latter terms for the specific clinical presentation. In the current classification of lymphoid neoplasms, diseases that typically produce tumor masses are called lymphomas, those that typically have only circulating cells are called leukemias, and those that often have both solid and circulating phases are designated lymphoma/leukemia. Finally, plasma cell neoplasms, including

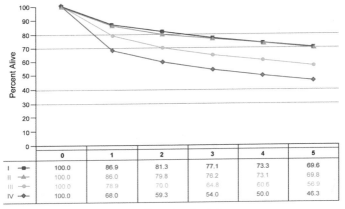

| | 0 | 1 | 2 | 3 | 4 | 5 |
|---|---|---|---|---|---|---|
| I ■ | 100.0 | 86.9 | 81.3 | 77.1 | 73.3 | 69.6 |
| II ▲ | 100.0 | 86.0 | 79.8 | 76.2 | 73.1 | 69.8 |
| III ● | 100.0 | 78.9 | 70.0 | 64.8 | 60.6 | 56.9 |
| IV ◆ | 100.0 | 68.0 | 59.3 | 54.0 | 50.0 | 46.3 |

Years from diagnosis

**FIGURE 1.** Observed survival rates for 57,596 patients with lymphomas classified by the current AJCC staging classification. Cases represent all lymphoma types and are not predictive of outcome for any particular lymphoma type. Data taken from the National Cancer Data Base (Commission of Cancer of the American College of Surgeons and the American Cancer Society) for the years 2001–2002. Stage I includes 17,674 patients; Stage II, 12,523; Stage III, 9,257; and Stage IV, 18,142.

multiple myeloma and plasmacytoma, have typically not been considered "lymphomas," but plasma cells are part of the B-cell lineage, and, thus, these tumors are B-cell neoplasms, which are now included in the classification of lymphoid neoplasms.

Lymphoid neoplasms are malignancies of lymphoid cells. Lymphoid cells include lymphoblasts, lymphocytes, follicle center cells (centrocytes and centroblasts), immunoblasts, and plasma cells. These cells are responsible for immune responses to infections. Immune responses involve recognition by lymphocytes of foreign molecules, followed by proliferation and differentiation to generate either specific cytotoxic cells (T or NK – natural killer – cells) or antibodies (B-cells and plasma cells). Lymphoid cells are normally found in greatest numbers in lymph nodes and in other lymphoid tissues such as Waldeyer's ring (which includes the palatine and lingual tonsils and adenoids), the thymus, Peyer's patches of the small intestine, the spleen, and the bone marrow (Figure 2). Lymphocytes also circulate in the peripheral blood and are found in small numbers in almost every organ of the body, where they either wait to encounter antigens or carry out specific immune reactions. Lymphoid neoplasms may occur in any site to which lymphocytes normally travel. Because lymphocytes normally circulate through the blood as well as the lymphatics – in contrast to epithelial cells, for example – it is often impossible to determine the "primary site" of a lymphoid neoplasm or to use a staging scheme that was developed for epithelial cancers, such as the TNM scheme.

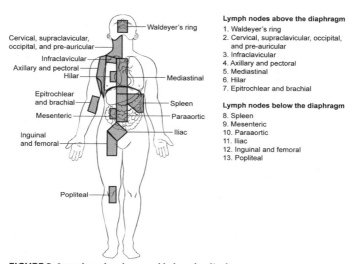

**FIGURE 2.** Lymph nodes above and below the diaphragm.

## RULES FOR CLASSIFICATION

Many different classification schemes have been proposed for lymphoid neoplasms, which has led to confusion on the part of both pathologists and oncologists. Between 1982 and 1994, in the USA, a classification called the Working Formulation was used. This scheme had the advantage of being simple, with only ten categories, and it did not require any special studies such as immunophenotyping or genetic studies. In addition, it provided simple clinical groupings for determining the approach to treatment (low, intermediate, and high clinical grades). Since its introduction, advances in understanding of the immune system and lymphoid neoplasms led to the recognition of many new categories of lymphoid neoplasms. The fact that several subtypes were in an incorrect category based on clinical behavior, and the development of better methods for diagnosis and classification – as well as for treatment – have caused the Working Formulation to become obsolete. In 1994 the International Lymphoma Study Group (ILSG) introduced a new classification, called the Revised European American Classification of Lymphoid Neoplasms (REAL), which incorporated not only morphology, but new information such as immunophenotype and genetic features, as well as clinical features, to define over 25 different categories of lymphoid neoplasms, including Hodgkin lymphoma.[1] More recently, the World Health Organization (WHO)[2] updated its Classification of Diseases of the Hematopoietic and Lymphoid Systems and adopted the REAL classification for lymphoid neoplasms with some modifications (the WHO classification also includes myeloid and histiocytic neoplasms). The WHO classification is now the standard for clinical trials in lymphoma (Table 1).

**TABLE 1.** WHO Classification of lymphoid neoplasms, 4th edition

*B-cell neoplasms*

**Precursor B-cell neoplasm**

- B-lymphoblastic leukemia/lymphoma (B-cell acute lymphoblastic leukemia)

**Mature (peripheral) B-cell neoplasms**

- Chronic lymphocytic leukemia/small lymphocytic lymphoma
- B-cell prolymphocytic leukemia
- Lymphoplasmacytic lymphoma
- Splenic marginal zone B-cell lymphoma (with or without villous lymphocytes)
- Hairy cell leukemia
- Splenic lymphoma/leukemia, unclassifiable
- Plasma cell myeloma/plasmacytoma
- Heavy chain diseases
- Extranodal marginal zone B-cell lymphoma of MALT type
- Nodal marginal zone B-cell lymphoma (with or without monocytoid B cells)
- Follicular lymphoma
- Primary cutaneous follicle center lymphoma
- Mantle cell lymphoma
- Diffuse large B-cell lymphoma (DLBCL)
  - Diffuse large B-cell lymphoma, not otherwise specified
  - T-cell/histiocyte rich large B-cell lymphoma
  - DLBCL associated with chronic inflammation
  - EBV positive DLBCL of the elderly
  - Lymphomatoid granulomatosis
  - Primary mediastinal (thymic) large B-cell lymphoma
  - Intravascular large B-cell lymphoma
  - Primary cutaneous DLBCL, leg type
  - ALK positive DLBCL
  - Plasmablastic lymphoma
  - Primary effusion lymphoma
  - Large B-cell lymphoma arising in HHV8-associated multicentric Castleman disease
- Burkitt lymphoma/Burkitt cell leukemia
- B-cell lymphoma, unclassifiable, with features intermediate between diffuse large B-cell lymphoma and Burkitt lymphoma
- B-cell lymphoma, unclassifiable, with features intermediate between diffuse large B-cell lymphoma and classical Hodgkin lymphoma

*T-cell and NK-cell neoplasms*

**Precursor T-cell neoplasm**

- T-lymphoblastic lymphoma/leukemia (T-cell acute lymphoblastic leukemia)

**Mature (peripheral) T/NK-cell neoplasms**

- T-cell prolymphocytic leukemia
- T-cell large granular lymphocytic leukemia

*continued*

- Aggressive NK-cell leukemia
- Systemic EBV positive T-cell lymphoproliferative disease of childhood (associated with chronic active EBV infection)
- Hydra vacciniforme-like lymphoma
- Adult T-cell lymphoma/leukemia (HTLV 1 +)
- Extranodal NK/T-cell lymphoma, nasal type
- Enteropathy-type T-cell lymphoma
- Hepatosplenic T-cell lymphoma
- Subcutaneous panniculitis-like T-cell lymphoma
- *Mycosis fungoides*/Sézary syndrome
- Primary cutaneous anaplastic large cell lymphoma
- Primary cutaneous aggressive epidermotropic CD8 positive cytotoxic T-cell lymphoma
- Primary cutaneous gamma-delta T-cell lymphoma
- Primary cutaneous small/medium CD4 positive T-cell lymphoma
- Peripheral T-cell lymphoma, not otherwise characterized
- Angioimmunoblastic T-cell lymphoma
- Anaplastic large cell lymphoma, ALK-positive
- Anaplastic large cell lymphoma, ALK-negative

From Swerdlow SH, Campo E, Harris NL, et al. WHO classification of Tumours of Haematopoietic and Lymphoid Tissues, 4th edition. Lyon: IARC, 2008, with permission.

The WHO classification is a list of distinct disease entities, which are defined by a combination of morphology, immunophenotypic, and genetic features and which have distinct clinical features.[3–6] The relative importance of each of these features varies among diseases, and there is no one gold standard. Morphology remains the first and most basic approach and is sufficient for both diagnosis and classification in many typical cases of lymphoma. Immunophenotyping and – particularly – molecular genetic studies are not needed in all cases, but they are very important in some diseases, are useful in difficult cases, and improve interobserver reproducibility. As mentioned previously, the WHO classification includes all lymphoid neoplasms: Hodgkin lymphoma, non-Hodgkin lymphomas, lymphoid leukemias, and plasma cell neoplasms. Both lymphomas and lymphoid leukemias are included, because both solid and circulating phases are present in many lymphoid neoplasms, and drawing a distinction between them is arbitrary. Thus, B-cell chronic lymphocytic leukemia and B-cell small lymphocytic lymphoma are simply different manifestations of the same neoplasm, as are lymphoblastic lymphomas and acute lymphoblastic leukemias. In addition, Hodgkin lymphoma and plasma cell myeloma are now recognized as lymphoid neoplasms of B-lineage and, therefore, belong in a compilation of lymphoid neoplasms.

The ability to study patterns of gene expression is providing new insights into these disorders. It is likely to change classification and might eventually supersede staging in the ability to predict outcome and the response to specific therapies.

# REFERENCES

1. Harris NL, Jaffe ES, Stein H, Banks PM, Chan JK, Cleary ML, et al. A revised European-American classification of lymphoid neoplasms: a proposal from the International Lymphoma Study Group [see comments]. Blood. 1994;84(5):1361–92.

2. Jaffe E, Harris N, Vardiman J, Stein H. Pathology and genetics: neoplasms of the haematopoietic and lymphoid tissues. In: Kleihaus P, Sobin L, editors. World Health Organization classification of tumours. Lyon: IARC; 2001.

3. Armitage JO, Weisenburger DD. New approach to classifying non-Hodgkin's lymphomas: clinical features of the major histologic subtypes. Non-Hodgkin's Lymphoma Classification Project. J Clin Oncol. 1998;16(8):2780–95.

4. Carbone PP, Kaplan HS, Musshoff K, Smithers DW, Tubiana M. Report of the Committee on Hodgkin's disease staging classification. Cancer Res. 1971;31(11):1860–1.

5. Lister TA, Crowther D, Sutcliffe SB, Glatstein E, Canellos GP, Young RC, et al. Report of a committee convened to discuss the evaluation and staging of patients with Hodgkin's disease: Cotswolds meeting. J Clin Oncol. 1989;7(11):1630–6.

6. Cheson BD, Pfistner B, Juweid ME, Gascoyne RD, Specht L, Horning SJ, et al. Revised response criteria for malignant lymphoma. J Clin Oncol. 2007;25(5): 579–86.

# Lymphoid Neoplasms

# Hodgkin and Non-Hodgkin Lymphomas

*(Excludes ocular adnexal lymphoma)*

## At-A-Glance

---

**SUMMARY OF CHANGES**

• There are no changes to the stage groups for the seventh edition

---

**ANATOMIC STAGE/PROGNOSTIC GROUPS**

Stage I    Involvement of a single lymphatic site (i.e., nodal region, Waldeyer's ring, thymus, or spleen) (I); or localized involvement of a single extralymphatic organ or site in the absence of any lymph node involvement (IE) (rare in Hodgkin lymphoma).

Stage II   Involvement of two or more lymph node regions on the same side of the diaphragm (II); or localized involvement of a single extralymphatic organ or site in association with regional lymph node involvement with or without involvement of other lymph node regions on the same side of the diaphragm (IIE). The number of regions involved may be indicated by a subscript, as in, for example, II3.

Stage III  Involvement of lymph node regions on both sides of the diaphragm (III), which also maybe accompanied by extralymphatic extension in association with adjacent lymph node involvement (IIIE) or by involvement of the spleen (IIIS) or both (IIIE,S). Splenic involvement is designated by the letter S.

Stage IV   Diffuse or disseminated involvement of one or more extralymphatic organs, with or without

**ICD-O-3 TOPOGRAPHY RANGES**
C00.0–C44.0,
C44.2–C68.9,
C69.1–C69.4,
C69.8–C80.9

**ICD-O-3 HISTOLOGY CODE RANGES**
9590–9699, 9702–9729,
9735, 9737, 9738
9811–9818, 9823, 9827,
9837 (excludes C42.0,
C42.1, C42.4)

57

---

associated lymph node involvement; or isolated extralymphatic organ involvement in the absence of adjacent regional lymph node involvement, but in conjunction with disease in distant site(s). Stage IV includes any involvement of the liver or bone marrow, lungs (other than by direct extension from another site), or cerebrospinal fluid.

## INTRODUCTION

All newly diagnosed patients with malignant lymphomas should have formal documentation of the anatomic disease extent prior to the initial therapeutic intervention; that is, clinical stage must be assigned and recorded. Patients with recurrent disease generally do not have a new clinical stage assigned at the time of relapse, although recording of the anatomic disease extent at the time of recurrence is recommended.

**Ann Arbor Staging System.** The current anatomic staging classification for lymphoma, known as the Ann Arbor classification, was originally developed over 30 years ago for Hodgkin lymphoma, as it better determined which patients might be suitable candidates for radiation therapy, and has subsequently been updated. It was subsequently applied to non-Hodgkin lymphoma as well. The pattern of disease spread in Hodgkin lymphoma tends to be more predictable compared to that encountered in non-Hodgkin lymphoma. The Ann Arbor classification has been accepted as the best means of describing the anatomic disease extent and has been found useful as a universal system for a variety of lymphomas. The AJCC and UICC have adopted the Ann Arbor classification as the official system for classifying the anatomic extent of disease in Hodgkin lymphoma and non-Hodgkin lymphoma, with the exception of cutaneous lymphomas (e.g., mycosis fungoides), which are dealt with later in this chapter.

For the purposes of coding and staging, lymph nodes, Waldeyer's ring, thymus, and spleen are considered *nodal* or *lymphatic* sites. *Extranodal* or *extralymphatic* sites include the bone marrow, the gastrointestinal tract, skin, bone, central nervous system, lung, gonads, ocular adnexae (conjunctiva, lacrimal glands, and orbital soft tissue), liver, kidneys, uterus, etc. Hodgkin lymphoma rarely presents in an extranodal site alone, but about 25% of non-Hodgkin lymphomas are extranodal at presentation. The frequency of extranodal presentation varies dramatically among different lymphomas, however, with some (mycosis fungoides and MALT lymphomas) being virtually always extranodal, except in advanced stages of the diseases, and some (follicular lymphoma, B-cell small lymphocytic lymphoma) seldom being extranodal, except for bone marrow involvement.

The Ann Arbor staging system also includes an E suffix for lymphomas presenting in extranodal sites. For example, lymphoma presenting in the thyroid gland with cervical lymph node involvement should be staged as IIE, while lymphoma presenting only in unilateral cervical lymph nodes would be Stage I. Frequently, extensive lymph node involvement is associated with extranodal extension of disease that may also directly invade other organs. Such extension may be described with an E suffix but should not be recorded as Stage IV. For example, mediastinal lymph nodes with *adjacent* lung extension should be classified as Stage IIE disease. Other examples of Stage IIE diseases include extension into the anterior chest wall *and* into the pericardium from a large mediastinal mass (two areas of extralymphatic involvement); involvement of the iliac bone in the presence of adjacent iliac lymph node involvement; involvement of a lumbar vertebral body in conjunction with para-aortic lymph node involvement; involvement of the pleura as an extension from adjacent internal mammary nodes. A pleural or pericardial effusion with negative (or unknown) cytology is not an E lesion. There are situations where the distinction between Stage IIE (or IIIE) and Stage IV can be problematic and where experts might disagree.

The extent of mediastinal disease is defined by a ratio between the maximum single width of the mediastinal mass on a standing PA chest radiograph and the maximum intrathoracic diameter on the same radiograph. A ratio greater than or equal to 1/3 defines a large (bulky) mediastinal mass. The presence of a large mediastinal mass or any other lesion with a greatest diameter of >10 cm is designated by the subscript letter X.

**Definition of Lymph Node Regions.** The staging classification for lymphoma uses the term *lymph node region*. The lymph node regions were defined at the Rye symposium in 1965 and have been used in the Ann Arbor classification. They are not based on any physiological principles but, rather, have been agreed upon by convention. The currently accepted classification of core nodal regions is as follows: right cervical (including cervical, supraclavicular, occipital, and preauricular lymph nodes) nodes and left cervical nodes, right axillary, left axillary, right infraclavicular, and left infraclavicular lymph nodes, mediastinal lymph nodes, right hilar lymph nodes, left hilar lymph nodes, para-aortic lymph nodes, mesenteric lymph nodes, right pelvic lymph nodes, left pelvic lymph nodes, right inguinofemoral lymph nodes, and left inguino-femoral lymph nodes. In addition to these core regions, non-Hodgkin lymphoma may involve epitrochlear lymph nodes, popliteal lymph nodes, internal mammary lymph nodes, occipital lymph nodes, submental lymph nodes, preauricular lymph nodes, and many other small nodal areas. The FLIPI prognostic scoring system has developed its own definition of nodal regions.

**A and B Classification (Symptoms).** Each stage should be classified as either A or B according to the absence or presence of defined constitutional symptoms. These are as follows:

1. *Fevers.* Unexplained fever with temperature above 38°C.
2. *Night sweats.* Drenching sweats (e.g., those that require change of bedclothes).

3. *Weight loss.* Unexplained weight loss of more than 10% of the usual body weight in the 6 months prior to diagnosis.

Other symptoms such as chills, pruritus, alcohol-induced pain or fatigue are recorded but are not included in the A or B designation.

**Criteria for Organ Involvement.** *Lymph node involvement* is demonstrated by (a) clinical or imaging enlargement of node when alternative pathology may reasonably be ruled out. Suspicious nodes should always be biopsied if treatment decisions are based on their involvement, preferably with an excisional biopsy; fine needle aspirations are strongly discouraged because of their high false-negative rate. Nodes larger than 1.5 cm are considered abnormal.

*Spleen involvement* is suggested by unequivocal palpable splenomegaly and demonstrated by radiologic confirmation (ultrasound or CT), by multiple focal defects that are neither cystic nor vascular (radiologic enlargement alone is inadequate).

*Liver involvement* is demonstrated by multiple focal defects that are neither cystic nor vascular. Clinical enlargement alone, with or without abnormalities of liver function tests, is not adequate. Liver biopsy may be used to confirm the presence of liver involvement in a patient with abnormal liver function tests or when imaging assessment is equivocal if treatment will be altered on the basis of those results.

*Lung involvement* is demonstrated by radiologic evidence of parenchymal involvement in the absence of other likely causes, especially infection. Lung biopsy may be required to clarify equivocal cases.

*Bone involvement* is demonstrated using appropriate imaging studies, and a bone biopsy from an involved area of bone may be necessary for a precise diagnosis, if treatment decisions depend on the findings.

*CNS involvement* is demonstrated by (a) a spinal intradural deposit or spinal cord or meningeal involvement, which may be diagnosed on the basis of the clinical history and findings supported by plain radiology, CSF examination, myelography, CT, and/or MRI (spinal extradural deposits should be carefully assessed, because they may be the result of soft tissue disease that represents extension from bone metastasis or disseminated disease) and (b) intracranial involvement, which will rarely be diagnosed clinically at presentation. It should be considered on the basis of a space-occupying lesion in the face of disease in additional extranodal sites.

*Bone marrow involvement* is assessed by an aspiration and bone marrow biopsy. Immunohistochemistry and/or flow cytometry may be useful adjuncts to histologic interpretation to determine if a lymphocytic infiltrate is malignant.

## RULES FOR CLASSIFICATION

**Clinical Staging.** Clinical staging includes the careful recording of medical history and physical examination; imaging of chest, abdomen, and pelvis; blood chemistry determination; complete blood count; and bone marrow biopsy (Table 57.1 and Figure 57.1).

**TABLE 57.1.** Recommendation for the diagnostic evaluation of patients with lymphoma

---

A. Mandatory procedures

  1. Biopsy (preferably excisional), with interpretation by a qualified pathologist

  2. History, with special attention to the presence and duration of fever, night sweats, and unexplained loss of 10% or more of body weight in the previous 6 months

  3. Physical examination

  4. Laboratory tests

     a. Complete blood cell count and platelet count

     b. Erythrocyte sedimentation rate or CRP (Hodgkin lymphoma patients)

     c. Chemistry panel (electrolytes, BUN, creatinine, calcium, phosphorus, uric acid, SGOT, SGPT, bilirubin, LDH, and alkaline phosphatase)

  5. Radiographic examination

     a. Chest X-ray

     b. CT of neck, chest, abdomen, and pelvis

     c. Metabolic imaging (FDG-PET) in appropriate indications

  6. Bone marrow examination[a]

  7. HIV testing in patients with an aggressive histology

  8. Hepatitis B serology in patients being considered for rituximab

B. Examples of ancillary procedures

  1. Radioisotopic bone scans, in selected patients with bone pain

  2. Gastroscopy and/or GI series in patients with GI presentations

  3. MRI of the spine in patients with suspected spinal cord involvement

  4. MRI of the brain in patients with cranial nerve palsy or suspected primary CNS lymphoma

  5. MRI of bone if nuclear imaging abnormality identified

  6. CSF cytology in patients with Stage IV disease and bone marrow involvement, testis involvement, or parameningeal involvement and in all children and all adults with lymphoblastic and Burkitt lymphoma. Flow cytometric analysis may be more sensitive than cytologic assessment.

---

[a] May include unilateral/bilateral bone marrow aspiration and biopsy in adults and children with NHL and unilateral/bilateral biopsies in children with Hodgkin lymphoma who present with B symptoms or advanced stage disease (III/IV).

The basic staging investigation in non-Hodgkin lymphoma includes physical examination, complete blood count, LDH, liver function tests, chest X-ray, and CT scan of the neck, chest, abdomen and pelvis, and bone marrow biopsy. In patients presenting with extranodal lymphoma, imaging of the presenting area with either CT or MRI is required to define local disease extent. 18-Fluorodeoxyglucose positron emission tomography (PET) scans are more sensitive and specific than CT scans; however, they have not yet been routinely incorporated into clinical staging. These studies are of greatest value in restaging and distinguishing lymphoma from scar tissue or fibrosis after treatment. The use of PET scans also varies with lymphoma histology and clinical situation. The use of PET in lymphoma clinical trials has recently been standardized by the International Harmonization Project.

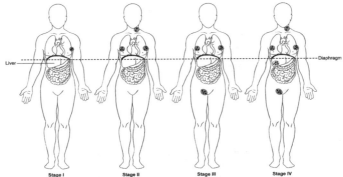

Stage I        Stage II        Stage III        Stage IV

**FIGURE 57.1.** Stage I: involvement of a single lymphatic site (i.e., nodal region, Waldeyer's ring, thymus, or spleen) (I), or localized involvement of a single extralymphatic organ or site in the absence of any lymph node involvement (IE) (rare in Hodgkin lymphoma). Stage II: involvement of two or more lymph node regions on the same side of the diaphragm (II), or localized involvement of a single extralymphatic organ or site in association with regional lymph node involvement with or without involvement of other lymph node regions on the same side of the diaphragm (IIE). The number of regions involved may be indicated by a subscript as in, for example, $II_3$. Stage III: involvement of lymph node regions on both sides of the diaphragm (III), which also may be accompanied by extralymphatic extension in association with adjacent lymph node involvement (IIIE) or by involvement of the spleen (IIIS) or both (IIIE,S). Splenic involvement is designated by the letter S. Stage IV: diffuse or disseminated involvement of one or more extralymphatic organs, with or without associated lymph node involvement, or isolated extralymphatic organ involvement in the absence of adjacent regional lymph node involvement, but in conjunction with disease in distant site(s). Stage IV includes any involvement of the liver or bone marrow, lungs (other than by direct extension from another site), or cerebrospinal fluid.

In patients at high risk for occult CNS involvement, CSF cytology is performed. Biopsies of any suspicious lesions may also be conducted as part of the initial clinical staging, especially if this would alter stage assignment. Bone marrow biopsy is a standard clinical staging investigation. However, liver biopsy is not required as part of clinical staging, unless abnormal liver function occurs in the presence of otherwise limited stage disease. Clinical staging is repeated at the end of therapy and forms the basis for defining response.

**Pathologic Staging.** The use of the term *pathologic staging* is reserved for patients who undergo staging laparotomy with an explicit intent to assess the presence of abdominal disease or to define histologic microscopic disease extent in the abdomen. As a result of improved diagnostic imaging, staging laparotomy and pathologic staging have been essentially abandoned as useful procedures.

## PROGNOSTIC FEATURES

**Prognostic Indices Used in Non-Hodgkin and Hodgkin Lymphoma.**
*International Prognostic Index (IPI).* The International Non-Hodgkin Lymphoma Prognostic Factors Project used pretreatment prognostic factors in a sample of several thousand patients with aggressive lymphomas treated with doxorubicin-based combination chemotherapy to develop a predictive model of outcome for aggressive non-Hodgkin lymphoma. The specific type of lymphoma and the IPI score are the major factors currently used in treatment decisions. On the basis of factors identified in multivariate analysis of the above data set, the International Prognostic Index (Table 57.2) was proposed. Five pretreatment characteristics were found to be independent statistically significant factors: age in years (<60 vs. >60); tumor stage I or II (localized) versus III or IV (advanced); number of extranodal sites of involvement (0–1 vs. > 1); patient's performance status (ECOG 0 or 1 vs. ≥2); and serum LDH level (normal vs. abnormal). With the use of these five pretreatment risk factors, patients could be assigned to one of the four risk groups on the basis of the number of presenting risk factors: low (0 or 1), low intermediate (2), high intermediate (3), and high (4 or 5). When patients were analyzed by risk factors, they were found to have very different outcomes with regard to complete response (CR), relapse-free survival (RFS), and overall survival (OS). The outcomes indicated that the low-risk

**57**

**TABLE 57.2.** Prognostic systems in common use for patients with lymphoma

| |
|---|
| *Risk factors in the International Prognostic Index (IPI) for NHL (APLES)*[9] |
| Age ≥ 60 years |
| Reduced performance status (such as ECOG ≥ 2) |
| Elevated LDH |
| ≥2 Extranodal sites of disease |
| Ann Arbor Stage III or IV |
| *Risk factors in the Follicular Lymphoma Prognostic Index (FLIPI) for follicular lymphoma (No LASH)*[10] |
| Number of nodal sites ≥ 5 |
| Elevated LDH |
| Age ≥ 60 years |
| Ann Arbor Stage III or IV |
| Hemoglobin (<12 g/dL) |
| *Risk factors in the International Prognostic Score for Hodgkin lymphoma*[11] |
| Serum albumin < 4 g/dL |
| Hemoglobin < 10.5 g/dL |
| Age ≥ 45 years |
| Male sex |
| Ann Arbor Stage IV |
| White blood cell count ≥ 15 × 10$^9$/L |
| Lymphocytopenia < 0.6 × 10$^9$/L or <8% |

patients had an 87% CR rate and an OS rate of 73% at 5 years in contrast to a 44% CR rate and 26% 5-year survival in patients in the high-risk group. A similar pattern of decreasing survival with a number of adverse factors was observed when younger patients only were considered.

The validity of the IPI is less clear in patients with T-cell lymphomas and other classifications have been proposed but none are yet universally accepted.

*The Follicular Lymphoma Prognostic Index (FLIPI).* The IPI was less useful in follicular lymphomas, and the FLIPI has been proposed. Factors that are included are the number of nodal sites ≤4 vs. > 4), serum LDH (normal vs. elevated), age (using 60 years as the cut-off), stage (I–II vs. III–IV), and serum hemoglobin concentration (≥12 vs. <12 g/dL). The three risk groups identified were 0–1 adverse factor, 2 factors, or 3 or more factors. Patients with low-risk disease had a 10-year survival of 71%, 51% with intermediate-risk disease, and only 36% for those with high-risk disease.

*The International Prognostic Score (IPS).* The International Prognostic Score (IPS) has been developed for Hodgkin lymphoma, which predicts outcome based on the following adverse factors: serum albumin < 4 g/dL, hemoglobin concentration < 10.5 g/dL, male sex, age ≥ 45 years, stage IV disease, white blood cell count ≥ 15,000/mm$^3$, and lymphocytopenia < 600/mm$^3$ or <8%. The rate of freedom from progression by risk category was: 0 factors 84%, 1 – 77%, 2 – 67%, 3 – 60%, 4 – 51%, 5 or higher – 42%. Other factors of note in Hodgkin lymphoma have included the number of sites of disease and the erythrocyte sedimentation rate.

## ANATOMIC STAGE/PROGNOSTIC GROUPS

| | |
|---|---|
| Stage I | Involvement of a single lymphatic site (i.e., nodal region, Waldeyer's ring, thymus or spleen) (I); or localized involvement of a single extralymphatic organ or site in the absence of any lymph node involvement (IE) (rare in Hodgkin lymphoma). |
| Stage II | Involvement of two or more lymph node regions on the same side of the diaphragm (II); or localized involvement of a single extralymphatic organ or site in association with regional lymph node involvement with or without involvement of other lymph node regions on the same side of the diaphragm (IIE). The number of regions involved may be indicated by an arabic numeral, as in, for example, II3. |
| Stage III | Involvement of lymph node regions on both sides of the diaphragm (III), which also maybe accompanied by extralymphatic extension in association with adjacent lymph node involvement (IIIE) or by involvement of the spleen (IIIS) or both (IIIE,S). Splenic involvement is designated by the letter S. |
| Stage IV | Diffuse or disseminated involvement of one or more extralymphatic organs, with or without associated lymph node involvement; or isolated extralymphatic organ involvement in the absence of adjacent regional lymph node involvement, but in conjunction with disease in distant site(s). Stage IV includes any involvement of the liver or bone marrow, lungs (other than by direct extension from another site), or cerebrospinal fluid. |

## PROGNOSTIC FACTORS (SITE-SPECIFIC FACTORS)
## (Recommended for Collection)

Required for staging    None

Clinically significant    Associated with HIV/AIDS
Symptoms at diagnosis (B symptoms)
International Prognostic Index (IPI) score
Follicular Lymphoma Prognostic Index (FLIPI) score
International Prognostic Score (IPS)

# Primary Cutaneous Lymphomas

## *At-A-Glance*

> **SUMMARY OF CHANGES**
>
> • There are no changes to the stage groups for the seventh edition

**ANATOMIC STAGE/PROGNOSTIC GROUPS**

| | T | N | M | Peripheral Blood Involvement |
|---|---|---|---|---|
| Stage IA | 1 | 0 | 0 | 0,1 |
| Stage IB | 2 | 0 | 0 | 0,1 |
| Stage IIA | 1,2 | 1,2 | 0 | 0,1 |
| Stage IIB | 3 | 0–2 | 0 | 0,1 |
| Stage III | 4 | 0–2 | 0 | 0,1 |
| Stage IIIA | 4 | 0–2 | 0 | 0 |
| Stage IIIB | 4 | 0–2 | 0 | 1 |
| Stage IVA1 | 1–4 | 0–2 | 0 | 2 |
| Stage IVA2 | 1–4 | 3 | 0 | 0–2 |
| Stave IVB | 1–4 | 0–3 | 1 | 0–2 |

ICD-O-3 TOPOGRAPHY RANGES

| | |
|---|---|
| C44.0–C44.9 | Skin |
| C51.0–C51.9 | Vulva |
| C60.0–C60.9 | Penis |
| C63.2 | Scrotum |

ICD-O-3 HISTOLOGY CODE RANGES
9700–9701

57

Primary cutaneous T- and B-cell lymphomas are a heterogeneous group of malignancies with varied clinical presentation and prognosis. The application of molecular, histological, and clinical criteria have allowed for a better characterization of defined entities with distinct features. The World Health Organization and European Organization of Research and Treatment of Cancer (WHO-EORTC) classification for cutaneous lymphomas provides a consensus categorization that allows for more uniform diagnosis and treatment of these disorders. Approximately 80% of the cutaneous lymphomas are of T cell origin. Mycosis fungoides and Sézary syndrome have a formal staging system proposed by the International Society for Cutaneous Lymphomas and EORTC.[1] The other cutaneous non-Hodgkin lymphomas are staged using the same system, described previously, for lymphomas presenting in other anatomic locations.

*Mycosis Fungoides. Mycosis fungoides* and its variants represent the most common form of cutaneous T cell lymphoma (CTCL). The malignant cell is derived from a post thymic T cell that typically bears a CD4+ helper/memory antigen profile. The disease is characterized by erythematous patches (usually in sun-protected areas) that progress to plaques or tumors. Initial evaluation should include delineation of skin involvement with photographs; skin biopsy (histopathology, immunophenotyping, and T-cell receptor (TCR) gene analysis); CBC with differential, Sézary cell count (peripheral blood); chemistry panel with LDH; and in select instances peripheral blood flow cytometric analysis of T-cell subsets (CD4/CD8 ratio); TCR gene analysis on peripheral blood; lymph node biopsy and bone marrow biopsies (histopathology, immunophenotyping and TCR gene analysis); CT/PET scans; and serologic tests (HTLV-1 and HIV). Skin directed and systemic therapies are determined by the patient's stage and symptoms. Prognosis is stage dependent.

*Sézary Syndrome.* Sézary syndrome is the aggressive leukemic, and erythrodermic form of CTCL, which is characterized by circulating atypical, malignant T lymphocytes with cerebriform nuclei (Sézary cells), and lymphadenopathy. The Sézary cells also have a mature memory T-cell phenotype (CD3+, CD4+) with loss of CD7 and CD26.

## DEFINITIONS OF TNM

### ISCL/EORTC Revision to the Classification of *Mycosis fungoides* and Sézary Syndrome

*Skin*

| | |
|---|---|
| T1 | Limited patches,* papules, and/or plaques** covering less than 10% of the skin surface. May further stratify into T1a (patch only) vs. T1b (plaque ± patch) |
| T2 | Patches, papules or plaques covering 10% or more of the skin surface. May further stratify into T2a (patch only) vs. T2b (plaque ± patch) |
| T3 | One or more tumors*** (≥1-cm diameter) |
| T4 | Confluence of erythema covering 80% or more of body surface area |

*Node*

| | |
|---|---|
| N0 | No clinically abnormal peripheral lymph nodes****; biopsy not required |
| N1 | Clinically abnormal peripheral lymph nodes; histopathology Dutch grade 1 or NCI LN0-2 |
| N1a | Clone negative***** |
| N1b | Clone positive***** |
| N2 | Clinically abnormal peripheral lymph nodes; histopathology Dutch grade 2 or NCI LN3 |
| N2a | Clone negative***** |
| N2b | Clone positive***** |
| N3 | Clinically abnormal peripheral lymph nodes; histopathology Dutch grades 3–4 or NCI LN4; clone positive or negative |
| Nx | Clinically abnormal peripheral lymph nodes; no histologic confirmation |

From Olsen E, Vonderheid E, Pimpinelli N, et al. Revisions to the staging and classification of mycosis fungoides and Sézary syndrome: a proposal of the International Society for Cutaneous Lymphomas (ISCL) and the cutaneous lymphoma task force of the European Organization of Research and Treatment of Cancer (EORTC). Blood. 2007;110(6):1713–22, with permission of the American Society of Hematology.

*For skin, patch indicates any size skin lesion without significant elevation or induration. Presence/absence of hypo- or hyperpigmentation, scale, crusting, and/or poikiloderma should be noted.

**For skin, plaque indicates any size skin lesion that is elevated or indurated. Presence or absence of scale, crusting, and/or poikiloderma should be noted. Histologic features such as folliculotropism or large-cell transformation (>25% large cells), CD30+ or CD30–, and clinical features such as ulceration are important to document.

***For skin, tumor indicates at least one 1-cm diameter solid or nodular lesion with evidence of depth and/or vertical growth. Note total number of lesions, total volume of lesions, largest size lesion, and region of body involved. Also note if histologic evidence of large-cell transformation has occurred. Phenotyping for CD30 is encouraged.

****For node, abnormal peripheral lymph node(s) indicates any palpable peripheral node that on physical examination is firm, irregular, clustered, fixed or 1.5 cm or larger in diameter. Node groups examined on physical examination include cervical, supraclavicular, epitrochlear, axillary, and inguinal. Central nodes, which are not generally amenable to pathologic assessment, are not currently considered in the nodal classification unless used to establish N3 histopathologically.

*****A T-cell clone is defined by PCR or Southern blot analysis of the T-cell receptor gene.

^For viscera, spleen and liver may be diagnosed by imaging criteria.

^^For blood, Sézary cells are defined as lymphocytes with hyperconvoluted cerebriform nuclei. If Sézary cells are not able to be used to determine tumor burden for B2, then one of the following modified ISCL criteria along with a positive clonal rearrangement of the TCR may be used instead: (1) expanded CD4+ or CD3+ cells with CD4/CD8 ratio of 10 or more, (2) expanded CD4+ cells with abnormal immunophenotype including loss of CD7 or CD26.

Histopathologic Staging of Lymph Nodes in *Mycosis fungoides* and Sézary Syndrome

| Updated ISCL/ EORTC classification | Dutch system[2] | NCI-VA classification[3]–[5] |
|---|---|---|
| N1 | Grade 1: dermatopathic lymphadenopathy (DL) | LN0: no atypical lymphocytes |
| | | LN1: occasional and isolated atypical lymphocytes (not arranged in clusters) |
| | | LN2: many atypical lymphocytes or in 3–6 cell clusters |
| N2 | Grade 2: DL; early involvement by MF (presence of cerebriform nuclei > 7.5 μm) | LN3: aggregates of atypical lymphocytes; nodal architecture preserved |
| N3 | Grade 3: partial effacement of LN architecture; many atypical cerebriform mononuclear cells (CMCs) | LN4: partial/complete effacement of nodal architecture by atypical lymphocytes or frankly neoplastic cells |
| | Grade 4: complete effacement | |

From Olsen E, Vonderheid E, Pimpinelli N, et al. Revisions to the staging and classification of mycosis fungoides and Sézary syndrome: a proposal of the International Society for Cutaneous Lymphomas (ISCL) and the cutaneous lymphoma task force of the European Organization of Research and Treatment of Cancer (EORTC). Blood. 2007;110(6):1713–22, with permission of the American Society of Hematology.

## ANATOMIC STAGE/PROGNOSTIC GROUPS

### ISCL/EORTC Revision to the Staging of *Mycosis fungoides* and Sézary Syndrome

| | T | N | M | Peripheral Blood Involvement |
|---|---|---|---|---|
| Stage IA | 1 | 0 | 0 | 0, 1 |
| Stage IB | 2 | 0 | 0 | 0, 1 |
| Stage IIA | 1, 2 | 1, 2 | 0 | 0, 1 |
| Stage IIB | 3 | 0–2 | 0 | 0, 1 |
| Stage III | 4 | 0–2 | 0 | 0, 1 |
| Stage IIIA | 4 | 0–2 | 0 | 0 |
| Stage IIIB | 4 | 0–2 | 0 | 1 |

| Stage IVA1 | 1–4 | 0–2 | 0 | 2 |
| Stage IVA2 | 1–4 | 3 | 0 | 0–2 |
| Stage IVB | 1–4 | 0–3 | 1 | 0–2 |

From Olsen E, Vonderheid E, Pimpinelli N, et al. Revisions to the staging and classification of mycosis fungoides and Sézary syndrome: a proposal of the International Society for Cutaneous Lymphomas (ISCL) and the cutaneous lymphoma task force of the European Organization of Research and Treatment of Cancer (EORTC). Blood. 2007;110(6):1713–22, with permission of the American Society of Hematology.

## PROGNOSTIC FACTORS (SITE-SPECIFIC FACTORS)
### (Recommended for Collection)

For *Mycosis fungoides* and Sézary Syndrome only

Required for staging    Peripheral blood involvement

Clinically significant    None

**Primary Cutaneous CD30+ Lymphoproliferative Disorders.** Primary cutaneous CD30+ lymphoproliferative disorders are the second most common group of CTCL. This spectrum of diseases includes lymphomatoid papulosis, anaplastic large cell lymphoma and borderline cases. The distinction between these entities can be challenging and is often determined by clinical behavior. Lymphomatoid papulosis represents a benign, chronic recurrent, self-healing, papulonodular, and papulonecrotic CD4+, CD30+ skin eruption. Primary cutaneous anaplastic large cell lymphoma typically presents with solitary or localized nodules.

**Follicle Center Cell Lymphoma.** Follicle center cell lymphoma is the most common cutaneous B cell lymphoma (CBCL). Erythematous nodules or plaques are comprised of a proliferation of centrocytes (small to large cleaved cells) and centroblasts (large round cells with prominent nuclei). The clinical course is usually indolent even when the infiltrate is composed of predominantly large cells.

**Marginal Zone Lymphoma.** Marginal zone lymphoma is an indolent CBCL. It has the histologic appearance of a MALT lymphoma and shows a nodular or diffuse dermal infiltrate with a heterogeneous cellular infiltrate of small lymphocytes, lymphoplasmacytoid cells, plasma cells, intranuclear inclusions (Dutcher bodies), and reactive germinal centers that may be infiltrated by neoplastic cells. They are often localized and usually follow an indolent course.

**Large B-Cell Lymphoma of the Leg.** Large B-cell lymphoma of the leg is an aggressive lymphoma most commonly seen in elderly women. Patients present with tumors that may ulcerate. The histologic evaluation shows a diffuse dermal infiltrate comprised of predominantly centroblasts often with multilobulated nuclei.

# Multiple Myeloma
# and Plasma Cell Disorders

## INTRODUCTION

Multiple myeloma is a neoplastic disorder characterized by the proliferation of a single clone of plasma cells derived from B cells. This clone of
plasma cells grows in the bone marrow and frequently invades the adjacent
bone, producing skeletal destruction that results in bone pain and fractures. Other common clinical findings include anemia, hypercalcemia, and
renal insufficiency. Recurrent bacterial infections and bleeding can occur,
but the hyperviscosity syndrome is rare. The clone of plasma cells produces
monoclonal (M-protein) of IgG or IgA and rarely IgD or IgE or free monoclonal light chains (kappa or lambda) (Bence Jones protein). The diagnosis
depends on identification of monoclonal plasma cells in the bone marrow,
M-protein in the serum or urine, osteolytic lesions, and a clinical picture
consistent with multiple myeloma.

## RULES FOR CLASSIFICATION

**Diagnosis.** Criteria for the diagnosis of multiple myeloma include the
presence of clonal bone marrow plasma cells or plasmacytoma, presence
of an M-protein in serum and/or urine, and the presence of related organ
or tissue impairment (CRAB: hypercalcemia, renal insufficiency, anemia,
or bony lesions) related to the underlying plasma cell disorder. Metastatic
carcinoma, lymphoma, leukemia, and connective tissue disorders must
be excluded. In addition, monoclonal gammopathy of undetermined significance (MGUS) and smoldering multiple myeloma (SMM) must be
excluded. MGUS is characterized by an M-protein <3 g/dL, fewer than
10% plasma cells in the bone marrow, and no end-organ involvement.
The plasma cell labeling index (PCLI) is helpful in differentiating MGUS
and SMM from multiple myeloma. An elevated PCLI is a strong indicator
of active multiple myeloma. However, 40% of patients with symptomatic
multiple myeloma have a normal PCLI. Monoclonal plasma cells of the
same isotype can be detected in the peripheral blood of 80% of patients
with active multiple myeloma. Circulating plasma cells either are absent or
are present in only small numbers in MGUS and SMM.

## PROGNOSTIC FEATURES

The median duration of survival in multiple myeloma is approximately
three to four years, but there is a great deal of variability from one patient
to another. Cytogenetic abnormalities are an important prognostic feature,

but are present in only 35% of patients. The deletion of chromosome 13 by cytogenetics or the presence of t(4;14), t(14;16), or -17p13 by FISH are all predictors of poor outcome. Hypodiploidy is an adverse prognostic feature. An elevated plasma cell labeling index, plasmablastic morphology, or circulating plasma cells in the peripheral blood are all associated with more aggressive disease. Age, levels of creatinine and calcium, and immunoglobulin class also have prognostic value. Novel agents such as lenalidamide and bortezomib show promise at overcoming these adverse prognostic factors for conventional and high dose therapies.

**Staging.** The Durie-Salmon staging system has been utilized for over 30 years.[6] Stage I requires hemoglobin >10.0 g/dL, serum calcium ≤ 12 mg/dL, normal bone x-rays or a solitary bone lesions, IgG < 5 g/dL, IgA < 3 g/dL, and urine M-protein < 4 g/24 h. Stage III includes one or more of the following: hemoglobin < 8.5 g/dL, serum calcium > 12 mg/dL, advanced lytic bone lesions, IgG > 7 g/dL, IgA > 5 g/dL, or urine M-protein > 12 g/24 h. Stage II patients fit neither Stage I nor Stage III. Patients are further subclassed as (A) serum creatinine < 2.0 mg/dL and (B) serum creatinine ≥ 2.0 mg/dL. The median survival is approximately 5 years for those with Stage 1A disease and is 15 months for those with Stage IIIB disease. This system primarily measures tumor cell burden and has major limitations. An international staging system (ISS) consisting of serum albumin and $\beta$-2 microglobulin is a useful measure of survival.[7] Patients with a serum albumin >3.5 g/dL and serum $\beta$-2 microglobulin < 3.5 mcg/mL had a median survival of 62 months, while those with a serum $\beta$-2 microglobulin ≥ 5.5 mcg/mL had a median survival of 29 months (Table 57.3).

**Monoclonal Gammopathy of Undetermined Significance.** The prevalence of monoclonal gammopathy of undetermined significance (MGUS) is 3% in persons 50 years or older, 5% in those over 70 years of age, and is higher in men than women. The rate of progression is approximately 1% per year. [The level of monoclonal protein and the subtype (i.e., IgA and IgM are at greater risk) along with the serum free light chain (FLC) level are important prognostic features.] Patients must continue to be observed throughout their life because the risk of progression persists.

**TABLE 57.3.** The international staging system for multiple myeloma

| Stage | Criteria | Median survival (months) |
|-------|----------|--------------------------|
| I | Serum $\beta_2$-microglobulin < 3.5 mg/L | 62 |
| | Serum albumin ≥ 3.5 g/dL | |
| II | Not stage I or III[a] | 44 |
| III | Serum $\beta_2$-microglobulin ≥ 6.6 mg/L | 29 |

From Greipp PR, San Miguel J, Durie BG, Crowley JJ, Barlogie B, Blade J, et al. International staging system for multiple myeloma. J Clin Oncol 2005;23(15):3412–20, with permission of the American Society of Clinical Oncology.

[a] There are two categories for stage II: serum $\beta_2$-microglobulin <3.5 mg/L but serum albumin <3.5 g/dL; or serum $\beta_2$-microglobulin 3.5 to <5.5 mg/L irrespective of the serum albumin level.

**Smoldering Multiple Myeloma.** Smoldering multiple myeloma (SMM) is characterized by the presence of an M-protein ≥3 g/dL and/or ≥10% plasma cells in the bone marrow but no end-organ damage. The risk of progression to multiple myeloma or AL amyloidosis is 10% per year for the first 5 years, approximately 3% per year for the next 5 years, and then 1% per year for the following 10 years.

**Waldenström's Macroglobulinemia.** This malignant lymphoplasmacytic cell proliferative disorder produces a high concentration of immunoglobulin M (IgM) paraprotein. Waldenström's macroglobulinemia (WM) cells express CD19, CD20, CD24, and only one light chain (kappa in about 75% of cases). Approximately 10% express CD5. The most common chromosomal abnormality is deletion of 6q21. In contrast to multiple myeloma, no translocations are found. Diagnostic criteria include an IgM paraprotein regardless of its size and bone marrow infiltration by small lymphocytes that exhibit plasmacytoid or plasma cell differentiation. Median survival is approximately 6 years. (Gender, age, hemoglobin, neutrophil, and platelet levels, serum albumin and β-2 microglobulin are all prognostic features.)

**57**

**Solitary Plasmacytoma (Solitary Myeloma) of Bone.** The diagnosis depends on histologic proof of a plasma cell tumor but no evidence of multiple myeloma. Complete skeletal radiographs, bone marrow aspiration and biopsy, and immunofixation of serum and urine should reveal no evidence of multiple myeloma.

A small monoclonal protein may be found in the serum or urine but it usually disappears after radiation of a solitary lesion. The persistence of a serum monoclonal protein ≥0.5 g/dL 1–2 years after diagnosis and an abnormal free light chain ratio at the time of diagnosis are indicative of disease progression. More than 50% of patients develop multiple myeloma.

**Extramedullary Plasmacytoma.** This is a plasma cell tumor that arises outside the bone marrow. The upper respiratory tract is involved in approximately 80% of cases. Approximately 15–20% of patients develop multiple myeloma.

# Pediatric Lymphoid
Malignancy

## DIAGNOSIS

Children with NHL usually have Burkitt lymphoma, lymphoblastic lymphoma, diffuse large B-cell lymphoma or anaplastic large cell lymphoma. The diagnosis of NHL is most readily established by examination of tissue obtained by open biopsy of the involved area. Histologic, immunophenotypic, cytogenetic, and molecular studies are all helpful in confirming the diagnosis. In cases in which the patient is too unstable for general anesthesia, as in the case of a child with a large anterior mediastinal mass, a parasternal fine-needle core biopsy of the mass may be sufficient to establish the diagnosis. In children with either pleural effusion or ascites, the diagnosis is often made by cytologic examination of fluid obtained by thoracentesis or paracentesis. Bone marrow and cerebrospinal fluid examination should be performed early in the workup of a child with suspected NHL because they may be diagnostic and may preclude the need for more invasive procedures. Children with Hodgkin lymphoma are staged using the same system as adults.

## WORKUP

The workup of a child with newly diagnosed NHL should include a history and physical examination, a complete blood count, and a chemistry panel. Diagnostic imaging studies should include CT scans of chest, abdomen and pelvis and nuclear imaging (PET or gallium scanning). MRI of the base of the skull should be considered in children with a cranial nerve palsy. Examination of the cerebrospinal fluid and bone marrow should be performed in all patients.

## PROGNOSTIC FEATURES

The degree of tumor burden, as reflected in both disease stage and serum lactate dehydrogenase (LDH), is the most important prognostic factor. Among certain histological subtypes, disease site also influences outcome. For example, central nervous system involvement is associated with a poorer outcome among children with Burkitt lymphoma, and involvement of mediastinum, viscera or skin is associated with a poorer outcome among those with anaplastic large cell lymphoma.

**TABLE 57.4.** St. Jude staging system

*Stage I*

A single tumor (extranodal) or single anatomic area (nodal), with the exclusion of mediastinum or abdomen

*Stage II*

A single tumor (extranodal) with regional node involvement

Two or more nodal areas on the same side of the diaphragm

Two single (extranodal) tumors with or without regional node involvement on the same side of the diaphragm

A primary gastrointestinal tract tumor, usually in the ileocecal area, with or without involvement of associated mesenteric nodes only[a]

*Stage III*

Two single tumors (extranodal) on opposite sides of the diaphragm

Two or more nodal areas above and below the diaphragm

All primary intrathoracic tumors (mediastinal, pleural, thymic)

All extensive primary intra-abdominal disease[a]

All paraspinal or epidural tumors, regardless of other tumor site(s)

*Stage IV*

Any of the above with initial CNS and/or bone marrow involvement[b]

From Murphy SB, Fairclough DL, Hutchison RE, Berard CW. Non-Hodgkin's lymphomas of childhood: an analysis of the histology, staging, and response to treatment of 338 cases at a single institution. J Clin Oncol 1989;7(2):186–93, with permission of the American Society of Clinical Oncology.

[a] A distinction is made between apparently localized GI tract lymphoma and more extensive intra-abdominal disease because of their quite different patterns of survival after appropriate therapy. Stage II disease typically is limited to one segment of the gut plus or minus the associated mesenteric nodes only and the primary tumor can be completely removed grossly by segmental excision. Stage III disease typically exhibits spread to para-aortic and retroperitoneal areas by implants and plaques in mesentery or peritoneum, or by direct infiltration of structures adjacent to the primary tumor. Ascites may be present, and complete resection of all gross tumor is not possible.

[b] If the marrow involvement is present initially, the number of abnormal cells must be 25% or less in an otherwise normal marrow aspirate with a normal peripheral blood picture.

## STAGING

Upon completion of the foregoing workup, the child is usually assigned a disease stage according to the St. Jude system described by Murphy (Table 57.4), which was designed to accommodate the noncontiguous nature of disease spread, predominant extra-nodal involvement and involvement of the central nervous system and bone marrow that characterize the pediatric NHLs.[8] Stages I and II are considered to represent limited stage disease whereas Stages III and IV are considered advanced stages.

## REFERENCES

1. Olsen E, Vonderheid E, Pimpinelli N, Willemze R, Kim Y, Knobler R et al. (2007) Revisions to the staging and classification of mycosis fungoides and Sézary syndrome: a proposal of the International Society for Cutaneous Lymphomas (ISCL) and the cutaneous lymphoma task force of the European Organization of Research and Treatment of Cancer (EORTC). Blood 110(6):1713–22

2. Scheffer E, Meijer CJLM, van Vloten WA (1980) Dermatopathic lymphadenopathy and lymph node involvement in mycosis fungoides. Cancer 45:137–48

3. Sausville EA, Worsham GF, Matthews MJ et al (1985) Histologic assessment of lymph nodes in mycosis fungoides/Sézary syndrome (cutaneous T-cell lymphoma): clinical correlations and prognostic import of a new classification system. Hum Pathol 16:1098–109

4. Clendenning WE, Rappaport HW (1979) Report of the committee on pathology of cutaneous T cell lymphomas. Cancer Treat Rep 63:719–24

5. Colby TV, Burke JS, Hoppe RT (1981) Lymph node biopsy in mycosis fungoides. Cancer 47:351–9

6. Durie BG, Salmon SE. A clinical staging system for multiple myeloma. Correlation of measured myeloma cell mass with presenting clinical features, response to treatment, and survival. Cancer. 1975;36(3):842–54.

7. Greipp PR, San Miguel J, Durie BG, Crowley JJ, Barlogie B, Blade J et al (2005) International staging system for multiple myeloma. J Clin Oncol 23(15):3412–20

8. Murphy SB, Fairclough DL, Hutchison RE, Berard CW (1989) Non-Hodgkin's lymphomas of childhood: an analysis of the histology, staging, and response to treatment of 338 cases at a single institution. J Clin Oncol 7(2):186–93

9. A predictive model for aggressive non-Hodgkin's lymphoma (1993) The International Non-Hodgkin's Lymphoma Prognostic Factors Project [see comments]. N Engl J Med 329(14):987–94

10. Solal-Celigny P, Roy P, Colombat P, White J, Armitage JO, Arranz-Saez R et al (2004) Follicular lymphoma international prognostic index. Blood 104(5):1258–65

11. Hasenclever D, Diehl V. A prognostic score for advanced Hodgkin's disease. International Prognostic Factors Project on Advanced Hodgkin's Disease [see comments]. N Engl J Med. 1998;339(21):1506–14.

**57**

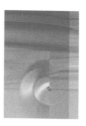

# PART XIII
# Personnel
# and Contributors

# AJCC Member Organizations

## FOUNDING ORGANIZATIONS
American Cancer Society
American College of Physicians
American College of Radiology
American College of Surgeons
College of American Pathologists
National Cancer Institute

## SPONSORING ORGANIZATIONS
American Cancer Society
American College of Surgeons
American Society of Clinical Oncology
Centers for Disease Control and Prevention
National Cancer Institute

## LIAISON ORGANIZATIONS
American Head and Neck Society
American Society of Colon and Rectal Surgeons
American Society for Therapeutic Radiology
American Urological Association
National Cancer Institute of Canada
National Cancer Registrars Association
National Comprehensive Cancer Network
North American Association of Central Cancer Registries
Society of Gynecologic Oncologists
Society of Surgical Oncology
Society of Urologic Oncology

## EXECUTIVE OFFICE
American Joint Committee on Cancer
633 North Saint Clair Street
Chicago, IL 60611-3211
PHONE: 312/202-5313
FAX: 312/202-5009
www.cancerstaging.org

# Seventh Edition Site
# Task Forces

## BONE

Jeffrey S. Kneisl, M.D., Chair
Carolinas Medical Center
Charlotte, North Carolina

Lee J. Helman, M.D.
National Cancer Institute
Bethesda, Maryland

Mark Krailo, Ph.D.
University of Southern California
Arcadia, California

Thomas Krausz, M.D.
University of Chicago
Chicago, Illinois

Ying Lu, Ph.D.
University of California
San Francisco, California

Brian O'Sullivan, M.D.
Princess Margaret Hospital
Toronto, Canada

Shreyaskumar Patel, M.D.
M.D. Anderson Cancer Center
Houston, Texas

Theola K. Rarick, C.T.R.
University of Iowa Hospital
and Clinics
Iowa City, Iowa

Andrew Rosenberg, M.D.
Massachusetts General Hospital
Boston, Massachusetts

Murali Sundaram, M.D.
Cleveland Clinic
Cleveland, Ohio

## BREAST

Daniel F. Hayes, M.D., Chair
University of Michigan
Ann Arbor, Michigan

Craig Allred, M.D.
Washington University
Saint Louis, Missouri

Benjamin O. Anderson, M.D.
University of Washington
Seattle, Washington

Stewart Anderson, Ph.D.
University of Pittsburgh
Pittsburgh, Pennsylvania

Pandora Ashley, C.T.R.
Scott and White Memorial
Hospital
Temple, Texas

William Barlow, Ph.D.
Cancer Research and Biostatistics
Seattle, Washington

Donald Berry, Ph.D.
M.D. Anderson Cancer Center
Houston, Texas

Robert W. Carlson, M.D.
Stanford University
Stanford, California

Rebecca Gelman, Ph.D.
Dana-Farber Cancer Institute
Boston, Massachusetts

Susan Hilsenbeck, Ph.D.
Baylor College of Medicine
Houston, Texas

Gabriel N. Hortobagyi, M.D.
M.D. Anderson Cancer Center
Houston, Texas

Michael Kattan, Ph.D., M.B.A.
Cleveland Clinic
Cleveland, Ohio

Susan Carole Lester, M.D., Ph.D.
Brigham and Women's Hospital
Boston, Massachusetts

Monica Morrow, M.D.
Memorial Sloan-Kettering
    Cancer Center
New York, New York

Peter M. Ravdin, M.D., Ph.D.
University of Texas
San Antonio, Texas

Lawrence J. Solin, M.D.
Albert Einstein Medical Center
Philadelphia, Pennsylvania

Sana O. Tabbara, M.D.
The George Washington
    University
Washington, DC

Ann Thor, M.D.
University of Colorado
Aurora, Colorado

Debasish Tripathy, M.D.
The University of Texas
Dallas, Texas

Giuseppe Viale, M.D.
University of Milan
Milan, Italy

Donald L. Weaver, M.D.
University of Vermont
Burlington, Vermont

Tim Whelan, B.M. B.ch., M.Sc.
Juravinski Cancer Centre
Hamilton, Canada

## CENTRAL NERVOUS SYSTEM

Edward R. Laws, Jr., M.D., Chair
Brigham & Women's Hospital
Boston, Massachusetts

James Brierley, M.B., M.S.
University of Toronto
Toronto, Canada

Susan M. Chang, M.D.
University of California
San Francisco, California

James E. Herndon II, Ph.D.
Duke University
Durham, North Carolina

M. Beatriz S. Lopes, M.D.
University of Virginia
Charlottesville, Virginia

Minesh Mehta, M.D.
University of Wisconsin
Madison, Wisconsin

Eileen J. Morgan, M.P.A., C.T.R.
Duke University
Durham, North Carolina

Angel Morris, R.N., B.S.N.
Psychiatric Alliance of
    the Blue Ridge
Charlottesville, Virginia

Joseph E. Parisi, M.D.
Mayo Clinic
Rochester, Minnesota

## FOREGUT

Mary Kay Washington, M.D., Ph.D.,
    Chair
Vanderbilt University
Nashville, Tennessee

Ross A. Abrams, M.D.
Rush University
Chicago, Illinois

Jacqueline Benedetti, Ph.D.
University of Washington
Seattle, Washington

Karl Bilimoria, M.D.
Northwestern University
Chicago, Illinois

Chuslip Charnsangavej, M.D.
M.D. Anderson Cancer Center
Houston, Texas

Daniel G. Coit, M.D.
Memorial Sloan-Kettering Cancer
    Center
New York, New York

Joseph P. Costantino, Dr.P.H.
University of Pittsburgh
Pittsburgh, Pennsylvania

Brian Czito, M.D.
Duke University
Durham, North Carolina

Deborah Etheridge, C.T.R.
American College of Surgeons
    Commission on Cancer
Chicago, Illinois

Douglas B. Evans, M.D.
M.D. Anderson Cancer
    Center
Houston, Texas

John P. Hoffman, M.D.
Temple University
Philadelphia, Pennsylvania

David Kelsen, M.D.
Memorial Sloan-Kettering
    Cancer Center
New York, New York

Markku Miettinen, M.D., Ph.D.
Armed Forces Institute
    of Pathology
Washington, DC

Irvin Modlin, M.D., Ph.D., D.Sc.
Yale University
New Haven, Connecticut

Eileen M. O'Reilly, M.D.
Memorial Sloan-Kettering Cancer
    Center
New York, New York

Tyvin Rich, M.D.
University of Virginia
Charlottesville, Virginia

Leslie H. Sobin, M.D.
Armed Forces Institute of Pathology
Washington, DC

Charles A. Staley, M.D.
Emory University
Atlanta, Georgia

Mark Talamonti, M.D.
NorthShore University Health
    System
Evanston, Illinois

Huamin Wang, M.D., Ph.D.
M.D. Anderson Cancer Center
Houston, Texas

Christian Wittekind, M.D.
Institut fur Patholgie der Universitat
Leipzig, Germany

## GENITOURINARY

Sam S. Chang, M.D., Chair
Vanderbilt University Medical Center
Nashville, Tennessee

James M. McKiernan, M.D., Vice-Chair
Herbert Irving Comprehensive
    Cancer Center
New York, New York

Mahul Amin, M.D.
Cedars-Sinai Medical Center
Los Angeles, California

Bernard H. Bochner, M.D.
Memorial Sloan-Kettering Cancer
    Center
New York, New York

Steven Campbell, M.D., Ph.D.
Cleveland Clinic
Cleveland, Ohio

Mary K. Gospodarowicz, M.D.
University of Toronto
Toronto, Ontario

Patti A. Groome, ph.d.
Queen's University
Kingston, Ontario

Celestia Higano, m.d.
University of Washington
Seattle, Washington

Peter A. Humphrey, m.d., ph.d.
Washington University
Saint Louis, Missouri

Michael Kattan, ph.d., m.b.a.
Cleveland Clinic
Cleveland, Ohio

Bradley Leibovich, m.d.
Mayo Clinic
Rochester, Minnesota

Curtis A. Pettaway, m.d.
M.D. Anderson Cancer Center
Houston, Texas

Alan Pollack, m.d., ph.d.
University of Miami
Miami, Florida

Mack Roach III, m.d.
University of California
San Francisco, California

Wael Sakr, m.d.
Wayne State University
Detroit, Michigan

Judith N. Shelby, r.h.i.t., c.t.r.
Vanderbilt University
Nashville, Tennessee

Walter M. Stadler, m.d.
University of Chicago
Chicago, Illinois

Valerie Vesich, r.h.i.t., c.t.r.
St. Joseph's Hospital and Medical
    Center
Phoenix, Arizona

Jacqueline Wieneke, m.d.
Armed Forces Institute of
    Pathology
Washington, DC

David P. Wood, m.d.
University of Michigan
Ann Arbor, Michigan

## GYNECOLOGIC

D. Scott McMeekin, m.d., Chair
University of Oklahoma
Oklahoma City, Oklahoma

J. L. Benedet, m.d.
Vancouver General Hospital
Vancouver, British Columbia

Russell Broaddus, m.d., ph.d.
M.D. Anderson Cancer Center
Houston, Texas

Dennis Chi, m.d.
Memorial Sloan-Kettering Cancer
    Center
New York, New York

Larry Copeland, m.d.
Ohio State University
Columbus, Ohio

Patricia J. Eifel, m.d.
M.D. Anderson Cancer Center
Houston, Texas

David M. Gershenson, m.d.
M.D. Anderson Cancer Center
Houston, Texas

Phyllis A. Gimotty, ph.d.
University of Pennsylvania
Philadelphia, Pennsylvania

Perry W. Grigsby, m.d.
Washington University
Saint Louis, Missouri

Lisa Landvogt, c.t.r.
American College of Surgeons
    Commission on Cancer
Chicago, Illinois

Karen H. Lu, m.d.
M. D. Anderson Cancer Center
Houston, Texas

Hextan Y. S. Ngan, m.d.
University of Hong Kong
Hong Kong, China

Esther Oliva, M.D.
Massachusetts General Hospital
Boston, Massachusetts

Edward E. Partridge, M.D.
University of Alabama
Birmingham, Alabama

Matthew A. Powell, M.D.
Washington University
Saint Louis, Missouri

William H. Rodgers, M.D., Ph.D.
University of Maryland
Baltimore, Maryland

Gustavo C. Rodriguez, M.D.
NorthShore University Health System
Evanston, Illinois

Charles W. Whitney, M.D.
Christiana Care
Newark, Delaware

## HEAD AND NECK

Jatin P. Shah, M.D., Chair
Memorial Sloan-Kettering Cancer
    Center
New York, New York

Kian Ang, M.D., Ph.D.
M.D. Anderson Cancer Center
Houston, Texas

Robert J. Baatenburg De Jong, M.D.
Erasmus Medical Center
Rotterdam, The Netherlands

Carol Bradford, M.D.
University of Michigan
Ann Arbor, Michigan

James Brierley, M.B., M.S.
University of Toronto
Toronto, Ontario

Joseph Califano, III, M.D.
Johns Hopkins University
Baltimore, Maryland

Amy Y. Chen, M.D., M.P.H.
Emory Healthcare
Atlanta, Georgia

Arlene A. Forastiere, M.D.
Johns Hopkins University
Baltimore, Maryland

Henry T. Hoffman, M.D.
University of Iowa
Iowa City, Iowa

J. Jack Lee, Ph.D., D.D.S.
M.D. Anderson Cancer Center
Houston, Texas

Nancy Lee, M.D.
Memorial Sloan-Kettering Cancer
    Center
New York, New York

William Lydiatt, M.D.
University of Nebraska
Omaha, Nebraska

Matthew S. Mayo, Ph.D.., M.B.A.
University of Kansas
Kansas City, Kansas

Bryan McIver, M.D.
Mayo Clinic
Rochester, Minnesota

Jesus Medina, M.D.
University of Oklahoma
Oklahoma City, Oklahoma

Suresh Mukherji, M.D.
University of Michigan
Ann Arbor, Michigan

Brian O'Sullivan, M.B. B.ch. B.A.O.
University of Toronto
Toronto, Ontario

Snehal Patel, M.D.
Memorial Sloan-Kettering Cancer
    Center
New York, New York

John A. Ridge, M.D., Ph.D.
Fox Chase Cancer Center
Philadelphia, Pennsylvania

Jennifer Seiffert, M.L.I.S., C.T.R.
Northrop Grumman
Warsaw, Indiana

Randal Weber, M.D.
M.D. Anderson Cancer Center
Houston, Texas

Bruce M. Wenig, M.D.
Beth Israel Medical Center
New York, New York

Bevan Yueh, M.D.
University of Washington
Seattle, Washington

## HEPATOBILIARY

J. Nicolas Vauthey, M.D., Chair
M.D. Anderson Cancer Center
Houston, Texas

Timothy M. Pawlik, M.D., M.P.H.,
    Vice-Chair
Johns Hopkins University
Baltimore, Maryland

Eddie K. Abdalla, M.D.
M.D. Anderson Cancer Center
Houston, Texas

Thomas A. Aloia, M.D.
The Methodist Hospital
Houston, Texas

Cynthia S. Boudreaux, L.P.N., C.T.R.
CB Professional Abstracting
    & Consulting Services
Raceland, Louisiana

Yun Shin Chun, M.D.
M.D. Anderson Cancer Center
Houston, Texas

Elijah Dixon, M.D.
University of Calgary
Calgary, Alberta

Yuman Fong, M.D.
Memorial Sloan-Kettering Cancer Center
New York, New York

David Kooby, M.D.
Emory University
Atlanta, Georgia

Gregory Y. Lauwers, M.D.
Massachusetts General Hospital
Boston, Massachusetts

Matthew S. Mayo, ph.D., M.B.A.
University of Kansas
Kansas City, Kansas

David M. Nagorney, M.D.
Mayo Clinic
Rochester, Minnesota

Kaye Reid Lombardo, M.D.
Mayo Clinic
Rochester, Minnesota

Bachir Taouli, M.D.
New York University
New York, New York

Mary Kay Washington, M.D., ph.D.
Vanderbilt University
Nashville, Tennessee

Christian Wittekind, M.D.
Institut fur Patholgie der
    Universitat
Leipzig, Germany

Tsung-Teh Wu, M.D., ph.D.
Mayo Clinic
Rochester, Minnesota

Andrew Zhu, M.D., ph.D.
Massachusetts General Hospital
Boston, Massachusetts

## HINDGUT

J. Milburn Jessup, M.D., Chair
National Cancer Institute
Bethesda, Maryland

Leonard Gunderson, M.D., Vice-Chair
Mayo Clinic
Scottsdale, Arizona

Jaffer Ajani, M.D.
M.D. Anderson Cancer Center
Houston, Texas

Robert W. Beart, Jr., M.D.
University of Southern California
Los Angeles, California

Al B. Benson III, M.D.
Northwestern University
Chicago, Illinois

James Brierley, M.B., M.S.
University of Toronto
Toronto, Ontario

John M. Carethers, M.D.
University of California
San Diego, California

Paul Catalano, SC.D.
Dana-Farber Cancer Institute
Boston, Massachusetts

George J. Chang, M.D.
M.D. Anderson Cancer Center
Houston, Texas

Julio Garcia-Aguilar, M.D., Ph.D.
City of Hope
Duarte, California

Richard M. Goldberg, M.D.
University of North Carolina
Chapel Hill, North Carolina

Daniel G. Haller, M.D.
University of Pennsylvania
Philadelphia, Pennsylvania

Stanley R. Hamilton, M.D.
M.D. Anderson Cancer Center
Houston, Texas

Donald E. Henson, M.D.
George Washington University
Washington, DC

Vencine Kelly, C.T.R.
Stony Brook University Medical
    Center
Stony Brook, New York

Bruce D. Minsky, M.D.
University of Chicago
Chicago, Illinois

Heidi Nelson, M.D.
Mayo Clinic
Rochester, Minnesota

Stephen Rubesin, M.D.
University of Pennsylvania
Philadelphia, Pennsylvania

Daniel J. Sargent, Ph.D.
Mayo Clinic
Rochester, Minnesota

Leslie H. Sobin, M.D.
Armed Forces Institute
    of Pathology
Washington, DC

Martin Weiser, M.D.
Sloan-Kettering Institute for Cancer
    Research
New York, New York

Mark Lane Welton, M.D.
Stanford University
Stanford, California

## LUNG AND ESOPHAGUS

Valerie W. Rusch, M.D., Chair
Memorial Sloan-Kettering Cancer
    Center
New York, New York

Henry D. Appelman, M.D.
University of Michigan
Ann Arbor, Michigan

Eugene Blackstone, M.D.
Cleveland Clinic
Cleveland, Ohio

Kelly J. Butnor, M.D.
University of Vermont
Burlington, Vermont

Daniel G. Coit, M.D.
Memorial Sloan-Kettering Cancer
    Center
New York, New York

John J. Crowley, Ph.D.
Cancer Research and Biostatistics
Seattle, Washington

Cynthia L. Dryer, B.A., C.T.R.
State Health Registry of Iowa
Iowa City, Iowa

Laurie Gaspar, M.D., M.B.A.
University of Colorado
Aurora, Colorado

Peter Goldstraw, M.D.
Royal Brompton Hospital
London, England

Patti A. Groome, ph.d.
Queen's Cancer Research
    Institute
Kingston, Ontario

James E. Herndon, II, ph.d.
Duke University
Durham, North Carolina

David H. Johnson, m.d.
Vanderbilt University
Nashville, Tennessee

David Kelsen, m.d.
Memorial Sloan-Kettering Cancer
    Center
New York, New York

Antoon Lerut, m.d.
University of Leuven
Leuven, Belgium

William Mackillop, m.b., ch.b.
Kingston Regional Cancer Center
Kingston, Canada

Steven J. Mentzer, m.d.
Brigham and Women's Hospital
Boston, Massachusetts

Mark B. Orringer, m.d.
University of Michigan
Ann Arbor, Michigan

Edward Patz, m.d.
Duke University
Durham, North Carolina

Tom Rice, m.d.
Cleveland Clinic
Cleveland, Ohio

Yu Shyr, ph.d.
Vanderbilt University
Nashville, Tennessee

William D. Travis, m.d.
Memorial Sloan-Kettering Cancer
    Center
New York, New York

Andrew Turrisi, m.d.
Wayne State University
Detroit, Michigan

## LYMPHOMA

James O. Armitage, m.d., Chair
University of Nebraska
Omaha, Nebraska

Bruce D. Cheson, m.d., Co-Chair
Georgetown University
Washington, DC

Kenneth C. Anderson, m.d.
Dana-Farber Cancer Institute
Boston, Massachusetts

Richard I. Fisher, m.d.
University of Rochester
Rochester, New York

Irene Ghobrial, m.d.
Dana-Farber Cancer Institute
Boston, Massachusetts

Mary Gospodarowicz, m.d.
University of Toronto
Toronto, Canada

Nancy Lee Harris, m.d.
Massachusetts General
    Hospital
Boston, Massachusetts

Richard T. Hoppe, m.d.
Stanford University
Stanford, California

Jerry W. Hussong, m.d., d.d.s.
Laboratory Medicine Consultants
Las Vegas, Nevada

Malik Juweid, m.d.
University of Iowa
Iowa City, Iowa

Robert A. Kyle, m.d.
Mayo Clinic
Rochester, Minnesota

Michael LeBlanc, ph.d.
Fred Hutchinson Cancer Research
    Center
Seattle, Washington

Andrew Lister, m.d.
St. Bartholomew's Hospital
London, England

Sharon Murphy, M.D.
University of Texas
San Antonio, Texas

Steven T. Rosen, M.D.
Northwestern University
Chicago, Illinois

John Sandlund, M.D.
St. Jude Children's Research
Hospital
Memphis, Tennesee

Krystyna Tybinkowski, B.A., C.T.R.
Princess Margaret Hospital
Toronto, Ontario

## MELANOMA

Charles M. Balch, M.D., FACS, Chair
Johns Hopkins University
Baltimore, Maryland

Jeffrey E. Gershenwald, M.D.,
Vice-Chair
M.D. Anderson Cancer Center
Houston, Texas

Michael B. Atkins, M.D.
Beth Israel Deaconess
Medical Center
Boston, Massachusetts

Antonio C. Buzaid, M.D.
Hospital Sirio Libanes
Sao Paulo, Brazil

Natale Cascinelli, M.D.
Istituto Nazionale dei Tumori
Milan, Italy

Alistair J. Cochran, M.D.
University of California
Los Angeles, California

Daniel G. Coit, M.D.
Memorial Sloan-Kettering Cancer
Center
New York, New York

Matthew Dickerson, B.S.
University of Alabama at
Birmingham
Birmingham, Alabama

Shouluan Ding, Ph.D.
University of Alabama at Birmingham
Birmingham, Alabama

Rush Elliott, B.S.
University of Alabama at Birmingham
Birmingham, Alabama

Alexander M. M. Eggermont, M.D., Ph.D.
Erasmus University Medical Center
Rotterdam, The Netherlands

Keith T. Flaherty, M.D.
University of Pennsylvania
Philadelphia, Pennsylvania

David Frishberg, M.D.
Cedars Sinai Medical Center
Los Angeles, California

Phyllis A. Gimotty, Ph.D.
University of Pennsylvania
Philadelphia, Pennsylvania

Allan C. Halpern, M.D., M.S.
Memorial Sloan-Kettering Cancer
Center
New York, New York

Alan N. Houghton, M.D.
Memorial Sloan-Kettering Cancer
Center
New York, New York

Marcella M. Johnson, M.S.
M.D. Anderson Cancer Center
Houston, Texas

John M. Kirkwood, M.D.
University of Pittsburgh
Pittsburgh, Pennsylvania

Kelly M. McMasters, M.D.
University of Louisville
Louisville, Kentucky

Martin C. Mihm, Jr., M.D.
Massachusetts General
Hospital
Boston, Massachusetts

Donald L. Morton, M.D.
John Wayne Cancer Institute
Santa Monica, California

Omgo E. Nieweg, M.D.
Netherlands Cancer Institute
Amsterdam, The Netherlands

Connie Pitts
University of Alabama
    at Birmingham
Birmingham, Alabama

Merrick I. Ross, M.D.
M.D. Anderson Cancer Center
Houston, Texas

Arthur Sober, M.D.
Massachusetts General Hospital
Boston, Massachusetts

Vernon Sondak, M.D.
H. Lee Moffitt Cancer Center
Tampa, Florida

John F. Thompson, M.D.
University of Sydney
Sydney, Australia

Seng-Jaw Soong, Ph.D.
University of Alabama at Birmingham
Birmingham, Alabama

Carla Warneke
M.D. Anderson Cancer Center
Houston, Texas

## NON-MELANOMA SKIN

Arthur Sober, M.D., Chair
Massachusetts General Hospital
Boston, Massachusetts

Joseph Califano, III, M.D.
Johns Hopkins University
Baltimore, Maryland

David Frishberg, M.D.
Cedars Sinai Medical Center
Los Angeles, California

Allan C. Halpern, M.D., M.S.
Memorial Sloan-Kettering Cancer
    Center
New York, New York

Timothy M. Johnson, M.D.
University of Michigan
Ann Arbor, Michigan

Bianca D. Lemos, M.D.
University of Washington
Seattle, Washington

Nanette J. Liegeois, M.D., Ph.D.
Johns Hopkins University
Baltimore, Maryland

Martin C. Mihm, Jr., M.D.
Massachusetts General
    Hospital
Boston, Massachusetts

Victor A. Neel, M.D., Ph.D.
Massachusetts General
    Hospital
Boston, Massachusetts

Kishwer S. Nehal, M.D.
Memorial Sloan-Kettering Cancer
    Center
New York, New York

Paul Nghiem, M.D., Ph.D.
University of Washington Medical
    Center
Seattle, Washington

Clark Otley, M.D.
Mayo Clinic
Rochester, Minnesota

Louise Schuman, M.A., C.T.R.
Clinical Data Systems
Fountain Valley, California

Seng-Jaw Soong, Ph.D.
University of Alabama
    at Birmingham
Birmingham, Alabama

Mark R. Wick, M.D.
University of Virginia
Charlottesville, Virginia

Siegrid Yu, M.D.
University of California
San Francisco, California

## OPHTHALMIC

Paul T. Finger, M.D., Chair
The New York Eye Cancer
    Center
New York, New York

Daniel Albert, M.D.
University of Wisconsin
Madison, Wisconsin

Darryl Ainbinder, M.D.
Madigan Army Medical Center
Tacoma, Washington

James J. Augsburger, M.D.
University of Cincinnati
Cincinnati, Ohio

Nikolas E. Bechrakis, M.D.
Universitatsklinik Fur
    Augenheilkunde und Optometrie
Innsbruck, Austria

Maj. John H. Boden, M.D.
Madigan Army Medical Center
Tacoma, Washington

Patricia Chevez-Barrios, M.D.
The Methodist Hospital
Houston, Texas

Sarah E. Coupland, M.B.B.S., Ph.D.,
    F.R.C.Path
Royal Liverpool Hospital
Liverpool, England

Bertil Damato, M.D.
Royal Liverpool University
    Hospital
Liverpool, England

Laurence Desjardins, M.D.
Institut Curie
Paris, France

Didi de Wolff-Rouendaal, M.D., Ph.D.
Leiden University
Leiden, The Netherlands

Ralph C. Eagle, M.D.
Wills Eye Hospital
Philadelphia, Pennsylvania

Deepak P. Edward, M.D.
Northeastern Ohio Universities
    College of Medicine
Akron, Ohio

Bita Esmaeli, M.D.
M.D. Anderson Cancer Center
Houston, Texas

James C. Fleming, M.D.
University of Tennessee
Memphis, Tennessee

Brenda L. Gallie, M.D.
University of Toronto
Toronto, Canada

Dan S. Gombos, M.D.
M.D. Anderson Cancer Center
Houston, Texas

Jean-Daniel Grange, M.D.
Croix-Rousse Hospital
Lyon, France

Hans Grossniklaus, M.D., M.B.A.
Emory University
Atlanta, Georgia

Barrett Haik, M.D.
The University of Tennessee
Memphis, Tennessee

Col. John B. Halligan, M.D.
Madigan Army Medical Center
Tacoma, Washington

J. William Harbour, M.D.
Washington University
St. Louis, Missouri

George J. Harocopos, M.D.
Washington University
St. Louis, Missouri

Leonard M Holbach, M.D.
University of Erlangen–Nuremberg
Erlangen, Germany

John L. Hungerford, M.D.
St. Bartholomew Hospital
London, England

Martine J. Jager, M.D., Ph.D.
Academisch Ziekenhuis Leiden
Afdeling Oogheelkunde
Leiden, The Netherlands

Zeynel A. Karcioglu, M.D.
University of Tennessee
Memphis, Tennessee

Tero Kivela, M.D.
Helsinki University Central Hospital
Helsinki, Finland

Emma Kujala, M.D.
Helsinki University Central Hospital
Helsinki, Finland

Ashwin C. Mallipatna, M.B.B.S.
Princess Margaret Hospital
Toronto, Ontario

Col. Robert A. Mazzoli, M.D.
Madigan Army Medical Center
Tacoma, Washington

Hugh McGowan, M.D.
University of Toronto
Toronto, Ontario

Tatyana Milman, M.D.
New York Eye and Ear Infirmary
New York, New York

A. Linn Murphree, M.D.
Children's Hospital
Los Angeles, California

Tim G. Murray, M.D., M.B.A.
Bascom Palmer Eye Institute
Miami, Florida

Jack Rootman, M.D., F.R.C.S.
University of British Columbia
Vancouver, British Columbia

Andrew P. Schachat, M.D.
Cleveland Clinic
Cleveland, Ohio

Stefan Seregard, M.D.
St. Erik's Eye Hospital
Stockholm, Sweden

E. Rand Simpson, M.D.
Princess Margaret Hospital
Toronto, Ontario

Arun D. Singh, M.D.
Cleveland Clinic
Cleveland, Ohio

Valerie A. White, M.D., MHSC
University of British Columbia
Vancouver, British Columbia

Matthew W. Wilson, M.D.
The University of Tennessee
Memphis, Tennessee

Christian W. Wittekind, M.D.
Institut fur Pathologie der Universitat
Leipzig, Germany

Guopei Yu, M.D., M.P.H.
The New York Eye and Ear Infirmary
New York, New York

## SOFT TISSUE SARCOMA

Raphael E. Pollock, M.D., Ph.D., Chair
M.D. Anderson Cancer Center
Houston, Texas

Laurence H. Baker, D.O.
University of Michigan
Ann Arbor, Michigan

Murray F. Brennan, M.D.
Memorial Sloan-Kettering Cancer
    Center
New York, New York

Kevin Coombes, Ph.D.
M.D. Anderson Cancer Center
Houston, Texas

Michael Kattan, Ph.D., M.B.A.
Cleveland Clinic
Cleveland, Ohio

Jeffrey S. Kneisl, M.D.
Carolinas Medical Center
Charlotte, North Carolina

Thomas Krausz, M.D.
University of Chicago
Chicago, Illinois

Alexander Lazar, M.D., Ph.D.
M.D. Anderson Cancer Center
Houston, Texas

Dina Chelouche Lev, M.D.
M.D. Anderson Cancer Center
Houston, Texas

Brian O'Sullivan, M.D.
Princess Margaret Hospital
Toronto, Ontario

David Panicek, M.D.
Memorial Sloan-Kettering Center
New York, New York

Peter W. T. Pisters, M.D.
M.D. Anderson Cancer Center
Houston, Texas

R. Lor Randall, M.D.
University of Utah
Salt Lake City, Utah

Chandrajit P. Raut, M.D., M.S.C.
Brigham and Women's Hospital
Boston, Massachusetts

Herman D. Suit, M.D., Ph.D.
Massachusetts General Hospital
Boston, Massachusetts

Carol Shaw Venuti, R.H.I.A., C.T.R.
Massachusetts General Hospital
Boston, Massachusetts

Sharon Weiss, M.D.
Emory University
Atlanta, Georgia

## OTHER CONTRIBUTORS

Cynthia S. Boudreaux, L.P.N., C.T.R.
CB Professional Abstracting &
    Consulting Services
Raceland, Louisiana

Iris Chilton
Alberta Cancer Registry
Edmonton, Alberta

Elaine Collins, R.H.I.A., C.T.R.
Minnesota Cancer Surveillance
    System
St. Paul, Minnesota

Michelle L. Esterly, R.H.I.A., C.T.R.
Pennsylvania Department of Health
Harrisburg, Pennsylvania

Greer Gay, Ph.D., M.P.H., R.N.
American College of Surgeons
    Commission on Cancer
Chicago, Illinois

Suzanna S. Hoyler, B.S., C.T.R.
Consultant
Austin, Texas

Katherine Mallin, Ph.D.
American College of Surgeons
    Commission on Cancer
Chicago, Illinois

Bryan Palis, M.A.
American College of Surgeons
    Commission on Cancer
Chicago, Illinois

Jerri Linn Phillips, M.A., C.T.R.
American College of Surgeons
    Commission on Cancer
Chicago, Illinois

Lynn Ries, M.S.
National Cancer Institute
Bethesda, Maryland

Jennifer Ruhl, R.H.I.T., C.T.R.
National Cancer Institute
Bethesda, Maryland

Jennifer Seiffert, M.L.I.S., C.T.R.
Northrop Grumman
Warsaw, Indiana

Colleen Sherman, R.H.I.A., C.T.R.
New York State Cancer Registry
Albany, New York

Karen Starratt
Nova Scotia Surveillance and
    Epidemiology Unit
Halifax, Nova Scotia

Andrew Stewart, M.A.
American College of Surgeons
    Commission on Cancer
Chicago, Illinois

Valerie Vesich, R.H.I.T., C.T.R.
St. Joseph's Hospital and Medical
    Center
Phoenix, Arizona

# Index

## A

Abdomen, 346. *See also* specific organs
Abdominal esophagus, 134
Acoustic/vestibular nerve, 651
Adamantinoma, 339
Adjusted survival rates, 33
Adnexa, 637
Adrenal gland, 585
Alpha-fetoprotein, 242, 496, 540, 541, 545
Alveolar ridges, 50
American Joint Committee on Cancer
    (AJCC)
    classification, 3
Ampulla of Vater, 272, 277–282
Anal canal, 207
Anaplastic astrocytoma, 653
Anaplastic carcinoma of the thyroid
    gland, 120
Anaplastic large T-cell lymphoma, 665
Anatomic stage/prognostic grouping
    rules, 20
Angiosarcoma, 339
Ann Arbor staging system, 670–671
Anorectal lymph nodes, 209
Anterior floor of mouth, 49
Anterior mediastinum, 345
Anterior (lingual) surface of epiglottis, 81
Anterior two-thirds of tongue, 49
Anterior wall of bladder, 569
Anterior wall of nasopharynx, 64
Anus, 207–217
Aortic lymph nodes, 301, 527, 549, 562
Aortopulmonary lymph nodes, 136
Appendix, 161–170
Armed Forces Institute of Pathology, 10
Articular cartilage, 333
Aryepiglottic folds, 64, 82
Arytenoids, 82
Ascending colon, 174, 175, 183, 193
*Atlas of Tumor Pathology*, 10
Autonomic nervous system, 345, 346
Autopsy classification, 19
Axillary lymph nodes, 421, 423, 424, 426

## B

Basal cell carcinomas, 360
Base of tongue, 63

B-cell lymphocytic leukemia/small
    lymphocytic lymphoma
    (B-cell CLL/SLL), 665
B-cell neoplasms, 664
Beta-2 microglobulin, 686
Bile ducts, extrahepatic, 271–272
Bile ducts, intrahepatic, 238
Biliary tract, 256
Bladder, 569
Bladder neck, 569
Bladder, urinary, 569–575
Body of pancreas, 285
Body of penis, 515
Body of stomach (other than
    proximal 5 cm), 145, 147
Body of stomach, proximal 5 cm only, 130
Bone, 333–340
Bone of limb, 333
Bones of skull and face, 333
Border of tongue, 49
Brain, 651–660
Brain stem, 651
Brain stem glioma, 651
Branchial cleft, 63
Breast, 419–456
Breast cancer
    cancer outcomes, 437–438
    SEER data, 29–32
    survival rates, 438, 448, 454
Bronchus, main, 299
Buccal mucosa, 50
Buccinator lymph nodes, 40

## C

CA-125, 496
Carcinomas
    anal canal, 215
    cervical, 474
    conjunctival, 599–602
    eyelid, 593–597
    hepatocellular, 241
    lacrimal gland, 631–634
    ovarian, 494, 498
    prostatic, 580
    skin, 359–373
    stomach, 145–152
    thyroid gland, 117–120

Mucosa of lip, 49
Mucosa of lower lip, 49
Mucosa of upper lip, 49
Multidrug resistance gene 1 (MDR1), 336
Multiple myeloma, 685–687
Multiple regression analysis, 34
Multiple tumors, 21
MX, 12, 13, 16
Mycosis fungoides, 670, 680–681
Myometrium, 481

# N

Nasal cavity, 93, 94, 98
Nasopharyngeal carcinoma, 77
Nasopharynx, 64–66, 69–73
National Cancer Data Base (NCDB), 45
National Cancer Institute Surveillance,
    Epidemiology, and End Results
    (SEER), 28
N classification rules, 17
Neck
    carcinoma of the skin, 360
    lymph nodes levels, 42–44
    melanoma of the skin, 388
    saggital view, 65
    soft-tissue sarcomas, 345, 346
Nerve sheath tumor, peripheral, 340
Nervous system, 651
Nipple, 421, 426, 430
NK-cell neoplasms, 664–665
Nomenclature, cancer morphology, 9–11
Non-Hodgkin lymphoma, 669–677
Non-small cell lung cancer (NSCLC),
    310–313, 315
    survival rates, 313
Nottingham combined histologic grade,
    445–446

# O

Obturator lymph nodes
    cervix uteri and, 474
    corpus uteri and, 483
    fallopian tubes and, 502
    ovaries and, 494
    prostate and, 527
    urethra and, 580
    urinary bladder and, 571
    vagina and, 469
Occipital lobe, 651
Olfactory nerve, 651
Oligodendroglioma, 653, 656
Omentum, 219–221
Optic nerve, 651
Oral cavity, 49–59
Orbit, 637–642
Orbit, sarcoma of, 637–639
Oropharynx, 63, 64, 66, 69, 70, 72, 74
    squamous cell carcinomas, 74

Osteosarcoma, 339
Ovary, 493–500
Overlapping lesion of palate, 50
Overlapping lesion of tongue, 49

# P

P53, 573
Palate, 50
Pancoast tumors, 319
Pancreas, 285–295
Pancreas, exocrine, 285–295
Pancreatic bile ducts, 278
Pancreatic ducts, 285
Pancreaticoduodenal lymph nodes, 155
Papillary adenocarcinoma of the thyroid
    gland, 117
Para-aortic lymph nodes
    corpus uteri and, 483
    fallopian tubes and, 502
    kidneys and, 549
    ovaries and, 494
    prostate and, 527
Paracardial lymph nodes, 137
Paracaval lymph nodes, 540, 549, 562
Paraesophageal lymph nodes, 137
Parametrial lymph nodes, 474, 483
Paranasal sinuses, 93–100
Parapharyngeal anatomy, 65
Parapharyngeal lymph nodes, 40
Paratracheal lymph nodes, 43, 136, 301
Parietal lobe, 651
Parotid gland, 103, 104
Parotid lymph nodes, 600, 638
Pathologic classification, 16–19
Pathologic M0, 18
Pathologic staging, 5, 6, 14, 15, 17, 19
Pediatric lymphoid malignancy, 689–690
Pelvic bones, 333
Pelvic lymph nodes
    corpus uteri and, 483
    fallopian tubes and, 502
    ovaries and, 494
    penis and, 516
    prostate and, 527
    ureter and, 562
    urethra and, 580
    urinary bladder and, 571
    vagina and, 469
Pelvis, 346
Penis, 388, 515–522
Periaortic lymph nodes, 540
Peribronchial lymph nodes, 317
Pericardial effusion, 317
Pericholedochal lymph nodes, 155
Pericolic lymph nodes, 176
Periduodenal lymph nodes, 257
Periesophageal lymph nodes, 135
Peripancreatic lymph nodes, 257, 278
Periparotid lymph nodes, 40
Peripheral nerves, 345

Peripheral T-cell lymphoma, 665
Perirectal lymph nodes, 209
Peritoneum, 346, 493
Peritoneum, NOS, 346
Periureteral lymph nodes, 562
Perivesical lymph nodes, 571
PET scan, 184
Peyer's patches, 662
P-glycoprotein, 336–337
Pharynx, 63–77
Phrenic nerve, 316
Pilocytic astrocytoma, 653, 656
Pineal gland, 651
Pituitary gland, 651
Placenta, 507
Plasmablasts, 664
Plasma cell disorders, 685–687
Plasma cell labeling index (PCLI), 685
Pleural effusion, 310
Pleural mesothelioma, 325–330
Pleura, 325, 345
pM0, 16, 18
PNET, 655
Postcricoid region, 64
Posterior cecal lymph nodes, 183
Posterior mediastinum, 345
Posterior pharyngeal wall, 63, 66
Posterior triangle lymph nodes, 43
Posterior wall of bladder, 569
Posterior wall of hypopharynx, 64
Posterior wall of nasopharynx, 64
Preaortic lymph nodes, 540
Preauricular lymph nodes, 40, 600, 605, 613, 624, 632
Precaval lymph nodes, 540
Prefixes, 22
Prelaryngeal lymph nodes, 43
Prepuce, 388, 515
Presacral lymph nodes, 474, 483, 571, 580
Pretracheal lymph nodes, 43, 301
Primary cutaneous lymphoma, 679–683
Primary tumors (T). See also specific sites
    definition of, 11
    T classification and survival, 241
Prostate gland, 525–535
Prostate-specific antigen (PSA), 531
Pulmonary ligament lymph nodes, 137
Pyloric lymph nodes, 155
Pylorus, 145
Pyriform sinus, 64

# R

Radiation Therapy Oncology Group (RTOG), 531
Rb, 573
Rectosigmoid junction, 174, 219, 227
Rectum, 173–200, 219, 227, 230, 233
Regional lymph nodes (N), 12. See also specific sites
Regression methods, 34

Relative survival rates, 33–34
Renal hilar lymph nodes, 549, 562
Renal pelvis, 561–566
Residual tumor (R), 23
Restaging, 191, 335, 351, 369, 673
Retina, 623
Retinoblastoma, 623–628
Retreatment classification, 19
Retroaortic lymph nodes, 540, 549
Retrocaval lymph nodes, 540
Retromolar area, 50
Retroperitoneal lymph nodes, 494, 528, 562
Retroperitoneum, 347
Retropharyngeal lymph nodes, 40
Revised European-American
        Classification of Lymphoid
        Neoplasms (REAL), 663
Rhabdomyosarcoma, 340
Right colic lymph nodes, 183
Right hepatic duct, 264
Rosenmuller's node, 64
Rounding tumor size, 16

# S

Sacral lymph nodes, 474, 527, 571, 580
Sacral promontory lymph nodes, 183
Sacrum, 333
Salivary glands, major, 103–108
Sarcomas
    bone, 334
    orbit, 637–640
    soft tissue, 345–354
Satellite nodules, 319
Scalene lymph nodes, 326, 528
Scalp, 360, 388
Scapula, 333
Schwannoma, 654, 657
Scrotum, 360, 388
Sentinel lymph nodes
    breast, 420, 428, 433, 438, 440–442
    melanoma, 387, 389, 391–393
Sézary syndrome, 680–683
Shoulders
    carcinoma of the skin, 360
    melanoma of the skin, 388
    soft-tissue sarcomas, 345, 346
Sigmoid colon, 174–176, 183, 193, 198
Sigmoid mesenteric lymph nodes, 183
Skeleton. See bone
Skin
    carcinoma of, 359–373
    melanoma of, 387–410
Skin of lip, 360
Small cell lung cancer (SCLC), 310, 312–315
Small intestine, 153–158, 220, 227, 229
Smoldering multiple myeloma (SMM), 687
Soft palate, 63
Soft tissues, 346, 347
Soft tissue sarcomas, 345–354

Special classification rules, 22
Spinal cord, 651–660
Spinal meninges, 651
Spleen, 672, 674, 676
Splenic flexure of colon, 174, 175, 183
Splenic lymph nodes, 137
Sputum, 315
Squamous cell carcinomas
    glottis, 88
    head and neck (SCCHN), 40
    hypopharyngeal, 75
    laryngeal, 87
    lip, 56
    nasopharyngeal, 73
    oropharyngeal, 74
    skin, 360
    subglottis, 89
    supraglottis, 90
Stage groupings, 3–9, 12, 20, 25, 241
Staging
    general rules of, 13
    philosophy of, 3
    principles of, 3–25
Staging classifications, 5–6, 15, 24
Standard error, 34–35
Starting points, survival studies,
    35–36
Sternum, 333
St. Jude staging system, 690
Stomach, 145–152, 219, 227, 229,
    231–233
Subcarinal lymph nodes, 137, 301
Subcutaneous tissues, 348–349
Subglottis, 81, 82, 85, 89
Sublingual glands, 103–107
Submandibular gland, 103
Submandibular lymph nodes, 42, 103–107,
    600, 605, 613, 624, 632, 638
Submental lymph nodes, 42
Sub-occipital lymph nodes, 40
Superficial inguinal lymph nodes, 516
Superior mesenteric lymph nodes, 247
Superior wall of nasopharynx, 64
Supraclavicular fossa, 70, 71
Supraclavicular lymph nodes, 136, 326,
    426, 427, 528
Supraglottis, 81, 84, 90
Supraglottis (laryngeal surface), 81
Suprahyoid epiglottis, 82
Surgical margins, 23
Surgical margins, pancreatic, 287
Survival analysis, 27–36
Survival curve, definition, 27
Survival rate analyses
    adjusted, 33
    breast cancer, 29
    calculation of, 28
    definition of, 27
    regression method, 34
    standard error of, 34–35
    starting points, 35–36
    statistical significance, 35–36

    subclassification, 30–32
    T classification and, 241
    time intervals, 36
Survival, relative, 33–34
*Systematized Nomenclature of Medicine*
    (SNOMED), 10

# T

Tail of pancreas, 285
T-cell lymphoma, peripheral, 665
T-cell neoplasms, 661, 664
T classification rules, 16
T, definition of, 348
Technitium scintigraphy, 335
Temporal lobe, 651
Terminal events, 36
Testis, 539–546
Thorax, soft-tissue sarcomas, 345
Thoracic esophagus, 129
Thyroid cartilage, 65
Thyroid gland, 111–120
    anaplastic carcinoma of, 120
    follicular adenocarcinoma of, 118
    medullary carcinoma of, 119
    papillary adenocarcinoma of, 117
Time period for staging, 14
TNM system, 11–12
    general rule of, 11–14
    philosophy of, 3
    subdivisions of, 21–23
Tongue, 49
    base of, 63
    oral, 51
Tonsillar fossa, 63
Tonsillar pillar, 63, 66
Tonsils, 63
Tracheobronchial lymph nodes, 137
Transverse colon, 174, 175, 183
Trigone of bladder, 569
Trophoblastic tumors, gestational,
    507–511
Trunk
    carcinoma of the skin, 359
    melanoma of the skin, 387
    soft-tissue sarcomas, 345
T1 tumor survival rates, 240
Tumor growth, 222, 248–253,
    573, 659

# U

Ulcerated tumors, 51, 52
Ulceration, melanoma, 394
Uncensored cases, 27–28
Undescended testis, 539
Upper gum, 49
Upper jugular lymph nodes, 42
Upper lobe lung, 299
Upper mediastinal lymph nodes, 43

---